Bariatric Surgery: Latest Advances and Prospects

Bariatric Surgery: Latest Advances and Prospects

Editor

David Benaiges Boix

Basel • Beijing • Wuhan • Barcelona • Belgrade • Novi Sad • Cluj • Manchester

Editor
David Benaiges Boix
Hospital del Mar
Barcelona, Spain

Editorial Office
MDPI
St. Alban-Anlage 66
4052 Basel, Switzerland

This is a reprint of articles from the Special Issue published online in the open access journal *Journal of Clinical Medicine* (ISSN 2077-0383) (available at: https://www.mdpi.com/journal/jcm/special_issues/bariatric_surgery).

For citation purposes, cite each article independently as indicated on the article page online and as indicated below:

Lastname, A.A.; Lastname, B.B. Article Title. *Journal Name* **Year**, *Volume Number*, Page Range.

ISBN 978-3-0365-9458-3 (Hbk)
ISBN 978-3-0365-9459-0 (PDF)
doi.org/10.3390/books978-3-0365-9459-0

Contents

Journal of
Clinical Medicine

MDPI

Article

A Longitudinal Study of the Antioxidant Barrier and Oxidative Stress in Morbidly Obese Patients after Bariatric Surgery. Does the Metabolic Syndrome Affect the Redox Homeostasis of Obese People?

Barbara Choromańska [1,*], Piotr Myśliwiec [1], Magdalena Łuba [1], Piotr Wojskowicz [1], Jacek Dadan [1], Hanna Myśliwiec [2], Katarzyna Choromańska [3], Anna Zalewska [4] and Mateusz Maciejczyk [5,*]

1. Department of General and Endocrine Surgery, Medical University of Bialystok, 24a M. Sklodowskiej-Curie Street, 15-276 Bialystok, Poland; piotr.a.mysliwiec@gmail.com (P.M.); ananau@wp.pl (M.Ł.); pwojsk@wp.pl (P.W.); jacdad@poczta.onet.pl (J.D.)
2. Department of Dermatology and Venereology, Medical University of Bialystok, 14 Żurawia Street, 15-540 Bialystok, Poland; hanna.mysliwiec@gmail.com
3. Department of Oral Surgery, Medical University of Gdansk, 7 Dębinki Street, 80-211 Gdansk, Poland; kasia24_89@o2.pl
4. Experimental Dentistry Laboratory, Medical University of Bialystok, 24a M. Sklodowskiej-Curie Street, 15-274 Bialystok, Poland; azalewska426@gmail.com
5. Department of Hygiene, Epidemiology and Ergonomics, Medical University of Bialystok, 2c Mickiewicza Street, 15-233 Bialystok, Poland

* Correspondence: barbara.choromanska@umb.edu.pl (B.C.); mat.maciejczyk@gmail.com (M.M.)

Received: 19 March 2020; Accepted: 31 March 2020; Published: 1 April 2020

Abstract: This is the first study to evaluate both the antioxidant barrier, glutathione metabolism, and oxidative damage to proteins and lipids in morbidly obese patients undergoing bariatric treatment. The study included 65 patients with class 3 obesity divided into two subgroups: morbidly obese patients without metabolic syndrome (OB) and obese patients with metabolic syndrome (OB + MS). Blood samples were collected before surgery as well as one, three, six, and twelve months after the bariatric treatment. Superoxide dismutase and reduced glutathione (GSH) were significantly decreased, whereas glutathione reductase and uric acid were enhanced in morbidly obese patients before bariatric surgery as compared to lean control. Moreover, in the OB group, we observed the increase of superoxide dismutase (SOD) and the decrease of uric acid (UA) after the bariatric treatment; however, these changes were not observed in the OB + MS group. The oxidative damage to proteins (advanced glycation end products, AGE; advanced oxidation protein products, AOPP) and lipids (8-isoprostanes, 8-isop; 4-hydroxynoneal) was higher in OB as well as OB + MS patients. We noticed that AGE and AOPP levels diminished after the bariatric treatment, whereas redox status (ratio of GSH to oxidized glutathione) was still reduced in the OB + MS group. Summarizing, morbid obesity is associated with disturbances in the antioxidant barrier and enhanced oxidative damage to proteins and lipids. Although bariatric surgery improves redox homeostasis in obese patients, those with metabolic syndrome show a continuous decrease in the antioxidant status. In patients undergoing bariatric treatment, antioxidant supplementation may be considered.

Keywords: oxidative stress; redox biomarkers; morbid obesity; bariatric surgery

1. Introduction

Morbid obesity (body mass index (BMI) > 40 kg/m^2) is one of the most serious health problems in the world. Many epidemiological studies have shown that obesity is frequently accompanied by metabolic disorders like hypertension, insulin resistance, type 2 diabetes (T2DM), ischemic heart disease, as well as cancer [1,2]. However, despite intensive research on morbid obesity, it remains unclear why some obese subjects develop the metabolic syndrome (MS), and some do not. It is well known that the development of obesity is caused by adipokine secretion like leptin, adipokine or resistin as well as an increased expression of fatty acid/cholesterol transporters in the target tissues [3–5]. Nevertheless, recent studies emphasize the critical role of oxidative stress (OS) in the development of obesity and its metabolic complications [6,7]. OS occurs when cellular components (e.g., lipids and proteins) are oxidized and cellular metabolism is disturbed. This condition is mainly due to the overproduction of reactive oxygen (ROS) and nitrogen (RNS) species [8]. The first sign of OS is lipid peroxidation because the cell membrane is the first to be exposed to ROS. Oxidative damage to lipids leads to the formation of peroxides such as 4-hydroxynonenal (4-HNE) and 8-isoprostanes (8-isoP); however, excessive formation of ROS also causes modifications of proteins and amino acid residues [9]. It was shown that protein/lipid oxidation products are very cytotoxic, leading to cell death by apoptosis and necrosis [10]. Therefore, in aerobic organisms, several antioxidant systems protect cells against OS. Antioxidants not only inhibit ROS-induced oxidation but also repair some forms of oxidative modification in biomolecules. The most important blood antioxidants include superoxide dismutase (SOD), catalase (CAT), glutathione peroxidase (GPx), glutathione reductase (GR), reduced glutathione (GSH) and uric acid (UA) [7,8,11]. It is suggested that antioxidant supplementation could reduce metabolic disorders and improve the condition of obese patients. However, little is still known about the efficiency of the antioxidant barrier in morbidly obese cases. Particularly, the unknown is the impact of metabolic syndrome on the redox homeostasis of these patients.

Nowadays, bariatric surgery is the most efficient method of obesity treatment [12]. Many studies have shown that bariatric surgery not only helps patients achieve long-term weight loss but also removes obesity-related complications, including T2DM and high blood pressure [13–16]. It has been demonstrated that weight-loss by laparoscopic sleeve gastrectomy leads to a 40%–65% reduction in excess weight. Moreover, 56% of obese patients achieve resolution of T2DM [17]. However, the exact reason for these changes is still unknown. It is postulated that the improvement of obese patients is associated with the reduction of oxidative stress levels [7,8,11]; however, there is no longitudinal data about the redox homeostasis of patients undergoing bariatric treatment. Therefore, the aim of our study was to evaluate the impact of morbid obesity as well as huge weight loss on the blood antioxidant systems/oxidative stress before as well as one, three, six and twelve months after bariatric surgery. For this purpose, we assessed the enzymatic and non-enzymatic antioxidant barrier, redox potential, as well as oxidative damage to proteins and lipids in the plasma and serum of both study groups and healthy controls. We are also the first to compare redox homeostasis in obese patients with metabolic syndrome to obese cases only.

2. Materials and Methods

The study was approved by the Ethics Committee of the Medical University of Bialystok (permission numbers: R-I-002/69/2012 and R-I-002/187/2017). All procedures were designed, conducted, and reported in compliance with the Declaration of Helsinki, according to the guidelines for Good Clinical Practice. All subjects gave their informed consent to participate in the study.

The study included 65 patients (women aged from 19 to 65 years) with class 3 obesity (BMI > 40 kg/m^2), who underwent elective bariatric surgery-laparoscopic sleeve gastrectomy. Patients were treated at the First Department of General and Endocrine Surgery at the University Hospital in Bialystok. The study group was divided into two subgroups: morbidly obese patients without metabolic syndrome (OB) (n = 34) and morbidly obese patients with metabolic syndrome (OB + MS) (n = 31). Material for testing was collected before surgery (OB 0; OB + MS 0) as well as one month (OB 1; OB + MS 1), three months (OB 3; OB + MS 3), six months (OB 6; OB + MS 6) and twelve months (OB 12; OB + MS 12) after bariatric treatment.

Thirteen patients were treated for type 2 diabetes mellitus (T2DM), and twenty-two patients were treated for hypertension. Patients with obesity had a mean weight loss of 5 ± 0.6 kg for a time interval of 10 to 30 days prior to surgery. It was associated with a low-calorie diet, which was a part of the preparation for the surgery.

Body weight, height and waist and hips circumferences were measured using standard methods. Waist circumference was measured halfway between the lower arch of the ribs and the upper edge of the iliac crest, and the circumference of the hips by the largest protrusion of the gluteal muscles, below the iliac plates. BMI was calculated as weight (kg) divided by the square of height (m^2). The metabolic syndrome (MS) was diagnosed in accordance with the International Diabetes Federation. A subject has metabolic syndrome if it satisfies three or more of the following traits: large waist circumference (at least 89 cm for women and 102 cm for men or waist circumference does not need to be measured if BMI is >30 kg/m^2, central obesity can be assumed), hypertriglyceridemia (150 mg/dL) or specific treatment of this lipid abnormality, reduced high-density lipoprotein (HDL) cholesterol (less than 40 mg/dL in men or less than 50 mg/dL), hypertension (130/85 mm Hg or higher) or treatment of previously diagnosed hypertension and elevated fasting blood glucose (100 mg/dL or higher) or previously diagnosed type 2 diabetes [18].

The control group consisted of 33 lean healthy women (aged from 19 to 65 years; BMI < 25 kg/m^2) attending follow-up visits at the Specialist Dental Clinic at the Medical University of Bialystok. Only patients with normal blood counts and biochemical blood tests (Na^+, K^+, creatinine, AST, ALT, INR) were included in the control group.

The exclusion criteria for both the study and control group comprised systemic diseases: metabolic diseases (type 1 diabetes, gout, osteoporosis, and mucopolysaccharidosis), autoimmune diseases (Hashimoto's disease, Crohn's disease, and ulcerative colitis), infectious diseases (hepatitis A, B, or C, HIV/AIDS), diseases of the cardiovascular (other than hypertension), respiratory, digestive (other than obstructive sleep apnea), and genitourinary systems.

Additional exclusion criteria for the control group were hypertension, insulin resistance and type 2 diabetes, and obstructive sleep apnea.

Within the three-month period preceding the study, patients and healthy controls declared not taking any antibiotics, nonsteroidal anti-inflammatory drugs, glucocorticosteroids, vitamins, and antioxidant supplements. The participants were non-smokers and did not drink alcohol more frequently than once a month. Pregnant women, patients with acute inflammatory infections and a history of malignancy were also excluded from the study.

The clinical characteristics of the control and study groups are shown in Table 1.

2.1. Blood Collection

All samples were collected from obese and lean patients in the overnight fasting state. Twenty-four hours before blood sampling, patients also did not practice intense physical activity. The blood was taken to serum and EDTA tubes (S-Monovette SARSTEDT). The blood samples were centrifuged for 10 min at 4000 rpm in 4 °C. The supernatant was retained for further testing. Butylated hydroxytoluene (BHT) was added to all samples to protect them against oxidation (10 μL 0.5 M BHT/1 mL serum/plasma) [19]. The samples were stored at −80 °C until final examinations.

2.2. Laboratory Measurements

Serum triglycerides, total cholesterol, low-density lipoprotein (LDL) and high-density lipoprotein (HDL) cholesterol, C-reactive protein (CRP), alanine transaminase (ALT), aspartate transaminase (AST), the full blood count, glucose, and insulin were quantified by using an Abbott analyzer (Abbott Diagnostics, Wiesbaden, Germany). Homeostatic model assessment (HOMA-IR = fasting glucose (mg/dl) x fasting insulin (mU/l)/405) index was calculated [20].

Table 1. Clinical characteristics of the control, patients with morbid obesity without metabolic syndrome (OB) and patients with morbid obesity and metabolic syndrome (OB + MS). Data given as median (minimum and maximum), * $p < 0.05$, ** $p < 0.01$, *** $p < 0.001$, **** $p < 0.0001$ indicate significant differences from the control, # $p < 0.05$, ## $p < 0.01$, ### $p < 0.001$, #### $p < 0.0001$ indicate significant differences from the morbid obesity without metabolic syndrome (OB 0) patients before bariatric surgery; ^ $p < 0.05$, ^^ $p < 0.01$ ^^^ $p < 0.001$ ^^^^ $p < 0.0001$ indicate significant differences from the morbid obesity with metabolic syndrome (OB + MS 0) patients before bariatric surgery, alanine transaminase (ALT), aspartate transaminase (AST), C-reactive protein (CRP), high-density lipoprotein (HDL), hemoglobin (HGB), homeostatic model assessment of insulin resistance (HOMA-IR), low-density lipoprotein (LDL), platelet count (PLT), red blood cell count (RBC), triacylglycerol (TG), white blood cell count (WBC), waist-hip ratio (WHR), morbidly obese patients without metabolic syndrome (OB) and morbidly obese patients with metabolic syndrome (OB + MS), before (OB 0; OB + MS 0) as well as one month (OB 1; OB + MS 1), three months (OB 3; OB + MS 3), six months (OB 6; OB + MS 6) and twelve months (OB 12; OB + MS 12) after bariatric surgery.

	C	OB 0	OB + MS 0	OB 1	OB + MS 1	OB 3	OB + MS 3	OB 6	OB + MS 6	OB 12	OB + MS 12
Age	42 (28–56)	39 (28–52)	49 (28–56)	-	-	-	-	-	-	-	-
Weight (kg)	62 (55–72)	118**** (99–169)	125**** (94–170)	107.5**** (90–156)	113.5**** (84–160)	95.5****## (80–124)	102**** (77–138)	85**#### (72–113)	92.5****^^^^ (70–125)	78#### (63–104)	85*^^^^ (64–112)
BMI (kg/m²)	23.04 (21.93–24.80)	44.87**** (40.16–61.34)	46.52**** (40.03–60.96)	40.39**** (30.34–58.01)	41.62**** (32.81–56.68)	36.19****## (28.34–46.86)	39.30**** (29.05–49.91)	32.03**#### (26.15–42.06)	34.41****^^^^ (26.21–47.62)	28.73#### (24.09–37.65)	31.23*^^^^ (22.67–40.15)
WHR	0.71 (0.64 – 0.74)	0.95**** (0.81–1.04)	0.97**** (0.84–1.15)	0.95**** (0.73–1.01)	0.98**** (0.87–1.15)	0.93**** (0.80–1.01)	0.98**** (0.83–1.12)	0.92*** (0.81–0.98)	0.96**** (0.86–1.13)	0.90*# (0.80–0.98)	0.93***^^ (0.84–0.99)
Waist circumference (cm)	73 (66–86)	132.5 (110–149)	140.5 (120–161)	125 (100–135)	134.5 (115–152)	112 (90–129)	121.5 (101–139)	101.5 (82–116)	110 (92–130)	92 (78–108)	100 (82–116)
CRP (mg/L)	5.5 (5.1–6.5)	8.8 (1.5–27.6)	11.7**** (5.3–18.2)	5.2 (0.5–26)	8.35 (1.5–13.6)	6.1 (0.3–16.5)	7.1 (0.6–16.5)	4.76 (0.3–19.5)	6.05^^ (0.5–11.05)	4.85## (0.2–7.8)	5.5^^^ (1.2–16.1)
Glucose (mg/dL)	76 (67–92)	98**** (76–122)	106*** (89–189)	94**** (69–115)	99**** (75–147)	88 (60–142)	97**** (79–116)	84.5# (68–109)	95**** (81–157)	84## (73–111)	90**^^^ (77–99)
Insulin (uIU/mL)	7.5 (7–9.4)	17.85**** (8.2–38.6)	22.25*** (9.3–40.7)	11.6**# (4–28)	15.15**** (5.8–35.3)	8.15#### (2.7–16.2)	10.5*^^^ (3.6–43.8)	8.9#### (4.1–12.3)	8.75^^^^ (4.5–17.1)	8.1#### (3–14.5)	8.5^^^^ (4.5–9.9)
HOMA-IR	1.44 (1.19–1.86)	4.15**** (1.78–9.34)	5.64*** (3.05–8.1)	2.77***# (0.73–6.56)	3.82**** (1.25–8.62)	1.94#### (0.46–3.8)	2.47****^^ (0.95–10.16)	1.88#### (0.75–2.91)	1.98*^^^^ (1.1–3.84)	1.67#### (0.58–3.50)	1.91^^^^ (1.07–2.17)
ALT (IU/L)	23 (16–35)	24 (6–93)	27 (12–54)	23.5 (6–52)	27.5 (14–56)	20 (6–43)	24 (13–59)	17 (6–51)	21 (12–31)	18 (8–37)	19 (8–43)

Table 1. *Cont.*

	C	OB 0	OB + MS 0	OB 1	OB + MS 1	OB 3	OB + MS 3	OB 6	OB + MS 6	OB 12	OB + MS 12
AST (IU/L)	22 (16–36)	19 (13–44)	21 (14–50)	23.5 (14–98)	27 (14–85)	19 (12–36)	21 (13–43)	17 (9–48)	20 (12–43)	18 (12–52)	19 (12–37.2)
Cholesterol (mg/dL)	175 (159–189)	195 (147–231)	211**** (167–268)	170.5 (124–210)	192* (126–235)	176 (120–217)	181^ (120–237)	178 (114–245)	188 (148–264)	176 (114–231)	174^^^ (138–295)
LDL (mg/dL)	119 (115–123)	124.5 (100–159)	144** (122–181)	110 (83–153)	122^^ (66–183)	106 (69–159)	116^^^ (50–189)	109 (61–166)	110^^^^ (83–157)	113# (59–134)	102^^^^ (64–164)
TG (mg/dL)	135 (119–145)	128.5 (62–197)	150 (104–289)	108.5 (66–209)	136 (75–367)	103.5** (46–182)	137 (78–240)	96****## (48–182)	130 (89–214)	98****## (36–182)	102**^^^^ (59–146)
HDL (mg/dL)	60 (45–68)	50** (33–62)	46**** (31–72)	47**** (30–106)	45**** (31–68)	47*** (27–141)	49*** (35–69)	50** (35–72)	52.5 (35–86)	53 (38–81)	56^^ (43–70)
WBC (10^3/µL)	7.5 (4.4–9.1)	8.295* (5.26–12.15)	9.53* (5.85–12.91)	6.53## (4.63–9.64)	7.16 (4.95–12.7)	5.78*#### (4.61–10.54)	6.9 (3.9–11.54)	5.98### (4.75–9.27)	7.195 (4.4–10.94)	5.92*#### (4.07–8.52)	6.96^^^ (4.21–10.26)
RBC (10^6/µL)	4.6 (3.9–5.2)	4.7 (3.51–5.78)	4.6 (4–5.46)	4.79 (4.11–6.03)	4.77 (4.31–6.01)	4.655 (4.11–5.13)	4.75 (4.11–5.45)	4.65 (3.98–5.69)	4.75 (4.02–5.66)	4.62 (4.03–5.4)	4.50 (3.33–5.65)
HGB (g/dL)	13.8 (11.5–14.7)	13.1 (11–15.2)	13.35 (12.1–16.2)	13.2 (10–15.9)	13.6 (11.2–16.6)	13.1 (11.5–15.7)	13.2 (10.9–16.3)	13.4 (9.7–15.4)	13.4 (10.6–16.3)	13.65 (9.1–15.8)	14.15 (8.7–16.2)
PLT (10^3/µL)	289 (265–315)	264.5 (141–417	258 (183–418)	261 (121–412)	229* (128–405)	265.5 (130–312)	247 (131–345)	273.5 (188–425)	251.5 (167–375)	214.5*** (130–345)	224** (164–378)

2.3. Redox Assays

For the redox assays, all reagents were obtained from Sigma-Aldrich (Nümbrecht, Germany/Saint Louis, MO, USA). Antioxidant enzymes were assessed in serum, whereas the non-enzymatic antioxidants, redox status, and oxidation products were assessed in the plasma. The absorbance/fluorescence was measured using a 96-well microplate reader Infinite M200 PRO Multimode (Tecan Group Ltd., Männedorf, Switzerland). All determinations were performed in duplicate samples and standardized to 1 mg of total protein. Total protein content was determined colorimetrically using the bicinchoninic acid assay with bovine serum albumin as a standard (Thermo Scientific PIERCE BCA Protein Assay Kit, Rockford, IL, USA).

2.3.1. Antioxidant Barrier

The activity of serum Cu-Zn-superoxide dismutase (SOD, EC 1.15.1.1) was assessed spectrophotometrically by measuring the inhibition rate of adrenaline oxidation at 480 nm [21]. One unit of SOD activity was defined as the quantity of enzyme inhibiting adrenaline oxidation by 50%. The activity of serum catalase (CAT, EC 1.11.1.6) was assessed spectrophotometrically by measuring hydrogen peroxide (H_2O_2) decomposition at 240 nm [22]. One unit of CAT activity was defined as the quantity of the enzyme catalyzing decomposition of 1 mM of H_2O_2 per 1 min. The activity of serum glutathione peroxidase (GPx, EC 1.11.1.9) was assessed spectrophotometrically at 340 nm based on the reduction of organic peroxides by GPx in the presence of reduced nicotinamide adenine dinucleotide phosphate (NADPH) [23]. The activity of serum glutathione reductase (GR, EC 1.8.1.7) was assessed spectrophotometrically at 340 nm by measuring the decrease in NADPH absorbance [24]. One unit of GR activity was defined as the amount of enzyme catalyzing the oxidation of 1 μM NADPH per 1 min.

The concentration of plasma glutathione was assessed colorimetrically using the enzymatic reaction with NADPH, 5,5′-dithiobis-(2-nitrobenzoic acid) (DTNB), and GR [25,26]. The absorbance was measured at 412 nm. The reduced glutathione (GSH) concentration was calculated from the difference between the concentration of total glutathione and oxidized glutathione (GSSG). Oxidation/reduction potential (redox status) was calculated based on the formula = $(GSH)^2/(GSSG)$ [27].

The concentration of plasma uric acid (UA) was assessed spectrophotometrically at 630 nm using the commercial kit (QuantiChromTM Uric Acid DIUA-250; BioAssay Systems, Harward, CA, USA), according to the manufacturer's instructions.

2.3.2. Oxidative Stress Products

The content of plasma advanced glycation end products (AGE) was assessed spectrofluorimetrically by measuring AGE-specific fluorescence at 350/440 nm [28]. Immediately before the assay, plasma samples were diluted (1:5, v:v) in 0.02 M phosphate-buffered saline (PBS), pH 7.4 [29]. The concentration of plasma advanced oxidation protein products (AOPP) was assessed spectrophotometrically at 340 nm by measuring the iodide ion oxidizing capacity of the plasma [28]. Immediately before the assay, plasma was diluted (1:5, v:v) in 0.02 M PBS [29]. The concentration of plasma 4-hydroxynoneal protein adducts (4-HNE) and 8-isoprostanes (8-isop) was evaluated using commercial ELISA kits (OxiSelect HNE Adducts Competitive ELISA Kit, Cell Biolabs, Inc., San Diego, CA; 8-Isoprostane ELISA Kit, Cayman Chemicals, Ann Arbor, MI, USA; respectively), according to the manufacturer's instructions.

2.3.3. Statistical Analysis

Statistical analysis was performed using GraphPad Prism 8.3.0 for MacOS (GraphPad Software, Inc. La Jolla, USA). The normality of the distribution was assessed using the Shapiro–Wilk test. For comparison of quantitative variables, the Kruskal–Wallis ANOVA test and Dunn's test were used. Multiplicity adjusted p-value was also calculated. The relationship between the assessed redox biomarkers was evaluated using the Spearman rank correlation. In order to determine the diagnostic utility of measured parameters, receiver operating characteristic (ROC) curves were drawn, and the area under the curve (AUC) was calculated. The statistical significance level was set at $p < 0.05$.

The number of subjects was determined based on our previous experiment, assuming that the power of the test would be equal to 0.9.

3. Results

Table 1 shows a comparison of the clinical and laboratory characteristics of the lean control (C), patients with morbid obesity without metabolic syndrome (OB 0) and patients with morbid obesity and metabolic syndrome (OB + MS 0) before and after the bariatric surgery. We found significantly higher values in BMI, waist-hip ratio (WHR), and waist circumference as well as in CRP, white blood cell, glucose, and insulin levels and HOMA-IR, in both groups of patients with obesity compared with lean patients, whereas HDL levels were decreased. Total cholesterol, low-density lipoprotein concentration, and blood pressure were greater in OB + MS 0 patients compared with controls. The body weight, BMI as well as WHR diminished after bariatric surgery in both studied groups at six and twelve months after bariatric surgery. Additionally, we noticed significant differences between OB 3 and OB + MS 3 as well as OB 6 and OB + MS 6 regarding the following: fasting plasma glucose and TAG (Table 1).

Individual data of metabolic parameters are presented in Supplementary Materials (Table S1).

3.1. *Antioxidant Barrier*

Both enzymatic (SOD, CAT, GPx, and GR) and non-enzymatic antioxidants (UA, GSH, and GSSG) were used to assess the antioxidant status. Redox potential $[GSH]^2/[GSSG]$ has also been calculated.

3.1.1. Superoxide Dismutase (SOD)

The activity of serum SOD was significantly decreased in both studied groups before the bariatric surgery: OB 0 (−23%, $p < 0.0001$) and OB + MS 0 (−27%, $p < 0.0001$) as compared to lean control. Interestingly, in morbidly obese patients with metabolic syndrome: OB + MS 1 (−19%, $p = 0.0064$), OB + MS 3 (−16%, $p = 0.0282$), OB + MS 6 (−18%, $p = 0.0085$) and OB + MS 12 (−21%, 0.0007), the activity of SOD was also lower in every time period after the surgery than in lean individuals, whereas we did not observe any changes in patients with morbid obesity without metabolic syndrome at the same time period. Furthermore, in OB 1 and OB 12 groups, we found the increase in SOD activity (+20%, $p = 0.0295$ +26%, $p = 0.003$, respectively) in comparison with OB 0 patients (Figure 1A).

3.1.2. Catalase (CAT) and Glutathione Peroxidase (GPx)

There were no statistically significant differences in the activity of serum CAT and GPx in the serum of studied groups (OB and OB + MS) compared with control. Also, the GPx activity did not change in OB and OB + MS patients after bariatric treatment (Figure 1B–D).

3.1.3. Glutathione Reductase (GR)

The activity of serum GR was significantly increased in the OB + MS 0 (+15%, $p = 0.05$) group as compared to healthy controls (+19%, $p = 0.05$) and the OB subgroup (+16%, $p = 0.05$).

3.1.4. Uric Acid (UA)

The plasma concentration of UA was significantly higher before (OB 0: +15%, $p = 0.0002$) as well as one month (OB 1: +13%, $p = 0.0029$) after the bariatric surgery in morbid obesity without metabolic syndrome patients compared to the control group. Furthermore, we observed a decrease in UA concentration in the OB 3 group (−17%, $p < 0.0001$) compared with OB 0. Interestingly, in plasma of morbidly obese subjects with metabolic syndrome, the UA concentration was greater in OB + MS 0 (+20%, $p < 0.0001$), OB +MS 1 (+14%, $p = 0.0003$), OB + MS 6 (+13%, $p = 0.0045$) and OB + MS 12 (+10%, $p = 0.0187$) as compared to lean individuals (Figure 1E).

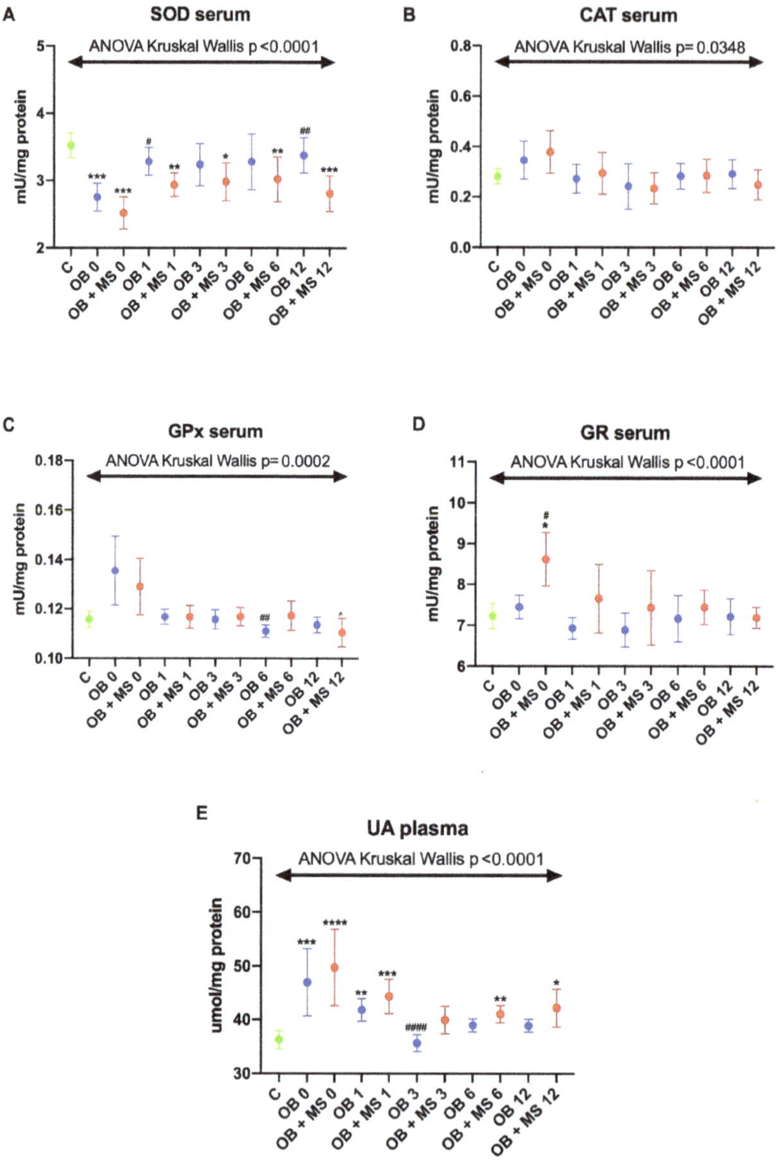

Figure 1. Activity of serum enzymatic (**A–D**) and plasma non-enzymatic antioxidants (**E**) of the control, morbid obesity without metabolic syndrome (OB) and morbid obesity with metabolic syndrome (OB + MS). Results are presented as median with 95% Cl. * $p < 0.05$, ** $p < 0.01$, *** $p < 0.001$, **** $p < 0.0001$ indicate significant differences from the control; # $p < 0.05$, ## $p < 0.01$, #### $p < 0.0001$ indicate significant differences from the morbid obesity without metabolic syndrome (OB 0) patients before bariatric surgery. Superoxide dismutase (SOD), catalase (CAT), glutathione peroxidase (GPx), glutathione reductase (GR) and uric acid (UA), morbidly obese patients without metabolic syndrome (OB) and morbidly obese patients with metabolic syndrome (OB + MS), before (OB 0; OB + MS 0) as well as one month (OB 1; OB + MS 1), three months (OB 3; OB + MS 3), six months (OB 6; OB + MS 6) and twelve months (OB 12; OB + MS 12) after bariatric surgery.

3.1.5. Reduced Glutathione (GSH)

The concentration of GSH was significantly lower in the plasma of both obese groups before the bariatric surgery: OB 0 (−26%, p = 0.0447) and OB + MS 0 (−33%, p = 0.0001) as compared to control. In addition, the GSH concentration was significantly decreased in the plasma of morbidly obese patients with metabolic syndrome in three (OB + MS 3: −31%, p = 0.0040) and six (OB + MS 6: −25%, p = 0.0108) months after bariatric treatment (Figure 2A).

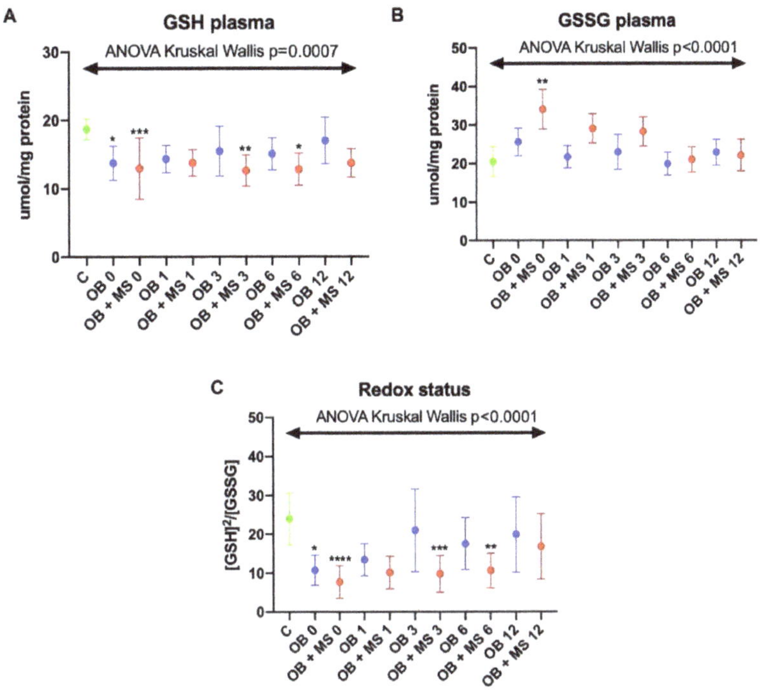

Figure 2. Plasma concentration of glutathione (GSH) (**A**), glutathione disulfide (GSSG) (**B**) and redox status (**C**) of the control, morbid obesity without metabolic syndrome (OB) and morbid obesity with metabolic syndrome (OB + MS). Results are presented as median with 95% Cl. *p < 0.05,** p < 0.01, *** p < 0.001, **** p < 0.0001 indicate significant differences from the control; glutathione (GSH), glutathione disulfide (GSSG), morbidly obese patients without metabolic syndrome (OB) and morbidly obese patients with metabolic syndrome (OB + MS), before (OB 0; OB + MS 0) as well as one month (OB 1; OB + MS 1), three months (OB 3; OB + MS 3), six months (OB 6; OB + MS 6) and twelve months (OB 12; OB + MS 12) after bariatric surgery.

3.1.6. Glutathione Disulfide (GSSG)

The concentration of plasma GSSG was only markedly higher in OB + MS 0 patients (+89%, p = 0.0015) as compared to the control group (Figure 2B).

3.1.7. Redox Status

Plasma redox status was significantly decreased in OB 0 (−46%, p = 0.0105) and OB + MS 0 (−82%, p < 0.0001) in comparison with the control group. Interestingly, in morbidly obese patients with metabolic syndrome it was still diminished after bariatric surgery: OB + MS 3 (−77%, p = 0.0004) and OB + MS 6 (−54%, p = 0.0088) (Figure 2C).

3.2. Oxidative Damage Products

Oxidative stress was assessed based on the protein (AGE, AOPP) and lipid (4-HNE, 8-isoP) oxidative damage.

3.2.1. Advanced Glycation End Products (AGE)

The AGE plasma content significantly increased in morbidly obese patients without metabolic syndrome OB 0 (+23%, p = 0.0026) as well as in those with metabolic syndrome OB + MS 0 (+31%, p < 0.0001) as compared to the control group. Moreover, we noticed that, the AGE content diminished in both obese groups twelve months after bariatric treatment OB 12 (−16%, p = 0.0041 vs. OB 0) and OB + MS 12 (−17%, p = 0.0018 vs. OB + MS 0) (Figure 3A).

3.2.2. Advanced Oxidation Protein Products (AOPP)

We found a markedly higher plasma concentration of AOPP in obese patients: OB 0 (+32%, p = 0.0099) and OB + MS 0 (+64%, p = 0.0001) as compared to lean ones. Similar to the AGE content, the AOPP concentration decreased after the bariatric surgery: OB 1 (−25%, p = 0.0323 vs. OB 0) and OB + MS 12 (−34%, p = 0.0417 vs. OB +MS 0) (Figure 3B).

3.2.3. 8-Isoprostanes (8-isop)

The 8-isop concentration was significantly greater in both morbidly obese groups before bariatric surgery as well as in every time period after the surgery compared to lean patients: OB 0 (+82%, p < 0.0001), OB 1 (+99%, p < 0.0001), OB 3 (+46%, p = 0.0002), OB 6 (+59%, p < 0.0001), OB 12 (+48%, p < 0.0001), OB + MS 0 (+77%, p < 0.0001), OB + MS 1 (+98%, p < 0.0001), OB + MS 3 (+49%, p = 0.0002), OB + MS 6 (+48%, p < 0.0001), and OB + MS 12 (+46%, p = 0.0002). Interestingly, in morbidly obese group with metabolic syndrome, the plasma concentration of 8-isop diminished three and twelve months after the bariatric surgery: OB + MS 3 (−17%, p = 0.014 vs. OB +MS 0) and OB + MS 12 (−18%, p = 0.0194 vs. OB + MS 0) (Figure 3C).

3.2.4. 4-Hydroxynoneal Protein Adducts (4-HNE)

We found differences in the plasma 4-HNE concentration of OB + MS 0 (+3%, p = 0.0053) and OB 6 (+4%, p = 0.0024) patients in comparison with the control group (Figure 3D).

3.2.5. Correlations

Correlations between the analyzed redox biomarkers and clinical parameters are presented in the heat maps (Figures 4 and 5).

In the OB subgroup, we found negative correlations between CAT and glucose (R = −0.432; p = 0.014) as well as GPx and HOMA-IR (R = −0.375; p = 0.049). Additionally, in OB patients there were positive correlations between GR and AOPP (R = 0.934; p < 0.0001) and GR and TG (R = 0.367; p = 0.046). A positive correlation was also revealed between UA and BMI (R = 0.371; p = 0.04). Moreover, serum GSSG concentration was associated with the plasma insulin (R = 0.616; p < 0.0001), HOMA-IR (R = 0.402; p = 0.028) and plasma CRP (R = 0.465; p = 0.006) of the OB subgroup. In OB patients, AOPP was positively correlated with TG (R = 0.402; p = 0.028) (Figure 4).

In the OB + MS subgroup, we showed high positive correlations between GR and AOPP (R = 0.93; p < 0.0001). The positive correlations were also demonstrated between UA and HDL (R = 0.507; p = 0.008) as well as AGE and LDL (R = 0.407; p = 0.031) (Figure 5).

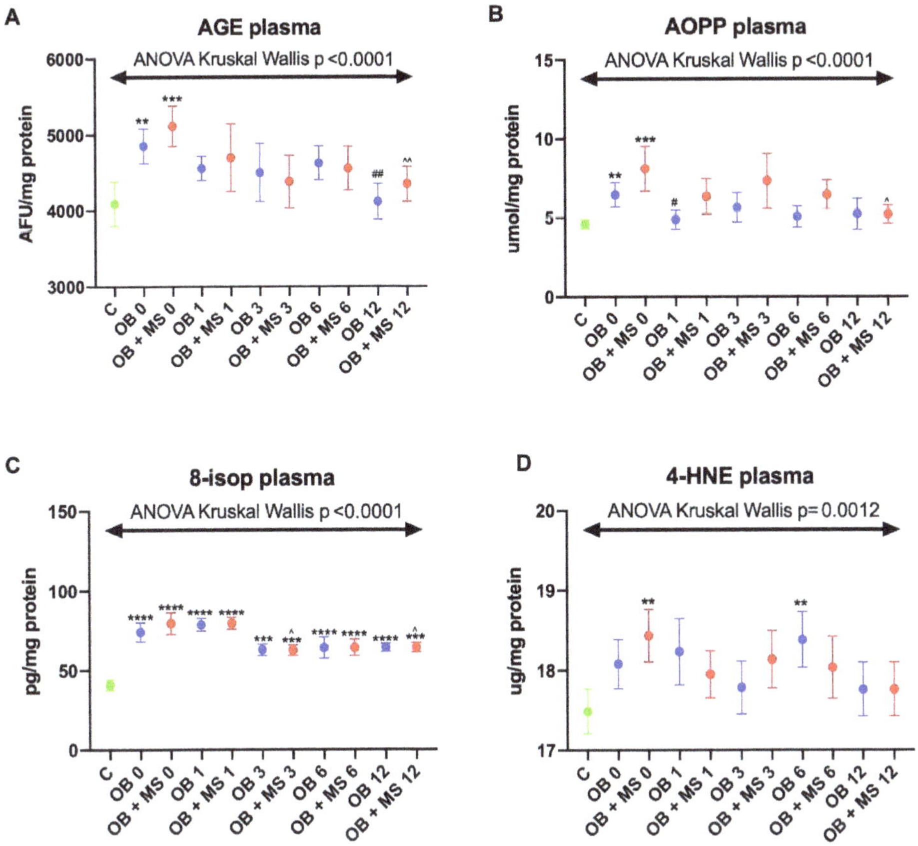

Figure 3. Plasma content of advanced glycation end products (AGE) (**A**), plasma concentration of advanced oxidation protein products (AOPP) (**B**), 8-isoprostanes (8-isop) (**C**) and 4-hydroxynoneal protein adducts (4-HNE) of the control (**D**), morbid obesity without metabolic syndrome (OB) and morbid obesity with metabolic syndrome (OB + MS). Results are presented as median with 95% Cl. ** $p < 0.01$, *** $p < 0.001$, **** $p < 0.0001$ indicate significant differences from the control; ## $p < 0.01$ indicate significant differences from the morbid obesity without metabolic syndrome (OB 0) patients before bariatric surgery; ^ $p < 0.05$, ^^ $p < 0.01$ indicate significant differences from the morbid obesity with metabolic syndrome (OB + MS 0) patients before bariatric surgery. Advanced glycation end products (AGE), advanced oxidation protein products (AOPP), 8-isoprostanes (8-isop) and 4-hydroxynoneal protein adducts (4-HNE), morbidly obese patients without metabolic syndrome (OB) and morbidly obese patients with metabolic syndrome (OB + MS), before (OB 0; OB + MS 0) as well as one month (OB 1; OB + MS 1), three months (OB 3; OB + MS 3), six months (OB 6; OB + MS 6) and twelve months (OB 12; OB + MS 12) after bariatric surgery.

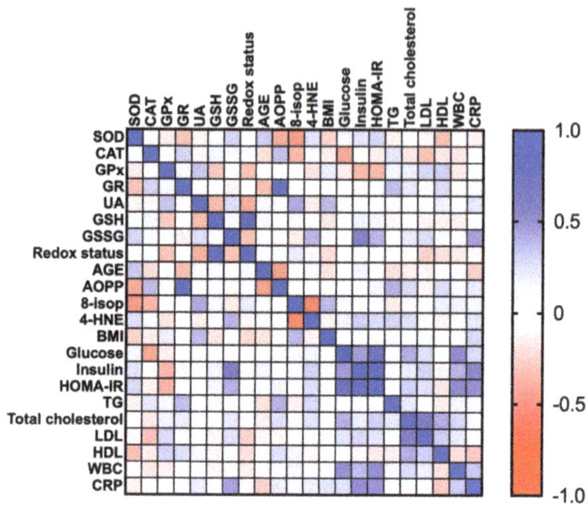

Figure 4. Correlations between the analyzed redox biomarkers and clinical parameters in patients with morbid obesity without metabolic syndrome (OB 0). Superoxide dismutase (SOD), catalase (CAT), glutathione peroxidase (GPx), glutathione reductase (GR) and uric acid (UA), glutathione (GSH), glutathione disulfide (GSSG) advanced glycation end products (AGE), advanced oxidation protein products (AOPP), 8-isoprostanes (8-isop) and 4-hydroxynoneal protein adducts (4-HNE), C-reactive protein (CRP), high-density lipoprotein (HDL), homeostatic model assessment of insulin resistance (HOMA-IR), low-density lipoprotein (LDL), triacylglycerol (TG), white blood cell count (WBC).

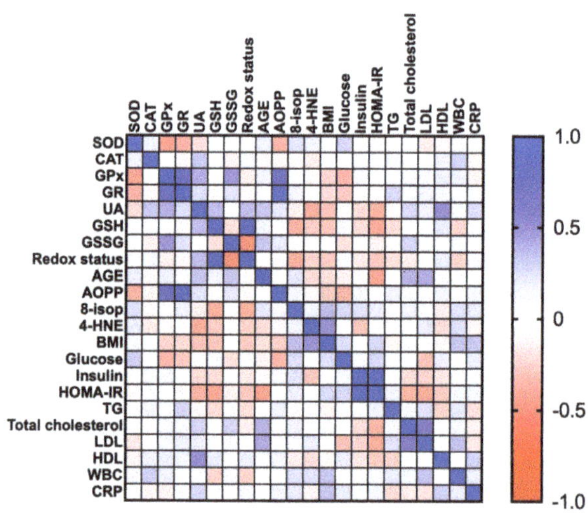

Figure 5. Correlations between the analyzed redox biomarkers and clinical parameters in patients with morbid obesity and metabolic syndrome (OB + MS 0). Superoxide dismutase (SOD), catalase (CAT), glutathione peroxidase (GPx), glutathione reductase (GR) and uric acid (UA), glutathione (GSH), glutathione disulfide (GSSG)advanced glycation end products (AGE), advanced oxidation protein products (AOPP), 8-isoprostanes (8-isop) and 4-hydroxynoneal protein adducts (4-HNE), C-reactive protein (CRP), high-density lipoprotein (HDL), homeostatic model assessment of insulin resistance (HOMA-IR), low-density lipoprotein (LDL), triacylglycerol (TG), white blood cell count (WBC).

3.2.6. ROC Analysis

We checked whether the assessed redox biomarkers differentiated cases with morbid obesity from obese cases with metabolic syndrome. Nevertheless, none of the biomarkers (with high specificity/sensitivity) distinguishes the tested groups. The best diagnostic utility has been demonstrated for the serum GR. This parameter with moderate sensitivity (71%) and specificity (61%) differentiates patients with morbid obesity from obese patients with MS (Figure 6). The optimal GR activity differentiating the two groups is >7.450 mU/mg protein at an AUC of 0.72 ($p = 0.003$).

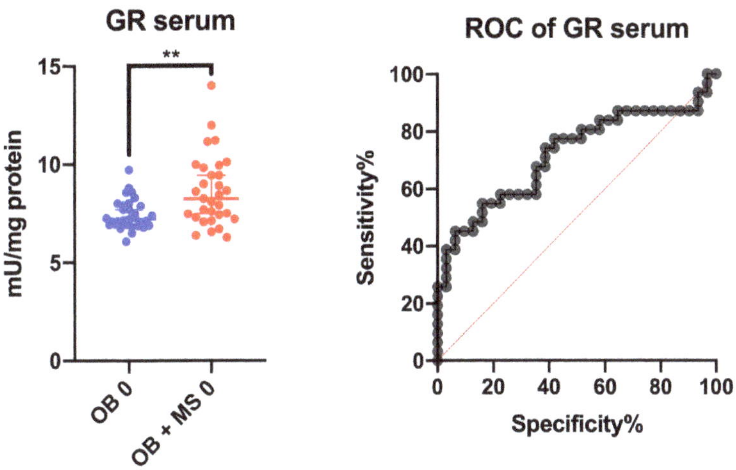

Figure 6. Area under the curve (AUC) of glutathione reductase (GR) activity between the obese patients and cases with obesity and metabolic syndrome. Glutathione reductase (GR), morbid obesity without metabolic syndrome (OB) and morbid obesity with metabolic syndrome (OB + MS). ** $p < 0.01$ indicate significant difference from the OB 0.

4. Discussion

Numerous studies indicate that visceral obesity is the main cause of insulin resistance and MS [30]; nevertheless, the causes of reduced insulin sensitivity in the target organs are not exactly known. It is suggested that the common denominator of these metabolic disturbances may be redox imbalance as well as increased oxidative stress [31]. Moreover, despite the proven effectiveness of bariatric surgery, it is unclear whether it improves the redox homeostasis of morbidly obese cases. According to our knowledge, this is the first study evaluating the redox balance, glutathione metabolism, and oxidative damage to proteins and lipids in the plasma and serum of morbidly obese patients not only before, but also one, three, six and twelve months after bariatric surgery. We are also the first to compare the redox homeostasis of obese patients with metabolic syndrome to obese cases only.

4.1. Antioxidant Barrier

Literature data unequivocally shows that bariatric surgery leads to a marked reduction in adipose tissue mass, followed by an improvement in systemic inflammation [32]. However, with respect to the antioxidant status and oxidative stress, there are some contradictions. Indeed, in obese patients, both increases and decreases in the antioxidant barrier are observed [33–35]. These differences may be associated with the duration of obesity as well as the age of obese patients. It is suggested that the antioxidant systems are prompted in the early stage of the disease, whereas in long-term obesity, the source of antioxidants depletes and causes decreased activity of the antioxidant enzymes [34,36]. In our study, the activity of antioxidant enzymes did not differ significantly. Nevertheless, SOD activity was reduced in obese patients both before as well as after the bariatric treatment. In obesity, an important source of ROS is an excessive increase in energetic substrates provided to the respiratory chain in mitochondria. This leads to the formation of considerable amounts of superoxide anions that exceed the antioxidant capacity of the body [37]. However, chronic inflammation is also associated with enhanced production of ROS in obese patients [38,39]. Adipokines secreted by adipose tissue activate the transcription factor NF-κB (nuclear factor-kappa B), which enhances NADPH oxidase (NOX) activity and stimulates phagocytes. Indeed, phagocytes are a rich source of superoxide radicals that produce their large quantities during respiratory burst [39,40]. Under these conditions, the active center of SOD can be inactivated by enhanced levels of free radicals. Although we have not directly evaluated the rate of ROS formation, decreased SOD activity may indicate the long-term overproduction of free radicals in obese patients. Interestingly, Mohseni et al. [41] found a positive correlation between SOD expression and BMI, insulin, HOMA-IR, LDL, total cholesterol and TG. In our study, the activity of SOD does not normalize after bariatric treatment, which suggests the persistence of redox imbalance in obese individuals. Indeed, although body weight has been significantly reduced after the surgery, all patients are still obese and their fat tissue may be an important source of ROS and inflammation.

The antioxidant reserves may also deplete with age. However, our patients were in a similar age range, so the effect of age on the evaluated redox biomarkers is limited [42].

The activity of CAT and GPx did not differ significantly. However, the activity of GR was statistically higher in patients with obesity and MS before bariatric surgery (as compared to controls and obese patients without MS). Considering that GR participates in the regeneration of GSH, an increase in enzyme activity may be an adaptive reaction related to a decrease in glutathione synthesis [24,36]. Indeed, GSH concentration was significantly lower in the plasma of both study groups as compared to healthy controls. Moreover, an increase in GR activity may respond to the overproduction of ROS and the enhanced oxidative damage in the cell. This hypothesis may be confirmed by the strong positive correlation between GR activity and protein oxidation products (AOPP) observed in the study group.

The glutathione level was also significantly reduced in obese patients with MS after the bariatric treatment. This indicates a higher depletion of glutathione reserves in patients with obesity and metabolic syndrome. It should be recalled that GSH is the most important intracellular antioxidant. Reduced glutathione can react with superoxide and hydroxyl radicals, leading to an accumulation of GSSG in the cytosol [43]. However, GSSG can also react with thiol groups of proteins, contributing to the induction of oxidative stress [43]. In our study, GSSG concentration was higher in obese patients with metabolic syndrome before the bariatric treatment (Figure 1B). The positive correlation between GSSG concentration and insulin level/HOMA-IR is also interesting, which may indicate a potential link between glutathione oxidation and disease progression. Importantly, the redox status of obese cases was significantly reduced before the surgery, similarly to obese patients with MS at 3 and 6 months after the surgery. The redox status (ratio of reduced and oxidized glutathione) is used to assess the oxidative-reduction potential of the sample and characterizes the resultant ability of the biological system to counteract oxidative stress [26]. Thus, the oxidant/antioxidant balance is disturbed in patients before the bariatric treatment. However, redox homeostasis is also impaired in obese patients with MS after the surgery. In opposition to our results, Bankoglu et al. [44] found greater GSH and GSSG content in erythrocytes from obese patients before bariatric surgery. Sarosiek et al. [17] observed an increase in oxidized forms of glutathione and cysteine in obese subjects after bariatric surgery.

Uric acid is the end-product of endogenous and dietary purine metabolism [45]. It is also the most important body antioxidant responsible for up to 70%–80% of plasma antioxidant capacity [40]. In low concentrations, UA effectively sweeps oxygen/nitrogen free radicals; nevertheless, at elevated concentrations, it also generates ROS and oxidizes cellular biomolecules [46]. It has been demonstrated that hyperuricemia is associated with obesity, especially with the accumulation of visceral fat [47]. Additionally, evaluated serum UA may imply an increased risk of various metabolic disorders, such as glucose intolerance, T2DM, high blood pressure, metabolic syndrome as well as cardiovascular disease [45,48,49]. Indeed, hyperuricemia is responsible for reducing the release of nitric oxide (NO) and the resulting endothelial dysfunction/platelet aggregation [46]. Although these reactions may be partially blocked by glutathione, when the concentration of GSH decreases, there is an increased production of nitrogen free radicals. However, how does bariatric treatment affect the blood UA levels? Liu et al. [45] observed a decrease in serum UA of women and men one year after bariatric surgery. However, in our study, a statistically significant change was found only in patients from the OB 3 group. No significant decrease of UA concentration after bariatric surgery, especially in the OB + MS group, may be associated with the very high weight of all patients (Figure 1E). Our patients had class 3 obesity (mean BMI > 40 kg/m^2), and those described by Liu et al. [45] had BMI < 35 kg/m^2 (class 1 obesity). This confirms our earlier hypothesis about the persistence of redox imbalance after bariatric surgery.

4.2. Oxidative Damage to Proteins and Lipids

Although changes in the concentration/activity of antioxidants may indicate a systemic redox imbalance, the evaluation of cellular oxidation products is necessary to demonstrate oxidative stress in the biological system [8]. In this study, we assessed the products of protein (AGE, AOPP) and lipid (4-HNE, 8-isop) plasma oxidation. AGEs are pro-oxidant compounds formed through the non-enzymatic glycation of proteins [50]. Their higher formation is caused mainly by hyperglycemia and, therefore, they are a recognized biomarker of protein carbonyl stress [51]. In our research, AGEs content was significantly increased in both studied groups as compared to the healthy control group. AGEs can bind to receptors on the cell surface and influence several intracellular processes. Indeed, by combining with a specific receptor (RAGE), AGEs increase the production of ROS (through NOX induction), but also enhance the expression of the NF-κB pathway. Under these conditions, other signal routes (MAP-kinases, NJK and p21RAS) can be activated [39,52]. It is suggested that AGEs may play a key role in the development of insulin resistance [39,52]. However, the AGE level was diminished twelve months after bariatric surgery. This is undoubtedly related to the improvement of metabolic status in obese people. Indeed, we observed a decrease in pro-inflammatory parameters such as CRP and WBC. Also, the plasma concentration of glucose and insulin, as well as total cholesterol and LDL diminished in both morbidly obese cases (Table 1). Given the key role of protein glycation in the progression of microvascular lesions, a decrease in AGEs after the surgery may explain the reduced incidence of retinopathy, nephropathy and neuropathy in patients undergoing treatment [52,53]. Indeed, the most common cause of microangiopathy is basement membrane thickening and extracellular matrix hypertrophy [53]. In our patients, the AOPPs concentration also decreased after the bariatric surgery. AOPPs are a family of dityrosine-containing products produced by the reaction of proteins with hypochlorous acid, resulting from myeloperoxidase activity [54]. AOPP appears to be superior to other redox markers due to its early formation, greater stability and longer half-life [55]. Increased accumulation of AOPP has been linked with oxidative stress-related diseases and impaired carbohydrate metabolism (obesity, T2DM as well as metabolic syndrome) [56–58]. Krzystek-Korpacka et al. [59] observed a reduction in the plasma AOPP levels after the weight loss caused by lifestyle modification (encompassing physical activity and low caloric diet). Nevertheless, so far, no one has examined the impact of bariatric surgery on AOPP levels in morbidly obese patients. Therefore, we have shown that bariatric surgery not only reduces protein glycation (carbonyl stress; AGE) but also decreases protein oxidation in obese cases (AOPP).

In our study we also evaluated lipid oxidation products: 8-isoprostanes and 4-hydroxynonneal protein adducts. Previously, greater levels of 8-isoP and 4-HNE have been shown in diabetes, atherosclerosis, cardiovascular diseases, and cancers [60–62]. However, knowledge of lipid oxidation in the course of bariatric treatment is still limited. In our previous study [7] we evaluated lipid oxidation products in the nonstimulated and stimulated saliva of patients with morbid obesity treated with bariatric surgery. We [7] found a significantly higher concentration of 8-isoP and 4-HNE in nonstimulated and stimulated saliva of obese cases before, as well as six months after the surgery. In this study, the 8-isop concentration was significantly greater in both obese groups before bariatric surgery as well as in every time period after the treatment (as compared to the control). This is not surprising because lipids, especially unsaturated ones, are relatively unstable compounds that are easily oxidized. Although lipid oxidation is a complex process, it occurs particularly when the antioxidant barrier is exhausted [26,40]. Thus, in our patients, changes in glutathione metabolism, reduced SOD activity as well as an increase in uric acid level may be crucial. It has been shown that lipid peroxidation products change the physical properties of cell membranes. Indeed, lipoperoxidation leads to a disturbance of cell membrane asymmetry as well as an inhibition of membrane enzymes and transporter proteins [26,40]. However, in morbidly obese cases, the plasma concentration of 8-isop diminished in three and twelve months after the surgery. This suggests a decrease in lipid peroxidation depending on the time of surgical treatment. Nevertheless, the level of 4-hydroxynonneal protein adducts was increased only in obese patients with metabolic syndrome before the bariatric surgery. Although lipid peroxides can react with proteins and nucleic acids, this occurs only under severe oxidative stress [26,40]. Additionally, of all lipid peroxidation products, 4-HNE is considered the most cytotoxic form of lipid damage [26].

4.3. Diagnostic Significance

Recently, there has been a growing interest in the use of redox biomarkers in the diagnosis of various systemic diseases [19,36,63–69]. This is not surprising because oxidative stress plays a key role not only in the pathogenesis of neurodegenerative diseases/cancers but also many metabolic diseases such as insulin resistance, hypertension, diabetes and metabolic syndrome [40]. We compared whether antioxidants/oxidation products can differentiate between patients with obesity and those with obesity and metabolic syndrome. Although the diagnostic criteria for MS are widely known and routinely used, we have checked whether the assessment of a single biomarker can help to diagnose metabolic syndrome. However, none of the parameters with high sensitivity/specificity differentiates the tested groups. The best diagnostic utility has been demonstrated for the serum GR. Interestingly, GR activity also correlates with TG content in obese cases. However, it is necessary to conduct further studies on a larger population of patients.

4.4. Study Limitations

Despite a carefully selected group of patients, our work has certain limitations. We are not able to eliminate the influence of hypotensive/antidiabetic drugs on the assessed redox biomarkers. Besides, the study was conducted exclusively on women. We have previously shown that blood redox homeostasis does not depend on sex in healthy controls [42]; however, it is still unclear whether sex does not affect oxidative stress in obese patients undergoing bariatric treatment. Finally, we evaluated only selected antioxidants and biomarkers of oxidative stress, so we cannot fully conclude on redox homeostasis in obese cases. Although the study should be conducted on a larger population of patients, it should be stressed that for long-term observation, we have included a relatively large number of obese patients cautiously selected for accompanying diseases. Thus, our study is the starting point for further basic and clinical research.

5. Conclusions

In obese patients, the antioxidant status is disturbed and protein/lipid oxidation is increased. Although bariatric surgery improves redox homeostasis in obese cases, enzymatic and non-enzymatic antioxidant barriers as well as oxidative stress are not found at the control group level. Although the redox homeostasis disorders seem to be similar in patients with obesity and MS as well as obesity itself, cases with metabolic syndrome showed a continuous decrease in the antioxidant status (GSH, $[GSH]^2/[GSSG]$), reduced SOD activity and an increase in UA plasma concentration. Given the persistence of glutathione alterations after the bariatric treatment, antioxidant supplementation should be considered in obese patients with MS. Additionally, further long-term studies are needed on a larger population of obese cases.

Supplementary Materials: The following are available online at http://www.mdpi.com/2077-0383/9/4/976/s1, Table S1: Individual data of metabolic parameters in the study group.

Author Contributions: Conceptualization, B.C., P.M., A.Z. and M.M.; Data curation, B.C. and M.M.; Formal analysis, B.C., H.M., K.C. and M.M.; Funding acquisition, B.C., A.Z. and M.M.; Investigation, B.C. and M.M.; Methodology, B.C. and M.M.; Project administration, B.C. and M.M.; Resources, B.C., P.M., M.Ł. and P.W.; Software, B.C.; Supervision, P.M., J.D. and A.Z.; Validation, B.C. and M.M.; Visualization, B.C. and M.M.; Writing—original draft, B.C. and M.M.; Writing—review and editing, P.M., A.Z. and M.M. All authors have read and agreed to the published version of the manuscript.

Funding: This work was supported by grants from the Medical University of Bialystok, Poland (grant numbers: SUB/1/DN/20/002/1209; SUB/1/DN/20/002/3330; SUB/1/DN/19/003/1140).

Conflicts of Interest: The authors declare no conflict of interest.

References

1. Andò, S.; Gelsomino, L.; Panza, S.; Giordano, C.; Bonofiglio, D.; Barone, I.; Catalano, S. Obesity, leptin and breast cancer: Epidemiological evidence and proposed mechanisms. *Cancers (Basel)* **2019**, *11*, E62. [CrossRef] [PubMed]
2. Zubrzycki, A.; Cierpka-Kmiec, K.; Kmiec, Z.; Wronska, A. The role of low-calorie diets and intermittent fasting in the treatment of obesity and type−2 diabetes. *J. Physiol. Pharmacol.* **2018**, *69*, 30683819.
3. Korybalska, K.; Luczak, J.; Swora-Cwynar, E.; Kanikowska, A.; Czepulis, N.; Kanikowska, D.; Skalisz, H.; Breborowicz, A.; Grzymislawski, M.; Witowski, J. Weight loss-dependent and -independent effects of moderate calorie restriction on endothelial cell markers in obesity. *J. Physiol. Pharmacol.* **2017**, *68*, 597–608.
4. Choromańska, B.; Myśliwiec, P.; Razak Hady, H.; Dadan, J.; Myśliwiec, H.; Chabowski, A.; Mikłosz, A. Metabolic Syndrome is Associated with Ceramide Accumulation in Visceral Adipose Tissue of Women with Morbid Obesity. *Obesity* **2019**. [CrossRef] [PubMed]
5. Choromanska, B.; Mysliwiec, P.; Hady, H.R.; Dadan, J.; Mysliwiec, H.; Bonda, T.; Chabowski, A.; Miklosz, A. The implication of adipocyte ATP-binding cassette A1 and G1 transporters in metabolic complications of obesity. *J. Physiol. Pharmacol.* **2019**. [CrossRef]
6. Barazzoni, R.; Gortan Cappellari, G.; Ragni, M.; Nisoli, E. Insulin resistance in obesity: An overview of fundamental alterations. *Eat. Weight Disord.* **2018**, *23*, 149–157. [CrossRef]
7. Fejfer, K.; Buczko, P.; Niczyporuk, M.; Ładny, J.R.; Hady, H.R.; Knaś, M.; Waszkiel, D.; Klimiuk, A.; Zalewska, A.; Maciejczyk, M. Oxidative Modification of Biomolecules in the Nonstimulated and Stimulated Saliva of Patients with Morbid Obesity Treated with Bariatric Surgery. *Biomed. Res. Int.* **2017**, *2017*. [CrossRef]
8. Lushchak, V.I. Free radicals, reactive oxygen species, oxidative stress and its classification. *Chem. Biol. Interact.* **2014**, *224*, 164–175. [CrossRef]
9. Maciejczyk, M.; Heropolitanska-Pliszka, E.; Pietrucha, B.; Sawicka-Powierza, J.; Bernatowska, E.; Wolska-Kusnierz, B.; Pac, M.; Car, H.; Zalewska, A.; Mikoluc, B. Antioxidant Defense, Redox Homeostasis, and Oxidative Damage in Children With Ataxia Telangiectasia and Nijmegen Breakage Syndrome. *Front. Immunol.* **2019**, *10*, 2322. [CrossRef]
10. Borys, J.; Maciejczyk, M.; Antonowicz, B.; Krętowski, A.; Sidun, J.; Domel, E.; Dąbrowski, J.R.; Ładny, J.R.; Morawska, K.; Zalewska, A. Glutathione Metabolism, Mitochondria Activity, and Nitrosative Stress in Patients Treated for Mandible Fractures. *J. Clin. Med.* **2019**, *8*, 127. [CrossRef]
11. Knaś, M.; Maciejczyk, M.; Sawicka, K.; Hady, H.R.; Niczyporuk, M.; Ładny, J.R.; Matczuk, J.; Waszkiel, D.; Żendzian-Piotrowska, M.; Zalewska, A. Impact of morbid obesity and bariatric surgery on antioxidant/oxidant balance of the unstimulated and stimulated human saliva. *J. Oral Pathol. Med.* **2016**, *45*, 455–464. [CrossRef] [PubMed]
12. Sudlow, A.; le Roux, C.; Pournaras, D. The metabolic benefits of different bariatric operations: What procedure to choose? *Endocr. Connect.* **2020**, *9*, R28–R35. [CrossRef] [PubMed]
13. Palleja, A.; Kashani, A.; Allin, K.H.; Nielsen, T.; Zhang, C.; Li, Y.; Brach, T.; Liang, S.; Feng, Q.; Jørgensen, N.B.; et al. Roux-en-Y gastric bypass surgery of morbidly obese patients induces swift and persistent changes of the individual gut microbiota. *Genome Med.* **2016**. [CrossRef] [PubMed]
14. Busetto, L.; Dicker, D.; Azran, C.; Batterham, R.L.; Farpour-Lambert, N.; Fried, M.; Hjelmesæth, J.; Kinzl, J.; Leitner, D.R.; Makaronidis, J.M.; et al. Practical Recommendations of the Obesity Management Task Force of the European Association for the Study of Obesity for the Post-Bariatric Surgery Medical Management. *Obes. Facts* **2018**, *28*, 2117–2121. [CrossRef] [PubMed]

15. Sjöström, L.; Peltonen, M.; Jacobson, P.; Ahlin, S.; Andersson-Assarsson, J.; Anveden, Å.; Bouchard, C.; Carlsson, B.; Karason, K.; Lönroth, H.; et al. Association of bariatric surgery with long-term remission of type 2 diabetes and with microvascular and macrovascular complications. *J. Am. Med. Assoc.* **2014**. [CrossRef] [PubMed]
16. Al Assal, K.; Prifti, E.; Belda, E.; Sala, P.; Clément, K.; Dao, M.C.; Doré, J.; Levenez, F.; Taddei, C.R.; Fonseca, D.C.; et al. Gut microbiota profile of obese diabetic women submitted to Roux-en-Y gastric bypass and its association with food intake and postoperative diabetes remission. *Nutrients* **2020**, 278. [CrossRef] [PubMed]
17. Sarosiek, K.; Pappan, K.L.; Gandhi, A.V.; Saxena, S.; Kang, C.Y.; McMahon, H.; Chipitsyna, G.I.; Tichansky, D.S.; Arafat, H.A. Conserved Metabolic Changes in Nondiabetic and Type 2 Diabetic Bariatric Surgery Patients: Global Metabolomic Pilot Study. *J. Diabetes Res.* **2016**. [CrossRef]
18. International Diabetes Federation. The IDF consensus worldwide definition of the metabolic syndrome. *IDF Commun.* **2006**, 1–23.
19. Zińczuk, J.; Maciejczyk, M.; Zaręba, K.; Romaniuk, W.; Markowski, A.; Kędra, B.; Zalewska, A.; Pryczynicz, A.; Matowicka-Karna, J.; Guzińska-Ustymowicz, K. Antioxidant Barrier, Redox Status, and Oxidative Damage to Biomolecules in Patients with Colorectal Cancer. Can Malondialdehyde and Catalase Be Markers of Colorectal Cancer Advancement? *Biomolecules* **2019**, *9*, 637. [CrossRef]
20. Matthews, D.R.; Hosker, J.P.; Rudenski, A.S.; Naylor, B.A.; Treacher, D.F.; Turner, R.C. Homeostasis model assessment: Insulin resistance and β-cell function from fasting plasma glucose and insulin concentrations in man. *Diabetologia* **1985**. [CrossRef]
21. Misra, H.P.; Fridovich, I. The role of superoxide anion in the autoxidation of epinephrine and a simple assay for superoxide dismutase. *J. Biol. Chem.* **1972**, *247*, 3170–3175. [PubMed]
22. Aebi, H. Catalase *in vitro*. In *Methods in Enzymology*; Sinauer Associates, Inc.: Sunderland, MA, USA, 1984; Volume 105, pp. 121–126.
23. Paglia, D.E.; Valentine, W.N. Studies on the quantitative and qualitative characterization of erythrocyte glutathione peroxidase. *J. Lab. Clin. Med.* **1967**, *70*, 158–169. [CrossRef]
24. Mize, C.E.; Longdon, R. Hepatic glutathione reductase. I. Purification and general kinetic properties. *J. Biol. Chem.* **1962**, *237*, 1589–1595.
25. Moron, M.; Depierre, J.; Mannervik, B. Levels of glutathione, glutathione reductase and glutathione S-transferase activities in rat lung and liver. *Biochim. Biophys. Acta Gen. Subj.* **1979**, *582*, 67–78. [CrossRef]
26. Zalewska, A.; Maciejczyk, M.; Szulimowska, J.; Imierska, M.; Błachnio-Zabielska, A. High-Fat Diet Affects Ceramide Content, Disturbs Mitochondrial Redox Balance, and Induces Apoptosis in the Submandibular Glands of Mice. *Biomolecules* **2019**, *9*, 877. [CrossRef] [PubMed]
27. Zalewska, A.; Ziembicka, D.; Żendzian-Piotrowska, M.; Maciejczyk, M. The Impact of High-Fat Diet on Mitochondrial Function, Free Radical Production, and Nitrosative Stress in the Salivary Glands of Wistar Rats. *Oxid. Med. Cell. Longev.* **2019**, *2019*, 2606120. [CrossRef] [PubMed]
28. Kalousová, M.; Skrha, J.; Zima, T. Advanced glycation end-products and advanced oxidation protein products in patients with diabetes mellitus. *Physiol. Res.* **2002**, *51*, 597–604.
29. Maciejczyk, M.; Skutnik-Radziszewska, A.; Zieniewska, I.; Matczuk, J.; Domel, E.; Waszkiel, D.; Żendzian-Piotrowska, M.; Szarmach, I.; Zalewska, A. Antioxidant Defense, Oxidative Modification, and Salivary Gland Function in an Early Phase of Cerulein Pancreatitis. *Oxid. Med. Cell. Longev.* **2019**, *2019*, 1–14. [CrossRef]
30. Tian, X.; Yan, C.; Liu, M.; Zhang, Q.; Liu, D.; Liu, Y.; Li, S.; Han, Y. Obesity and insulin resistance. *PLoS ONE* **2017**. [CrossRef]
31. Yazıcı, D.; Sezer, H. Insulin resistance, obesity and lipotoxicity. In *Advances in Experimental Medicine and Biology*; Springer: Berlin, Germany, 2017; Volume 960, pp. 277–304.
32. Illán-Gómez, F.; Gonzálvez-Ortega, M.; Orea-Soler, I.; Alcaraz-Tafalla, M.S.; Aragón-Alonso, A.; Pascual-Díaz, M.; Pérez-Paredes, M.; Lozano-Almela, M.L. Obesity and inflammation: Change in adiponectin, C-reactive protein, tumour necrosis factor-alpha and interleukin-6 after bariatric surgery. *Obes. Surg.* **2012**. [CrossRef]
33. Molnár, D.; Decsi, T.; Koletzko, B. Reduced antioxidant status in obese children with multimetabolic syndrome. *Int. J. Obes.* **2004**. [CrossRef] [PubMed]
34. Sfar, S.; Boussoffara, R.; Sfar, M.T.; Kerkeni, A. Antioxidant enzymes activities in obese Tunisian children. *Nutr. J.* **2013**. [CrossRef] [PubMed]

35. Zalewska, A.; Kossakowska, A.; Taranta-Janusz, K.; Zięba, S.; Fejfer, K.; Salamonowicz, M.; Kostecka-Sochoń, P.; Wasilewska, A.; Maciejczyk, M. Dysfunction of Salivary Glands, Disturbances in Salivary Antioxidants and Increased Oxidative Damage in Saliva of Overweight and Obese Adolescents. *J. Clin. Med.* **2020**, *9*, 548. [CrossRef]
36. Świderska, M.; Maciejczyk, M.; Zalewska, A.; Pogorzelska, J.; Flisiak, R.; Chabowski, A. Oxidative stress biomarkers in the serum and plasma of patients with non-alcoholic fatty liver disease (NAFLD). Can plasma AGE be a marker of NAFLD? *Free Radic. Res.* **2019**. [CrossRef]
37. Styskal, J.; Van Remmen, H.; Richardson, A.; Salmon, A.B. Oxidative stress and diabetes: What can we learn about insulin resistance from antioxidant mutant mouse models? *Free Radic. Biol. Med.* **2012**, *52*, 46–58. [CrossRef] [PubMed]
38. Solinas, G.; Karin, M. JNK1 and IKKβ: Molecular links between obesity and metabolic dysfunction. *FASEB J.* **2010**. [CrossRef]
39. Maciejczyk, M.; Żebrowska, E.; Chabowski, A. Insulin Resistance and Oxidative Stress in the Brain: What's New? *Int. J. Mol. Sci.* **2019**, *20*, 874. [CrossRef]
40. Valko, M.; Leibfritz, D.; Moncol, J.; Cronin, M.T.D.; Mazur, M.; Telser, J. Free radicals and antioxidants in normal physiological functions and human disease. *Int. J. Biochem. Cell Biol.* **2007**, *39*, 44–84. [CrossRef]
41. Mohseni, R.; Sadeghabadi, Z.A.; Goodarzi, M.T.; Teimouri, M.; Nourbakhsh, M.; Razzaghy Azar, M. Evaluation of Mn-superoxide dismutase and catalase gene expression in childhood obesity: Its association with insulin resistance. *J. Pediatr. Endocrinol. Metab.* **2018**. [CrossRef]
42. Maciejczyk, M.; Zalewska, A.; Ładny, J.R. Salivary Antioxidant Barrier, Redox Status, and Oxidative Damage to Proteins and Lipids in Healthy Children, Adults, and the Elderly. *Oxid. Med. Cell. Longev.* **2019**, *2019*, 1–12. [CrossRef]
43. Aquilano, K.; Baldelli, S.; Ciriolo, M.R. Glutathione: New roles in redox signalling for an old antioxidant. *Front. Pharmacol.* **2014**, *5*, 196. [CrossRef]
44. Bankoglu, E.E.; Seyfried, F.; Arnold, C.; Soliman, A.; Jurowich, C.; Germer, C.T.; Otto, C.; Stopper, H. Reduction of DNA damage in peripheral lymphocytes of obese patients after bariatric surgery-mediated weight loss. *Mutagenesis* **2018**. [CrossRef] [PubMed]
45. Liu, W.; Zhang, H.; Han, X.; Zhang, P.; Mao, Z. Uric acid level changes after bariatric surgery in obese subjects with type 2 diabetes mellitus. *Ann. Transl. Med.* **2019**, *7*, 332. [CrossRef] [PubMed]
46. Sautin, Y.Y.; Johnson, R.J. Uric Acid: The Oxidant-Antioxidant Paradox. *Nucleosides Nucleotides Nucleic Acids* **2008**, *27*, 608–619. [CrossRef] [PubMed]
47. Kim, T.; Lee, S.; Yoo, J.; Kim, S.; Yoo, S.; Song, H.; Kim, Y.S.; Choi, E.; Kim, Y.K. The relationship between the regional abdominal adipose tissue distribution and the serum uric acid levels in people with type 2 diabetes mellitus. *Diabetol. Metab. Syndr.* **2012**. [CrossRef] [PubMed]
48. Nejatinamini, S.; Ataie-Jafari, A.; Qorbani, M.; Nikoohemat, S.; Kelishadi, R.; Asayesh, H.; Hosseini, S. Association between serum uric acid level and metabolic syndrome components. *J. Diabetes Metab. Disord.* **2015**. [CrossRef]
49. Wei, F.; Chang, B.; Yang, X.; Wang, Y.; Chen, L.; Li, W.D. Serum Uric Acid Levels were Dynamically Coupled with Hemoglobin A1c in the Development of Type 2 Diabetes. *Sci. Rep.* **2016**. [CrossRef]
50. Schmidt, A.M.; Hori, O.; Brett, J.; Du Yan, S.; Wautier, J.L.; Stern, D. Cellular receptors for advanced glycation end products: Implications for induction of oxidant stress and cellular dysfunction in the pathogenesis of vascular lesions. *Arterioscler. Thromb.* **1994**, *14*, 1521–1528. [CrossRef]
51. Goldin, A.; Beckman, J.A.; Schmidt, A.M.; Creager, M.A. Advanced glycation end products: Sparking the development of diabetic vascular injury. *Circulation* **2006**, *114*, 597–605. [CrossRef]
52. Ott, C.; Jacobs, K.; Haucke, E.; Navarrete Santos, A.; Grune, T.; Simm, A. Role of advanced glycation end products in cellular signaling. *Redox Biol.* **2014**, *2*, 411–429. [CrossRef]
53. Rains, J.L.; Jain, S.K. Oxidative stress, insulin signaling, and diabetes. *Free Radic. Biol. Med.* **2011**, *50*, 567–575. [CrossRef] [PubMed]
54. Çakatay, U.; Kayali, R.; Uzun, H. Relation of plasma protein oxidation parameters and paraoxonase activity in the ageing population. *Clin. Exp. Med.* **2008**. [CrossRef] [PubMed]
55. Dalle-Donne, I.; Rossi, R.; Giustarini, D.; Milzani, A.; Colombo, R. Protein carbonyl groups as biomarkers of oxidative stress. *Clin. Chim. Acta* **2003**, *329*, 23–28. [CrossRef]

56. Atabek, M.; Keskin, M.; Yazici, C.; Kendirci, M.; Hatipoglu, N.; Koklu, E.; Kurtoglu, S. Protein oxidation in obesity and insulin resistance. *Eur. J. Pediatr.* **2006**, *165*, 753–756. [CrossRef]
57. Korkmaz, G.G.; Altinoglu, E.; Civelek, S.; Sozer, V.; Erdenen, F.; Tabak, O.; Uzun, H. The association of oxidative stress markers with conventional risk factors in the metabolic syndrome. *Metabolism* **2013**. [CrossRef]
58. Maciejczyk, M.; Matczuk, J.; Żendzian-Piotrowska, M.; Niklińska, W.; Fejfer, K.; Szarmach, I.; Ładny, J.R.; Zieniewska, I.; Zalewska, A. Eight-Week Consumption of High-Sucrose Diet Has a Pro-Oxidant Effect and Alters the Function of the Salivary Glands of Rats. *Nutrients* **2018**, *10*, 1530. [CrossRef]
59. Krzystek-Korpacka, M.; Patryn, E.; Boehm, D.; Berdowska, I.; Zielinski, B.; Noczynska, A. Advanced oxidation protein products (AOPPs) in juvenile overweight and obesity prior to and following weight reduction. *Clin. Biochem.* **2008**. [CrossRef]
60. Kanaya, A.M.; Wassel, C.L.; Stoddard, P.J.; Harris, T.B.; Cummings, S.R.; Kritchevsky, S.B.; Goodpaster, B.H.; Green, C.; Satterfield, S.; Gross, M.D. F 2-isoprostanes and adiposity in older adults. *Obesity* **2011**. [CrossRef]
61. Cohen, G.; Riahi, Y.; Sunda, V.; Deplano, S.; Chatgilialoglu, C.; Ferreri, C.; Kaiser, N.; Sasson, S. Signaling properties of 4-hydroxyalkenals formed by lipid peroxidation in diabetes. *Free Radic. Biol. Med.* **2013**, *65*, 978–987. [CrossRef]
62. Gargiulo, S.; Gamba, P.; Testa, G.; Rossin, D.; Biasi, F.; Poli, G.; Leonarduzzi, G. Relation between TLR4/NF-κB signaling pathway activation by 27-hydroxycholesterol and 4-hydroxynonenal, and atherosclerotic plaque instability. *Aging Cell* **2015**, *14*, 569–581. [CrossRef]
63. Maciejczyk, M.; Zalewska, A.; Gerreth, K. Karolina Salivary Redox Biomarkers in Selected Neurodegenerative Diseases. *J. Clin. Med.* **2020**, *9*, 497. [CrossRef] [PubMed]
64. Maciejczyk, M.; Szulimowska, J.; Taranta-Janusz, K.; Werbel, K.; Wasilewska, A.; Zalewska, A. Salivary FRAP as A Marker of Chronic Kidney Disease Progression in Children. *Antioxidants* **2019**, *8*, 409. [CrossRef] [PubMed]
65. Maciejczyk, M.; Szulimowska, J.; Skutnik, A.; Taranta-Janusz, K.; Wasilewska, A.; Wiśniewska, N.; Zalewska, A. Salivary Biomarkers of Oxidative Stress in Children with Chronic Kidney Disease. *J. Clin. Med.* **2018**, *7*, 209. [CrossRef] [PubMed]
66. Sawczuk, B.; Maciejczyk, M.; Sawczuk-Siemieniuk, M.; Posmyk, R.; Zalewska, A.; Car, H. Salivary Gland Function, Antioxidant Defence and Oxidative Damage in the Saliva of Patients with Breast Cancer: Does the BRCA1 Mutation Disturb the Salivary Redox Profile? *Cancers (Basel)* **2019**, *11*, 1501. [CrossRef]
67. Skutnik-Radziszewska, A.; Maciejczyk, M.; Fejfer, K.; Krahel, J.; Flisiak, I.; Kołodziej, U.; Zalewska, A. Salivary Antioxidants and Oxidative Stress in Psoriatic Patients: Can Salivary Total Oxidant Status and Oxidative Status Index Be a Plaque Psoriasis Biomarker? *Oxid. Med. Cell. Longev.* **2020**, *2020*, 9086024. [CrossRef] [PubMed]
68. Klimiuk, A.; Zalewska, A.; Sawicki, R.; Knapp, M.; Maciejczyk, M. Salivary Oxidative Stress Increases With the Progression of Chronic Heart Failure. *J. Clin. Med.* **2020**, *9*, 769. [CrossRef]
69. Maciejczyk, M.; Taranta-Janusz, K.; Wasilewska, A.; Kossakowska, A.; Zalewska, A. A Case-Control Study of Salivary Redox Homeostasis in Hypertensive Children. Can Salivary Uric Acid be a Marker of Hypertension? *J. Clin. Med.* **2020**, *9*, 837. [CrossRef]

Journal of *Clinical Medicine*

MDPI

Article

New Metrics to Assess Type 2 Diabetes after Bariatric Surgery: The "Time-Within-Remission Range"

Ana de Hollanda [1,2,3,*], Albert Lecube [4,5,*], Miguel Angel Rubio [6], Enric Sánchez [4], Núria Vilarrasa [5,7], José Gregorio Oliva [8], María Luisa Fernández-Soto [9], Jordi Salas-Salvadó [3,10], María D. Ballesteros-Pomar [11], Andreea Ciudin [12], Ferran Torres [13,14], Concepción Vidal [15], María José Morales [16], Sergio Valdés [5,17], Silvia Pellitero [5,18], Inka Miñambres [19], Lluís Masmiquel [20], Albert Goday [3,21], Lorena Suarez [22], Liliam Flores [1,2,5], Marta Bueno [4], Assumpta Caixàs [23], Irene Bretón [24], Rosa Cámara [25], Romina Olbeyra [2], Rona Penso [26], María José de la Cruz [27], Andreu Simó-Servat [28], Francisca María Pereyra-García [8], Elena Teresa López-Mezquita [9], Anna Gils [10], Enzamaria Fidilio [12], Orosia Bandrés [15], Ángel Martínez [16], Jose Abuín [17], Montserrat Marques-Pamies [18], Laura Tuneu [19], Magdalena Arteaga [20], Olga Castañer [21], Fernando Goñi [29], Cristina Arrizabalaga [29], Manuel Antonio Botana [30], Alfonso Calañas [31] and Ángel Rebollo [31]

1 Hospital Clínic de Barcelona, 08036 Barcelona, Spain; LFLORES@clinic.cat
2 Institut d'Investigacions Biomèdiques August Pi i Sunyer (IDIBAPS), 08036 Barcelona, Spain; rominaolbeyra@gmail.com
3 CIBER de Obesidad y Nutrición (CIBEROBN), Instituto de Salud Carlos III (ISCIII), 28029 Madrid, Spain; jordi.salas@urv.cat (J.S.-S.); Agoday@parcdesalutmar.cat (A.G.)
4 Hospital Universitari Arnau de Vilanova, Grup de Recerca en Obesitat, Diabetes i Metabolisme (ODIM), Institut de Recerca Biomèdica de Lleida (IRBLleida), Universitat de Lleida, 25198 Lleida, Spain; esanchez@irblleida.cat (E.S.); mbuenodiez@gmail.com (M.B.)
5 CIBER de Diabetes y Enfermedades Metabólicas Asociadas (CIBERDEM), Instituto de Salud Carlos III (ISCIII), 28029 Madrid, Spain; nuriavilarrasa@yahoo.es (N.V.); sergio.valdes@hotmail.es (S.V.); spelli75@gmail.com (S.P.)
6 Hospital Clínico San Carlos IDISSC, 28040 Madrid, Spain; marubioh@gmail.com
7 Hospital Universitari de Bellvitge, Institut d'Investigació Biomèdica de Bellvitge (IDIBELL), L'Hospitalet de Llobregat, 08907 Barcelona, Spain
8 Hospital Universitario Nuestra Señora de Candelaria, 38010 Santa Cruz de Tenerife, Spain; olivajg@gmail.com (J.G.O.); francispereyra@telefonica.net (F.M.P.-G.)
9 Hospital Universitario San Cecilio, 18016 Granada, Spain; marisafsoto@gmail.com (M.L.F.-S.); elopezmt@gmail.com (E.T.L.-M.)
10 Hospital Universitari Sant Joan de Reus, Institut d'Investigació Sanitària Pere Virgili (IISPV), Universitat Rovita i Virgili Reus, 43204 Tarragona, Spain; annagilsc@gmail.com
11 Hospital de León, 24008 León, Spain; mdballesteros@telefonica.net
12 Hospital Universitari Vall d'Hebron, 08035 Barcelona, Spain; aciudin@vhebron.net (A.C.); enzamariafidilio@gmail.com (E.F.)
13 Medical Statistics Core Facility, Clinical Pharmacology Deparment, Hospital Clínic Barcelona, 08036 Barcelona, Spain; Ferran.Torres@uab.cat
14 Biostatistics Unit, Faculty of Medicine, Universitat Autònoma de Barcelona, 08193 Barcelona, Spain
15 Hospital Royo Villanova, 50015 Zaragoza, Spain; cvidal@unizar.es (C.V.); orosiabandres@gmail.com (O.B.)
16 Complejo Hospitalario Universitario de Vigo, 36312 Vigo, Spain; maria.jose.morales.gorria@sergas.es (M.J.M.); angelmg88@hotmail.com (Á.M.)
17 Hospital Regional Universitario de Málaga, Instituto de Investigación Biomédica de Málaga (IBIMA), Universidad de Málaga, 29010 Málaga, Spain; jose.abuin.fdez@gmail.com
18 Hospital Universitari Germans Trias i Pujol, Institut d'Investigació Germans Trias (IGTP), 08916 Badalona, Spain; montse98.89@gmail.com
19 Hospital de la Santa Creu i Sant Pau, Universitat Autònoma de Barcelona, 08041 Barcelona, Spain; iminambres@santpau.cat (I.M.); laura.tuneu@quironsalud.es (L.T.)
20 Hospital Universitario Son Llàtzer, Instituto de Investigación Sanitaria de las Islas Baleares (IdISBa), 07198 Palma de Mallorca, Spain; lmasmiquel@gmail.com (L.M.); marteagao@gmail.com (M.A.)

[21] Parc de Salut Mar, Institut Hospital del Mar d'Investigacions Mèdiques (IMIM), Universitat Autònoma de Barcelona, 08003 Barcelona, Spain; ocastaner@imim.es
[22] Hospital Universitario Central de Asturias, 33011 Oviedo, Spain; loresuarezgu@gmail.com
[23] Hospital Universitari Parc Taulí, Universitat Autònoma de Barcelona, Institut d'Investigació i Innovació Parc Taulí (I3PT), 08208 Sabadell, Spain; acaixas@gmail.com
[24] Hospital General Universitario Gregorio Marañón, Instituto de Investigación Sanitaria Gregorio Marañón (IISGM), 28007 Madrid, Spain; irenebreton@gmail.com
[25] Hospital Universitari i Politècnic La Fe, 46026 Valencia, Spain; rosacamaragomez@gmail.com
[26] Hospital Central de la Defensa Gómez Ulla, 28047 Madrid, Spain; ronapenso@hotmail.com
[27] Hospital Universitario Fundación Jiménez Díaz, 28040 Madrid, Spain; mariajocf@gmail.com
[28] Hospital Mútua de Terrassa, 08221 Terrassa, Spain; andreusimoservat@gmail.com
[29] Hospital de Basurto, 48013 Bilbao, Spain; fgonigoicoechea@gmail.com (F.G.); cristinarri@hotmail.com (C.A.)
[30] Hospital Universitario Lucus Augusti, 27003 Lugo, Spain; manuelbotanal@gmail.com
[31] Hospital Universitario Reina Sofia, 14004 Córdoba, Spain; contentine@yahoo.es (A.C.); rebollo.ang@gmail.com (Á.R.)
* Correspondence: anidehollanda@gmail.com (A.d.H.); alecube@gmail.com (A.L.); Tel.: +34-932-279-846 (A.d.H.); +34-973-705-183 (A.L.); Fax: +34-973-705-189 (A.L.)

Received: 12 March 2020; Accepted: 7 April 2020; Published: 9 April 2020

Abstract: Almost one third of patients do not achieve type 2 diabetes remission after bariatric surgery or are unable to sustain this effect long term. Our objective was to delve further into the dynamic responses of diabetes after bariatric surgery and to evaluate the "time-within-remission range" as a variable of metabolic control. A descriptive cohort study was done using a computerised multicentre and multidisciplinary registry. All data were adjusted by propensity score. A total of 1186 subjects with a follow-up of 4.5 ± 2.5 years were included. Type of surgery, diabetes remission, recurrence of diabetes, "time-within-remission range" and key predictors of diabetes outcomes were assessed. All patients (70% women, 51.4 ± 9.2 years old, body mass index (BMI) 46.3 ± 6.9 kg/m^2) underwent primary bariatric procedures. "Time-within-remission range" were 83.3% (33.3–91.6) after gastric bypass, 68.7% (7.1–87.5) after sleeve gastrectomy and 90% (83.3–92.8) after malabsorptive techniques ($p < 0.001$ for all). Duration of diabetes, baseline HbA1c and insulin treatment were significantly negatively correlated with the "time-within-remission range". The association of bariatric techniques with "time-within-remission range", using gastric bypass as a reference, were: odds ratio (OR) 3.70 (2.34–5.84), $p < 0.001$ for malabsorptive techniques and OR 0.55 (0.40–0.75), $p < 0.001$ for sleeve gastrectomy. Characteristics of type 2 diabetes powerfully influence the outcomes of bariatric surgery. The "time-within-remission range" unveils a superiority of gastric bypass compared to sleeve gastrectomy.

Keywords: bariatric surgery; time-within-remission range; type 2 diabetes; metabolic control

1. Introduction

There is no doubt that obesity has reached pandemic trends during the latter half of the century [1]. This evidence goes in parallel with another concern, the finding of higher waist circumference at increasing body mass index (BMI) levels, further accelerating the cardiometabolic health consequences of abdominal adiposity [2]. In fact, obesity increases the risk of comorbid conditions, including type 2 diabetes, cardiovascular diseases, obstructive sleep apnea, non-alcoholic fatty liver disease and cancer. Therefore, obesity impairs quality of life and life expectancy of the world's population, becoming a major public health challenge that requires strategies at many levels, not only on prevention but also on monitoring and management. However, the discouraging long-term results achieved with dietary and behavioural interventions and the up-till-now few safe and effective drugs available for the treatment of obesity have led to a marked increase in the use of bariatric surgery (BS) in Western countries [3].

Nowadays, BS is the most effective treatment for weight loss and remission of comorbidities in subjects with severe obesity. Regarding type 2 diabetes, BS results in superior short- and long-term outcomes compared to the best medical treatment. These outcomes include diabetes remission, and improvement in microvascular complications, together with favourable consequences in hard endpoints such as macrovascular complications and death [4–6]. However, a growing number of patients (25%–40%) with diabetes do not achieve "biochemical remission" after BS or are unable to sustain this effect in the long term despite initial success [7–9]. High baseline HbA1c, low C-peptide values, preoperative use of insulin, long diabetes duration and low magnitude of weight loss have been negatively related to type 2 diabetes remission [10].

There is still no conclusive evidence about which is the best type of surgery to treat obesity and diabetes. Three randomised clinical trials (RCT) have been carried out to assess diabetes' short-term outcomes comparing gastric bypass (GBP) and sleeve gastrectomy (SG), with similar results [11–13]. In addition, the RCT from Mingrone et al. clearly showed better glycaemic control and weight loss results after biliopancreatic diversion compared to GBP and medical treatment [14]. However, the limited number of participants assigned to each arm precluded definitive conclusions. Also, there is no data available from RCT about the impact of BS on other metrics of glycaemic control beyond glycaemia and HbA1c. Data from the continuous glucose monitoring (CGM) studies in patients with type 1 diabetes suggest that time within glucose target range ("time-in-range") provides more suitable information than fasting plasma glucose or HbA1c for medical care [15]. This kind of metric approximation has not been previously applied to BS studies.

In May 2011, the Obesity Group of the Spanish Endocrinology and Nutrition Society (GOSEEN) created a non-exhaustive computerised multicentre and multidisciplinary registry of patients with obesity undergoing bariatric procedures in Spanish public hospitals since 2000 [16]. The RICIBA (Registro Informatizado de Cirugía Bariátrica) tries to better understand the baseline characteristics and surgical outcomes of BS [17]. Therefore, our objective was to delve further into the dynamic responses of diabetes in 1186 patients with morbid obesity and type 2 diabetes included in the RICIBA-DM (diabetes mellitus) study who underwent bariatric procedures between 2000 and 2016 in Spain.

2. Methods

2.1. Study Design and Description of the Study Population

In this study, we have investigated the dynamic responses of diabetes following bariatric surgery in a large cohort of Spanish subjects according the "Strengthening the Reporting of Observational Studies in Epidemiology" guidelines for reporting cohort studies [18]. The RICIBA-DM was created in August 2017 with the main objective to register patients with type 2 diabetes, who underwent primary BS in 25 public Spanish hospitals between the years 2000 and 2016. The initial database was designed by a specific board from GOSEEN, and every health professional willing to participate obtained an access password. Each researcher had access only to their own patients according to the Spanish data protection law.

Only subjects with complete and documented baseline data and at least a 1-year follow-up period were included in the final analysis. Subjects who underwent revisional surgeries finished the follow-up at that moment.

2.2. Assessed Variables in the RICIBA-DM

The following information was recorded at baseline and every six months until the end of the follow-up: demographic and anthropometric data (gender, age, weight and height), analytical data (triglycerides, high-density lipoprotein cholesterol (HDLc) and low-density lipoprotein cholesterol (LDLc)), morbidity related to the obesity state (high blood pressure, dyslipidaemia), data related with diabetes (fasting plasma glucose, HbA1c, antidiabetic treatment, need for insulin, disease duration) and type of surgical procedure performed.

2.3. Study Size for the RICIBA-DM

By January 2019, a total of 1637 registers had been summited to the RICIBA-DM database. The database including the required clinical, analytical and anthropometric information of 1337 patients with obesity and type 2 diabetes was closed in February 2019. Finally, the 1186 subjects with no missing data and who had a minimum follow-up of 12 months after BS were included in the analysis (Figure S1).

2.4. Diagnostic Criteria to Define Metabolic and Weight Responses After Bariatric Surgery

Diabetes was diagnosed according to the American Diabetes Association criteria [19]. We defined diabetes remission as HbA1c < 6.5% and fasting plasma glucose (FPG) < 126 mg/dl in the absence of diabetic medication, including both complete and partial remission within this description. Recurrence of diabetes was defined as a new diagnosis of diabetes once remission had been achieved. Good metabolic control was defined as HbA1c < 7%, irrespective of diabetes medication [19]. A novel variable, "time-within-remission range", was created: the time that subjects were in diabetes remission during the follow-up after BS, expressed as median percentage (25th–75th percentiles). The aim of this variable was to include all the periods of time during follow-up during which subjects met the diabetes remission criteria, taking into account that subjects could switch from one glycaemic category to another several times during the follow-up.

Hypertension was defined as blood pressure ≥ 140/90 mmHg or taking antihypertensive treatment. Dyslipidaemia was based on the presence of fasting LDLc ≥ 160 mg/dL, HDLc ≤ 40 mg/dL, fasting triglyceride ≥ 200 mg/dL or active use of lipid lowering therapy [19]. Weight regain was calculated as the difference between the weight lost at nadir and the weight on the last observation expressed as percentage [20].

2.5. Statistical Analysis

Given the diversity of surgical techniques, in particular, malabsorptive surgeries, we grouped surgeries into three main groups: GBP, SG and the malabsorptive techniques' group (MAs), which includes biliopancreatic diversion with or without duodenal switch, and single anastomosis duodenal-ileal bypass with sleeve gastrectomy (SADI-S).

Categorical variables were described as frequencies and percentages and continuous variables as mean (standard deviation, SD). The survival function was described using the Kaplan–Meier function.

Standardised differences, defined as differences between groups divided by pooled standard deviation, were used to assess heterogeneity between the three cohorts for baseline covariables. To address potential sources of bias, the Inverse Probability of the Treatment Weights (IPTW) approach [21] was used to create a pseudo-population, in which the 3 surgery groups were balanced across baseline covariates. The stabilised weights were calculated using propensity scores (PS) obtained from a logistic regression model aimed at minimising the standardised differences between arms [22]. The covariates included in the final model were age, gender, BMI, weight, glucose, LDLc, HDLc, triglycerides, HbA1c, type of diabetes treatment, diabetes duration, hypertension and dyslipidaemia. Almost all are key predictors of diabetes outcomes that might be imbalanced in non-randomised comparisons.

Post-baseline variables and outcomes were available only after the definition of the final model for the IPTW approach. Covariate balance was assessed using the standardised differences with the initial goal to achieve values <0.10. The IPTW approach was used to define insignificant differences in potential confounders. For baseline comparisons between GBP and SG, this cut-off target was always achieved. For comparisons between GBP or SG and MAs, since it was unfeasible to achieve <0.1 for all variables and that for some authors, <0.2 might also be acceptable, the cut-off value for this comparison was redefined to 0.15 [23].

Baseline categorical data were compared using the chi-square test and continuous variables using analysis of variance (ANOVA) with rank-transformed data for raw and IPTW-adjusted analyses. Raw and IPTW-adjusted logistic and Cox regression models were used to estimate risks: odds ratio (OR) and hazard ratio (HR) with 95% confidence interval (CI) for binary and time to event variables, respectively.

Since a number of variables were different at baseline among the types of surgery performed, all data shown in this paper were adjusted by propensity score using the IPTW method, unless specified otherwise. In all statistical analyses, a two-sided type-I error of 5% was applied. The software SPSS v25 (IBM) and SAS v9.4 (Cary, NC, USA) were used.

2.6. Ethics Statement

A non-written informed consent was defined in the RICIBA-DM protocol and was obtained from all participants. The human ethics committee of Hospital Clínic de Barcelona approved the study and the procedure outlined for the verbal consent obtainment. The entire process was documented in the clinical history of each participant. Each researcher had access only to their own patients, as the system prevented unauthorised access by third parties, according to the Spanish data protection law. Finally, all patient records and information were anonymised and de-identified prior to analysis.

3. Results

3.1. Baseline Characteristics of the Whole Cohort and According to Bariatric Surgery

A total of 1186 individuals with type 2 diabetes who underwent BS between the years 2000–2016 in 25 public Spanish hospitals were included. The average age was 51.4 ± 9.2 years, presurgical BMI was 46.3 ± 6.9 kg/m^2 and 70.0% were women. The known duration of diabetes was 6.3 ± 5.7 years and baseline mean HbA1c was 7.4% ± 1.8%. Two-hundred and nineteen individuals (18.5%) were treated only with diet, 604 (50%) with non-insulin medications, 229 (19.3%) with both insulin and non-insulin medications and 134 (11.3%) exclusively with insulin.

Of all patients, 47.5% underwent GBP, 35.8% SG and 16.5%, MAs. The length of follow-up for the whole cohort was 4.5 ± 2.5 years (4.4 ± 2.4 in GBP, 4.0 ± 2.0 in SG and 4.1 ± 3.0 in MAs). The rate of follow-up was 100% at 1 year, 93.6% at 2 years and 49% after 5 years of BS, without differences between surgical techniques. The main baseline clinical and biochemical characteristics, including comorbidities, for the whole cohort and according to BS technique, before and after propensity score-IPTW approach, are shown in Table S1 and Table 1, respectively.

Table 1. Baseline main clinical and metabolic characteristics of participants in the study after propensity score adjustment.

	Treatment			*p*-Value			Standardised Difference		
	GBP (n = 562)	SG (n = 423)	MAs (n = 196)	GBP Versus SG	GBP Versus MAs	SG Versus MAs	GBP Versus SG	GBP Versus MAs	SG Versus MAs
Gender (%females)	69.2	70.0	74.4	0.797	0.173	0.262	−0.017	−0.114	−0.098
Age (years)	51.3 (8.4)	51.3 (9.9)	52.1 (10.2)	0.909	0.176	0.209	−0.005	0.089	0.087
Weight (Kg)	121(20)	121(22)	121 (22)	0.633	0.944	0.784	−0.008	0.006	0.014
BMI (Kg/m^2)	46.1 (6.7)	46.0 (6.9)	46.4 (6.5)	0.949	0.453	0.508	−0.011	0.043	0.053
Dyslipidaemia (%)	48.3	49.2	48.6	0.771	0.944	0.881	0.019	0.006	−0.013
Hypertension (%)	70.4	72.5	76.8	0.481	0.089	0.261	0.045	0.144	0.098
Diabetes duration (years)	6.2 (5.5)	6.1 (5.6)	6.3 (6.0)	0.625	0.846	0.781	−0.021	0.016	0.036
On Insulin (%)	11.3	10.5	8.5	0.981	0.714	0.843	0.027	0.104	0.108
Good control (%)	50.9	51.6	55.4	0.838	0.283	0.380	0.013	0.089	0.076
HbA1c (%)	7.3 (1.7)	7.3 (1.8)	7.3 (1.6)	0.891	0.906	0.977	0.007	−0.026	−0.032
HbA1c (mmol/mol)	56 (18.6)	56 (19.7)	56 (17.5)	0.891	0.906	0.977	0.007	−0.026	−0.032
FPG (mg/dL)	159 (59)	159 (65)	157 (53)	0.388	0.857	0.387	−0.001	−0.033	−0.030
Triglycerides (mg/dl)	183 (128)	183 (128)	175 (138)	0.974	0.343	0.274	0.003	−0.056	−0.059
LDLc (mg/dl)	106 (34)	106 (36)	105 (35)	0.822	0.917	0.938	−0.008	−0.031	−0.023
HDLc (mg/dl)	45 (14)	45 (13)	46 (11)	0.545	0.340	0.148	−0.005	0.057	0.065

Data are expressed as median (standard deviation) or percentage. BMI: body mass index; FPG: fasting plasma glucose; HbA1c: glycated haemoglobin; LDLc: low-density lipoprotein cholesterol; HDLc: high-density lipoprotein cholesterol; GBP: gastric bypass; SG: sleeve gastrectomy; MAs: malabsorptive surgeries.

3.2. Diabetes Remission

Diabetes remission rates in the whole cohort were: 72% (95%CI: 69–74) at 1 year of surgery, 76% (74–79) at 2 years and 80.3% (78–82) at 5 years. Remission rates by type of surgery were as follows: after GBP, the remission rate was 73% (69–76) at 1 year, 79% (75–82) at 2 years and 83% (79–86) at 5 years, after SG, 64% (60–69), 68% (64–73) and 74% (69–78) and after MAs, 84% (78–89), 87% (82–91) and 89% (84–93) at 1, 2 and 5 years, respectively.

Multivariate analysis for diabetes remission at one year after BS shows that remission was associated with: age at the time of BS (OR 0.97, (0.96–0.99), $p = 0.006$), diabetes duration (OR 0.89, (0.86–0.92), $p < 0.0001$), presurgical BMI (OR 0.97, (0.94–0.99), $p = 0.004$), baseline HbA1c (OR 0.72, (0.65–0.79), $p < 0.0001$), insulin treatment (OR 0.23, (0.12–0.42), $p < 0.0001$) and weight loss 1 year after BS (OR 1.05, (1.03–1.07), $p < 0.0001$). Regarding the type of BS, using GBP as the reference, associations with remission rates were as follows: (OR 3.69 (2.14–6.35), $p < 0.0001$) for MAs and (OR 0.73 (0.52–1.02), $p = 0.068$) for SG.

Multivariate IPTW Cox survival analysis (Concordance statistic (95%CI): 0.80 (0.78–0.82)) shows that type of surgery, diabetes duration, baseline insulin treatment, baseline HbA1c and percentage of weight loss at 1 year were independent factors associated to diabetes remission along the follow-up. HR were 0.91 (0.78–1.05) for SG and 1.19 (1.00–1.42) for MAs (GBP as reference), 0.96 (0.95–0.97) for diabetes duration, 0.58 (0.43–0.79) for insulin treatment, 0.92 (0.90–0.96) for HbA1c and 1.01 (1.02–1.20) for weight loss at 1 year. Figure 1 shows survival curves for diabetes remission by type of surgery.

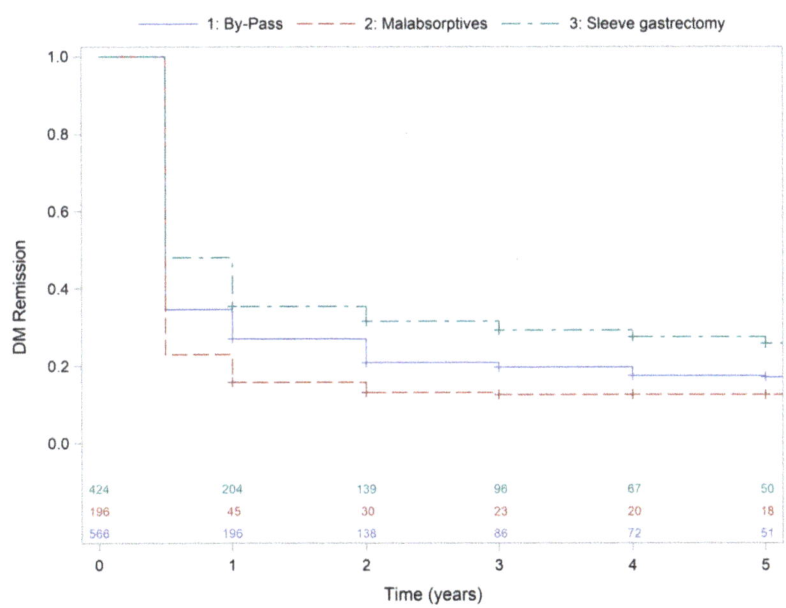

Figure 1. Kaplan–Meier for type 2 diabetes remission according to type of bariatric surgery.

3.3. Time-in-Remission Range

"Time-within-remission range" expressing the percentages of persistence of diabetes remission during all the follow-up periods, were 83.3% (33.3–91.6) after GBP, 68.7% (7.1–87.5) after SG and 90% (83.3–92.8) after MAs ($p < 0.001$ for comparisons between the three groups).

Previous duration of diabetes was negatively correlated with the percentage of "time-within-remission range", OR 0.89, (0.86–0.92), $p < 0.0001$, as was baseline HbA1c, OR 0.85, (0.74–0.97), $p = 0.0184$ and treatment with insulin, OR 0.24, (0.17–0.35), $p < 0.0001$. However, age and baseline BMI were not related with this parameter. Weight lost at 1 year after BS was positively correlated, OR 1.06, (1.04–1.08), $p < 0.0001$, with the "time-within-remission range". The association of BS type with "time-within-remission range", using GBP as a reference, were: OR 3.70 (2.34–5.84), $p < 0.0001$ for MAs and OR 0.55 (0.40–0.75), $p = 0.0002$ for SG.

3.4. Good Metabolic Control

Good metabolic control was presented in 92%, 89% and 86% patients in the whole cohort at 1, 2 and 5 years of follow-up after BS, respectively. Good metabolic control at 1 year was negatively associated with age, OR 0.96 (0.93–0.99), $p = 0.003$, diabetes duration, OR 0.93, (0.90–0.97), $p < 0.0001$, baseline treatment with insulin, OR 0.12 (0.03–0.43), $p = 0.001$ and baseline HbA1c, OR 0.71 (0.63–0.80), $p < 0.001$. Regarding the type of surgery, compared to GBP, the associations were: OR 4.91 (1.67–14.45), $p = 0.004$ for MAs, and OR 0.53 (0.32–0.86), $p = 0.011$ for SG.

3.5. Diabetes Recurrence

After diabetes remission, recurrence occurred in 16% (12–19, 95%CI) of patients after GBP, 24% (18–28, 95%CI) after SG and 12% (12–19, 95%CI) after MAs. Recurrence was associated with diabetes duration (hazard ratio (HR) 1.04, (1.02–1.07), $p = 0.001$), baseline HbA1c (HR 1.14, (1.11–1.25), $p = 0.002$), insulin treatment (HR 2.35, (1.38–4.0), $p < 0.0001$), weight regain (HR 1.01, (1.01–1.02), $p = 0.03$) and type of BS (HR 0.48 (0.29–0.82), $p = 0.007$ for MAs and HR 1.56 (1.13–2.16), $p = 0.006$ for SG, using GBP as reference).

3.6. Weight Loss and Weight Regain

One year after BS, the estimated weight loss was 30.7% (29.9–31.4) after GBP, 27.52% (26.72–28.32) after SG and 32.93% (31.76–34.10) after MAs. After 1 year of follow-up, weight loss was statistically different between the three types of surgery included in our cohort. Figure 2 shows the weight loss evolution.

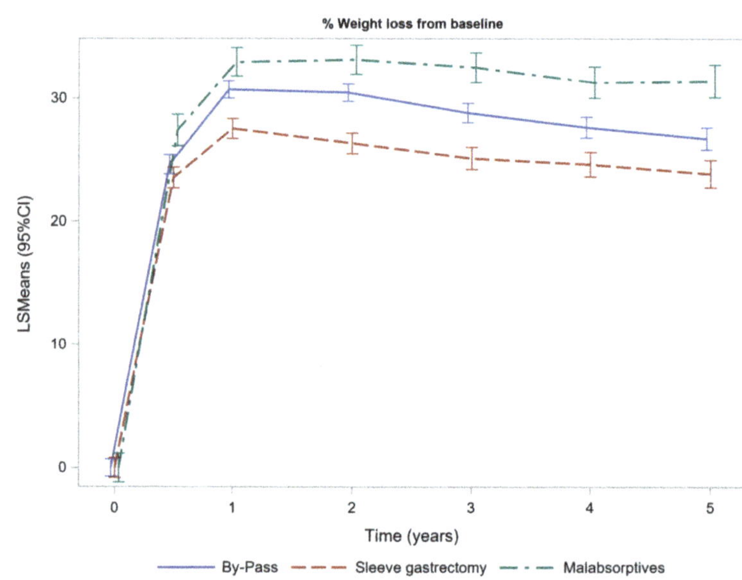

Figure 2. Weight loss evolution of patients with type 2 diabetes, expressed as percentage of initial body weight.

Weight regain at three years was 14.78% (13.2–16.37) after GBP, 10.87% (8.41–13.3) after MAs and 18.99% (17.14–20.84) after SG. Weight regain was statistically different between the three types of BS. A 20% weight regain at three years after BS was observed in 18.9% after GBP, 26.7% after SG and 13.8% after MAs. All comparisons between type of BS were statistically different, $p < 0.05$. Table 2 shows the data regarding weight loss and weight regain.

Table 2. Weight loss and weight regain evolution bariatric surgery according to the surgical technique, Inverse Probability of the Treatment Weights (IPTW) analysis.

	Time After BS	Treatment			*p*-Value		
		GBP	SG	MAs	GBP Versus SG	GBP Versus MAs	SG Versus MAs
Weight loss * (%)	0.5 year	24.6 (23.8–25.4)	23.5 (22.6–24.4)	27.4 (26.1–28.7)	0.064	0.003	<0.001
	1 year	30.6 (30.0–31.4)	27.5 (26.7–28.3)	32.9 (31.7–34.1)	<0.001	0.012	<0.001
	2 years	30.4 (29.7–31.2)	26.3 (25.5–27.1)	33.1 (31.9–34.3)	<0.001	0.001	<0.001
	3 years	28.8 (28.0–29.6)	25.2 (24.2–26.0)	32.5 (31.3–33.7)	<0.001	<0.001	<0.001
	4 years	27.6 (26.7–28.5)	24.6 (23.6–25.6)	31.2 (30.0–32.7)	<0.001	<0.001	<0.001
	5 years	26.7 (25.8–27.6)	23.8 (22.7–25.0)	31.4 (30.1–32.7)	<0.001	<0.001	<0.001
Weight regain & (%)	2 years	6.5 (5.0–7.9)	10.8 (9.1–12.6)	5.9 (3.5–8.5)	0.002	0.734	0.02
	3 years	14.7 (13.2–16.4)	18.9 (17.1–20.8)	10.8 (8.4–13.3)	0.007	0.008	<0.001
	4 years	19.7 (17.9–21.4)	24.7 (22.7–26.8)	14.7 (12.1–17.2)	0.002	0.001	<0.001
	5 years	22.4 (20.6–24.2)	28.7 (26.6–31.0)	15.2 (12.7–17.8)	<0.001	<0.001	<0.001

Data are expressed as mean (95%CI). * Expressed as percentage of initial body weight. & Expressed as percentage of weight lost at nadir point. BS: bariatric surgery; GBP: gastric bypass; SG: sleeve gastrectomy; MAs: malabsorptive surgeries.

4. Discussion

This study involved a large cohort of post-bariatric patients with type 2 diabetes from public hospitals in a Mediterranean area. After matching using the PS and the IPTW methods, we examined the diabetes and weight loss outcomes of the three main types of surgical techniques used in BS. In our cohort, MAs was the group with higher diabetes remission, a major percentage of "time-within-remission range", less diabetes recurrence, more weight loss and less weight regain compared to GBP. On the other side, subjects who had undergone SG obtained similar diabetes remission rates but spent less "time-within-remission range", achieved less percentage of good metabolic control and had more recurrences, together with a smaller weight loss and more weight regain compared to GBP.

This study has several strengths. First, the use of data obtained from clinical registries, albeit in a retrospective way, may better reflect the daily clinical practice compared to results from randomised control trials, which permits the generalisation of the results to our population. Another strong point is the excellent adjustment for covariates, performed taking into consideration several known variables relevant to the prediction of diabetes outcomes, thus allowing the different types of surgeries to be compared without the interference of confounding factors. Also, it is extremely interesting that we have included a considerable number of patients operated on using malabsorptive techniques. Finally, we introduced a new approach to measure the metabolic beneficial effects of BS, the percentage of time during the follow-up period that diabetes remains under remission. Taking into account that the legacy effect also occurs in type 2 diabetes [24], our study attempts to transpose the glucose parameter "percentage of time-in-range" used in CGM in type 1 diabetes to BS results. Given that, this variable considers all the time during which the subject remains in each glycaemic category and not just the time until the first diabetes recurrence, while encompassing the different patterns of weight loss and weight recovery. The "time-within-remission range" emerges as a relevant parameter to evaluate the long-term diabetes outcomes, a chronic disease largely conditioned by the fluctuations in weight that occur throughout the life of the subjects after BS. However, we acknowledge that the potential implications for daily clinical practice still need further evaluation.

Two population-based cohorts that were matched with no surgical management show results from real world settings in Europe, using stricter diabetes remission criteria [25,26]. A Danish cohort, with 1111 patients with diabetes, found a one-year diabetes remission rate of 74% and a relapse rate of 27% after 5 years of follow-up. However, GBP was the only surgical technique included [25]. In another cohort from the United Kingdom, Yska et al. found greater remission of diabetes after GBP (n = 280) than after SG (n = 83) or gastric band (n = 200) [26]. Neither of the two studies analysed other relevant issues, such as the duration of diabetes remission, the recurrence or the percentage of good metabolic control. A third real world setting study, focussing only on medication discontinuation in the short term, showed that GBP (n = 922) was more effective than SG (n = 1111) in achieving this primary outcome [27]. None of these studies evaluated the factors associated with diabetes outcomes exhaustively. On the other hand, our cohort, like others, showed that MAs has the greatest efficacy regarding weight loss and diabetes remission. But, given the concern about nutritional consequences, it requires a very personalised indication [28,29].

In our Spanish cohort, characteristics related with type 2 diabetes, such as longer diabetes duration, need for insulin therapy and higher baseline HbA1c values, were strongly associated with all assessed outcomes (remission, good metabolic control, time-within-remission range and recurrence). In addition, some features of the patient such as older age and higher BMI were also negatively related with diabetes remission. Finally, weight response after BS was also able to influence type 2 diabetes remission (weight loss) and recurrence (weight regain). The same predictors were described in previous studies [30,31].

Our results regarding weight loss were comparable to a recently published US large PS-matched bariatric cohort (n = 8493 GBP and n = 4387 SG). Their results showed that individuals with diabetes lost more weight after GBP than SG, but diabetes outcomes results were not published [32]. Our data shows a greater weight regain after SG than GBP and MAs, in the same direction as an Indian cohort (n = 9617), although their data were not adjusted for baseline differences and data on the percentage of diabetes was not provided [33]. On the other hand, a Spanish cohort recently reported a high percentage of reoperations after SG, expressly 23%, due to issues regarding gastroesophageal reflux or insufficient weight loss; however, this may be an advantage of GBP over SG [31].

Our study has some limitations. First, patients were not randomly assigned to the procedures, so there was a risk of unobserved confounding that may have persisted despite covariate and PS adjustment in our pair-wise comparisons. Second, the short duration of follow-up and attrition could preclude recognition of diabetes relapse that could hinder long-term generalisation. Lastly, the adverse effects occurring with the three types of surgery included in the study have not been assessed, precluding an accurate assessment of cost effectiveness ratio.

5. Conclusions

In conclusion, our results from a large multicentre Spanish cohort showed that diabetes outcomes and weight evolution were better after MAs surgeries compared to GBP and SG. Although SG showed remission rates like GBP, patients undergoing SG experienced a greater recurrence of diabetes, a shorter time-within-remission range and a lower percentage of good metabolic control. Furthermore, SG was also associated with less weight loss and greater weight recovery than GBP. Based on our findings, we propose choosing the bariatric technique that achieves the best metabolic effect, the greatest weight loss and the longest time of diabetes remission, carefully weighed with the adverse effects and the inherent surgical risk. For this selection, it is imperative to assess the characteristics of type 2 diabetes, as they will powerfully influence the outcomes of BS.

Supplementary Materials: The following are available online at http://www.mdpi.com/2077-0383/9/4/1070/s1: Table S1: Baseline main clinical and metabolic characteristics of participants in the study before propensity score adjustment. Figure S1: Flow chart of the study population.

Author Contributions: A.d.H., A.L., M.A.R., E.S., N.V., J.G.O., M.L.F.-S., J.S.-S., M.D.B.-P., A.C. (Andreea Ciudin), F.T., C.V., M.J.M., S.V., S.P., I.M., L.M., A.G., L.S., L.F., M.B., A.C. (Assumpta Caixàs), I.B., R.C., R.O., R.P., M.J.d.l.C., A.S.-S., F.M.P.-G., E.T.L.-M., A.G., E.F., O.B., Á.M., J.A., M.M.-P., L.T., M.A., O.C., F.G., C.A., M.A.B., A.C. (Alfonso Calañas), and Á.R. recruited patients, collected data, critically reviewed the draft of the article and had final approval of the version for publication; A.L. designed the study; A.d.H. and A.L. supervised the research, interpreted data and wrote the first draft of the manuscript; A.d.H. and F.T. analysed data and supervised the statistical analysis; A.d.H., A.L., M.A.R., E.S., N.V., J.G.O., M.L.F.-S., J.S.-S., M.D.B.-P. and A.C. (Andreea Ciudin) contributed to the discussion. All authors have read and agreed to the published version of the manuscript.

Funding: This study was supported by the Spanish Society of Endocrinology and Nutrition (SEEN). The RICIBA and RICIBA-DM are property of the Spanish Society of Endocrinology and Nutrition (SEEN). J.S.S. gratefully acknowledges the financial support by ICREA under the ICREA Academia programme.

Conflicts of Interest: The authors declare no conflicts of interest.

References

1. Blüher, M. Obesity: Global epidemiology and pathogenesis. *Nat. Rev. Endocrinol.* **2019**, *15*, 288–298. [CrossRef] [PubMed]
2. Popkin, B.M.; Slining, M.M. New dynamics in global obesity facing low- and middle-income countries. *Obes. Rev.* **2013**, *14* (Suppl. 2), 11–20. [CrossRef] [PubMed]
3. Angrisani, L.; Santonicola, A.; Iovino, P.; Vitiello, A.; Higa, K.; Himpens, J.; Buchwald, H.; Scopinaro, N. IFSO worldwide survey 2016: Primary, endoluminal, and revisional procedures. *Obes Surg.* **2018**, *28*, 3783–3794. [CrossRef] [PubMed]
4. Gloy, V.L.; Briel, M.; Bhatt, D.L.; Kashyap, S.R.; Schauer, P.R.; Mingrone, G.; Bucher, H.C.; Nordmann, A.J. Bariatric surgery versus non-surgical treatment for obesity: A systematic review and meta-analysis of randomised controlled trials. *BMJ* **2013**, *347*, f5934. [CrossRef] [PubMed]
5. Schauer, P.R.; Nor Hanipah, Z.; Rubino, F. Metabolic surgery for treating type 2 diabetes mellitus: Now supported by the world's leading diabetes organizations. *Cleve Clin. J. Med.* **2017**, *84* (Suppl. 1), S47–S56. [CrossRef]
6. Sheng, B.; Truong, K.; Spitler, H.; Zhang, L.; Tong, X. The long-term effects of bariatric surgery on type 2 diabetes remission, microvascular and macrovascular complications, and mortality: A systematic. *Rev. Meta Anal.* **2017**, *27*, 2724–2732. [CrossRef]
7. Buse, J.B.; Caprio, S.; Cefalu, W.T.; Ceriello, A.; Del Prato, S.; Inzucchi, S.E.; McLauglin, S.; Phillips, G.L., 2nd; Robertson, R.P.; Rubino, F.; et al. How do we define cure of diabetes? *Diabetes Care* **2009**, *32*, 2133–2135. [CrossRef]
8. Ahuja, A.; Tantia, O.; Chaudhuri, T.; Khanna, S.; Seetharamaiah, S.; Majumdar, K.; Goyal, G. Predicting remission of diabetes post metabolic surgery: A comparison of ABCD, diarem, and DRS scores. *Obes. Surg.* **2018**, *28*, 2025–2031. [CrossRef]
9. Chikunguwo, S.M.; Wolfe, L.G.; Dodson, P.; Meador, J.G.; Baugh, N.; Clore, J.N.; Kellum, J.M.; Maher, J.W. Analysis of factors associated with durable remission of diabetes after Roux-en-Y gastric bypass. *Surg. Obes. Relat. Dis.* **2010**, *6*, 254–259. [CrossRef]
10. Still, C.D.; Wood, G.C.; Benotti, P.; Petrick, A.T.; Gabrielsen, J.; Strodel, W.E.; Ibele, A.; Seiler, J.; Irving, B.A.; Celaya, M.P.; et al. Preoperative prediction of type 2 diabetes remission following Roux-en-Y gastric bypass surgery: A retrospective cohort study. *Lancet Diabetes Endocrinol.* **2014**, *2*, 38–45. [CrossRef]
11. Salminen, P.; Helmiö, M.; Ovaska, J.; Juuti, A.; Leivonen, M.; Peromaa-Haavisto, P.; Hurme, S.; Soinio, M.; Nuutila, P.; Victorzon, M. Effect of laparoscopic sleeve gastrectomy vs. laparoscopic Roux-en-Y gastric bypass on weight loss at 5 years among patients with morbid obesity. *JAMA* **2018**, *319*, 241–254. [CrossRef] [PubMed]
12. Peterli, R.; Wölnerhanssen, B.K.; Vetter, D.; Nett, P.; Gass, M.; Borbély, Y.; Peters, T.; Schiesser, M.; Schultes, B.; Beglinger, C.; et al. Laparoscopic sleeve gastrectomy versus Roux-Y-Gastric bypass for morbid obesity-3-year outcomes of the prospective randomized swiss multicenter bypass or sleeve study (SM-BOSS). *Ann. Surg.* **2017**, *265*, 466–473. [CrossRef] [PubMed]

13. Schauer, P.R.; Bhatt, D.L.; Kirwan, J.P.; Wolski, K.; Aminian, A.; Brethauer, S.A.; Navaneethan, S.D.; Singh, R.P.; Pothier, C.E.; Nissen, S.E.; et al. Bariatric surgery versus intensive medical therapy for diabetes—5-year outcomes. *N. Engl. J. Med.* **2017**, *376*, 641–651. [CrossRef] [PubMed]
14. Mingrone, G.; Panunzi, S.; De Gaetano, A.; Guidone, C.; Iaconelli, A.; Nanni, G.; Castagneto, M.; Bornstein, S.; Rubino, F. Bariatric-metabolic surgery versus conventional medical treatment in obese patients with type 2 diabetes: 5 year follow-up of an open-label, single-centre, randomised controlled trial. *Lancet* **2015**, *386*, 964–973. [CrossRef]
15. Battelino, T.; Danne, T.; Bergenstal, R.M.; Amiel, S.A.; Beck, R.; Biester, T.; Bosi, E.; Buckingham, B.A.; Cefalu, W.T.; Close, K.L.; et al. Clinical targets for continuous glucose monitoring data interpretation: Recommendations from the international consensus on time in range. *Diabetes Care* **2019**, *42*, 1593–1603. [CrossRef]
16. Lecube, A.; Monereo, S. RICIBA, what do we know about bariatric surgery in Spain? *Endocrinol. Nutr.* **2011**, *58*, 323–324. [CrossRef]
17. Lecube, A.; de Hollanda, A.; Calañas, A.; Vilarrasa, N.; Rubio, M.A.; Breton, I.; Goday, A.; Vidal, J.; Iglesias, P.; Fernández-Soto, M.L.; et al. Trends in bariatric surgery in spain in the twenty-first century: Baseline results and 1-month follow up of the RICIBA, a national registry. *Obes. Surg.* **2016**, *26*, 1836–1842. [CrossRef]
18. Von Elm, E.; Altman, D.G.; Egger, M.; Pocock, S.J.; Gøtzsche, P.C.; Vandenbroucke, J.P.; STROBE Initiative. The Strengthening the Reporting of Observational Studies in Epidemiology (STROBE) statement: Guidelines for reporting observational studies. *Lancet* **2007**, *370*, 1453–1457. [CrossRef]
19. American Diabetes Association. Standards of medical care in diabetes-2018. *Diabetes Care* **2018**, *41* (Suppl. 1), 13–27. [CrossRef]
20. King, W.C.; Hinerman, A.S.; Belle, S.H.; Wahed, A.S.; Courcoulas, A.P. Comparison of the performance of common measures of weight regain after bariatric surgery for association with clinical outcomes. *JAMA* **2018**, *320*, 1560–1569. [CrossRef]
21. D'Agostino, R.B., Jr. Propensity score methods for bias reduction in the comparison of a treatment to a non-randomized control group. *Stat Med.* **1998**, *17*, 2265–2281. [CrossRef]
22. Austin, P.C. An introduction to propensity score methods for reducing the effects of confounding in observational studies. *Multivar. Behav. Res.* **2011**, *46*, 399–424. [CrossRef] [PubMed]
23. Cohen, J. *Statistical Power Analysis for the Bahavioral Sciences*, 2nd ed.; Academic Press: New York, NY, USA, 1977; pp. 19–66. [CrossRef]
24. Laiteerapong, N.; Ham, S.A.; Gao, Y.; Moffet, H.H.; Liu, J.Y.; Huang, E.S.; Karter, A.J. The legacy effect in type 2 diabetes:impactofearlyglycemic control on future complications (the Diabetes & Aging study). *Diabetes Care* **2019**, *42*, 416–426. [PubMed]
25. Madsen, L.R.; Baggesen, L.M.; Richelsen, B.; Thomsen, R.W. Effect of Roux-en-Y gastric bypass surgery on diabetes remission and complications in individuals with type 2 diabetes: A Danish population-based matched cohort study. *Diabetologia* **2019**, *62*, 611–620. [CrossRef]
26. Yska, J.P.; van Roon, E.N.; de Boer, A.; Leufkens, H.G.M.; Wilffert, B.; de Heide, L.J.; de Vries, F.; Lalmohamed, A. Remission of type 2 diabetes mellitus in patients after different types of bariatric surgery. *JAMA Surg.* **2015**, *150*, 1126. [CrossRef]
27. Lewis, K.H.; Arterburn, D.E.; Zhang, F.; Callaway, K.; Wallace, J.; Fernandez, A.; Ross-Degnan, D.; Wharam, J.F. Comparative effectiveness of vertical sleeve gastrectomy versus roux en y gastric bypass for diabetes treatment. *Ann Surg.* **2019**. [CrossRef]
28. Carlsson, L.M.S.; Sjöholm, K.; Karlsson, C.; Jacobson, P.; Andersson-Assarsson, J.C.; Svensson, P.A.; Larsson, I.; Hjorth, S.; Neovius, M.; Taube, M.; et al. Long-term incidence of microvascular disease after bariatric surgery or usual care in patients with obesity stratified by baseline glucose status: A post-hoc analysis of participants from the swedish obese subjects study. *Lancet Diabetes Endocrinol.* **2017**, *5*, 271–279. [CrossRef]
29. Topart, P.A.; Becouarn, G. Revision and reversal after biliopancreatic diversion for excessive side effects or ineffective weight loss: A review of the current literature on indications and procedures. *Surg. Obes. Relat. Dis.* **2015**, *11*, 965–972. [CrossRef]
30. Ramos-Levi, A.M.; Matia, P.; Cabrerizo, L.; Barabash, A.; Sanchez-Pernaute, A.; Calle-Pascual, A.L.; Torres, A.J.; Rubio, M.A. Statistical models to predict type 2 diabetes remission after bariatric surgery. *J. Diabetes* **2014**, *6*, 472–477. [CrossRef]

31. Jiménez, A.; Ibarzabal, A.; Moizé, V.; Pané, A.; Andreu, A.; Molero, J.; de Hollanda, A.; Flores, L.; Ortega, E.; Lacy, A.; et al. Ten-year outcomes after Roux-en-Y gastric bypass and sleeve gastrectomy: An observational nonrandomized cohort study. *Surg. Obes. Relat. Dis.* **2019**, *15*, 382–388. [CrossRef]
32. Arterburn, D.; Wellman, R.; Emiliano, A.; Smith, S.R.; Odegaard, A.O.; Murali, S.; Williams, N.; Coleman, K.J.; Courcoulas, A.; Coley, R.Y.; et al. Comparative effectiveness and safety of bariatric procedures for weight loss a PCORnet cohort study. *Ann. Int. Med.* **2018**, *169*, 741–750. [CrossRef] [PubMed]
33. Baig, S.J.; Priya, P.; Mahawar, K.K.; Shah, S.; Indian Bariatric Surgery Outcome Reporting (IBSOR) Group. Weight regain after bariatric surgery—A multicentre study of 9617 patients from indian bariatric surgery outcome reporting group. *Obes. Surg.* **2019**, *29*, 1583–1592. [CrossRef] [PubMed]

Journal of
Clinical Medicine

MDPI

Article

The Influence of Bariatric Surgery on Pregnancy and Perinatal Outcomes—A Case-Control Study

Anna Różańska-Walędziak [1], Maciej Walędziak [2,*], Paweł Bartnik [1], Joanna Kacperczyk-Bartnik [1], Michał Janik [2], Piotr Kowalewski [2], Andrzej Kwiatkowski [2] and Krzysztof Czajkowski [1]

[1] 2nd Department of Obstetrics and Gynecology, Medical University of Warsaw, Karowa 2 St., 00-315 Warsaw, Poland; aniaroza@tlen.pl (A.R.-W.); bartnik.pawel@gmail.com (P.B.); asiakacperczyk@gmail.com (J.K.-B.); krzysztof.czajkowski@wum.edu.pl (K.C.)

[2] Department of General, Oncological, Metabolic and Thoracic Surgery, Military Institute of Medicine, Szaserów 128 St., 04-141 Warsaw, Poland; mjanik@wim.mil.pl (M.J.); pkowalewski@wim.mil.pl (P.K.); akwiatkowski@wim.mil.pl (A.K.)

* Correspondence: maciej.waledziak@gmail.com

Received: 21 April 2020; Accepted: 29 April 2020; Published: 2 May 2020

Abstract: Introduction: Obesity in pregnant women increases the incidence of pregnancy-induced comorbidities and the rate of operative deliveries. Purpose of the Study: As bariatric surgery is the reference method of treatment of obesity, we wanted to evaluate its influence on the course of pregnancy and perinatal outcomes. Material and Methods: Data was collected from 627 female patients after bariatric surgery, of whom 107 had a history of pregnancy after the surgery, and 345 non-bariatric patients who had a delivery at a tertiary perinatal center. Sixty-one cases were matched (1:1) with controls for age, pre-pregnancy BMI and presence of pre-pregnancy comorbidities. The main endpoints were gestational diabetes mellitus (GDM), pregnancy-induced hypertension (PIH), small (SGA) and large for gestational age infants (LGA) and cesarean sections (CS). Results: Patients after bariatric procedures were significantly less likely to have GDM (19.67%/37.7%; $p = 0.0433$), PIH (11.47%/16.39%; $p = 0.6072$) and preterm delivery (13.11%/37.7%; $p = 0.0026$). The CS rate was higher (57.38%/40.98%; $p = 0.0987$). There was an increased risk of SGA (18.03%/13.11%; $p = 0.6072$) and a decreased risk of LGA (6.56%/16.39%; $p = 0.146$). Conclusions: Patients after bariatric surgery have a decreased risk of pregnancy-induced comorbidities, preterm deliveries and LGA infants, with an increase in rate of CS and SGA infants compared to general population matched for pre-pregnancy BMI, age and presence of pre-pregnancy comorbidities.

Keywords: bariatric surgery; pregnancy; gestational diabetes mellitus; pregnancy-induced hypertension

---

1. Introduction

Obesity is a major healthcare problem with an increasing global prevalence, having reached 650 million people in 2016, which represents 13% of the world population [1]. Obesity is a well-known risk factor for many concomitant diseases, distinctively diabetes mellitus type 2, hypertension, heart disease and obstructive sleep apnea syndrome (OSAS). It can also lead to sexual dysfunctions in both sexes. Obese women of reproductive age can suffer from infertility due to hormonally related ovulation dysfunction. Obesity in pregnant women increases the incidence of gestational diabetes mellitus (GDM), pregnancy-induced hypertension (PIH), which also influences the way of delivery, with an increase in number of vacuum deliveries and cesarean sections [2,3]. Bariatric surgery is the reference method of treatment for obesity, because of the durability and pace of the weight loss, reduction of symptoms and remission of concomitant diseases. As the prevalence of obesity in women of reproductive age is rising every year, the number of pregnancies after bariatric surgery is also increasing, creating a demand for knowledge among obstetricians about the influence of the bariatric surgery on the course of pregnancy. Women constitute up to 80% of bariatric patients, most of them being of reproductive age [4–6]. Bariatric surgery leads to various micronutrient deficiencies in pregnant women, with possible influence on fetal development, though further studies are needed on the subject [3,7–9]. Bariatric surgery and the resulting weight loss, reduction in adipose tissue as well as alteration of the gastrointestinal absorption lead to hormonal and metabolic changes that may affect the well-being of the woman and the fetus. They can also influence the incidence and course of pregnancy-induced co-morbidities. Bariatric surgery is known to have influence on the pregnancy and neonatal outcomes, increasing the rate of small for gestational age (SGA) infants and maternal anemia and decreasing the risk of GDM, PIH and large for gestational age infants (LGA) infants [10–13].

2. Purpose of the Study

In our study, we analyzed a group of patients with a history of pregnancy after bariatric surgery and compared them with a matched group of controls to examine the influence of restrictive and malabsorptive procedures on the course of pregnancy, pregnancy-induced diseases and perinatal outcomes. The study was designed as a retrospective case-control. The patients in the study group had a history of previous bariatric surgery, the mean time-to-conception interval after the surgery was 23.25 (± 16.9) months. The control group included patients without a history of bariatric surgery, matched for: age, BMI at the beginning of the pregnancy, presence of pre-pregnancy diabetes mellitus type 2 (PGDM) and pre-pregnancy hypertension (PPH). The primary end-points of our study were the occurrence of GDM, PIH, intrauterinal growth restriction (IUGR), small for gestational age (SGA) and large for gestational age (LGA) infants, neonatal intensive care unit (NICU) admission as well as premature deliveries, vacuum deliveries (VE) and cesarean sections (CS). We also analyzed the gestational weight gain (GWG) and the body mass index (BMI) at the moment of the delivery.

3. Material and Method

3.1. Participants—Subjects

We collected data from 627 female patients with a history of bariatric surgery, using paper and internet original survey. The recruitment was based on the bariatric center register and cooperation with Polish Bariatric Patients Society. There were 107 patients with a history of at least one pregnancy after bariatric surgery, out of whom 74 patients had laparoscopic sleeve gastrectomy (LSG), 21 laparoscopic Roux-en-Y gastric bypass (LRYGB), 9 adjustable silicone gastric banding (ASGB) and 3 other bariatric procedures. There were 77 patients from the group who met the inclusion criteria—having had at least one pregnancy ended with a delivery of a single live-born neonate after the bariatric surgery. The exclusion criteria were: multiple pregnancies, stillbirth and no sufficient data for the matching process. They were further surveyed for the data about the course of the pregnancy, maternal and neonatal outcomes. The vast majority of patients had spontaneous pregnancies, only one patient became pregnant after using methods of reproductive assistance. The approval from Military Institute of Medicine Ethics Committee was obtained on 22nd August 2018 (no. 117/WIM/2018).

3.2. Participants—Controls

We analyzed pregnancy and perinatal outcomes of 345 patients who were hospitalized and had a delivery at a tertiary perinatal center. The preliminary collected data included patients' age, BMI at the beginning of the pregnancy, PGDM and PPH. They were further surveyed for data about the course of the pregnancy, and maternal and neonatal outcomes.

3.3. Matching

Propensity scores (i.e., the estimated probability of undergoing bariatric surgery before pregnancy on the basis of the preoperative values) were estimated for each patient by use of logistic regression.

Potential confounding variables were considered and included age, body mass index, hypertension and diabetes type 2. We used a greedy matching algorithm (developed by Mayo Clinic group—http://bioinformaticstools.mayo.edu/research/gmatch/) to match each case to a control, restricting successful matches to those for whom the propensity scores did not differ by more than 0.2 units. Balance on potential confounding variables between the matched controls and cases were evaluated with standard univariable summary statistics and absolute standardized difference scores (absolute value of difference in means or proportions, divided by a combined estimate of standard deviation among the groups being compared). Variables with an absolute standardized difference score of less than 0.10 were considered adequately balanced. McNemar test was used to assess effect of exposure on dichotomous outcomes. The Cochran–Mantel–Haenszel test was used in the analysis of matched data. Continuous outcomes were assessed using the Wilcoxon signed-rank test.

3.4. Study Design

The study group and the control group were compared for the following variables: occurrence of GDM and PIH, premature delivery (defined as delivery before 37th week of pregnancy), method of delivery (vaginal spontaneous delivery, vacuum delivery, scheduled or urgent cesarean section due to pathological cardiotocography tracings or other indications), pregnancy duration and neonatal data, with strong emphasis on SGA and LGA neonates. Neonatal data included birth weight, birth length, ponderal index and Apgar score. SGA was defined as below the 10th percentile and LGA as over 90th percentile using population adjusted birth weight scores.

Pregnancy-induced hypertension was defined as de novo onset of hypertension (>140 mmHg systolic or >90 mmHg diastolic) after 20th week of gestation. Gestational diabetes mellitus was diagnosed with the oral glucose tolerance test with 75 g glucose (OGTT), administered after 8 h of fasting. GDM was identified in case of fasting blood glucose level of ≥5.1 mmol/L up to 6.9 mmol/L, ≥10 mmol/L after first hour of glucose administration and/or ≥ 8.5 mmol/L up to 11.0 mmol/L after the second hour. OGTT was recommended between 24th and 28th week of gestation in the general population and in the 1st trimester in case of BMI ≥ 30 kg/m^2, history of GDM in previous pregnancies, family history of diabetes mellitus type 2 and having given birth to a child of ≥4500 g birth weight [14]. Though our national guidelines suggest an alternative form of screening—home glucose monitoring—for patients after bariatric surgery with dumping syndrome, the vast majority patients included in the study had OGTT administered [15].

4. Results

Sixty-one pairs were created, matched for age, BMI at the beginning of pregnancy and presence of pre-pregnancy comorbidities, such as diabetes mellitus and hypertension. Standardized differences in the propensity score matched sample are shown in Table 1 and demographic characteristics in Table 2.

Table 1. Standardized differences in propensity score.

	d
Age	0.070
Body Mass Index	0.088
Diabetes	0.063
Hypertension	0.047

d: standardized differences.

Table 2. Demographic characteristics.

Characteristic	Original Cohort			Matched Cohort		
	Cases	Controls		Cases	Controls	
	$N = 77$	$N = 345$	p-Value	$N = 61$	$N = 61$	p-Value
	Mean (SD) or %			Mean (SD) or %		
Age (years)	34.92 (± 5.77)	30.76 (± 4.3)	<0.001	34.03 (± 5.56)	33.69 (± 4.19)	0.783
BMI (kg/m^2)	29.27 (± 5.65)	23.86 (±5.05)	<0.001	28.17 (± 4.15)	28.63 (± 6.11)	0.822
Pre-Op Hypertension	11.69%	13.04%	0.852	13.11%	14.75%	1.000
Pre-Op Diabetes Mellitus	6.49%	16.81%	0.022	6.56%	8.2%	1.000

BMI: Body Mass Index.

The general characteristics about the pregnancy length and neonatal data is presented in Table 3.

Table 3. Pregnancy length and neonatal data.

	Cases (Median (Q_1–Q_3))	Controls (Median (Q_1–Q_3))	p-Value
5th minute Apgar	10 (10–10)	10 (9–10)	0.0027
Birth weight (g)	3200 (2860–3550)	3140 (2830–3540)	0.9495
Birth length (cm)	54 (52–56)	54 (50–55)	0.2057
Ponderal index (kg/cm^3) (1000 × weight/(length × length × length))	19.91 (18.51–22.99)	20.64 (19.06–21.52)	0.3695
Pregnancy duration (days)	273 (266–280)	259 (255–269)	0.0002
Week of gestation at the delivery (weeks)	39 (38–40)	37 (36–38)	<0.0001

The mean pregnancy duration was 39 weeks in the study group and 37 weeks in the control group. Patients who had undergone bariatric surgery before the pregnancy had longer pregnancies, the difference being statistically significant ($p < 0.0001$). The Apgar score (5th minute after the delivery) used to evaluate neonates' condition was higher in the study group than in the control group ($p = 0.0027$) with a statistically significant difference present in the distribution of the results.

Statistically significant differences were observed neither in the neonates' birth weight nor in the birth length between the study group and the control group. The ponderal index was slightly lower in the study group, although the difference observed was not statistically significant.

We did not observe either maternal nor neonatal fatal cases in either study or control groups.

Patients after bariatric procedures were significantly less likely to have GDM than the control group (19.67% vs. 37.7%; $p = 0.0433$). Preterm delivery was less likely in the bariatric group than in the control group (13.11% vs. 37.7%; $p = 0.0026$). The differences found in the incidence of GDM and premature delivery were both statistically significant.

The incidence of pregnancy-induced hypertension was lower in the study group; however, it was not observed to be of statistical significance (11.47% vs. 16.39%; $p = 0.6072$).

Patients after bariatric procedures were less likely to have a vaginal spontaneous delivery (40.98% vs. 59.02%; $p = 0.0708$). Forceps and vacuum delivery were observed in only two cases in the study group (3.28%).

The proportion of CS was higher in the bariatric group than in the control group (57.38% vs. 40.98%; $p = 0.0987$). Patients after bariatric procedures most often had scheduled CS, followed by urgent CTG indications and other urgent indications (22 vs. 10 vs. 3).

Neonates in the bariatric group were more likely to be classified to be SGA and less likely to be LGA (SGA—18.03% vs. 13.11%; $p = 0.6072$/LGA—6.56% vs. 16.39%; $p = 0.146$).

The results are summarized in Table 4.

Table 4. Influence of bariatric surgery on pregnancy.

Characteristics	Cases	Controls	p-Value
gestational diabetes mellitus	19.67%	37.7%	0.0433
preterm delivery	13.11%	37.7%	0.0026
pregnancy-induced hypertension	11.47%	16.39%	0.6072
vaginal spontaneous delivery	40.98%	59.02%	0.0708
forceps or vacuum delivery	3.28%	0	
cesarean section	57.38%	40.98%	0.0987
small for gestational	18.03%	13.11%	0.6072
large for gestational	6.56%	16.39%	0.146

5. Discussion

Our principal findings indicate lower incidence of GDM and PIH in patients after bariatric surgery when compared to general population matched for pre-pregnancy BMI, age and presence of pre-pregnancy comorbidities. Similar to the literature, we found a lower rate of preterm deliveries and LGA infants with an increase in rate of SGA infants in the bariatric surgery group. We also observed an increase in number of scheduled CS with a decrease in proportion of urgent CS in bariatric patients.

Compared to other studies, our analysis includes a higher number of patients, making it possible to present results of statistical significance. The uniqueness of our study is the comparison between patients after bariatric surgery and patients matched for BMI at the beginning of pregnancy, age and pre-pregnancy co-morbidities. Most case-control studies about the influence of bariatric surgery on the course of pregnancy and neonatal outcomes include controls matched for BMI from before the operation and often lack information about pre-pregnancy co-morbidities. This makes it possible to see an increased positive impact of bariatric surgery on the pregnancy adverse outcomes, but also leads to interpretation bias, as obese patients in the control group are more likely to have pregnancy complications due to obesity. This emphasizes the positive influence of bariatric surgery on reduction of obesity-related complications, but excludes the possibility of comparison of bariatric patients with general population. In our study, we compare patients after bariatric surgery to patients from the general population, not only those who are obese. Pre-existing hypertension can strongly influence the birth weight of the neonate and further the evaluation of the correlation between bariatric surgery and the risk of LGA and IUGR. Pre-pregnancy diabetes mellitus, especially with poor control of blood glucose levels can lead to LGA and also influence the results of the analysis. Both PPH and PGDM may cause the necessity of ending the pregnancy preterm and can lead to pregnancy and neonatal complications, non-attributable to bariatric surgery, hence the importance of including them in the matching process.

Johansson et al. presented a study based on the Swedish Birth Register, in which they matched patients after bariatric surgery and controls for the pre-surgery BMI, age, parity, smoking and educational level [16]. They observed a reduction in the incidence of GDM (1.9% in the study group vs. 6.8% in the control group) and LGA (8.4% vs. 22.4%). There was an increased risk of SGA in the bariatric group—15.6% vs. 7.6% and a reduction in the pregnancy length—273.0 days vs. 277.5 days. We matched the patients for BMI at the beginning of pregnancy, which may be the reason for the differences in the results. In our study, 19.67% patients after bariatric procedures were diagnosed with GDM compared with 37.7% in the study group. The higher incidence of GDM may be result of population disparity, but also of different GDM diagnosis criteria. We did not observe a reduction in the pregnancy length in patients after bariatric surgery and furthermore, preterm delivery was less likely in the bariatric group than in the control group—13.11% vs. 37.7%. Our analysis presented a higher proportion of SGA among neonates of bariatric patients, and lower proportion of LGA neonates. A major limitation of the Johansson's study was that 98% of bariatric procedures were gastric bypass surgery. The increase in the rate of SGA infants after bariatric surgery has been widely discussed in the literature, with some studies indicating that the increase is comparable in pregnancies after SG to those after GB [10,13,17], while others suggest that the increase is mostly observed after LRYBG [8], or even determine no increase in the rate of SGA [18].

Aricha-Tamir et al. analyzed a group of patients with a history of delivery before and after bariatric surgery [19]. The study mostly included patients after LSG and vertical banded gastroplasty (VGB) with only 3.8% patients after LRYGB. The study presented a decrease in proportion of hypertension (without determining whether pre-pregnancy or pregnancy-induced hypertension) after the surgery from 31.9% to 16.7% and of GDM—from 19.3% to 3.5%. The analysis presented an increase in the number of CS, from 24.3% to 31.9%, with a decrease in urgent CS of 5%. Most studies present an increase in the rate of CS after bariatric surgery [12,20], although some researchers observed the opposite [2]. In our study, we also observed an increase in number of scheduled CS with a decrease in proportion of urgent CS. The difference between pre-surgery and after-surgery pregnancies in Aricha-Tamir's study was not statistically significant in the proportion of LGA neonates or the birth weight as general.

Galazis et al. presented a meta-analysis of the perinatal outcomes after bariatric surgery, based on 17 studies [21]. The primary endpoints were preeclampsia, GDM, maternal anemia, premature delivery, LGA and SGA neonates, NICU admission and perinatal mortality. The risk of preeclampsia, GDM and LGA neonates was 50% lower after bariatric surgery, unlike the rate of SGA neonates, which was 80% higher and of premature delivery—28% higher. The analysis did not reveal any differences in the proportion of CS. The results obtained in our study were comparable in terms of GDM. We cannot compare the data about hypertension, as we included all cases of PIH and Galazis et al. analyzed only cases of preeclampsia (PIH followed by additional proteinuria or other maternal organ dysfunction). In our study, we observed a lower rate of premature deliveries in the bariatric group than in the control group.

A more than three-fold decrease in the incidence of GDM was observed in a study by Burke et al., who compared a group of women with a delivery before and after bariatric surgery, having based on a private insurance claims database [22]. Kwong et al. presented a meta-analysis about the influence of bariatric surgery on pregnancy course and perinatal outcomes. The analysis showed that bariatric surgery led to reduced rates of GDM (OR 0.20), LGA infants (OR 0.32) and all hypertensive disorders (OR 0.38) and an increase in SGA infants (OR 2.16) and preterm deliveries (OR 1.35) [20]. The meta-analysis included studies comparing bariatric patients with control subjects matched for pre-surgery BMI. In our study, we compared bariatric patients matched with controls for BMI at the beginning of the pregnancy, age, presence of PGDM and PPH. The impact of bariatric procedures on the reduction of the rate of GDM and LGA, together with an increased rate of SGA infants was also observed in a case-control study by Chevrot et al. [23].

The question about the incidence of GDM in pregnant patients after bariatric surgery is whether the result of OGTT, performed with liquid glucose solution is reliable and whereas the absorption changes after the operation do or do not influence blood sugar results and therefore the result of OGTT. A reduction in the glucose absorption might lead to lower blood sugar levels after the glucose intake, so it remains to be analyzed whether the real proportion of GDM is the one found with OGTT screening. Home glucose monitoring is more reliable and is advised in the guidelines.

Home glucose monitoring with evaluation of fasting and postprandial blood sugar levels is suggested in our national guidelines as an alternative form of GDM screening in patients after bariatric surgery with dumping syndrome [15]. The American College of Obstetricians and Gynecologists recommends home glucose monitoring with evaluation of fasting blood glucose levels and two hours postprandial, whereas our recommendations suggest after one hour [24]. However, the differences between countries in diagnostic algorithms and blood glucose thresholds lead to heterogeneity in study results [25]. The suggested period of monitoring in both guidelines is of one week between 24th and 28th week of gestation [26], which is repetitively emphasized in other studies and recommendations [4,27,28]. Even though the recommendations remain clear, the vast majority patients included in the study admitted having had OGTT administered. The problem of introduction and adherence to the guidelines remains to be ameliorated. Rottenstreich emphasizes the problem of hypoglycemia after OGTT in bariatric patients as it affects almost 50% of pregnant patients after bariatric surgery with incidence of 83% in patients after LRYGB [29]. Hypoglycemia in OGTT is correlated with a higher proportion of SGA infants and patients after bariatric surgery may experience hypoglycemia during a substantial portion of time, which may be the reason for the increased risk of IUGR and SGA.

6. Limitations of the Study

The main limitation of our study is its retrospective nature and the possibility of recall and selection bias. Having collected data with a paper and internet survey resulted in the impossibility of obtaining all the necessary data about all pregnant women and their newborns. Additionally, there is a possibility of sample bias, as patients from the control group were hospitalized in a 3rd degree perinatal center and the percentage of patients with high risk pregnancies was higher than in general population.

7. Conclusions

Bariatric surgery is well known to reduce the risk of GDM, PIH, LGA infants, with an increase in the number of SGA infants. Most studies compare pregnancy complications and neonatal outcomes in bariatric patients with obese control groups, matched for preoperational BMI. As obesity is an independent risk factor of many comorbidities, those studies mostly show the positive influence of bariatric procedures and the following reduction of body weight on reduction of obesity-dependent pregnancy complications and neonatal outcomes. In our study, we presented a comparison of patients after bariatric procedures with a group of controls matched for BMI at the beginning of pregnancy. Our results show that bariatric patients have a decreased risk of pregnancy comorbidities and LGA even when compared with non-obese population. Additionally, we included in our matching presence of pre-pregnancy diabetes mellitus and hypertension, to exclude their influence on incidence of LGA, SGA and perinatal complications.

Although all types of bariatric operations are meant to lead to a similar therapeutic effect, their influence on the physiology of digestion and absorption of nutrients is based on different mechanisms. We acknowledge the importance of heterogeneity of bariatric procedures and the need for comparing the influence of restrictive and malabsorptive procedures on the pregnancy and neonatal adverse outcomes, which will be subject of our further studies.

Author Contributions: A.R.-W., M.W., P.B., J.K.-B., M.J., P.K., A.K., K.C. Conceptualization, A.R.-W. and M.W.; methodology, A.R.-W., M.W. and M.J.; validation, M.J. and M.W.; formal analysis, A.R.-W., M.W., P.B., J.K.-B. and M.J.; investigation, A.R.-W., M.W., P.B., J.K.-B.; writing—original draft preparation, A.R.-W. and M.W.; writing—review and editing, A.R.-W. and M.W.; supervision, A.K., K.C. and A.R.-W.; funding acquisition, M.W. and A.K.; Resources, A.R.-W., M.W., P.B., J.K.-B., M.J., P.K. and A.K. All authors have read and agreed to the published version of the manuscript.

Funding: The APC was funded by Military Institute of Medicine.

Conflicts of Interest: The authors declare no conflict of interest.

Abbreviations

OSAS	obstructive sleep apnea syndrome
GDM	pregnancy diabetes mellitus
PIH	pregnancy-induced hypertension
PGDM	pre-pregnancy diabetes mellitus type 2
PPH	pre-pregnancy hypertension
IUGR	intrauterine fetal growth restriction
SGA	small for gestational age
LGA	large for gestational age
NICU	neonatal intensive unit
VE	vacuum extractor
CS	cesarean section
GWG	gestational weight gain

BMI	body mass index
LSG	laparoscopic sleeve gastrectomy
LRYGB	laparoscopic Roux-en-Y gastric bypass
ASGB	adjustable silicone gastric banding
LGB	laparoscopic gastric banding
OGTT	oral glucose tolerance test

References

1. Neylan, C.; Kannan, U.; Dempsey, D.T.; Williams, N.N.; Dumon, K.R. The Surgical Management of Obesity. *Gastroenterol. Clin. N. Am.* **2016**, *45*, 689–703. [CrossRef] [PubMed]
2. Costa, M.M.; Belo, S.; Souteiro, P.; Neves, J.S.; Magalhaes, D.; Silva, R.B.; Oliveira, S.C.; Freitas, P.; Varela, A.; Queiros, J.; et al. Pregnancy after bariatric surgery: Maternal and fetal outcomes of 39 pregnancies and a literature review. *J. Obstet. Gynaecol. Res.* **2018**, *44*, 681–690. [CrossRef] [PubMed]
3. Slater, C.; Morris, L.; Ellison, J.; Syed, A.A. Nutrition in Pregnancy Following Bariatric Surgery. *Nutr.* **2017**, *9*, 1338. [CrossRef] [PubMed]
4. Shawe, J.; Ceulemans, D.; Akhter, Z.; Neff, K.; Hart, K.; Heslehurst, N.; Štotl, I.; Agrawal, S.; Steegers-Theunissen, R.; Taheri, S.; et al. Pregnancy after bariatric surgery: Consensus recommendations for periconception, antenatal and postnatal care. *Obes. Rev.* **2019**, *20*, 1507–1522. [CrossRef] [PubMed]
5. Rottenstreich, A.; Elazary, R.; Levin, G. Pregnancy after bariatric surgery and the risk of fetal growth restriction. *Surg. Obes. Relat. Dis.* **2018**, *14*, 1919–1920. [CrossRef] [PubMed]
6. Carreau, A.-M.; Nadeau, M.; Marceau, S.; Marceau, P.; Weisnagel, S.J. Pregnancy after Bariatric Surgery: Balancing Risks and Benefits. *Can. J. Diabetes* **2017**, *41*, 432–438. [CrossRef] [PubMed]
7. Rottenstreich, A.; Elazary, R.; Goldenshluger, A.; Pikarsky, A.J.; Elchalal, U.; Porat, T.B.-. Maternal nutritional status and related pregnancy outcomes following bariatric surgery: A systematic review. *Surg. Obes. Relat. Dis.* **2019**, *15*, 324–332. [CrossRef]
8. Coupaye, M.; Legardeur, H.; Sami, O.; Calabrese, D.; Mandelbrot, L.; LeDoux, S. Impact of Roux-en-Y gastric bypass and sleeve gastrectomy on fetal growth and relationship with maternal nutritional status. *Surg. Obes. Relat. Dis.* **2018**, *14*, 1488–1494. [CrossRef]
9. Yau, P.O.; Parikh, M.; Saunders, J.K.; Chui, P.; Zablocki, T.; Welcome, A.U. Pregnancy after bariatric surgery: The effect of time-to-conception on pregnancy outcomes. *Surg. Obes. Relat. Dis.* **2017**, *13*, 1899–1905. [CrossRef]
10. Akhter, Z.; Rankin, J.; Ceulemans, D.; Ngongalah, L.; Ackroyd, R.; Devlieger, R.; Vieira, R.; Heslehurst, N. Pregnancy after bariatric surgery and adverse perinatal outcomes: A systematic review and meta-analysis. *PLoS Med.* **2019**, *16*, e1002866. [CrossRef]
11. Watanabe, A.; Seki, Y.; Haruta, H.; Kikkawa, E.; Kasama, K. Maternal impacts and perinatal outcomes after three types of bariatric surgery at a single institution. *Arch. Gynecol. Obstet.* **2019**, *300*, 145–152. [CrossRef] [PubMed]
12. Haseeb, Y.A. A Review of Obstetrical Outcomes and Complications in Pregnant Women after Bariatric Surgery. *Sultan Qaboos Univ. Med. J. [SQUMJ]* **2019**, *19*, 284–290. [CrossRef] [PubMed]
13. Malik, S.; Teh, J.L.; Lomanto, D.; Kim, G.; So, J.B.-Y.; Shabbir, A.; Guowei, K. Maternal and fetal outcomes of Asian pregnancies after bariatric surgery. *Surg. Obes. Relat. Dis.* **2020**, *16*, 529–535. [CrossRef] [PubMed]
14. Wender-Ożegowska, E.; Bomba-Opoń, D.; Brązert, J.; Celewicz, Z.; Czajkowski, K.; Gutaj, P.; Malinowska-Polubiec, A.; Zawiejska, A.; Wielgoś, M. Polish Society of Gynaecologists and Obstetricians Standards for the management of patients with diabetes. *Ginekol Pol.* **2018**, *89*, 341–350. [CrossRef]
15. Wender-Ożegowska, E.; Bomba-Opoń, D.; Brązert, J.; Celewicz, Z.; Czajkowski, K.; Karowicz-Bilińska, A.; Malinowska-Polubiec, A.; Meczekalski, B.; Zawiejska, A.; Polish Gynecological Society. Polish Society of Gynaecologists and Obstetricians Standards: Management of obese patients. *Ginekol. Pol.* **2012**, *83*, 795–799.
16. Johansson, K.; Cnattingius, S.; Näslund, I.; Roos, N.; Lagerros, Y.T.; Granath, F.; Stephansson, O.; Neovius, M. Outcomes of Pregnancy After Bariatric Surgery. *Surv. Anesthesiol.* **2016**, *60*, 62. [CrossRef]
17. Rottenstreich, A.; Elchalal, U.; Kleinstern, G.; Beglaibter, N.; Khalaileh, A.; Elazary, R. Maternal and Perinatal Outcomes After Laparoscopic Sleeve Gastrectomy. *Obstet. Gynecol.* **2018**, *131*, 451–456. [CrossRef]

18. Dolin, C.D.; Chervenak, J.; Pivo, S.; Welcome, A.U.; Kominiarek, M.A. Association between time interval from bariatric surgery to pregnancy and maternal weight outcomes. *J. Matern. Neonatal Med.* **2019**, 1–7. [CrossRef]
19. Aricha-Tamir, B.; Weintraub, A.Y.; Levi, I.; Sheiner, E. Downsizing pregnancy complications: A study of paired pregnancy outcomes before and after bariatric surgery. *Surg. Obes. Relat. Dis.* **2012**, *8*, 434–439. [CrossRef]
20. Kwong, W.; Tomlinson, G.; Feig, D.S. Maternal and neonatal outcomes after bariatric surgery; a systematic review and meta-analysis: Do the benefits outweigh the risks? *Am. J. Obstet. Gynecol.* **2018**, *218*, 573–580. [CrossRef]
21. Galazis, N.; Docheva, N.; Simillis, C.; Nicolaides, K.H. Maternal and neonatal outcomes in women undergoing bariatric surgery: A systematic review and meta-analysis. *Eur. J. Obstet. Gynecol. Reprod. Boil.* **2014**, *181*, 45–53. [CrossRef] [PubMed]
22. Burke, A.E.; Bennett, W.L.; Jamshidi, R.M.; Gilson, M.M.; Clark, J.M.; Segal, J.B.; Shore, A.D.; Magnuson, T.H.; Dominici, F.; Wu, A.W.; et al. Reduced Incidence of Gestational Diabetes with Bariatric Surgery. *J. Am. Coll. Surg.* **2010**, *211*, 169–175. [CrossRef] [PubMed]
23. Chevrot, A.; Kayem, G.; Coupaye, M.; Lesage, N.; Msika, S.; Mandelbrot, L.; Information, P.E.K.F.C. Impact of bariatric surgery on fetal growth restriction: Experience of a perinatal and bariatric surgery center. *Am. J. Obstet. Gynecol.* **2016**, *214*, 655.e1–655.e7. [CrossRef] [PubMed]
24. American College of Obstetricians and Gynecologists. ACOG Practice Bulletin. Clinical Management Guidelines for Obstetrician-Gynecologists. *Obstetrics Gynecol.* **2009**, *113*, 1405–1413.
25. Falcone, V.; Stopp, T.; Feichtinger, M.; Kiss, H.; Eppel, W.; Husslein, P.; Prager, G.; Göbl, C.S. Pregnancy after bariatric surgery: A narrative literature review and discussion of impact on pregnancy management and outcome. *BMC Pregnancy Childbirth* **2018**, *18*, 507. [CrossRef]
26. Kominiarek, M.A. Preparing for and managing a pregnancy after bariatric surgery. *Semin. Perinatol.* **2011**, *35*, 356–361. [CrossRef]
27. Adam, S.; Ammori, B.; Soran, H. Pregnancy after bariatric surgery: Screening for gestational diabetes. *BMJ* **2017**, *356*, j533. [CrossRef]
28. Narayanan, R.P.; Syed, A.A. Pregnancy Following Bariatric Surgery–Medical Complications and Management. *Obes Surg.* **2016**, *26*, 2523–2529. [CrossRef]
29. Rottenstreich, A.; Elazary, R.; Ezra, Y.; Kleinstern, G.; Beglaibter, N.; Elchalal, U. Hypoglycemia during oral glucose tolerance test among post-bariatric surgery pregnant patients: Incidence and perinatal significance. *Surg. Obes. Relat. Dis.* **2018**, *14*, 347–353. [CrossRef]

Journal of
Clinical Medicine

MDPI

Article

Bariatric Surgery during COVID-19 Pandemic from Patients' Point of View—The Results of a National Survey

Maciej Walędziak [1], Anna Różańska-Walędziak [2], Michał Pędziwiatr [3], Jacek Szeliga [4], Monika Proczko-Stepaniak [5], Michał Wysocki [3], Tomasz Stefura [3] and Piotr Major [3,*]

1 Department of General, Oncological, Metabolic and Thoracic Surgery, Military Institute of Medicine, 04-141 Warsaw, Poland; maciej.waledziak@gmail.com
2 2nd Department of Obstetrics and Gynecology, Medical University of Warsaw, 00-315 Warsaw, Poland; aniaroza@tlen.pl
3 2nd Department of General Surgery, Jagiellonian University Medical College, 31-008 Kraków, Poland; mpedziwiatr@googlemail.com (M.P.); m.wysocki@doctoral.uj.edu.pl (M.W.); tomasz.stefura@gmail.com (T.S.)
4 Department of General, Gastroenterological, and Oncological Surgery, Collegium Medicum Nicolaus Copernicus University, 85-067 Torun, Poland; jacky2@wp.pl
5 Department of General, Endocrine and Transplant Surgery, Medical University of Gdansk, 80-210 Gdansk, Poland; monika.proczko-stepaniak@gumed.edu.pl
* Correspondence: piotr.major@uj.edu.pl; Tel.: +48-12-400-26-01

Received: 5 May 2020; Accepted: 29 May 2020; Published: 2 June 2020

Abstract: Introduction: The aim of the study was to investigate the impact of the COVID-19 pandemic on bariatric care from the patients' point of view. The COVID-19 pandemic has perturbed the functioning of healthcare systems around the world and led to changes in elective surgical care, with bariatric procedures being postponed until the end of pandemic. There is no data in the literature about the effect of a new epidemiological situation on bariatric patients. Methods: The study was designed as an online survey containing multiple open questions about bariatric care during the COVID-19 pandemic. The survey was conducted among pre- and postoperative bariatric patients. Results: Out of 800 respondents, 74.53% felt anxiety about their health in regard to the present epidemiologic state. Some (72.25%) were aware of the fact that obesity was an important risk factor that could impair the course of the COVID-19 disease. Almost 30% of respondents admitted having put on weight, significantly more in the group of preoperative patients (43.8% vs. 22.69%; $p < 0.001$). Only 20.92% of patients had a possibility of continuing direct bariatric care; 67.3% of patients had an opportunity of remote contact with a bariatric specialist, including online consultations, teleconsultations and social media meetings. Conclusions: Limited access to medical care and quarantine lockdown may result in a deterioration of long-time operation outcomes and lower weight losses. Patients should be encouraged to profit from online consultations with specialists and telemedicine to reduce the negative effects of the pandemic on their health.

Keywords: bariatric surgery; COVID

1. Introduction

Obesity has reached epidemic proportions worldwide, and all evidence suggests that the situation is likely to get worse [1]. It is estimated that 65% of the adult population in the USA is overweight or obese [2]. Bariatric surgery is a mainstay treatment of obesity [3]. It is essential that patients receive long-term follow-up and monitoring to help them achieve the estimated weight loss, reduction of comorbidities and to prevent long-term problems that may arise following surgery [4].

A new disease appeared in the last quarter of the year 2019, causing a wide range of symptoms, from mild influenza-like illness to severe, life-threatening pneumonia. The infectious agent was found to be severe acute respiratory syndrome coronavirus 2 (SARS-CoV-2). In February 2020, the disease was designated by the World Health Organization (WHO) COVID-19, which stands for Coronavirus Disease 2019. On 11th March 2020, WHO declared COVID-19 a pandemic [5,6]. Until 22th April 2020, more than 2.61 million cases were reported across 185 countries, resulting in more than 182,000 deaths. In the same time, there were more than 10,000 COVID-19 cases reported and 400 people died because of COVID-19 pneumonia, but this data is most likely underestimated.

The new epidemiological situation has perturbed the functioning of healthcare systems around the world and led to changes in elective surgical care. It has not been confirmed yet that there is an increased incidence of COVID-19 pneumonia in obese patients. However, it is known that the process of treatment is less effective in people with comorbidities such as hypertension and diabetes mellitus, which are common in obese patients [7,8]. The International Federation for the Surgery of Obesity and Metabolic Disorders (IFSO) recommended that all elective metabolic and bariatric procedures, both surgical and endoscopic, should be postponed until the end of the pandemic [9]. The delay of operation may affect patients' health in different ways, regardless if in the case of oncological or bariatric patients. While some data have already been gathered on the condition of surgery in a time of pandemic [10–12], there is hardly any data specifically about bariatric surgery and practically none about the effects of the COVID-19 pandemic on bariatric patients' wellbeing.

The aim of the study was to investigate the impact of the COVID-19 pandemic on bariatric care from the patients' point of view.

2. Methods

This study was designed as an online survey with the aim to collect data about bariatric care during the COVID-19 pandemic from patients in the course of qualification for bariatric surgery and patients after bariatric surgery. Survey contains 46 (multiple choice, open and Likert scale) questions. The questionnaire was evaluated and approved of by several independent experts in the field of bariatric surgery. The online survey was published and distributed via social media in cooperation with the Polish bariatric patients' society, which integrates more than 1500 bariatric patients. The survey started on 9th April 2020 and was open until 17th April 2020. It was divided into four chapters: general information about the patient, life during the COVID-19 pandemic, bariatric care during the COVID-19 pandemic and life after the COVID-19 pandemic. Survey is shown in Appendix A. The project was supported by the Metabolic and Bariatric Chapter of Polish Surgeons' Association (SCMiB). The data was completely anonymized and contained no patient identification data.

2.1. Statistical Analysis

Results are presented as means with standard deviation or medians with interquartile range. We performed the statistical analysis using StatSoft Statistica version 6.1 PL (StatSoft Inc., Tulsa, OK, USA). Normality of the data was tested with Shapiro–Wilk test. Continuous variables were compared with the Student's *t*-test for normally distributed or Mann–Whitney U test for non-normally distributed data. Categorical variables were compared using the chi-square or Fisher test. Statistical significance was set at $p < 0.05$.

2.2. Ethical Considerations

The study was anonymous, performed in accordance with the ethical standards laid down in the 1964 Declaration of Helsinki and its latter amendments (Fortaleza). Participants were informed about the aim of the study, and informed consent was obtained electronically prior to the beginning of the survey. The study was approved by the Bioethics Committee of Jagiellonian University (1072.6120.103.2020).

3. Results

3.1. Basic Characteristics of the Patients

There were 800 participants, with the median age 39 (33–45) and body mass index (BMI) 34.26 (29.05–40.81) and mostly female (88%). The basic characteristics of the cases and the incidences of comorbidities are shown in Table 1. IQR: interquartile range. n/a: not applicable.

Table 1. Basic characteristics.

	All	Preoperative Patients	Postoperative Patients	*p*-Value
n (%)	800 (100%)	258 (32%)	542 (68%)	n/a
Median age, years (IQR)	39 (33–45)	37 (32–43)	39 (33–46)	0.005
Males/Females, *n* (%)	97/703 (12%/88%)	33/225 (12%/88%)	64/478 (12%/88%)	0.647
Median BMI, kg/m^2 (IQR)	34.26 (29.05–40.81)	42.24 (38.64–47.75)	31.18 (27.36–35.43)	<0.001
Insulin resistance, *n* (%)	224 (28%)	86 (33.33%)	138 (25.46%)	0.020
Type 2 diabetes mellitus, *n* (%)	93 (11.63%)	31 (12.02%)	62 (11.44%)	0.812
Obstructive sleep apnea, *n* (%)	63 (7.88%)	23 (8.91%)	40 (7.38%)	0.451
Arterial hypertension, *n* (%)	265 (33.13%)	86 (33.33%)	179 (33.03%)	0.931
Dyslipidemia, *n* (%)	68 (8.5%)	27 (10.47%)	41 (7.56%)	0.169
Arthritis/Joint pain, *n* (%)	272 (34%)	106 (41.09%)	166 (30.63%)	0.003

3.2. Life During the COVID-19 Pandemic

Only 6.64% of respondents had contact with patients with confirmed COVID-19 or were staying in quarantine. Some (21.9%) patients were treated in bariatric centers that currently manage COVID-19 patients. The majority (74.53%) of patients felt more anxiety/fear about their health in regard to the present epidemiologic state. Many (72.25%) were aware of the fact that obesity was an important risk factor that could impair the course of COVID-19. More than one-third of patients changed their eating habits during the epidemic, significantly less often after bariatric surgery. More than nine in ten patients did not increase physical activity. Half of patients did not gain weight, but almost 30% of respondents admitted to having put on weight, significantly more in the group of preoperative patients (43.8% vs. 22.69%; $p < 0.001$).

3.3. Bariatric Care During the COVID-19 Pandemic

Only 20.92% of patients had a possibility of continuing direct bariatric care during the COVID-19 pandemic, significantly less often in the group of preoperative patients (10.2% vs. 26.09%; $p < 0.001$). In 172 cases (69.36%), the date of bariatric surgery was postponed due to the COVID-19 pandemic; in 3.63% cases, it was the patient's decision; in 65.73% cases, it was the decision of the bariatric center; in 30.65% cases, the date of the surgery did not change. In the present situation, 50.33% of respondents decided to undergo bariatric surgery in spite of the pandemic, considerably more likely in the preoperative group (67.72% vs. 41.62%; $p < 0.001$). Some (60.67%) patients, both from the preoperative and postoperative groups, had their control visits postponed by the bariatric centers. A number (67.3%) of patients had an opportunity of remote contact with a bariatric specialist, including online consultations, teleconsultations and social media meetings. Regardless of the risk of becoming infected with COVID-19, 42.69% of patients would like to have a visit in a bariatric clinic, for the most part in the preoperative group (57.59% vs. 35.47%; $p < 0.001$). Most patients affirmed the necessity of the continuous support of bariatric surgeons, dietician nutritionists and psychologists. The vast majority of patients accept and are satisfied with teleconsultations as a form of contact with a specialist or qualification for bariatric treatment. More than 60% of patients did not have the possibility of doing diagnostic tests related to bariatric care, and more than 90% had problems with their availability. Almost 20% of patients admitted to having anxiety about health problems that might have resulted from the limited access to bariatric care, mostly in the postoperative group (43.61% vs. 29.07%; $p < 0.001$).

3.4. Life after the COVID-19 Pandemic

An important question that was part of the last chapter of the survey was when the bariatric procedures should be restarted. Preoperative patients compared with postoperative patients significantly more often declared that bariatric procedures should be resumed as soon as the daily number of COVID-19 infections would start to decrease (51.75% vs. 15.9%). Other possible answers were: as soon as the WHO would declare the end of the pandemic (30.74% of the preoperative group vs. 54.93% of the postoperative group), the discharge from the hospital of the last COVID-19 patient (13.23% vs. 14.89%) and after the introduction of a COVID-19 vaccine (4.28% vs. 14.29%).

Some (47.14%) patients recognized the priority in treating patients with cancer before bariatric patients. A number (67.93%) of patients stated that patients whose operations were postponed due to the COVID-19 pandemic should be treated first when the bariatric procedures are resumed. A number (52.80%) of patients accepted the possibility of a requalification for bariatric treatment and repeated diagnostic tests after the pandemic.

The majority of patients still wanted to undergo surgery (88.01%) after the pandemic and did not consider changing their bariatric center (87.59%). Only 2.55% of patients were thinking about changing the type of bariatric procedure planned.

The majority of patients (93.99%) planned to increase their physical activity after the pandemic, more often in the preoperative group (97.29% vs. 92.37%; $p = 0.006$). Some (63.6%) patients considered changing their eating habits after the pandemic, significantly more often in the preoperative group (85.77% vs. 52.79%; $p < 0.001$). Detailed data is presented in Table 2.

Table 2. Results of the questionnaire.

Questions	Answers	All	Preoperative Patients	Postoperative Patients	*p*-Value
Life During the COVID-19 Pandemic					
Have any of your relatives or friends currently contracted COVID-19 or are in quarantine?	Yes	53 (6.64%)	8 (3.1%)	45 (8.33%)	0.021
	No	721 (90.35%)	242 (93.80%)	479 (88.70%)	
	I do not know	24 (3.01%)	8 (3.1%)	16 (2.96%)	
Do you feel more anxiety/fear about your health/life in regards to the current epidemiologic state?	Yes	594 (74.53%)	201 (78.21%)	393 (72.78%)	0.099
Are you aware of the fact that obesity is important risk factor impairing the course of infection of COVID-19?	Yes	578 (72.25%)	195 (75.58%)	383 (70.66%)	0.147
Did you change eating habits due to the epidemy?	Yes	274 (34.29%)	120 (46.51%)	154 (28.47%)	<0.001
Has your physical activity changed due to the limited possibilities of going outside, closing places of recreation and sports facilities?	Yes—increased	63 (7.88%)	22 (8.53%)	41 (7.56%)	0.789
	Yes—decreased	481 (60.13%)	151 (58.53%)	330 (60.89%)	
	No	256 (32%)	85 (32.95%)	171 (31.55%)	
Are you exercising at home by your own?	Yes	582 (72.75%)	173 (67.05%)	409 (75.46%)	0.013
How has the pandemic influenced your body weight?	Increase	236 (29.5%)	113 (43.8%)	123 (22.69%)	<0.001
	Decrease	154 (19.25%)	24 (9.3%)	130 (23.99%)	
	No changes	410 (51.25%)	121 (46.9%)	289 (53.32%)	
Bariatric Care During the COVID-19 Pandemic					
Do you currently have the option of continuing bariatric treatment?	Yes	164 (20.92%)	26 (10.20%)	138 (26.09%)	<0.001
Has the date of bariatric surgery been postponed due to the COVID-19 pandemic?	Yes—my own decision	15 (2.68%)	9 (3.63%)	6 (1.93%)	<0.001
	Yes—decision of the hospital administration	188 (33.63%)	163 (65.73%)	25 (8.04%)	
	No	356 (63.69%)	76 (30.65%)	280 (90.03%)	
In spite of the pandemic and the associated risk of developing COVID-19, would you undergo bariatric surgery in the current situation?	Yes	383 (50.33%)	172 (67.72%)	211 (41.62%)	<0.001
Has the date of the visit to the surgery center been moved due to the COVID-19 pandemic?	Yes—my own decision	45 (6.86%)	14 (5.58%)	31 (7.65%)	<0.001
	Yes—decision of the hospital administration	353 (53.81%)	166 (66.14%)	187 (46.17%)	
	No	258 (39.33%)	71 (28.29%)	187 (46.17%)	

Table 2. *Cont.*

Questions	Answers	All	Preoperative Patients	Postoperative Patients	p-Value
Do you have the opportunity to contact doctors providing bariatric treatment, e.g., online consultations, teleconsultations and social media?	Yes	529 (67.30%)	149 (58.2%)	380 (71.7%)	<0.001
In spite of the pandemic and the associated risk of developing COVID-19, would you visit a bariatric clinic in the current situation?	Yes	336 (42.69%)	148 (57.59%)	188 (35.47%)	<0.001
How do you assess the safety of meetings in a bariatric clinic in terms of the possibility of developing COVID-19?	Median score (IQR)	5 (3-8)	5 (2-7)	6 (4-8)	<0.001
Do you think that remote advice for bariatric patients during a pandemic is needed?	Median score (IQR)	10 (8-10)	10 (8-10)	10 (8-10)	0.216
Do you think that remote advice of bariatric surgeons for bariatric patients during a pandemic is needed?	Median score (IQR)	9 (7-10)	9 (7-10)	9 (7-10)	0.438
Do you think that remote advice of dieticians for bariatric patients during a pandemic is needed?	Median score (IQR)	10 (8-10)	10 (8-10)	10 (8-10)	0.036
Do you think that remote advice of psychologists for bariatric patients during a pandemic is needed?	Median score (IQR)	10 (8-10)	10 (8-10)	10 (8-10)	0.016
Have you used online support groups during a pandemic?	Yes	422 (53.28%)	140 (54.69%)	282 (52.61%)	0.584
I consider the participation of support groups and patient organizations during a pandemic to be:	Median score (IQR)	9 (7-10)	9 (7-10)	8 (6-10)	0.016
Do you accept teleconsultations as a form of treatment or qualification for bariatric treatment?	Median score (IQR)	9 (6-10)	9 (6-10)	10 (6-10)	0.082
How satisfied are you with teleconsultations?	Median score (IQR)	8 (5-10)	8 (5-10)	7 (5-10)	0.018
Do you have the opportunity to perform the tests recommended by the attending physician?	Yes	69 (8.96%)	19 (7.45%)	49 (9.72%)	0.560
	Yes—but limited	232 (30.57%)	81 (31.76%)	151 (29.96%)	
	No	459 (60.47%)	155 (60.78%)	304 (60.32%)	
Has the situation of limited access to bariatric care caused any health problems for you?	Yes	133 (17.05%)	75 (29.07%)	58 (43.61%)	<0.001
	Life after the COVID-19 Pandemic				
After the pandemic, will you still want to undergo surgery?	Yes	499 (88.01%)	258 (100%)	241 (77.99%)	n/a

Table 2. *Cont.*

Questions	Answers	All	Preoperative Patients	Postoperative Patients	p-Value
Do you intend to undergo surgery at the same unit?	Yes	494 (87.59%)	254 (98.45%)	240 (78.43%)	<0.001
Have you changed your decision about the type of surgery after the pandemic?	Yes	20 (2.55%)	3 (1.17%)	17 (5.52%)	0.005
At what point should bariatric procedures resume?	As soon as the daily number of COVID-19 infections start to decrease	212 (28.12%)	133 (51.75%)	79 (15.90%)	<0.001
	After the introduction of a COVID-19 vaccine	82 (10.88%)	11 (4.28%)	71 (14.29%)	
	As soon as the WHO will declare the end of the pandemic	352 (46.68%)	79 (30.74%)	273 (54.93%)	
	After discharge of the last COVID-19 patient from the hospital	108 (14.32%)	34 (13.23%)	74 (14.89%)	
After what time should bariatric procedures be resumed?	After the waiting list for oncologic procedures will be shortened	363 (47.14%)	82 (31.78%)	281 (54.88%)	<0.001
	At the same time of the oncologic procedures	122 (15.84%)	62 (24.03%)	60 (11.72%)	
	Due to a low risk before the oncologic procedures	75 (9.74%)	47 (18.22%)	28 (5.47%)	
	No opinion	210 (27.27%)	67 (25.97%)	143 (27.93%)	
Are you ready to undergo a requalification and examination cycle due to postponed surgery?	Yes	349 (52.80%)	174 (67.44%)	175 (43.42%)	<0.001
	No	86 (13.01%)	54 (20.93%)	32 (7.94%)	
	No opinion	226 (34.19%)	30 (11.63%)	196 (48.64%)	
Do you consider it necessary to postpone the dates of new qualifications and bariatric surgeries in the period after the pandemic ends so that postponed patients due to a pandemic could be treated first?	Yes	494 (67.39%)	168 (65.37%)	326 (68.49%)	<0.001
	No	76 (10.37%)	47 (18.29%)	29 (5.09%)	
	No opinion	163 (22.24%)	42 (16.34%)	121 (25.42%)	
Do you have a plan to increase physical activity after the pandemic?	Yes	735 (93.99%)	251 (97.29%)	484 (92.37%)	0.006
Do you have a plan to change your eating habits after the pandemic?	Yes	491 (63.60%)	217 (85.77%)	274 (52.79%)	<0.001

4. Discussion

Our study based on a national range survey among pre- and postoperative bariatric patients presents the impact of the COVID-19 pandemic on the life of bariatric patients. The novelty of our study was the analysis of the impact of the COVID-19 pandemic on bariatric care from the patients' point of view. The fact of postponing elective bariatric surgery procedures has affected the lives of many patients waiting for the operation. The quarantine lockdown has influenced lifestyles and dietary regimens of pre- and postoperative patients. Although the vast majority of responders did not have contact with COVID-19 infected patients, most patients felt anxious about their health in regards to the present epidemiologic state. The majority of responders were aware of the fact that obesity was an important risk factor that could impair the course of COVID-19 disease. More than two-thirds of preoperative patients had their operation postponed and, more than a half, their control visits. Almost 70% of patients had a possibility of online consultations with a specialist and the use of telemedicine. Most patients before surgery wanted to undergo surgical treatment after the pandemic. Only less than half the patients recognized the priority of treating oncological patients; the others preferred a simultaneous restart of all kinds of surgical procedures. The majority of patients planned on increasing their physical activity and changing eating habits after the pandemic.

The COVID-19 pandemic has a tremendous impact on the daily routine and quality of life of billions of people worldwide. Self-isolation and quarantine lockdown cause additional distress and increase the levels of fear and anxiety [13]. Bariatric patients are in a high-risk group of increased eating psychopathology and trouble in self-management in such a situation of emotional distress. Followed by a reduction of physical activity due to lockdown, possible financial difficulties and trouble with food availability, the pandemic may result in difficulties with optimum weight losses, possible weight gains and the deterioration of long-term outcomes [14].

The importance of a multidisciplinary team in bariatric care has been well-established [15,16]. The success of an operation is mostly determined by postoperative care, and patients must remain in regular contact not only with their bariatric surgeon but, also, dietitian, psychologist and a specialist in internal medicine or endocrinologist [4,17]. Our study showed that the present state of the pandemic is a major obstacle for the patients with maintaining contact and getting help from their bariatric team. As patients have limited access to ambulatory clinics, new ways of communication have had to be quickly developed. Before the era of pandemics, telemedicine was used in our country only in very limited situations, mostly for teleconferences between specialists and the live consulting of test results. Due to the lockdown, it had to develop quickly as the most important tool of present communication between patients, doctors, dietitians and psychologists. Telemedicine and remote consultations are proven to be effective in fighting distress and reducing the level of psychological disorders in bariatric patients [14]. According to the data from the Central Statistical Office from 2019, 86.7% of Polish households had internet access. Therefore, the general majority of patients after bariatric procedures have internet access, and the results of the study should not be influenced by the problem of internet and telemedicine availability [18].

There have been no surveys about COVID-19 conducted among bariatric patients yet, so we can compare our study to only similar studies in other fields, though they are also scarce at this time. Wolf et al. conducted a survey in a group of 630 patients with at least one chronic disease [19]. Only 24.6% patients were "very worried" about getting COVID-19, and 12.95% of patients were "not worried at all". More than half the patients (58.6%) admitted that coronavirus had a high impact on their daily routine, and only 20.8% of respondents felt "very prepared" for the outbreak. The study by Wolf et al. revealed profound gaps in the patients' knowledge and level of concern about the virus. In our study, most patients (more than 74%) were worried about the risk brought by the COVID-19 pandemic. Another survey-based report regarding patients' awareness, attitudes and actions related to COVID-19 was published about people living with HIV in China [20]. The majority of the respondents felt well-informed; they were concerned about specific protective measures, and 64.15% reported difficulties in accessing antiretroviral medicines due to lockdown. Almost 30% of respondents declared a need for sociopsychological support. There also was a report published basing on a survey among Indian ophthalmologists regarding the effects of the pandemic on their practice and patient care, 77.5% of whom decided to use different forms of telemedicine [21].

Limitations of the Study

The possible limitations of our study can be the recall bias and the subjectivity of patients' opinions. Another limitation was that the survey was conducted only among Polish bariatric patients who were able to fill it out by means of the internet. All respondents were voluntary members of the bariatric patient support group, which introduced them to the purpose and methodology of the study. Moreover, there was no incentive to introduce dishonesty into the responses. However, direct control of the respondents was currently not possible due to the ongoing pandemic, and it is unfortunately a limitation of the study. Additionally, in order to obtain the highest possible number of responders in a considerably short period of time, we decided to post the questionnaire on the Polish bariatric patients' society website, and we were not able to calculate the response rate.

5. Conclusions

The COVID-19 pandemic affected the functioning of Polish bariatric surgery, as elective procedures were postponed until the end of the pandemic. Patients have problems with access to bariatric surgeons, dieticians, nutritionists and psychologists, who together form teams taking care of bariatric patients. Limited access to medical care and quarantine lockdown may result in patients' bad eating habits, lack of physical exercise and psychological distress and lead to the deterioration of long-time operation outcomes and lower weight losses. Patients should be encouraged to profit from online consultations with specialists and telemedicine to reduce the negative effects of the pandemic on their health.

Author Contributions: Conceptualization, M.W., A.R.-W., M.P., J.S., M.P.-S., M.W., T.S. and P.M.; data curation, M.W. and P.M.; investigation, M.W.; methodology, M.W. and A.R.-W.; validation, M.P.; writing—original draft, M.W., A.R.-W. and P.M. and writing—review and editing, M.W., A.R.-W. and P.M. All authors have read and agreed to the published version of the manuscript.

Funding: The publication was funded by subvention of the Ministry of Science and Higher Education of Poland.

Conflicts of Interest: The authors declare no conflicts of interest.

Appendix A. Questionnaire for Bariatric Patients

Questions	Answers
Basic Characteristics	
Age	(Number)
Sex	Male/Female
Weight	(Number)
Height	(Number)
Co-morbidities	Insulin resistance
	Type 2 diabetes mellitus
	Obstructive sleep apnea
	Arterial hypertension
	Dyslipidemia
	Arthritis/Joint pain
What is your bariatric status	Pre-operative
	Post-operative

Life During COVID-19 Pandemic	
Do any of your relatives or friends is currently contracted with COVID-19 or in quarantine?	Yes
	No
	I do not know
Do you feel more anxiety/fear about your health/life in regards to current epidemiologic state?	Yes
	No
Are you aware of the fact that obesity is important risk factor impairing the course of infection of COVID-19?	Yes
	No
Did you changed eating habits due to the epidemy?	Yes
	No
Has your physical activity changed due to the limited possibilities of going outside, closing places of recreation and sports facilities?	Yes—increased
	Yes—decreased
	No
Are you exercising at home by your own?	Yes
	No
How the pandemic influenced your body weight?	Increase
	Decrease
	No changes
Bariatric Care During COVID-19 Pandemic	
Do you currently have the option of continuing bariatric treatment?	Yes
	No
Has the date of bariatric surgery been postponed due to the COVID-19 pandemic?	Yes—my own decision
	Yes—decision of the hospital administration
	No
In spite of the pandemic and the associated risk of developing COVID-19, would you undergo bariatric surgery in the current situation?	Yes
	No
Has the date of the visit to the surgery center been moved due to the COVID-19 pandemic?	Yes—my own decision
	Yes—decision of the hospital administration
	No
Do you have the opportunity to contact doctors providing bariatric treatment, e.g., online consultations, tele-consultations, social media?	Yes
	No
In spite of the pandemic and the associated risk of developing COVID-19, would you visit a Bariatric Clinic in the current situation?	Yes
	No
How do you assess the safety of meetings in the Bariatric Clinic in terms of the possibility of developing COVID-19?	From 1 to 10
Do you think that remote advice for bariatric patients during a pandemic is needed?	From 1 to 10
Do you think that remote advice of bariatric surgeon for bariatric patients during a pandemic is needed?	From 1 to 10
Do you think that remote advice of dietician for bariatric patients during a pandemic is needed?	From 1 to 10
Do you think that remote advice of psychologist for bariatric patients during a pandemic is needed?	From 1 to 10
Have you used online support groups during a pandemic?	Yes
	No

I consider the participation of support groups and patient organizations during a pandemic to be:	From 1 to 10
Do you accept tele-consultations as a form of treatment or qualification for bariatric treatment?	From 1 to 10
How satisfied are you with tele-consultations?	From 1 to 10
Do you have the opportunity to perform the tests recommended by the attending physician?	Yes
	Yes—but limited
	No
Has the situation of limited access to bariatric care caused any health problems to you?	Yes
	No
Life after COVID-19 Pandemic	
After the pandemic, will you still want to undergo surgery?	Yes
	No
Do you intend to undergo surgery in the same unit?	Yes
	No
Have you changed your decision about the type of surgery after the pandemic?	Yes
	No
At what point should bariatric procedures resume?	As soon as daily number of COVID-19 infections start to decrease
	After introduction of COVID-19 vaccine
	As soon as WHO will declare end of pandemic
	After discharge of the last COVID-19 patient from hospital
After what time should bariatric procedures be resumed?	After the waiting list for oncologic procedures will be shortened
	At the same time of oncologic procedures
	Due to low risk before oncologic procedures
	No opinion
Are you ready to undergo a re-qualification and examination cycle due to postponed surgery?	Yes
	No
	No opinion
Do you consider it necessary to postpone the dates of new qualifications and bariatric surgeries in the period after the pandemic ends so that postponed patients due to a pandemic could be treated first?	Yes
	No
	No opinion
Do you have a plan to increase physical activity after the pandemic?	Yes
	No
Do you have a plan to change your eating habits after the pandemic?	Yes
	No

References

1. World Health Organization. *International Obesity Task Force. The Asian-Pacific Perspective: Redefining Obesity and Its Treatment*; WHO Western Pacific Region: Geneva, Switzerland, 2000.
2. Flegal, K.M.; Carroll, M.D.; Ogden, C.L.; Johnson, C.L. Prevalence and Trends in Obesity Among US Adults, 1999–2000. *JAMA* **2002**, *288*, 1723–1727. [CrossRef] [PubMed]
3. Gloy, V.L.; Briel, M.; Bhatt, D.L.; Kashyap, S.R.; Schauer, P.R.; Mingrone, G.; Bucher, H.C.; Nordmann, A.J. Bariatric surgery versus non-surgical treatment for obesity: A systematic review and meta-analysis of randomised controlled trials. *BMJ* **2013**, *347*, f5934. [CrossRef] [PubMed]

4. O'Kane, M.; Parretti, H.M.; Hughes, C.A.; Sharma, M.; Woodcock, S.; Puplampu, T.; Blakemore, A.I.; Clare, K.; MacMillan, I.; Joyce, J.; et al. Guidelines for the follow-up of patients undergoing bariatric surgery. *Clin. Obes.* **2016**, *6*, 210–224. [CrossRef] [PubMed]
5. World Health Organization. Director-General's Remarks at the Media Briefing on 2019-nCoV on 11 February 2020. Available online: https://www.who.int/dg/speeches/detail/who-director-general-s-remarks-at-the-media-briefing-on-2019-ncov-on-11-february-2020 (accessed on 20 April 2020).
6. WHO Director-General's Opening Remarks at the Media Briefing on COVID-19—11 March 2020. Available online: https://www.who.int/dg/speeches/detail/who-director-general-s-opening-remarks-at-the-media-briefing-on-covid-19---11-march-2020 (accessed on 20 April 2020).
7. Yang, J.; Zheng, Y.; Gou, X.; Pu, K.; Chen, Z.; Guo, Q.; Ji, R.; Wang, H.; Wang, Y.; Zhou, Y. Prevalence of comorbidities in the novel Wuhan coronavirus (COVID-19) infection: A systematic review and meta-analysis. *Int. J. Infect. Dis.* **2020**, *94*, 91–95. [CrossRef] [PubMed]
8. Emami, A.; Javanmardi, F.; Pirbonyeh, N.; Akbari, A. Prevalence of Underlying Diseases in Hospitalized Patients with COVID-19: A Systematic Review and Meta-Analysis. *Arch. Acad. Emerg. Med.* **2020**, *8*, e35. [PubMed]
9. Yang, W.; Wang, C.; Shikora, S.; Kow, L. Recommendations for Metabolic and Bariatric Surgery During the COVID-19 Pandemic from IFSO. *Obes. Surg.* **2020**, 1–3. [CrossRef] [PubMed]
10. Liu, Z.; Zhang, Y.; Wang, X.; Zhang, D.; Diao, D.; Chandramohan, K.; Booth, C.M. Recommendations for Surgery During the Novel Coronavirus (COVID-19) Epidemic. *Indian J Surg.* **2020**, 1–5. [CrossRef] [PubMed]
11. Correia, M.I.T.D.; Ramos, R.F.; Bahten, L.C.V. The surgeons and the COVID-19 pandemic. Os cirurgiões e a pandemia do COVID-19. *Revista Colégio Brasileiro Cirurgiões* **2020**, *47*, e20202536. [CrossRef] [PubMed]
12. Diaz, A.; Sarac, B.A.; Schoenbrunner, A.R.; Janis, J.E.; Pawlik, T.M. Elective surgery in the time of COVID-19. *Am. J. Surg.* **2020**. [CrossRef]
13. Montemurro, N. The emotional impact of COVID-19: From medical staff to common people. *Brain Behav. Immun.* **2020**. [CrossRef] [PubMed]
14. Sockalingam, S.; Leung, S.E.; Cassin, S.E. The Impact of COVID-19 on Bariatric Surgery: Re-Defining Psychosocial Care. *Obesity* **2020**. [CrossRef]
15. Mechanick, J.I.; Apovian, C.; Brethauer, S.; Garvey, W.T.; Joffe, A.M.; Kim, J.; Kushner, R.F.; Lindquist, R.; Pessah-Pollack, R.; Seger, J.; et al. Clinical practice guidelines for the perioperative nutrition, metabolic, and nonsurgical support of patients undergoing bariatric procedures—2019 update: Cosponsored by American association of clinical endocrinologists/American college of endocrinology, the obesity society, American society for metabolic & bariatric surgery, obesity medicine association, and American society of anesthesiologists. *Surg. Obes. Relat. Dis.* **2019**, *25*, 1346–1359. [CrossRef]
16. Li, Z.J.; Yu, J.C. Multidisciplinary Team and Nutrition Management for Bariatric Surgery. *Zhongguo yi xue ke xue yuan xue bao. Acta Academiae Medicinae Sinicae* **2018**, *40*, 577–580. [CrossRef] [PubMed]
17. Verkindt, H.; Verhelst, C.; Skorupinski, J. Le chemin clinique du patient obèse sévère candidat à une chirurgie bariatrique [Bariatric surgery: The clinical pathway of the patient with a severe obesity surgery]. *Presse Med.* **2018**, *47*, 439–443. [CrossRef] [PubMed]
18. Central Statistical Office. Polish Informative Society in 2019. Available online: https://stat.gov.pl/obszary-tematyczne/nauka-i-technika-spoleczenstwo-informacyjne/spoleczenstwo-informacyjne/spoleczenstwo-informacyjne-w-polsce-w-2019-roku,2,9.html (accessed on 26 May 2020).
19. Wolf, M.S.; Serper, M.; Opsasnick, L.; O'Conor, R.M.; Curtis, L.M.; Benavente, J.Y.; Wismer, G.; Batio, S.; Eifler, M.; Zheng, P.; et al. Awareness, attitudes and actions related to COVID-19 among adults with chronic conditions at the onset of the U.S. outbreak. *Ann Intern Med.* **2020**. [CrossRef] [PubMed]
20. Guo, W.; Weng, H.L.; Bai, H.; Liu, J.; Wei, X.N.; Zhou, K.; Sande, A. Quick community survey on the impact of COVID-19 outbreak for the healthcare of people living with HIV. *Zhonghua liu Xing Bing xue za zhi Zhonghua Liuxingbingxue Zazhi* **2020**, *41*, 663–667. [CrossRef]
21. Nair, A.G.; Gandhi, R.A.; Natarajan, S. Effect of COVID-19 related lockdown on ophthalmic practice and patient care in India: Results of a survey. *Indian J. Ophthalmol.* **2020**, *68*, 725–730. [CrossRef] [PubMed]

Journal of
Clinical Medicine

MDPI

Article

Long-Term Effects in Bone Mineral Density after Different Bariatric Procedures in Patients with Type 2 Diabetes: Outcomes of a Randomized Clinical Trial

Fernando Guerrero-Pérez [1], Anna Casajoana [2], Carmen Gómez-Vaquero [3], Nuria Virgili [1], Rafael López-Urdiales [1], Laura Hernández-Montoliu [1], Jordi Pujol-Gebelli [2], Javier Osorio [2], Anna Prats [4], Anna Vidal-Alabró [5], Manuel Pérez-Maraver [1,5,6], Sonia Fernández-Veledo [6,7], Joan Vendrell [6,7] and Nuria Vilarrasa [1,6,*]

1 Department of Endocrinology and Nutrition, Bellvitge University Hospital-IDIBELL, L'Hospitalet de Llobregat, 08907 Barcelona, Spain; fguerrerop@bellvitgehospital.cat (F.G.-P.); mvirgili@bellvitgehospital.cat (N.V.); rafaellopez@bellvitgehospital.cat (R.L.-U.); laura.hermont@gmail.com (L.H.-M.); mmperez@bellvitgehospital.cat (M.P.-M.)
2 Bariatric Surgery Unit, Bellvitge University Hospital-IDIBELL, L'Hospitalet de Llobregat, 08907 Barcelona, Spain; acbadia@bellvitgehospital.cat (A.C.); jpujol@bellvitgehospital.cat (J.P.-G.); josorio@bellvitgehospital.cat (J.O.)
3 Department of Rheumatology, Bellvitge University Hospital-IDIBELL, L'Hospitalet de Llobregat, 08907 Barcelona, Spain; cgomezvaq@ambitcp.catsalut.net
4 Clinical Nutrition Unit, Bellvitge University Hospital-IDIBELL, L'Hospitalet de Llobregat, 08907 Barcelona, Spain; apratsf@bellvitgehospital.cat
5 Instituto de Investigación Biomédica-IDIBELL, L'Hospitalet de Llobregat, 08907 Barcelona, Spain; avidala@idibell.cat
6 CIBERDEM-CIBER de Diabetes y Enfermedades Metabólicas Asociadas, Instituto de Salud Carlos III, 28014 Madrid, Spain; sonia.fernandezveledo@gmail.com (S.F.-V.); jvortega2002@gmail.com (J.V.)
7 Pere Virgili Research Institute (IISPV), University Hospital Joan XXIII, 43005and Rovira i Virgili University, 43003 Tarragona, Spain
* Correspondence: nuriavilarrasa@yahoo.es; Tel.: +34-932-602-784

Received: 8 May 2020; Accepted: 8 June 2020; Published: 11 June 2020

Abstract: There is scant evidence of the long-term effects of bariatric surgery on bone mineral density (BMD). We compared BMD changes in patients with severe obesity and type 2 diabetes (T2D) 5 years after randomization to metabolic gastric bypass (mRYGB), sleeve gastrectomy (SG) and greater curvature plication (GCP). We studied the influence of first year gastrointestinal hormone changes on final bone outcomes. Forty-five patients, averaging 49.4 (7.8) years old and body mass index (BMI) 39.4 (1.9) kg/m^2, were included. BMD at lumbar spine (LS) was lower after mRYGB compared to SG and GCP: 0.89 [0.82;0.94] vs. 1.04 [0.91;1.16] vs. 0.99 [0.89;1.12], $p = 0.020$. A higher percentage of LS osteopenia was present after mRYGB 78.6% vs. 33.3% vs. 50.0%, respectively. BMD reduction was greater in T2D remitters vs. non-remitters. Weight at fifth year predicted BMD changes at the femoral neck (FN) (adjusted R^2: 0.3218; $p = 0.002$), and type of surgery (mRYGB) and menopause predicted BMD changes at LS (adjusted R^2: 0.2507; $p < 0.015$). In conclusion, mRYGB produces higher deleterious effects on bone at LS compared to SG and GCP in the long-term. Women in menopause undergoing mRYGB are at highest risk of bone deterioration. Gastrointestinal hormone changes after surgery do not play a major role in BMD outcomes.

Keywords: bone mineral density; bariatric surgery; gastrointestinal hormones

---

1. Introduction

Bariatric surgery has become an increasingly common treatment for severe obesity due to its outstanding results in long-term weight loss and sustained improvement in obesity-related comorbidities, mortality and quality of life [1,2]. However, there is arising evidence of negative effects on bone health and risk of bone fractures at long-term in patients with surgically induced weight loss [3–5]. Patients with obesity and type 2 diabetes (T2D), before undergoing bariatric surgery, could have an increased risk of bone fracture. Contrary to what was believed, although obese individuals usually have higher bone mineral density (BMD) compared to non-obese individuals [6,7], obesity per se is not protective and there is a site- and gender-specific relationship between body mass index (BMI) and fracture risk [8–11]. On the other hand, individuals with T2D have normal or higher BMD in comparison with those without diabetes [12,13], but their bone quality is diminished and their risk of fracture is also increased [14]. Hence, patients with obesity and T2D whom undergo bariatric surgery meet many potentially deleterious factors on bone health that should be taken into consideration.

The negative skeletal effects of bariatric surgery are multifactorial and probably procedure-specific [15]. Several mechanisms seem to be involved in postoperative bone loss, including mechanical unloading induced by weight reduction and nutrient deficiencies, such as protein, calcium, vitamin D and the subsequent secondary hyperparathyroidism [15,16]. Furthermore, gastrointestinal hormonal changes caused by anatomical shift and weight loss could affect bone health [16,17]. Data coming from animal models [18–20] and a few human studies [21,22] have shown a relationship between changes in gastric inhibitory polypeptide (GIP), ghrelin, glucagon-like peptide-1 (GLP-1) or peptide YY (PYY) and changes in bone remodeling markers. Other factors like adipokines (leptin, adiponectin), muscle mass loss and bone marrow fat could be implicated [23–26]. All these modifications and their impact on bone might vary between different surgical procedures and are probably more pronounced after malabsorptive or, more accurately named, hypoabsortive techniques [15,17,27]. Some studies have compared BMD outcomes after different surgical procedures, although most of them in a non-randomized manner and at short-term (1–3 years of follow-up) [21,24,28–32].

Our aim in the present study was to compare BMD changes in patients with obesity and T2D, 5 years after being randomized to: metabolic gastric bypass (mRYGB), sleeve gastrectomy (SG), and greater curvature plication (GCP) in the setting of a randomized controlled trial (RCT). We have also analyzed the relationship between changes in gastrointestinal hormones during the first year after surgery with 5 years skeletal outcome.

2. Materials and Methods

This research was part of a prospective, single center and non-blinded RCT, including patients with T2D and obesity. Participants were consecutively recruited from a morbid obesity outpatient clinic. Inclusion criteria were as follows: age between 18 and 60 years, BMI 35–43 kg/m^2, T2D on hypoglycemic agents alone, insulin or both. Exclusion criteria were type 1 diabetes or positivity for GAD autoantibodies, secondary forms of diabetes, acute metabolic complications, liver disease, renal dysfunction or patients under anticoagulant treatment, previous bariatric surgery, congenital or acquired abnormalities of the digestive tract, pregnancy, nursing or desired pregnancy in the 12 months following inclusion, and corticoid use by the oral or intravenous route for more than 14 consecutive days in the last three months.

The study protocol was previously published [33]. We used Buse criteria to define T2D remission at 5 year of follow-up [34]. There were no changes to methods after the commencement of the study. The study was carried out according to the principles of the Declaration of Helsinki, and all patients signed an informed consent. This manuscript has been approved for its publication by the Research Ethics Committee of our institution (reference PR144/20). The trial was registered at www.controlledtrials.com as ISRCTN14104758.

2.1. Randomization

The randomization process was performed by the statistic department using a computer software program that generated the random sequence. The allocation of patients was assigned by simple randomization 1:1:1 to undergo mRYGB, SG or GCP, using opaque sealed sequentially numbered envelopes with stratification according to baseline levels of HbA1c (greater or lower/equal to 7%). After signing informed consent, patients were allocated to a specific surgery. The study was therefore not blinded and the patients, endocrinologist and surgeon were informed about the type of surgery procedure the patient had been allocated to. After surgical intervention, a multivitamin pill once daily and calcium/vitamin D (1000 mg/800 IU) was prescribed in all participants. In addition, patients undergoing mRYGB received 16.000 IU of vitamin D every 15 days. All patients were managed by the same endocrinologist and two dietitians. They were given the same diet, physical activity and behavioral counseling during the follow-up.

2.2. Anthropometric Parameters

Weight change after surgery was referred to as total weight loss percentage (TWL%). Body composition (fat and lean mass) (Kg), whole body bone mineral content (BMC) (g) and BMD (g/cm^2) at lumbar spine (LS) L2-L4 and femoral neck (FN) were measured by DXA (Hologic QDR 4500; Hologic Inc., Waltham, MA, USA) before and 5 years after surgery. World Health Organization (WHO) criteria were used to defined osteoporosis (T-score below −2.5) and osteopenia (T-score between −1.0 and −2.5) [35]. Trabecular bone score (TBS) was calculated using LS DXA scans. As proposed by manufacturers MedImaps [36], we evaluated TBS in patients with BMI between 15 and 35 kg/m^2. TBS $\geq$ 1.350 was considered normal; TBS between 1.200 and 1.350 as partially degraded and TBS $\leq$ 1.200 was defined as degraded [36]. The Spanish classic fracture risk assessment system (FRAX®) (Centre for Metabolic Bone Diseases, University of Sheffield, UK) corrected by TBS was used to evaluate the 10-year probability of hip fracture and major osteoporotic fractures [37,38]. High risk of major osteoporotic fractures was calculated including BMD and defined as a probability ≥7.5% or ≥5% and osteoporosis [39].

2.3. Standard Meal Test

A standard meal test (SMT) was performed before and 1 and 12 months after bariatric surgery. The SMT consisted of 200 mL of a liquid meal (Edanec®, NACE, Paris, France). Blood was drawn immediately before and 15, 30, 60 and 120 min following the SMT for GLP-1 and insulin determination. Fasting ghrelin, PYY and glucagon levels were measured before the SMT.

2.4. Laboratory Determinations

Phospho-calcium metabolism was determined before and 1 and 5 years after bariatric intervention. Glucose, calcium, phosphorus and alkaline phosphatase were determined using standard enzymatic methods. 25-hydroxyvitamin D (25(OH)D_3) concentrations were determined using a radioimmunoassay (DiaSorin, Stillwater, MN, USA). Intact serum parathyroid hormone (PTH) was measured by a two-site immunoradiometric assay (Diagnostic System Laboratories, Webster, TX, USA). Plasma insulin was analyzed by immunoassay (Coat-A-Count Insulin, Diagnostic Products Corp., Los Angeles, CA, USA). GLP-1 was measured by radioimmunoassay (Millipore, Saint Charles, MO, USA) and plasma ghrelin by enzyme immunoassay (CUSABIO biotech, Wuhan, China). Glucagon and PYY were measured by enzyme immunoassay (Yanahaira Institute Inc., Awakura, Fujinomiya-shi Shizuoka, Japan).

2.5. Surgical Procedures

mRYGB combines both restriction (a small gastric pouch) and malabsorption (a 200 cm biliopancreatic limb with an alimentary limb of 100 cm). SG is a restrictive technique with a

75–80% of gastric volume reduction (stomach resection beginning 4 cm from the pylorus and ending at the angle of His). GCP is a restrictive and reversible procedure in which an invagination of the greater gastric curvature is performed instead of gastric resection.

2.6. Statistical Analysis

Based on preliminary data, the study design and sample size was calculated to detect a 20% difference in GLP-1 secretion (measured by the area under the curve (AUC) after (SMT) before and 1 year after bariatric surgery, with a power of 80% and α risk of 0.05 [33]. The primary outcome of the study was the predictive value of gut hormone dynamics (GLP-1, glucagon, PYY and ghrelin) on glucose metabolism improvement at 1 and 12 months after surgery for each procedure. A secondary outcome was the comparison of changes in BMD at 1 and 5 years between surgical techniques and their relationship with gastrointestinal hormones. There were no changes to trial outcomes after commencement of the study. Normally distributed variables were expressed as the mean (standard deviation) and non-normally distributed variables were expressed as the median (first and third quartile). Categorical variables were compared using Chi-square test and quantitative variables using ANOVA test for normally distributed variables and Kruskal–Wallis test was applied for non-normally distributed variables. GLP-1 area under the curve (AUC) was calculated by the trapezoidal method [40]. Two-way ANOVA with repeated measures was performed to analyze BMD changes throughout the observation period. Bivariate (Pearson or Spearman) and multivariate linear regression analyses and a mixed model were employed to determine associated and predicting factors of BMD decrease after bariatric surgery. Relevant clinical variables previously associated were included in the model (type of surgery, changes in weight, gastrointestinal hormones concentrations, phospho-calcium metabolism, metabolic parameters and the presence of T2D remission). Statistical analysis was performed using R software version 3.4.0 (R Foundation for Statistical Computing, Vienna, Austria). A p-value < 0.05 was considered statistically significant.

3. Results

Forty-five morbidly obese patients with T2D, aged 49.4 (7.8) years, BMI 39.4 (1.9) kg/m^2, initial HbA$_{1c}$ 7.7 (1.9) %, were consecutively randomized to mRYGB (n = 15), SG (n = 15), or GCP (n = 15) from May 2012 to February 2014. Follow up compliance was 97.78% (n = 44) at year 1 and 86.6% (n = 39) at year 5. Therefore, the 5-year evaluation was performed in patients undergoing mRYGB (n = 14), SG (n = 12) and GCP (n = 13); the rest of participants refused the BMD evaluation for personal reasons. Sixty-six percent of patients were women equally distributed between groups and menopause was present in 62% of those undergoing mRYGB, 60% in SG, and 75% in GCP, p = 0.704. Initial clinical, biochemical, and body composition characteristics were comparable between groups, except BMI, which was higher in GCP (Table 1). One-year outcomes and procedure complications, stratified according to the Clavien-Dindo classification, were previously described [33]. As a summary of earlier published data [27,33], at year one, TWL% was significantly greater in the mRYGB group compared to SG and GCP. At the end of the study, TWL% in the mRYGB group was −27.32 (7.87) vs. −18.00 (10.6) and −14.83 (7.84) in SG and GCP, respectively, p = 0.001. Regarding metabolic outcomes, at 5 year follow up, complete T2D remission was observed in 46.7% of patients undergoing mRYGB vs. 20.0% after SG and 6.6% after GCP, $p < 0.001$. Changes in biochemical parameters and body composition are shown in Table 2. Of note, mRYGB showed a better metabolic improvement and higher weight loss at an expense of fat mass. Serum calcium, phosphate and vitamin D levels were within normal concentrations and similar in all groups at the end of the study. PTH concentrations were slightly higher after mRYGB, but without reaching statistical significance (Table 2).

Table 1. Patient's baseline characteristics.

Parameter	Metabolic Gastric Bypass	Sleeve Gastrectomy	Greater Curvature Plication	p
Sex (male/female)	7/8	5/10	3/12	0.301
Age (years)	51.1 (7.70)	49.2 (9.16)	49.7 (8.12)	0.827
Weight (kg)	103.01 (10.8)	102.30 (10.7)	105.53 (11.8)	0.301
BMI (kg/m^2)	38.73 (2.01)	39.02 (1.68)	40.90 (1.44)	0.004 *
HbA$_{1c}$ (%)	7.39 (1.95)	7.89 (1.71)	8.05 (2.15)	0.498
Calcium (mmol/L)	2.35 (0.12)	2.37 (0.12)	2.6 (0.12)	0.978
Phosphate (mmol/L)	1.06 (0.16)	1.09 (0.18)	1.08 (0.15)	0.856
PTH (pmol/L)	4.75 (4.46)	3.66 (1.58)	5.05 (4.45)	0.803
Vitamin D (nmol/L)	54.99 (21.35)	52.67 (29.78)	52.78 (25.97	0.606
Fat Mass (kg)	36.53 (8.09)	34.22 (5.57)	35.01 (12.27)	0.414
Lean Mass (kg)	57.39 (10.80)	53.78 (8.29)	50.82 (17.33)	0.670
FNBMD	0.89 [0.84;0.96]	0.90 [0.81;0.96]	0.95 [0.84;1.07]	0.344
FN T-score	−0.05 [−0.50;0.40]	0.08 [−0.40;0.50]	0.85 [−0.25;1.55]	0.077
FN Z-score	0.81 [0.48;1.37]	0.96 [0.10;1.60]	1.54 [0.73;2.00]	0.134
LSBMD	1.03 [0.98;1.09]	1.11 [1.04;1.21]	1.08 [0.99;1.14]	0.255
LS T-score	−0.59 [−1.15;0.05]	0.28 [−0.40;1.10]	0.09 [−0.45;0.50]	0.082
LS Z-score	0.01 [−0.50;0.50]	0.79 [0.10;1.80]	0.62 [−0.05;1.03]	0.239

Data are expressed as mean (standard deviation) for normal distributed variables and median (first and third quartiles) for non-normal distributed variables. BMD, bone mineral density; BMI, body mass index; FN, femoral neck; HbA$_{1c}$, glycated hemoglobin, LS, lumbar spine; p, statistical significance; PTH, parathyroid hormone; *, $p < 0.05$ was considered statistically significant.

Table 2. Patient's characteristics 5 years after bariatric surgery.

Parameter	Metabolic Gastric Bypass	Sleeve Gastrectomy	Greater Curvature Plication	p
Sex (male/female)	6/8	4/8	3/10	0.552
Age (years)	55.2 (7.40)	55.2 (8.30)	53.6 (8.54)	0.700
Weight (kg)	74.7 (9.97)	84.4 (17.0)	89.2 (11.7)	0.014 *
BMI (kg/m^2)	28.1(2.99)	32.0 (4.56)	34.7 (3.68)	<0.001 *
HbA$_{1c}$ (%)	5.43 (0.69)	6.97 (1.32)	7.07 (1.66)	0.002 *
Calcium (mmol/L)	2.32 (0.10)	2.38 (0.10)	2.38 (0.10)	0.221
Phosphate (mmol/L)	1.13 (0.21)	1.08 (0.22)	1.08 (0.15)	0.722
PTH (pmol/L)	8.39 (3.50)	5.66 (2.19)	6.73 (2.63)	0.059
Vitamin D (nmol/L)	61.9 (46.7)	65.3 (33.6)	73.4 (52.3)	0.801
Fat Mass (kg)	31.2 (6.37)	40.0 (8.82)	41.9 (6.86)	0.001 *
Lean Mass (kg)	39.4 (6.74)	43.4 (8.91)	43.1 (7.98)	0.352
FNBMD	0.77 [0.72;0.82]	0.83 [0.78;0.92]	0.85 [0.74;0.98]	0.259
FN T-score	−1.08 [−1.68;−0.80]	−0.50 [−0.92;0.23]	−0.40 [−1.07;0.38]	0.186
FN Z-score	−0.08 [−0.40;0.20]	0.60 [−0.05;1.15]	0.78 [0.00;1.40]	0.081
LSBMD	0.89 [0.82;0.94]	1.04 [0.91;1.16]	0.99 [0.89;1.12]	0.020 *
LS T-score	−1.55 [−2.05;−1.20]	−0.04 [−1.12;1.21]	−0.83 [−1.68;0.23]	0.011 *
LS Z-score	−0.82 [−1.30;−0.40]	0.93 [0.15;1.83]	0.34 [−0.80;1.40]	0.004 *

Data are expressed as mean (standard deviation) for normal distributed variables and median [first and third quartiles]) for non-normal distributed variables. BMD, bone mineral density; BMI, body mass index; FN, femoral neck; HbA$_{1c}$, glycated hemoglobin, LS, lumbar spine; p, statistical significance; PTH, parathyroid hormone; *, $p < 0.05$ was considered statistically significant.

3.1. Changes in BMD after Bariatric Surgery

From baseline to year one, a similar reduction in the FNBMD percentage was observed after mRYGB compared to SG and GCP: −10.34 (6.05) vs. −5.30 (6.17) vs. −6.69 (5.68), $p = 0.118$. However, a greater decrease at LS BMD percentage was detected after mRYGB compared to SG and GCP: −7.29 (4.6) vs. −0.48 (3.9) vs. −1.2 (2.7), $p < 0.001$). The overall percentage descent from baseline to year five at the FN was −12.10 (11) vs. −4.19 (10) vs. −7.0 (7.96), $p = 0.159$ (Figure 1) and at LS: −11.64 (15.0) vs. −3.87 (7.91) vs. −4.34 (4.07), $p = 0.158$ (Figure 2). Thus, BMD at LS was significantly lower at

5 years after mRYGB (Table 2). We performed a two-way ANOVA analysis with repeated measures. At FN, no differences were observed between surgical techniques. Only after mRYGB, we observed effect of time that was significant between baseline and one year ($p < 0.001$), but not between one to 5 years, indicating that changes at this site took place during the first year after mRYGB. Regarding LS, the mixed model found significant differences in mRYGB compared to SG and GCP; and only after mRYGB was the effect of time significant in each observation period, $p < 0.001$, indicating an ongoing process along the 5 year follow-up.

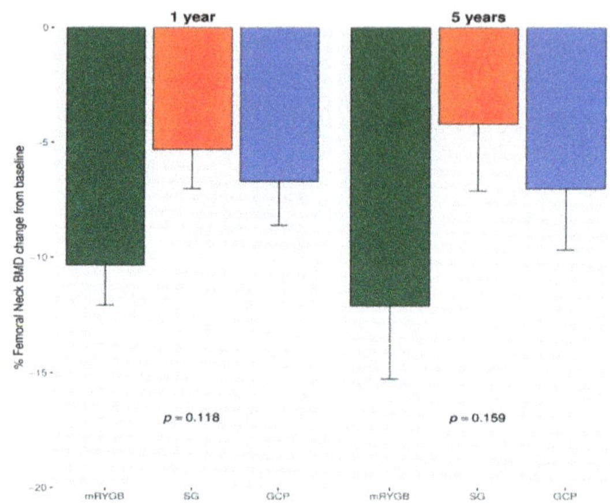

Figure 1. Percentage femoral neck BMD change at year 1 and 5 from baseline. BMD, bone mineral density; mRYGB, metabolic gastric bypass; SG, sleeve gastrectomy; GCP, greater curvature plication. p value result from comparing mRYGB with SG and GCP.

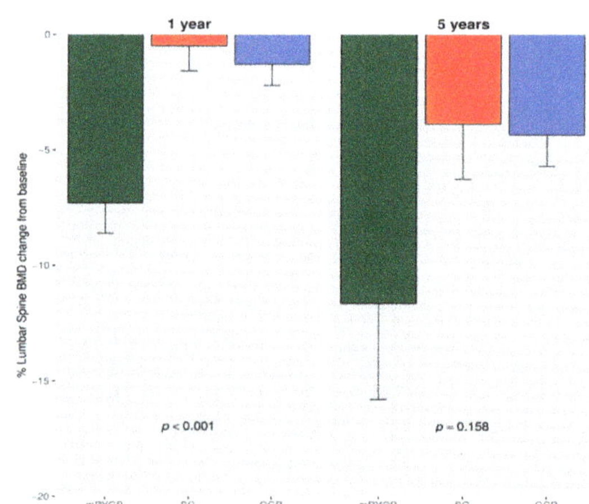

Figure 2. Percentage lumbar spine BMD change at year 1 and 5 from baseline. mRYGB, metabolic gastric bypass; SG, sleeve gastrectomy; GCP, greater curvature plication. p-value result from comparing mRYGB with SG and GCP.

At the end of the study, FN osteopenia was present in 50.0% ($n = 7$) after mRYGB, 25.0% ($n = 3$) in SG and 25.0% ($n = 3$) in GCP participants; while osteoporosis only affected one patient in the GCP group, $p = 0.365$. At LS, osteopenia was present in 78.6% ($n = 11$) of the mRYGB group vs. 33.3% ($n = 4$) and 50.0% ($n = 6$) in SG and GCP, respectively, and osteoporosis affected two patients (one in each mRYGB and GCP groups), $p = 0.030$. No bone fractures were observed during the study. At year 5,

TBS values did not show statistical differences when comparing mRYGB with SG and GCP: 1.288 (0.09) vs. 1.320 (0.11) vs. 1.311 (0.12), $p = 0.759$. However, 85% of patients had partially or totally degraded microarchitecture after mRYGB compared to 66.7% after SG and 58.3% in GCP, without reaching significant differences among groups, $p = 0.291$. The ten year risk of major osteoporotic fracture was 2.5% (1.20) in mRYGB vs. 2.1% (1.28) and 2.6% (1.50) in SG and GCP, respectively, $p = 0.74$. Risk of hip fracture was 0.30% (0.20) in mRYGB vs. 0.20% (0.56) in SG and 0.10% (0.63) in GCP, $p = 0.995$.

3.2. Correlation of BMD with Anthropometrics, Biochemical and Hormonal Parameters

Bivariate correlations between BMD changes at FN and LS with body composition, biochemical parameters and hormonal changes after surgery are shown in Table 3.

Table 3. Correlations of BMD changes at the femoral neck and lumbar spine with body composition, biochemical parameters and hormonal changes after surgery.

Characteristic	ΔFN BMD		ΔLS BMD	
	R	*p*-Value	*R*	*p*-Value
$Weight_b$ (kg)	0.450	0.009 *	0.507	0.003 *
BMI_b	0.104	0.563	0.061	0.733
$Weight_5$ (kg)	0.661	<0.001 *	0.656	<0.001 *
BMI_5	0.588	<0.001 *	0.499	0.003 *
Fat $mass_5$ (kg)	0.596	<0.001 *	0.509	0.003 *
Lean $mass_5$ (kg)	0.408	0.021 *	0.565	<0.001 *
Vitamin D_5 (nmol/L)	−0.58	0.753	0.009	0.963
PTH_5 (pmol/L)	−0.224	0.217	−0.251	0.166
APh_5 (μkat/L)	−0.260	0.143	−0.418	0.016 *
$\Delta Osteocalcin_{b-1a}$ (μg/L)	−0.241	0.191	−0.360	0.047 *
HbA_{1c5} (%)	0.452	0.008 *	0.495	0.003 *
$\Delta GLP\text{-}1AUC_{b-1a}$	−0.337	0.080	−0.528	0.004 *
ΔPYY_{b-1a}	−0.114	0.586	−0.124	0.553
$\Delta Glucagon_{b-1a}$	−0.096	0.646	0.045	0.830
$\Delta Ghrelin_{b-1a}$	0.142	0.453	0.241	0.199
ΔAUC $Insulin_{b-1a}$	−0.110	0.547	0.116	0.553

Spearman and Pearson analysis were performed. APh, alkaline phosphatase; AUC, area under the curve; BMD, bone mineral density; FN, femoral neck; GLP-1, glucagon like-peptide 1; HbA_{1c}, glycated hemoglobin; LS, lumbar spine; PTH, parathyroid hormone; PYY, peptide YY; b, baseline; 5, values at 5 years; Δ changes from baselines to 5 years; Δ b−1, changes from baselines to year 1; *, $p < 0.05$ was considered statistically significant.

When analyzing variables associated with the reduction in BMD after surgery, the decrease at FN and LS correlated positively with reduction in body weight, fat mass, lean mass and HbA_{1c} values at 5 year follow-up. Additionally, BMD decline at LS correlated inversely with alkaline phosphatase and the increase from baselines to one year in osteocalcin and the AUC for GLP-1. No correlations were found between BMD changes and phospho-calcium parameters at the fifth year nor with other gastrointestinal hormones.

3.3. Changes in BMD Regarding 5 Year T2D Outcomes after Surgery

Considering the possible influence of metabolic effects in skeleton metabolism, we compared BMD changes in patients with persistent T2D remission vs. non-remitters five years after surgery. BMD reduction was greater among remitters vs. non-remitters. At FN, the percentage of reduction was −4.37 (9.90) in non-remitters, −16.08 (1.98) in partial remitters and −10.57 (10.7) in complete remitters, $p = 0.042$. At LS, the percentage of reduction was −2.12 (10.7) in non-remitters, −16.15 (6.57) in partial remitters and −11.97 (8.01) in complete remitters, $p = 0.005$. No significant differences were observed in TBS values regarding T2D remission. Of note, no significant differences between groups were observed in antidiabetic agents used before surgery. Patients requiring pharmacological treatment after surgery were mainly treated with metformin and DPP-IV inhibitors.

3.4. Predicting Factors of BMD Reduction after Surgery

We performed a multiple regression analysis to better determinate BMD predictors. Weight at 5 year was found to be the only variable that predicted BMD changes at FN (adjusted R-squared: 0.3218, p-value: 0.00247). On the other hand, the type of surgery (mRYGB) and menopause were the variables that predicted BMD changes at LS (adjusted R-squared for the model: 0.2507, $p < 0.005$. Other variables such as changes in HbA_{1c}, phospho-calcium parameters and gastro-intestinal hormones including GLP-1 AUC were not final predictors of bone outcomes at either location. Coefficients of the regression model are shown in Table 4. We completed the analysis with a mixed model obtaining similar results; with this model, the effect of time was also significant, in agreement with the results of two-way ANOVA analysis.

Table 4. Coefficients of the regression model.

ΔFN BMD	Estimate	Std. Error	p-Value
(Intercept)	−40.439	8.301	<0.001 *
mRYGB	(1 Ref.)		
SG	3.584	3.636	0.333
GCP	−0.559	4.028	0.891
weight	0.379	0.106	<0.001 *
ΔLS BMD	**Estimate**	**Std. Error**	**p-Value**
Intercept	−5.825	3.268	0.086
mRYGB	(Ref.)		
SG	9.113	4.005	0.031
GCP	9.881	4.228	0.027
Male	(Ref.)		
Female No Menop	-9.916	4.660	0.042
Female Menop	−11.463	3.831	0.006

BMD, bone mineral density; FN, femoral neck; GCP, greater curvature plication; LS, lumbar spine; mRYGB, metabolic gastric bypass; SG, sleeve gastrectomy; Menop, menopause; Δ, changes from baseline to year 5, *, $p < 0.05$ was considered statistically significant.

4. Discussion

To our knowledge, this is the first study that has compared 5 year BMD outcomes between three different bariatric procedures (mRYGB, SG, and GCP) in the setting of a RCT. We found that mRYGB, characterized by a hypoabsortive component, showed a greater deleterious effect on LS at long-term compared to SG and GCP. Women with menopause had the greatest risk of bone loss at LS.

Bariatric surgery produces detrimental effects on bone health and there is a significant and non-uniform reduction in BMD across different bone sites [3,16,41,42]. In the short-term, the preferential bone loss at FN and weight-bearing sites suggests that this could be a response to unloading after weight loss [43,44]. Only a few previous studies, mainly focusing on standard RYGB, have evaluated long-term BMD outcomes. In this sense, two observational studies have reported bone deterioration 5 years after RYGB. Raoof et al. [45] found a linear and significant decline in BMD at FN (25%) and LS (19%) among 32 women that had not received calcium and vitamin D supplementation. Lindeman et al. [46] also detected a greater reduction in BMD at total hip (15.3%) and less reduction at LS (7.8%), although the majority of bone loss occurred within the first 2 years. Recently, Hansen et al. analyzed BMD changes 7 years after RYGB [47]. Among 17 participants, a BMD decline of 17% at total hip and 8% at LS was observed. Changes at LS occurred during the first 2 years, although there was a continuous decline in total hip BMD between the second and seventh year after surgery. In our cohort, we observed an overall reduction around 12% after mRYGB (FN and LS) and between 4 and 7% (FN) and 3.8 and 4.3% (LS) after restrictive procedures. FN BMD loss was more pronounced during the first year after surgery when maximum weight loss was achieved, probably due to the effects of skeletal unloading. On the other hand, LSBMD decline was not as pronounced during the first year but it was an ongoing process, especially after mRYGB. The differences observed when compared to former studies could be explained by the heterogeneity in the patient's characteristics (proportion of women, menopausal status), calcium and vitamin D supplementation and type of surgery; particularly in our cohort where mRYGB with a greater hypoabsortive component was performed.

There is a lack of studies comparing long-term BMD outcomes after different surgical procedures. In a meta-analysis, comparing BMD changes after RYGB and SG, bone outcomes were similar [48]. However, in only one of 13 studies included, the follow-up time was greater than 2 years. The STAMPEDE study compared bone changes after RYGB and SG versus intensive medical treatment in patients with T2D in the setting of a RCT. At 2 years, BMD changes were similar between groups, but at 5 years, RYGB showed a greater increase in bone metabolism markers compared to SG, thus supporting our findings [23,49]. No previous data have been published analyzing BMD changes after GCP.

Bone loss after bariatric surgery is complex and many predicting factors have been proposed. Changes like weight loss, especially at weight bearing sites [50], and the lean mass decline have been associated to the BMD reduction [51,52]. We found a positive correlation between whole BMD, FN and LS, 5 years after surgery with final weight; fat mass and lean mass. Our results therefore support the influence of body composition variations on BMD changes after bariatric surgery and highlight the importance of preserving lean mass to reduce the risk of osteosarcopenia [53]. Interestingly, in the multiple regression analysis, FN decline was influenced mainly by weight loss, supporting the hypothesis of a direct effect of weight unloading. However, at LS, other predicting factors such as menopause and hypoabsortive techniques were found. In this sense, it has been suggested that LS trabecular bone is metabolically more active and therefore more reactive to hormonal changes [54]. Moreover, the peripheral conversion of androgens to estrogens by adipose aromatase can be compromised with body fat reduction and this could negatively influence LS BMD, mainly in older menopausal women [24]. Also, body fat secretes many adipokines, such as leptin and adiponectin, which have been implicated in bone metabolism [21,55].

Micronutrient absorption is commonly affected after bariatric surgery. Significantly lower vitamin D and higher PTH levels have been reported in surgically treated obese patients compared to nonsurgical obese patients [52]. Carrasco et al. [56] reported a similar calcium reduction in both SG and RYGB 2 years after surgery compared to baseline, and it was not associated with changes in BMD. Our findings go in the same direction, and we did not find a relationship between 5 year postsurgical levels of calcium, vitamin D, PTH or PTH variation from the baseline values with BMD reduction. However, we should consider that our patients were given proper calcium and vitamin D supplementation and normal mean values of calcium and vitamin D were maintained across the study. However, as mRYGB has a greater malabsortive component compared to classic RYGB, we cannot discard deficiencies in other micronutrients and minerals that could affect bone health.

The influence of gastrointestinal hormone changes after bariatric surgery in bone metabolism is still unclear. While some studies in mice suggest that incretins like GLP-1 and GIP may have a beneficial effect on bone [18,57], a negative association between bone formation markers and PYY has been reported among adolescents with anorexia nervosa [58]. Carrasco et al. [21] observed that ghrelin reduction was associated with BMD loss after RYGB and SG. Another study in patients with obesity and T2D showed that fluctuation in a ghrelin gene product (unacylated ghrelin) after RYGB was associated with the reduction in BMD [59]. In our cohort, as we described previously [33], we observed a significantly higher increase in the AUC for GLP-1, as well as fasting values of PYY and ghrelin one year after mRYGB compared to restrictive procedures. At the fifth year, we found a negative correlation between BMD reductions at LS with an increase in AUC for GLP-1 observed one year after surgery. This can be explained by the fact that the patients undergoing RYGB who experienced the greatest LS loss showed the greatest increase in AUC for GLP-1. We also found correlation between whole BMD changes at the end of the study with other hormones one year after surgery, such as ghrelin (negative), and glucagon and insulin (positive). Nevertheless, in the multiple regression analysis, gastrointestinal hormones, particularly GLP-1, lost statistical significance, casting doubts on their key role on BMD changes after bariatric surgery.

Recently, BMD has been related to glucose tolerance status [60]. It has been suggested that chronic hyperglycaemia could degrade bone quality through the inhibition of osteocalcin, increased reactive oxygen species, bone accumulation of advanced glycation end products or the inhibition of GLP-1 [40]. In a cross-sectional matched cohort study including individuals with BMI > 35kg/m^2 and T2D (treated by RYGB and non-operated), the authors did not observe a relation between T2D status at the end of the study (remission vs. non-remission) with bone loss [61]. Conversely, in our study, LSBMD at 5 year follow-up correlated positively with HbA_{1c} values and we found a significantly lower BMD at FN as well as at LS among T2D remitters compared to non-remitters. However, although a better bone quality could be expected in T2D remitters, similar bone microarchitecture measured with TBS values was observed in remitters and non-remitters. Probably, the fact that patients undergoing RYGB were those with greater T2D remission and greater weight loss could explain our findings. Also, we cannot underestimate the effect of oral antidiabetic agents on bone. However, no significant differences in anti-diabetic agents were observed at the beginning of the study. Those patients where T2D persisted or recurred after surgery were mostly treated with metformin and DPP-IV inhibitors. No patient received glitazones or SGLT-2 that might negatively affect bone.

Surgically induced weight loss is associated with an increased risk of vertebral and non-vertebral fractures that starts in the second year, but becomes significant at the fifth year after surgery [62,63]. In a meta-analysis, the highest possibility of fracture was found after malabsortive procedures (biliopancreatic diversion) followed by the mixed techniques (RYGB) without an increased risk after restrictive procedures (adjustable gastric banding and SG) compared to the nonsurgical population [64]. Recently, the 26 year results of the S.O.S study [65] observed the highest incidence rate for first fracture after RYGB compared to restrictive procedures. In our cohort, the small size and time of observation were probably the reason why we had no bone fractures. Nonetheless, at 5 years, we observed a high percentage of patients with osteopenia, reaching 70% at LS after mRYGB, but a low percentage of osteoporosis. Of note, mean Z-scores (which compare BMD with same-aged healthy population) were below 0 after mRYGB but no patient was ≤ -2, the threshold for BMD below the expected range for the age. It is also unsettling that the fracture risk calculated with the FRAX algorithm was low in our patients and none of our patients fulfilled the criteria for treatment. The fact that age is the factor that counts the most in the algorithm along with previous fractures, and that our patients were relatively young, can probably explain the low values obtained. Nevertheless, in our cohort, we analyzed TBS which is a simple, non-invasive and inexpensive method to assess bone microarchitecture. To date, very few studies have evaluated TBS after bariatric surgery [42,66]. In a previous study reported by us including 38 obese women with an initially normal TBS score, 26.3% of patients had abnormal TBS values 3 years after RYGB [67]. In the present cohort, abnormal TBS at 5 years (partial or totally degraded) reached 85% of patients after mRYGB, but also about 50% of those undergoing restrictive procedures. This supports the hypothesis of a continuous bone microarchitecture declining over time which could increase the risk of fracture in the longer term.

The findings of our study cannot be generalized to all patients undergoing bariatric surgery as only three types of procedure were analyzed in a selected population with T2D. Our results should be understood taking into consideration several limitations. Firstly, the size of the study group is small and the diversity of participants (gender, menopause status, metabolic improvement after surgery) could influence the final BMD. In addition, we cannot discard the effect of antidiabetic drugs on bone. Secondly, the DEXA scan has limited accuracy in obese individuals because of the excess fat overlying bone and the heterogeneity of its distribution [68]. Also, BMD at LS can be altered by the presence of degenerative disk disease and osteophytes which can lead to falsely elevated measurements. Lastly, the small number of gastrointestinal hormones determined that were only evaluated during the first year after bariatric surgery.

5. Conclusions

In summary, our results show that mRYGB induces higher deleterious effects, especially at LS compared to SG and GCP. Elderly women with menopause undergoing mRYGB are at a higher risk of bone deterioration. Phospho-calcium metabolism and gastrointestinal hormone changes do not seem to have a major role in BMD outcomes 5 years later. Our findings reinforce the importance of long-life bone surveillance in bariatric patients and the need to select the bariatric technique according to the patient's risk for fractures. Restrictive procedures should be preferable over mRYGB, especially in those who are susceptible to osteoporosis.

Author Contributions: Conceived the study, N.V., J.V., J.P.-G.; acquisition data, N.V., R.L.-U., L.H.-M., A.P., A.V.-A.; curation data, F.G.-P., A.C.; N.V.; analysis and interpretation data, F.G.-P., A.C., C.G.-V., N.V.; writing-original draft preparation, F.G.-P., N.V.; contributed to writing and final revision of the manuscript, A.C., N.V., R.L.-U., C.G.-V.; critical revision of the manuscript, M.P.-M., J.O., J.P.-G., S.F.-V., J.V.; validation: all authors. All authors have read and agreed to the published version of the manuscript.

Funding: N.V. is the recipient of grants "Ajuts per a projectes de recerca clínica de l'Hospital Universitari de Bellvitge (2011-PR143/11)" and of the project "PI11/01960; PI14/01997 and PI17/01556" funded by the Instituto de Salud Carlos III and co-funded by the European Union (ERDF, "A way to build Europe"). J.V. has funding from the Instituto de Salud Carlos III through the project PI14/00228 and PI17/01503 co-funded by the European Union (ERDF, "A way to build Europe"). S.F.-V. has funding from the Spanish Ministry of Economy and Competitiveness and the European Regional Development Fund (ERDF) (SAF2015-65019-R). The Spanish Biomedical Research Center in Diabetes and Associated Metabolic Disorders (CIBERDEM) (CB07708/0012) is an initiative of the Instituto de Salud Carlos III. SFV acknowledges support from the Miguel Servet tenure-track program (CP10/00438 and CPII16/0008) from the Fondo de Investigación Sanitaria (FIS) co-financed by the ERDF.

Acknowledgments: The authors thank Jonathan Rogerson and Georgia Konstandakopoulou for helpful discussions on the manuscript and Bernat Miguel Huguet for statistical analysis. We thank CERCA Programme Generalitat de Catalunya for institutional support.

Conflicts of Interest: The authors declare no conflict of interest.

References

1. Kuno, T.; Tanimoto, E.; Morita, S.; Shimada, Y.J. Effects of bariatric surgery on cardiovascular disease: A concise update of recent advances. *Front. Cardiovasc. Med.* **2019**, *6*, 94. [CrossRef] [PubMed]
2. Castanha, C.R.; Tcbc-Pe, Á.A.B.F.; Castanha, A.R.; Belo, G.Q.M.B.; Lacerda, R.M.R.; Vilar, L. Evaluation of quality of life, weight loss and comorbidities of patients undergoing bariatric surgery. *Rev. Col. Bras. Cir.* **2018**, *45*, e1864. [PubMed]
3. Yu, E.W.; Kim, S.C.; Sturgeon, D.J.; Lindeman, K.G.; Weissman, J.S. Fracture risk after Roux-en-Y gastric bypass vs adjustable gastric banding among medicare beneficiaries. *JAMA Surg.* **2019**, *154*, 746–753. [CrossRef] [PubMed]
4. Nakamura, K.M.; Haglind, E.G.C.; Clowes, J.A.; Achenbach, S.J.; Atkinson, E.J.; Melton, L.J.; Kennel, K.A. Fracture risk following bariatric surgery: A population-based study. *Osteoporos. Int.* **2013**, *25*, 151–158. [CrossRef] [PubMed]
5. Rousseau, C.; Jean, S.; Gamache, P.; Lebel, S.; Mac-Way, F.; Biertho, L.; Michou, L.; Gagnon, C. Change in fracture risk and fracture pattern after bariatric surgery: Nested Case-Control study. *BMJ* **2016**, *354*, i3794. [CrossRef]
6. Compston, J. Obesity and bone. *Curr. Osteoporos. Rep.* **2013**, *11*, 30–35. [CrossRef]
7. Gnudi, S.; Sitta, E.; Lisi, L. Relationship of body mass index with main limb fragility fractures in postmenopausal women. *J. Bone Miner. Metab.* **2009**, *27*, 479–484. [CrossRef]
8. Ong, T.; Sahota, O.; Tan, W.; Marshall, L. A United Kingdom perspective on the relationship between body mass index (BMI) and bone health: A cross sectional analysis of data from the Nottingham Fracture Liaison Service. *Bone* **2014**, *59*, 207–210. [CrossRef] [PubMed]
9. Premaor, M.O.; Pilbrow, L.; Tonkin, C.; A Parker, R.; Compston, J. Obesity and fractures in postmenopausal women. *J. Bone Miner. Res.* **2009**, *25*, 292–297. [CrossRef]
10. Compston, J.E.; Watts, N.B.; Chapurlat, R.; Cooper, C.; Boonen, S.; Greenspan, S.; Pfeilschifter, J.; Silverman, S.; Diez-Perez, A.; Lindsay, R.; et al. Obesity is not protective against fracture in postmenopausal women: Glow. *Am. J. Med.* **2011**, *124*, 1043–1050. [CrossRef]

11. Lespessailles, E.; Paccou, J.; Javier, R.-M.; Thomas, T.; Cortet, B. GRIO scientific committee obesity, bariatric surgery, and fractures. *J. Clin. Endocrinol. Metab.* **2019**, *104*, 4756–4768. [CrossRef] [PubMed]
12. Compston, J.E. Type 2 diabetes mellitus and bone. *J. Intern. Med.* **2018**, *283*, 140–153. [CrossRef]
13. Ferrari, S. Diabetes and bone. *Calcif. Tissue Int.* **2017**, *100*, 107–108. [CrossRef] [PubMed]
14. Ferrari, S.; Abrahamsen, B.; Napoli, N.; Akesson, K.; Chandran, M.; Eastell, R.; Fuleihan, G.E.-H.; Josse, R.; Kendler, D.; Kraenzlin, M.; et al. Diagnosis and management of bone fragility in diabetes: An emerging challenge. *Osteoporos. Int.* **2018**, *29*, 2585–2596. [CrossRef] [PubMed]
15. Gagnon, C.; Schafer, A.L. Bone health after bariatric surgery. *JBMR Plus* **2018**, *2*, 121–133. [CrossRef] [PubMed]
16. Stein, E.M.; Silverberg, S.J. Bone loss after bariatric surgery: Causes, consequences, and management. *Lancet Diabetes Endocrinol.* **2014**, *2*, 165–174. [CrossRef]
17. Martínez, S.B.; Jauregui, E.P.; Martín, J.E.S. Impact of bariatric surgery on bone tissue. *Endocrinol. Diabetes Nutr.* **2019**, *66*, 62–68.
18. Mieczkowska, A.; Irwin, N.; Flatt, P.; Chappard, D.; Mabilleau, G. Glucose-Dependent insulinotropic polypeptide (GIP) receptor deletion leads to reduced bone strength and quality. *Bone* **2013**, *56*, 337–342. [CrossRef]
19. Wong, I.P.L.; Driessler, F.; Khor, E.C.; Shi, Y.-C.; Hörmer, B.; Nguyen, A.D.; Enriquez, R.F.; Eisman, J.A.; Sainsbury, A.; Herzog, H.; et al. Peptide YY regulates bone remodeling in mice: A link between gut and skeletal biology. *PLoS ONE* **2012**, *7*, e40038. [CrossRef]
20. Nuche-Berenguer, B.; Moreno, P.; Esbrit, P.; Dapía, S.; Caeiro, J.R.; Cancelas, J.; Haro-Mora, J.J.; Villanueva-Peñacarrillo, M.L. Effect of GLP-1 treatment on bone turnover in normal, type 2 diabetic, and insulin-resistant states. *Calcif. Tissue Int.* **2009**, *84*, 453–461. [CrossRef]
21. Carrasco, F.; Basfi-Fer, K.; Rojas, P.; Valencia, A.; Csendes, A.; Codoceo, J.; Inostroza, J.; Ruz, M. Changes in bone mineral density after sleeve gastrectomy or gastric bypass: Relationships with variations in vitamin d, ghrelin, and adiponectin levels. *Obes. Surg.* **2014**, *24*, 877–884. [CrossRef] [PubMed]
22. Yu, E.W.; Wewalka, M.; Ding, S.-A.; Simonson, D.C.; Foster, K.; Holst, J.J.; Vernon, A.; Goldfine, A.B.; Halperin, F. Effects of gastric bypass and gastric banding on bone remodeling in obese patients with type 2 diabetes. *J. Clin. Endocrinol. Metab.* **2015**, *101*, 714–722. [CrossRef] [PubMed]
23. Maghrabi, A.H.; Wolski, K.; Abood, B.; Licata, A.; Pothier, C.; Bhatt, D.L.; Nissen, S.; Brethauer, S.A.; Kirwan, J.P.; Schauer, P.R.; et al. Two-Year outcomes on bone density and fracture incidence in patients with T2DM randomized to bariatric surgery versus intensive medical therapy. *Obesity (Silver Spring)* **2015**, *23*, 2344–2348. [CrossRef] [PubMed]
24. Vilarrasa, N.; José, P.S.; Garcia, I.; Gomez-Vaquero, C.; Miras, P.M.; De Gordejuela, A.G.R.; Masdevall, C.; Pujol, J.; Soler, J.; Gómez, J.M. Evaluation of bone mineral density loss in morbidly obese women after gastric bypass: 3-Year Follow-Up. *Obes. Surg.* **2010**, *21*, 465–472. [CrossRef]
25. Muschitz, C.; Kocijan, R.; Marterer, C.; Nia, A.R.; Muschitz, G.K.; Resch, H.; Pietschmann, P. Sclerostin levels and changes in bone metabolism after bariatric surgery. *J. Clin. Endocrinol. Metab.* **2015**, *100*, 891–901. [CrossRef] [PubMed]
26. Sheu, Y.; Cauley, J.A. The role of bone marrow and visceral fat on bone metabolism. *Curr. Osteoporos. Rep.* **2011**, *9*, 67–75. [CrossRef]
27. Guerrero-Pérez, F.; Casajoana, A.; Gómez-Vaquero, C.; Virgili, N.; López-Urdiales, R.; Hernández-Montoliu, L.; Pujol-Gebelli, J.; Osorio, J.; Alves, C.; Perez-Maraver, M.; et al. Changes in bone mineral density in patients with type 2 diabetes after different bariatric surgery procedures and the role of gastrointestinal hormones. *Obes. Surg.* **2019**, *30*, 180–188. [CrossRef]
28. Bredella, M.A.; Greenblatt, L.; Eajazi, A.; Torriani, M.; Yu, E.W. Effects of Roux-En-Y gastric bypass and sleeve gastrectomy on bone mineral density and marrow adipose tissue. *Bone* **2016**, *95*, 85–90. [CrossRef]
29. Coupaye, M.; Rivière, P.; Breuil, M.C.; Castel, B.; Bogard, C.; Dupré, T.; Flamant, M.; Msika, S.; LeDoux, S. Comparison of nutritional status during the first year after sleeve gastrectomy and Roux-En-Y gastric bypass. *Obes. Surg.* **2013**, *24*, 276–283. [CrossRef]
30. Hsin, M.-C.; Huang, C.-K.; Tai, C.-M.; Yeh, L.-R.; Kuo, H.-C.; Garg, A. A Case-Matched study of the differences in bone mineral density 1 year after 3 different bariatric procedures. *Surg. Obes. Relat. Dis.* **2015**, *11*, 181–185. [CrossRef]

31. Lanzarini, E.; Nogues, X.; Goday, A.; Benaiges, D.; De Ramón, M.; Villatoro, M.; Pera, M.; Grande, L.; Ramón, J.M. High-Dose vitamin D supplementation is necessary after bariatric surgery: A prospective 2-Year Follow-up study. *Obes. Surg.* **2015**, *25*, 1633–1638. [CrossRef] [PubMed]
32. Vix, M.; Liu, K.-H.; Diana, M.; D'Urso, A.; Mutter, D.; Marescaux, J. Impact of Roux-En-Y gastric bypass versus sleeve gastrectomy on vitamin D metabolism: Short-Term results from a prospective randomized clinical trial. *Surg. Endosc.* **2013**, *28*, 821–826. [CrossRef]
33. Casajoana, A.; Pujol, J.; Garcia, A.; Elvira, J.; Virgili, N.; De Oca, F.J.; Duran, X.; Fernández-Veledo, S.; Vendrell, J.; Vilarrasa, N. Predictive value of gut peptides in T2D remission: Randomized controlled trial comparing metabolic gastric bypass, sleeve gastrectomy and greater curvature plication. *Obes. Surg.* **2017**, *27*, 2235–2245. [CrossRef]
34. Buse, J.B.; Caprio, S.; Cefalu, W.T.; Ceriello, A.; Del Prato, S.; Inzucchi, S.E.; McLaughlin, S.; Phillips, G.L., 2nd; Robertson, R.P.; Rubino, F.; et al. How do we define cure of diabetes? *Diabetes Care* **2009**, *32*, 2133–2135. [CrossRef] [PubMed]
35. Kanis, J.A. Assessment of fracture risk and its application to screening for postmenopausal osteoporosis: Synopsis of a WHO report. *Osteoporos. Int.* **1994**, *4*, 368–381. [CrossRef] [PubMed]
36. Pothuaud, L.; Barthe, N.; Krieg, M.-A.; Mehsen, N.; Carceller, P.; Hans, D. Evaluation of the potential use of trabecular bone score to complement bone mineral density in the diagnosis of osteoporosis: A preliminary spine BMD–Matched, Case-Control study. *J. Clin. Densitom.* **2009**, *12*, 170–176. [CrossRef]
37. Kanis, J.; McCloskey, E.V.; Johansson, H.; Oden, A.; Strom, O.; Borgström, F. Development and use of FRAX®in osteoporosis. *Osteoporos. Int.* **2010**, *21*, 407–413. [CrossRef]
38. McCloskey, E.V.; Odén, A.; Harvey, N.C.; Leslie, W.D.; Hans, D.; Johansson, H.; Kanis, J. Adjusting fracture probability by trabecular bone score. *Calcif. Tissue Int.* **2015**, *96*, 500–509. [CrossRef]
39. Azagra, R.; Zwart, M.; Aguyé, A.; Martín-Sánchez, J.C.; Casado, E.; Díaz-Herrera, M.A.; Moriña, D.; Cooper, C.; Díez-Pérez, A.; Dennison, E.M.; et al. Fracture experience among participants from the FROCAT study: What thresholding is appropriate using the FRAX tool? *Maturitas* **2016**, *83*, 65–71. [CrossRef]
40. Wolever, T.M.; Jenkins, D.J.; Jenkins, A.L.; Josse, R.G. The glycemic index: Methodology and clinical implications. *Am. J. Clin. Nutr.* **1991**, *54*, 846–854. [CrossRef]
41. Brzozowska, M.; Sainsbury, A.; Eisman, J.A.; Baldock, P.A.; Center, J.R. Bariatric surgery, bone loss, obesity and possible mechanisms. *Obes. Rev.* **2012**, *14*, 52–67. [CrossRef] [PubMed]
42. Muschitz, C.; Kocijan, R.; Haschka, J.; Zendeli, A.; Pirker, T.; Geiger, C.; Müller, A.; Tschinder, B.; Kocijan, A.; Marterer, C.; et al. The impact of vitamin d, calcium, protein supplementation, and physical exercise on bone metabolism after bariatric surgery: The BABS study. *J. Bone Miner. Res.* **2015**, *31*, 672–682. [CrossRef] [PubMed]
43. Tangalakis, L.L.; Tabone, L.; Spagnoli, A.; Muehlbauer, M.; Omotosho, P.; Torquati, A. Effects of Roux-En-Y gastric bypass on osteoclast activity and bone density in morbidly obese patients with type 2 diabetes. *Obes. Surg.* **2019**, *30*, 290–295. [CrossRef]
44. Liu, C.; Wu, D.; Zhang, J.-F.; Xu, D.; Xu, W.-F.; Chen, Y.; Liu, B.-Y.; Li, P.; Li, L. Changes in bone metabolism in morbidly obese patients after bariatric surgery: A Meta-Analysis. *Obes. Surg.* **2015**, *26*, 91–97. [CrossRef] [PubMed]
45. Raoof, M.; Näslund, I.; Rask, E.; Szabo, E. Effect of gastric bypass on bone mineral density, parathyroid hormone and vitamin d: 5 Years Follow-up. *Obes. Surg.* **2016**, *26*, 1141–1145. [CrossRef]
46. Lindeman, K.G.; Greenblatt, L.; Rourke, C.; Bouxsein, M.L.; Finkelstein, J.S.; Yu, E.W. Longitudinal 5-Year evaluation of bone density and microarchitecture after Roux-En-Y gastric bypass surgery. *J. Clin. Endocrinol. Metab.* **2018**, *103*, 4104–4112. [CrossRef]
47. Hansen, S.; Jørgensen, N.R.; Hermann, A.P.; Støving, R.K. Continuos decline in bone mineral density and deterioration of bone microarchitecture 7 years after Roux-En-Y gastric bypass surgery. *Eur. J. Endocrinol.* **2020**, *182*, 303–311. [CrossRef]

48. Tian, Z.; Fan, X.-T.; Li, S.-Z.; Zhai, T.; Dong, J. Changes in bone metabolism after sleeve gastrectomy versus gastric bypass: A Meta-Analysis. *Obes. Surg.* **2019**, *30*, 77–86. [CrossRef]
49. Crawford, M.R.; Pham, N.; Khan, L.; Bena, J.F.; Schauer, P.R.; Kashyap, S.R. Increased bone turnover in type 2 diabetes patients randomized to bariatric surgery versus medical therapy at 5 years. *Endocr. Pract.* **2018**, *24*, 256–264. [CrossRef]
50. Scibora, L.M.; Ikramuddin, S.; Buchwald, H.; Petit, M.A. Examining the link between bariatric surgery, bone loss, and osteoporosis: A review of bone density studies. *Obes. Surg.* **2012**, *22*, 654–667. [CrossRef]
51. Vilarrasa, N.; Gómez, J.M.; Elio, I.; Gómez-Vaquero, C.; Masdevall, C.; Pujol, J.; Virgili, N.; Burgos, R.; Sánchez-Santos, R.; de Gordejuela, A.G.; et al. Evaluation of bone disease in morbidily obese women after gastric bypass and risk factors implicated in bone loss. *Obes. Surg.* **2009**, *19*, 860–866. [CrossRef] [PubMed]
52. Costa, T.L.; Paganotto, M.; Radominski, R.B.; Kulak, C.M.; Borba, V.C. Calcium metabolism, vitamin D and bone mineral density after bariatric surgery. *Osteoporos. Int.* **2014**, *26*, 757–764. [CrossRef]
53. Coen, P.M.; Carnero, E.A.; Goodpaster, B.H. Exercise and bariatric surgery. *Exerc. Sport Sci. Rev.* **2018**, *46*, 262–270. [CrossRef] [PubMed]
54. Chen, H.; Zhou, X.; Fujita, H.; Onozuka, M.; Kubo, K.-Y. Age-Related changes in trabecular and cortical bone microstructure. *Int. J. Endocrinol.* **2013**, *2013*, 213234. [CrossRef] [PubMed]
55. Korner, J.; Inabnet, W.; Febres, G.; Conwell, I.M.; McMahon, N.J.; Salas, R.; Taveras, C.; Schrope, B.; Bessler, M. Prospective study of gut hormone and metabolic changes after adjustable gastric banding and Roux-En-Y gastric bypass. *Int. J. Obes.* **2009**, *33*, 786–795. [CrossRef] [PubMed]
56. Carrasco, F.; Basfi-Fer, K.; Rojas, P.; Csendes, A.; Papapietro, K.; Codoceo, J.; Inostroza, J.; Krebs, N.F.; Westcott, J.L.; Miller, L.V.; et al. Calcium absorption may be affected after either sleeve gastrectomy or Roux-En-Y gastric bypass in premenopausal women: A 2-Y prospective study. *Am. J. Clin. Nutr.* **2018**, *108*, 24–32. [CrossRef]
57. Ma, X.; Meng, J.; Jia, M.; Bi, L.; Zhou, Y.; Wang, Y.; Hu, J.; He, G.; Luo, X. Exendin-4, a Glucagon-Like Peptide-1 receptor agonist, prevents osteopenia by promoting bone formation and suppressing bone resorption in aged ovariectomized rats. *J. Bone Miner. Res.* **2013**, *28*, 1641–1652. [CrossRef]
58. Misra, M.; Miller, K.K.; Tsai, P.; Gallagher, K.; Lin, A.; Lee, N.; Herzog, D.B.; Klibanski, A. Elevated peptide YY levels in adolescent girls with anorexia nervosa. *J. Clin. Endocrinol. Metab.* **2006**, *91*, 1027–1033. [CrossRef]
59. Wang, J.; Ma, J.; Yu, H.; Zhang, P.; Han, J.; Bao, Y. Unacylated ghrelin is correlated with the decline of bone mineral density after Roux-En-Y gastric bypass in obese Chinese with type 2 diabetes. *Surg. Obes. Relat. Dis.* **2019**, *15*, 1473–1480. [CrossRef]
60. Li, Y.; Zhao, Z.; Wang, L.; Fu, Z.; Ji, L.; Wu, X. The prevalence of osteoporosis tested by quantitative computed tomography in patients with different glucose tolerances. *J. Clin. Endocrinol. Metab.* **2019**, *105*, dgz036. [CrossRef]
61. Madsen, L.R.; Espersen, R.; Ornstrup, M.J.; Jørgensen, N.R.; Langdahl, B.L.; Richelsen, B. Bone health in patients with type 2 diabetes treated by Roux-En-Y gastric bypass and the role of diabetes remission. *Obes. Surg.* **2019**, *29*, 1823–1831. [CrossRef]
62. Zhang, Q.; Chen, Y.; Li, J.; Chen, D.; Cheng, Z.; Xu, S.; Huang, Y.; Wang, Q. A Meta-Analysis of the effects of bariatric surgery on fracture risk. *Obes. Rev.* **2018**, *19*, 728–736. [CrossRef]
63. Ablett, A.D.; Boyle, B.R.; Avenell, A. Fractures in adults after weight loss from bariatric surgery and weight management programs for obesity: Systematic review and Meta-analysis. *Obes. Surg.* **2019**, *29*, 1327–1342. [CrossRef]
64. Zhang, Q.; Dong, J.; Zhou, D.; Liu, F. Comparative risk of fracture for bariatric procedures in patients with obesity: A systematic review and Bayesian network Meta-Analysis. *Int. J. Surg.* **2020**, *75*, 13–23. [CrossRef]
65. Ahlin, S.; Peltonen, M.; Sjöholm, K.; Anveden, Å.; Jacobson, P.; Andersson-Assarsson, J.C.; Taube, M.; Larsson, I.; Lohmander, L.S.; Näslund, I.; et al. Fracture risk after three bariatric surgery procedures in Swedish obese subjects: Up to 26 years Follow-Up of a controlled intervention study. *J. Intern. Med.* **2020**, *287*, 546–557. [CrossRef] [PubMed]
66. Leib, E.; Winzenrieth, R.; Lamy, O.; Hans, D. Comparing bone microarchitecture by trabecular bone score (TBS) in Caucasian American women with and without osteoporotic fractures. *Calcif. Tissue Int.* **2014**, *95*, 201–208. [CrossRef]

67. Marengo, A.P.; Pérez, F.G.; Martín, L.S.; Monseny, R.; Casajoana, A.; Yepes, R.V.; Virgili, N.; Simó-Servat, A.; Prats, A.; Gómez-Vaquero, C.; et al. Is trabecular bone score valuable in bone microstructure assessment after gastric bypass in women with morbid obesity? *Nutrients* **2017**, *9*, 1314. [CrossRef]
68. Tothill, P.; Hannan, W.J.; Cowen, S.; Freeman, C.P. Anomalies in the measurement of changes in Total-Body bone mineral by Dual-Energy X-Ray absorptiometry during weight change. *J. Bone Miner. Res.* **1997**, *12*, 1908–1921. [CrossRef]

Journal of
Clinical Medicine

MDPI

Article

Amino Acid Metabolites and Slow Weight Loss in the Early Postoperative Period after Sleeve Gastrectomy

Yeongkeun Kwon [1,2,†], Mi Jang [3,†], Youngsun Lee [4], Jane Ha [2,5] and Sungsoo Park [1,2,*]

1 Division of Foregut Surgery, Korea University College of Medicine, Seoul 02841, Korea; kukwon@korea.ac.kr
2 Center for Obesity and Metabolic Diseases, Korea University Anam Hospital, Seoul 02841, Korea; janehapti@korea.ac.kr
3 Department of Biotechnology and Food Science, Norwegian University of Science and Technology, 7491 Trondheim, Norway; kia3111@gmail.com
4 Advanced Analysis Center, Korea Institute of Science and Technology, Seoul 02792, Korea; youngsunlee@snu.ac.kr
5 Department of Medicine, Korea University College of Medicine, Seoul 02841, Korea
* Correspondence: kugspss@korea.ac.kr; Tel.: +82-2-920-6772
† Authors contributed equally.

Received: 24 June 2020; Accepted: 22 July 2020; Published: 23 July 2020

Abstract: Background: Profiles of amino acid metabolites (AAMs) have been linked to obesity and energy homeostasis. We investigated whether baseline obesity-related AAMs were associated with weight status in the early postoperative period after sleeve gastrectomy. Methods: In this prospective, single-arm, longitudinal study, 27 bariatric patients underwent sleeve gastrectomy. Twenty obesity-related AAMs were comprehensively quantified prior to surgery, and slow weight loss was defined as the lowest 40% of the percentage excess weight loss (%EWL) at three and six months postoperatively. Linear regression models were used to assess the association between baseline obesity-related AAMs and %EWL, and receiver operating characteristic curves were assessed. Results: Isoleucine and metabolites from the serotonin pathway were significantly associated with the %EWL at three and six months after sleeve gastrectomy. Among the metabolites identified to be significant in the regression analyses, serotonin (area under receiver operating characteristic curves (AUROC): 0.79, 95% confidence interval (CI): 0.59–0.97) and serotonin/5-hydroxytryptophan ratio (AUROC: 0.80, 95% CI: 0.58–1.00) showed superior performance in predicting slow weight loss six months after sleeve gastrectomy. Conclusions: Our findings underscore the importance of baseline AAM profiles, especially serotonin and serotonin/5-hydroxytryptophan ratio, in predicting slow weight loss in the early postoperative period after sleeve gastrectomy.

Keywords: amino acid; metabolomics; sleeve gastrectomy; bariatric surgery; weight loss

1. Introduction

Bariatric surgery is currently the most successful and durable treatment for the morbidly obese [1–3]; however, there is wide variability in the weight loss response to bariatric surgery [4–6] and over 20% of bariatric patients experience long-term postoperative weight regain [2,7,8]. Although suboptimal weight loss after bariatric surgery has been known to be associated with the recurrence of obesity-related comorbidities and a deterioration in the health-related quality of life [9–11], there currently exist few effective methods for predicting postoperative weight status. Recently, weight loss in the early postoperative period has been suggested to be able to predict long-term weight outcomes [12,13]. Indicators such as the percentage excess weight loss (%EWL) or weight loss velocity up to six months after bariatric surgery have been suggested to predict long-term weight response to bariatric surgery [12,13]. Given that postoperative behavioral or intensive lifestyle interventions improve weight loss after bariatric surgery [14,15], early identification of slow weight loss responders is an important focus area for individualized postoperative care.

Interestingly, circulating concentrations of branched-chain amino acids (BCAAs), aromatic amino acids (AAAs), and various tryptophan-derived metabolites (TDMs) have been highlighted as potential biomarkers for obesity-related medical conditions. BCAAs, AAAs, and various TDMs as signaling molecules participate in nutritional metabolism and energy homeostasis and the adipose tissue has been known to regulate these circulating metabolites [16–19]. Levels of circulating BCAAs and AAAs tend to be elevated in individuals with obesity and appear to be closely related to an individual's metabolic health and future insulin resistance or type 2 diabetes [20,21]. Although several mechanisms (e.g., activation of mammalian target of rapamycin complex 1, mitochondrial dysfunction induced by amino acids dysmetabolism) have been proposed to explain the increased amino acid and insulin resistance and obesity, the exact causative associations have not been investigated [20]. Among various TDMs, peripheral serotonin has been well known as affecting organismal energy homeostasis [22,23], and inhibition of peripheral serotonin synthesis protects against diet-induced obesity [24]. Serotonin metabolism has been known to regulate glucose levels and in turn obesity through its effects on hepatocyte and adipocyte functions [25].

Sleeve gastrectomy is one of the most commonly performed bariatric surgeries and appears to be similar in achieve weight loss compared with the Roux-en-Y gastric bypass, which has been considered the gold standard procedure for morbidly obese patients [26]. To elucidate the role of AAMs as potential predictors for early postoperative weight status after sleeve gastrectomy, we performed a comprehensive metabolomic study targeting 20 obesity-related AAMs in bariatric patients and investigated whether pre-operative AAMs are associated with weight loss in the early postoperative period after sleeve gastrectomy.

2. Methods

2.1. Study Participants

In January 2019, a prospective, single-arm, longitudinal study to assess the effect of bariatric surgery on energy homeostasis began at a university hospital. The original study was designed to perform follow ups until 12 months postoperative, and this study details the interim results at six months postoperative (Institutional Review Board approval number: 2019AN0055). Following the general criteria for bariatric surgery in Korea, eligibility criteria included body mass index (BMI) ≥ 35 kg/m^2, or BMI ≥ 30 kg/m^2 and at least one or more obesity-related co-morbidities, and age ≥ 20. Patients were excluded if they had previous bariatric surgeries, other complex abdominal surgeries, or had poorly controlled medical or psychiatric disorders (details of eligibility criteria are presented in Supplementary Table S1). Because of the lack of literature on the association between AAMs and weight status after bariatric surgery, sample size calculation was not performed. We designed this study with a sample size of 30 participants out of whom three failed to report during follow-ups. Patients providing written informed consent entered a screening process for study eligibility and underwent physical and laboratory evaluations to confirm eligibility.

2.2. Pre-operative Education of Bariatric Patients

Following study enrollment, all patients received nutritional evaluations including weight-loss expectations, eating behaviors and patterns, physical activity habits, and psychosocial assessments. To achieve optimal weight loss after sleeve gastrectomy, a bariatric physician and registered dietitian provided dietary and lifestyle recommendations including dietary principles, such as macro- and micro-nutrient compositions, carbohydrate counting, and advice regarding regular aerobic exercise (if medically approved by the physician who provided their medical care). All patients began guideline-based micronutrient (vitamin and mineral) supplementation after enrollment in this study [27].

2.3. Surgical Procedures

Sleeve gastrectomies were performed laparoscopically by a single bariatric surgeon and involved a gastric volume reduction of 80% to 85% using a 30-French endoscope to perform stomach resections beginning 3 cm from the pylorus and terminating at the angle of His.

2.4. Postoperative Care Regarding Nutrition and Exercise

Postoperatively, patients received education via a protocol-driven staged-meal progression. If tolerable, a low-sugar clear liquid meal was initiated within 24 h after sleeve gastrectomy, and soft and regular diets were recommended to begin at three–four weeks and nine weeks, respectively. A protein intake of 50 g/day and up to 1.5 g/kg ideal body weight per day was recommended with oral supplementation of amino acids including BCAAs and AAAs: leucine 5.55 g/day, isoleucine 2.65 g/day, valine 2.7 g/day, phenylalanine 1.75 g/day, tyrosine 1.75 g/day, and tryptophan 1.35 g/day. Promax® (Korea Medical Foods Co., Seoul, South Korea) was used for amino acid supplements.

In the first four weeks postoperatively, patients exercised by walking and gradually increased speed in their tolerated threshold. Patients were asked to walk 150 min per week. In 5–26 weeks postoperatively the patient's total walking time increased to ≥ 200 min per week and ≥ 4 days per week. Additionally, patients were asked to perform three ≥ 20 min strength exercise sessions including shoulder and hip strengthening exercises ≥ 3 days per week. The intensity of the exercises was a perceived exertion rating between 12 to 14 on the Borg Scale [28]. All participants were followed-up every two weeks via telephone and by text message to confirm compliance with their nutritional and exercise recommendations.

2.5. Measurements of Serum AAMs

Pre-operative blood samples of patients were obtained within two weeks prior to surgery. Blood sampling was performed eight h after fasting when patients were not on a pre-operative calorie-restricted diet. Amino acid profiling was performed using liquid chromatography-mass spectrometry in the College of Life Sciences & Biotechnology, Korea University, Seoul, Korea. We selected 20 obesity-related AAMs based on the results of previous studies relating AAMs and obesity or energy homeostasis (Supplementary Figure S1): (1) BCAAs (leucine, isoleucine, valine); (2) AAAs (phenylalanine, tyrosine, tryptophan); (3) TDMs including kynurenine pathway metabolites (kynurenine, anthranilic acid, 3-hydroxykynurenine, 3-hydroxyanthranilic acid, kynurenic acid, xanthurenic acid); indole pathway metabolites (indoxyl sulfate, indole-3-acetic acid, indole-3-lactic acid, indole-3-propionic acid); serotonin pathway metabolites (5-hydroxytryptophan (5-HTrp), serotonin, 5-hydroxyindoleacetic acid (5-HIAA)); and tyrosine pathway metabolites (L-dihydroxyphenylalanine). We also calculated the ratios between adjacent metabolites (downstream metabolites/upstream metabolites) to compare the enzymatic activity among participants. A detailed protocol for serum metabolite measurements and enzymes corresponding to the metabolite ratios are presented in Supplementary Tables S2 and S3.

2.6. Outcome Measures

The primary outcomes were the associations between baseline obesity-related AAMs and changes in weight status three and six months post sleeve gastrectomy. Changes in weight status were calculated with %EWL by dividing the number of kilograms lost by the number of kilograms in the patient's excess body weight.

2.7. Statistical Analysis

Summary data are presented as percentages for categorical variables and as means with standard deviations (SDs) for continuous variables. Patients' characteristics at baseline and three or six months postoperatively were compared using the paired t-test or Wilcoxon signed rank test for continuous variables. Serum metabolite concentrations were log-transformed to improve the normality of their distributions based on the Shapiro-Wilk test results. First, we examined associations of %EWL with baseline obesity-related AAMs three and six months postoperatively using linear regression models adjusted for baseline BMIs. Sensitivity analyses were also performed to determine the consistency of the statistical significance according to the following baseline characteristics: age ≥ 45 years, female sex, BMI ≥ 35 kg/m2, hypertension, diabetes, and non-smoker status. Secondly, using AAMs identified as significant in the regression analyses, receiver operating characteristic (ROC) curves were generated to analyze individual AAM performances to predict slow weight loss three and six months postoperatively. Considering that about 40% of the bariatric patients at our hospital do not attain 50% EWL at 6 months postoperative, slow weight loss was defined as the lowest 40% of the %EWL at three and six months postoperative. Statistical analyses were performed using Stata12 (Stata Corp., College Station, TX, USA), and a two-sided p-value of < 0.05 was considered statistically significant.

3. Results

3.1. Patients' Characteristics at Baseline

The mean age of the 27 study participants was 42.1 years (SD: 12.9), and 63% of the patients were women (Table 1). The mean BMI and mean waist circumference were 38.7 kg/m^2 (SD: 5.2) and 120.5 cm (SD: 19.9), respectively. Among the study participants, 78% had metabolic syndromes and 15% were current smokers. Participants with hypertension, diabetes, and dyslipidemia were 52%, 74%, and 74%, respectively.

Table 1. Baseline characteristics.

Variables	Values (n = 27)
Age, years	42.1 ± 12.9
Female sex, n (%)	17 (63)
Body mass index[1], kg/m^2	38.7 ± 5.2
Body weight, kg	105.1 ± 17.0
Waist circumference, cm	120.5 ± 19.9
Current smoker, n (%)	4 (15)
Metabolic syndrome, n (%)	21 (78)
Hypertension, n (%)	14 (52)
Diabetes, n (%)	20 (74)
Dyslipidemia, n (%)	20 (74)

Values are given as mean ± standard deviation [1] The body mass index is the weight in kilograms divided by the square of the height in meters.

3.2. Changes in Patients' Characteristics after Bariatric Surgery

All patients experienced a significant decrease in BMI and body weight (BMI at three months: 31.5 kg/m^2 (SD: 5.1), $p < 0.001$; body weight at three months: 85.1 kg (SD: 15.3), $p < 0.001$; BMI at six months: 27.9 kg/m^2 (SD: 4.6), $p < 0.001$; and body weight at six months: 73.9 kg (SD: 11.5), $p < 0.001$) (Table 2). Patients presented with a mean of 62.5% (SD: 35.1) and 92.3% (SD: 49.8) %EWL at three and six months after bariatric surgery, respectively. Body fat mass (BFM) and fat free mass (FFM) also showed significant postoperative decreases at three months (BFM: $p < 0.001$; FFM: $p < 0.001$) and six months (BFM: $p = 0.002$; FFM: $p = 0.007$). Fasting plasma glucose levels decreased to 14.5% of the baseline at three months ($p = 0.028$), and 17.0% of the baseline at six months ($p = 0.034$). Patients' homeostatic model assessment of insulin resistance (HOMA-IR) improved at three months (2.8 (SD: 1.6), $p = 0.033$) and at six months (2.2 (SD: 0.6), $p = 0.044$) compared to the baseline. Mean systolic and diastolic blood pressures at six months were 126.1 mmHg and 83.1 mmHg, respectively, which represented a decrease of 11.6% and 14.9% from the baseline, respectively. Mean high-density lipoprotein (HDL) cholesterol and triglyceride levels at six months were 54.6 mg/dL and 115.6 mg/dL, respectively, which represented a 15.6% increase from the baseline (p = 0.041) and a decrease of 23.6% from the baseline (p = 0.016), respectively.

Table 2. Average values and percentage changes at three and six months after sleeve gastrectomy.

Variables	Measurement Time						
	Baseline (n = 27)	3 Months after Surgery (n = 27)			6 Months after Surgery (n = 27)		
	Values	Values	Change from Baseline, %	p	Values	Change from Baseline, %	p
Body-mass index, kg/m^2	38.7 ± 5.2	31.5 ± 5.1	−18.8 ± 4.2	<0.001	27.9 ± 4.6	−26.1 ± 4.6	<0.001
Body weight, kg	105.1 ± 17.0	85.1 ± 15.3	−18.8 ± 4.2	<0.001	73.9 ± 11.5	−26.1 ± 4.6	<0.001
% Excess weight loss		62.5 ± 35.1			92.3 ± 49.8		
Waist circumference, cm	120.5 ± 19.9	102.3 ± 13.6	−14.9 ± 7.4	<0.001 *	94.4 ± 13.5	−21.7 ± 7.3	<0.001 *
Body fat mass, kg	54.4 ± 12.0	35.5 ± 10.0	−28.7 ± 8.0	<0.001	26.0 ± 6.7	−46.5 ± 8.1	0.002
Fat free mass, kg	57.5 ± 9.9	50.3 ± 8.3	−10.3 ± 4.2	<0.001	48.6 ± 9.8	−12.0 ± 6.5	0.007
Fasting plasma glucose, mg/dL	131.6 ± 54.4	104.2 ± 17.6	−14.5 ± 33.3	0.028*	100.6 ± 18.6	−17.0 ± 29.2	0.034 *
HOMA-IR	6.4 ± 10.0	2.8 ± 1.6	−50.6 ± 36.4	0.033	2.2 ± 0.6	−47.1 ± 50.8	0.044
Systolic blood pressure, mmHg	142.6 ± 5.8	134.3 ± 6.3	5.7 ± 2.2	<0.001	126.1 ± 4.8	11.6 ± 2.2	<0.001
Diastolic blood pressure, mmHg	97.6 ± 6.2	89.3 ± 5.4	8.4 ± 3.2	<0.001	83.1 ± 5.7	14.9 ± 3.2	<0.001
High-density lipoprotein cholesterol, mg/dL	46.0 ± 10.4	49.2 ± 10.0	9.9 ± 31.6	0.792 *	54.6 ± 14.4	15.6 ± 20.9	0.041 *
Triglycerides, mg/dL	173.6 ± 82.2	131.3 ± 37.1	−10.7 ± 42.3	0.042 *	115.6 ± 37.0	−23.6 ± 31.7	0.016 *

HOMA-IR, Homeostasis model assessment-insulin resistance. Values are given as mean ± standard deviation. Body fat mass and fat free mass were measured with bioimpedance analyses. * p-Value was calculated with Wilcoxon signed rank test.

3.3. *Baseline AAMs and Weight Loss after Sleeve Gastrectomy*

Several baseline AAMs were associated with %EWL at three and six months after sleeve gastrectomy (Table 3). Baseline isoleucine was significantly associated with %EWL at three months (β (standard error (SE)): 0.67 (0.27); p = 0.026) and six months (β (SE): 1.02 (0.36); p = 0.016) postoperatively. Among metabolites from the serotonin pathway, 5-HIAA and 5-HIAA/serotonin ratio were significantly associated with %EWL at three months (serotonin: β (SE), −39.7 (13.5); p = 0.009; 5-HIAA: β (SE), 106.7 (32.5); p = 0.004; and 5-HIAA/serotonin ratio: β (SE), 54.7 (12.4); p < 0.001), and at six months (serotonin: β (SE), −50.8 (21.1); p = 0.032; 5-HIAA: β (SE), 125.2 (54.7)O; p = 0.040; and 5-HIAA/serotonin ratio: β (SE), 54.5 (21.6); p = 0.026) post bariatric surgery. The 5-HTrp/tryptophan ratio (β (SE): 64.6 (30.6); p = 0.049) and the serotonin/5-HTrp ratio (β (SE): −45.7 (14.1); p = 0.005) were significantly associated with %EWL at three months, but not at six months post bariatric surgery. The results of other AAMs are presented in Supplementary Table S4. Sensitivity analyses showed that the statistical significance did not change in the various patient groups (Supplementary Table S5).

Table 3. Association between baseline amino acid metabolites and %EWL at three and six months after sleeve gastrectomy.

	%EWL at 3 Months (n = 27)		%EWL at 6 Months (n = 27)	
	β (SE)	p	β (SE)	p
Branched-chain amino acids				
Leucine	0.24 (0.32)	0.455	0.26 (0.47)	0.576
Isoleucine	0.67 (0.27)	0.026	1.02 (0.36)	0.016
Valine	0.17 (0.19)	0.378	0.31 (0.28)	0.281
Aromatic amino acids				
Tryptophan	−0.57 (0.40)	0.169	−1.21 (0.59)	0.061
Phenylalanine	0.04 (0.48)	0.921	0.02 (0.76)	0.973
Tyrosine	−0.37 (0.26)	0.171	−0.52 (0.39)	0.208

Table 3. *Cont.*

	%EWL at 3 Months (n = 27)		%EWL at 6 Months (n = 27)	
	β (SE)	p	β (SE)	p
Sum of branched-chain amino acids	0.13 (0.09)	0.181	0.20 (0.13)	0.155
Sum of large neutral amino acids	−0.15 (0.13)	0.273	0.04 (0.10)	0.673
Metabolites from serotonin pathway				
5-hydroxytryptophan *	61.0 (37.8)	0.124	71.7 (62.6)	0.273
Serotonin	−39.7 (13.5)	0.009	−50.8 (21.1)	0.032
5-hydroxyindoleacetic acid *	106.7 (32.5)	0.004	125.2 (54.7)	0.040
Ratios of metabolites from serotonin pathway				
5-hydroxytryptophan / Tryptophan †	64.6 (30.6)	0.049	83.2 (45.8)	0.093
Serotonin / 5-hydroxytryptophan ‡	−45.7 (14.1)	0.005	−45.2 (23.1)	0.073
5- hydroxy-indoleacetic acid / Serotonin §	54.7 (12.4)	<0.001	54.5 (21.6)	0.026

%EWL, % excess weight loss; SE, standard error. Linear regression models were adjusted for baseline body mass index. %EWL was calculated by dividing the number of kilograms lost by the number of kilograms in a patient's excess body weight. Large neutral amino acids are a sum of branched-chain amino acids and aromatic amino acids. Results of metabolites from kynurenine, indole, and tyrosine pathway are shown in Supplemental Table S4. All simbols mean the same and significant association with %EWL

3.4. *Prediction for Slow Weight Loss after Sleeve Gastrectomy*

ROC curves were generated with isoleucine and metabolites from the serotonin pathway, which were significantly associated with %EWL after sleeve gastrectomy (Table 3). Serotonin and serotonin/5-HTrp ratio showed superior performance in predicting slow weight loss at three and six months postoperatively (Figure 1). The values of the AUROCs were, serotonin, 0.78 (95% CI: 0.58–0.97) at three months and 0.79 (95% CI: 0.59–0.97) at six months; serotonin/5-HTrp ratio, 0.81 (95% CI: 0.61–1.00) at three months and 0.80 (95% CI: 0.58–1.00) at six months.

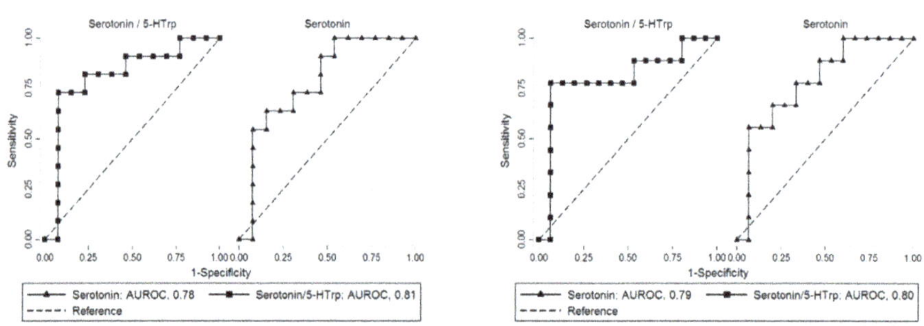

(A) (B)

Figure 1. Performance of baseline serotonin and serotonin/5-HTrp ratio in predicting slow weight loss at: (**A**) three months and (**B**) six months after sleeve gastrectomy. AUROCs were calculated using amino acid metabolites proven to be significant (Table 3). Among the test metabolites, serotonin and serotonin/5-HTrp ratio showed superior prognostic performance with the best discriminatory ability for predicting slow weight loss three and six months after sleeve gastrectomy. AUROC values included: serotonin, 0.78 (95% CI: 0.58–0.97) at three months and 0.79 (95% CI: 0.59–0.97) at six months; serotonin/5-HTrp ratio, 0.81 (95% CI: 0.61–1.00) at three months and 0.80 (95% CI: 0.58–1.00) at six months. 5-HTrp: 5-hydroxytryptophan, AUROC: area under receiver operating characteristic curves, CI: confidence interval.

4. Discussion

In this study, we showed that the profiles of obesity-related AAMs before sleeve gastrectomy were significantly associated with %EWL at three and six months postoperatively. Among the AAMs which proved to be significant, serotonin and the serotonin/5-HTrp ratio showed superior prognostic performance with the best discriminatory ability for slow weight loss at three and six months after sleeve gastrectomy. To our knowledge, these results are the first to suggest that pre-operative AAM profiles are useful biomarkers for predicting early postoperative weight status after sleeve gastrectomy.

Our findings, which highlight BCAAs, are noteworthy in the context of experimental and clinical data which suggest that BCAAs may be markers of insulin resistance in obesity [21,29,30]. Although changes in the levels of amino acids, including BCAAs and AAAs were observed in patients who underwent bariatric surgery [31–33], less knowledge is available regarding how pre-bariatric surgery amino acid profiles affect weight loss after bariatric surgery. Our data showed that pre-operative BCAA profiles, especially higher levels of serum isoleucine, were associated with more successful weight loss in the relatively early postoperative period (three and six months postoperatively) (Table 3). Given that isoleucine has been known to have a role in the improvement of visceral obesity and hyperinsulinemia and lipid metabolism in white adipose tissue [34,35], our findings support the opinion that hyper-isoleucinemia could be a pre-operative manifestation to predict optimal weight loss after sleeve gastrectomy.

Our results, which underscore serum metabolites from the serotonin pathway for predicting slow weight loss after sleeve gastrectomy, should also be viewed in the context of previous studies suggesting peripheral serotonin as a potential biological mediator in energy homeostasis [4,24]. Since serotonin cannot cross the blood-brain barrier, central and peripheral serotonin systems are functionally separated and serotonin is synthesized from the essential amino acid tryptophan by the sequential actions of tryptophan hydroxylase (TPH) and aromatic L-amino acid decarboxylase (AADC) (Supplementary Figure S1). Increased circulating serotonin levels are observed in mice with diet-induced obesity [22,36] and humans with obesity [37]. Additionally, gain-of-function polymorphisms in TPH, which promote hyperserotonemia, were associated with BMI and waist circumference in a genome-wide association study of nondiabetic individuals [38]. However, the absence of serotonin through a genetic or pharmacological block of peripheral TPH protects against the development of metabolic syndrome in mice on a high-fat diet [24,39].

Our results showed that lower levels of serotonin and higher levels of 5-HIAA before surgery were associated with higher %EWL at three and six months postoperatively (Table 3). In accordance with these results, lower level of serotonin/5-HTrp ratio (representing AADC activity) and higher level of 5-HIAA/serotonin ratio (representing monoamine oxidase A (MAO-A) activity), which promote hyposerotonemia, were associated with higher %EWL at three months postoperatively. Serotonin and serotonin/5-HTrp ratio in particular showed superior performance in predicting slow weight loss three and six months after sleeve gastrectomy (Figure 1). Circulating serotonin has been known to interact with multiple organs and stimulate insulin secretion and lipogenesis, thereby accelerating the energy storage process of the body [40]. Our findings on the association between hyposerotonemia and rapid postoperative weight loss is in line with previous studies that have demonstrated that peripheral serotonin can promote efficient energy storage. Our results are the first to suggest that serum metabolites from the serotonin pathway predict weight loss after sleeve gastrectomy and further studies are warranted to assess whether the serotonin pathway contributes to a variability in the weight loss response.

This study had several limitations. First, our results did not preclude that other serum metabolites may also predict weight status after sleeve gastrectomies. For example, analyzing downstream kynurenine pathway metabolites such as quinolinic acid and nicotinamide adenine dinucleotide, and BCAA metabolites such as alanine, glutamine, and glutamate would require further evaluation. Secondly, postoperative energy balance, mainly determined by caloric intake and expenditure, could also affect postoperative weight status. Although we monitored compliance and postoperative diet and exercise recommendations every two weeks, bias could occur due to indirect supervision via telephone or text messages. Thirdly, supplementation of amino acids may also modify the alteration in postoperative weight status [41,42]. However, we followed and monitored the equivalent intake of oral amino acid supplements during the study and various sensitivity analyses showed a consistency of statistical significance for the overall results. Fourthly, our study was conducted on a small number of Asian patients with relatively low BMIs and high rates of metabolic syndrome (the mean BMI was 38.7 kg/m^2 and 78% of the patients had metabolic syndrome). Caution is advised in applying our results to patients of other ethnicities, patients with higher BMIs, or patients with lower rates of metabolic syndrome. Our results should be further validated in studies with more patients. Fifthly, as an early postoperative study, our results preclude the usefulness of preoperative AAM profile for predicting long term weight status after sleeve gastrectomy. Sixthly, our results should be interpreted with caution for a potential type I error induced by multiple comparisons.

5. Conclusions

In conclusion, pre-operative profiles of AAMs (especially those of serotonin and serotonin/5-HTrp ratio) showed superior predictive performances for weight status three and six months after sleeve gastrectomy. Further studies are warranted to assess whether measurements of serum AAMs might assist in the identification of patients who maintain successful weight loss in long-term follow-ups and to elucidate the biological mechanisms by which certain AAMs might mediate successful weight loss after sleeve gastrectomy.

Supplementary Materials: The following are available online at http://www.mdpi.com/2077-0383/9/8/2348/s1, Figure S1: Amino acid metabolites analyzed in the current study, Table S1: Inclusion and exclusion criteria, Table S2: Protocol for measurement of serum amino acids metabolites, Table S3: Chromatographic Retention time (RT), selected MRM parameters, DP, EP, CE, CXP for each analyte measured, Table S4: Association between baseline amino acid metabolites and %EWL at 3 and 6 month after sleeve gastrectomy, Table S5: Sensitivity analyses: association between baseline serotonin and serotonin/5-hydroxytryptophan ratio, and %EWL after sleeve gastrectomy.

Author Contributions: Conceptualization, Y.K. and M.J.; methodology, Y.K. and M.J.; formal analysis, Y.K., M.J. and Y.L.; investigation, Y.K. and M.J.; writing-original draft preparation, Y.K. and J.H.; writing-review and editing, Y.K. and S.P.; visualization, Y.K. and S.P. All authors have read and agreed to the published version of the manuscript

Funding: This research was supported by Korea University Grant (K1912791), and Basic Science Research Program through the National Research Foundation of Korea (NRF) funded by the Ministry of Education (2020R1I1A1A01070106)

Conflicts of Interest: The authors declare no conflict of interest.

References

1. Gloy, V.L.; Briel, M.; Bhatt, D.L.; Kashyap, S.R.; Schauer, P.R.; Mingrone, G.; Bucher, H.C.; Nordmann, A.J. Bariatric surgery versus non-surgical treatment for obesity: A systematic review and meta-analysis of randomised controlled trials. *BMJ* **2013**, *347*, f5934. [CrossRef]
2. Adams, T.D.; Davidson, L.E.; Litwin, S.E.; Kim, J.; Kolotkin, R.L.; Nanjee, M.N.; Gutierrez, J.M.; Frogley, S.J.; Ibele, A.R.; Brinton, E.A.; et al. Weight and metabolic outcomes 12 years after gastric bypass. *N. Engl. J. Med.* **2017**, *377*, 1143–1155. [CrossRef] [PubMed]
3. Sjöström, L.; Narbro, K.; Sjöström, C.D.; Karason, K.; Larsson, B.; Wedel, H.; Lystig, T.; Sullivan, M.; Bouchard, C.; Carlsson, B.; et al. Effects of bariatric surgery on mortality in Swedish obese subjects. *N. Engl. J. Med.* **2007**, *357*, 741–752. [CrossRef] [PubMed]
4. Oh, C.M.; Namkung, J.; Go, Y.; Shong, K.E.; Kim, K.; Kim, H.; Park, B.Y.; Lee, H.W.; Jeon, Y.H.; Song, J.; et al. Regulation of systemic energy homeostasis by serotonin in adipose tissues. *Nat. Commun.* **2015**, *6*, 6794. [CrossRef] [PubMed]
5. Courcoulas, A.P.; Christian, N.J.; Belle, S.H.; Berk, P.D.; Flum, D.R.; Garcia, L.; Horlick, M.; Kalarchian, M.A.; King, W.C.; Mitchell, J.E.; et al. Weight change and health outcomes at 3 years after bariatric surgery among individuals with severe obesity. *JAMA* **2013**, *310*, 2416–2425. [CrossRef]

6. Puzziferri, N.; Nakonezny, P.A.; Livingston, E.H.; Carmody, T.J.; Provost, D.A.; Rush, A.J. Variations of weight loss following gastric bypass and gastric band. *Ann. Surg.* **2008**, *248*, 233. [CrossRef]
7. Sjöström, L. Review of the key results from the Swedish Obese Subjects (SOS) trial—A prospective controlled intervention study of bariatric surgery. *J. Intern. Med.* **2013**, *273*, 219–234. [CrossRef]
8. Courcoulas, A.P.; King, W.C.; Belle, S.H.; Berk, P.; Flum, D.R.; Garcia, L.; Gourash, W.; Horlick, M.; Mitchell, J.E.; Pomp, A.; et al. Seven-year weight trajectories and health outcomes in the Longitudinal Assessment of Bariatric Surgery (LABS) study. *JAMA Surg.* **2018**, *153*, 427–434. [CrossRef]
9. Karlsson, J.; Taft, C.; Ryden, A.; Sjöström, L.; Sullivan, M. Ten-year trends in health-related quality of life after surgical and conventional treatment for severe obesity: The SOS intervention study. *Int. J. Obes.* **2007**, *31*, 1248. [CrossRef]
10. Karmali, S.; Brar, B.; Shi, X.; Sharma, A.M.; de Gara, C.; Birch, D.W. Weight recidivism post-bariatric surgery: A systematic review. *Obes. Surg.* **2013**, *23*, 1922–1933. [CrossRef]
11. Laurino Neto, R.M.; Herbella, F.A.; Tauil, R.M.; Silva, F.S.; de Lima, S.E., Jr. Comorbidities remission after Roux-en-Y Gastric Bypass for morbid obesity is sustained in a long-term follow-up and correlates with weight regain. *Obes. Surg.* **2012**, *22*, 1580–1585. [CrossRef] [PubMed]
12. Mor, A.; Sharp, L.; Portenier, D.; Sudan, R.; Torquati, A. Weight loss at first postoperative visit predicts long-term outcome of Roux-en-Y gastric bypass using Duke weight loss surgery chart. *Surg. Obes. Relat. Dis.* **2012**, *8*, 556–560. [CrossRef] [PubMed]
13. Manning, S.; Pucci, A.; Carter, N.C.; Elkalaawy, M.; Querci, G.; Magno, S.; Tamberi, A.; Finer, N.; Fiennes, A.G.; Hashemi, M.; et al. Early postoperative weight loss predicts maximal weight loss after sleeve gastrectomy and Roux-en-Y gastric bypass. *Surg. Endosc.* **2015**, *29*, 1484–1491. [CrossRef] [PubMed]
14. Rudolph, A.; Hilbert, A. Post-operative behavioural management in bariatric surgery: A systematic review and meta-analysis of randomized controlled trials. *Obes. Rev.* **2013**, *14*, 292–302. [CrossRef]
15. Nijamkin, M.P.; Campa, A.; Sosa, J.; Baum, M.; Himburg, S.; Johnson, P. Comprehensive nutrition and lifestyle education improves weight loss and physical activity in Hispanic Americans following gastric bypass surgery: A randomized controlled trial. *J. Acad. Nutr. Diet.* **2012**, *112*, 382–390. [CrossRef]
16. Stipanuk, M.H. Leucine and protein synthesis: mTOR and beyond. *Nutr. Rev.* **2007**, *65*, 122–129. [CrossRef]
17. Dadvar, S.; Ferreira, D.M.; Cervenka, I.; Ruas, J.L. The weight of nutrients: Kynurenine metabolites in obesity and exercise. *J. Intern. Med.* **2018**, *284*, 519–533. [CrossRef]
18. Herman, M.A.; She, P.; Peroni, O.D.; Lynch, C.J.; Kahn, B.B. Adipose tissue branched chain amino acid (BCAA) metabolism modulates circulating BCAA levels. *J. Boil. Chem.* **2010**, *285*, 11348–11356. [CrossRef]
19. Namkung, J.; Kim, H.; Park, S. Peripheral serotonin: A new player in systemic energy homeostasis. *Mol. Cells* **2015**, *38*, 1023.
20. Lynch, C.J.; Adams, S.H. Branched-chain amino acids in metabolic signalling and insulin resistance. *Nat. Rev. Endocrinol.* **2014**, *10*, 723. [CrossRef]
21. Newgard, C.B.; An, J.; Bain, J.R.; Muehlbauer, M.J.; Stevens, R.D.; Lien, L.F.; Haqq, A.M.; Shah, S.H.; Arlotto, M.; Slentz, C.A.; et al. A branched-chain amino acid-related metabolic signature that differentiates obese and lean humans and contributes to insulin resistance. *Cell Metab.* **2009**, *9*, 311–326. [CrossRef] [PubMed]
22. Kim, H.J.; Kim, J.H.; Noh, S.; Hur, H.J.; Sung, M.J.; Hwang, J.T.; Park, J.H.; Yang, H.J.; Kim, M.S.; Kwon, D.Y.; et al. Metabolomic analysis of livers and serum from high-fat diet induced obese mice. *J. Proteome Res.* **2011**, *10*, 722–731. [CrossRef] [PubMed]
23. Haub, S.; Ritze, Y.; Ladel, I.; Saum, K.; Hubert, A.; Spruss, A.; Trautwein, C.; Bischoff, S.C. Serotonin receptor type 3 antagonists improve obesity-associated fatty liver disease in mice. *J. Pharmacol. Exp. Ther.* **2011**, *339*, 790–798. [CrossRef] [PubMed]
24. Crane, J.D.; Palanivel, R.; Mottillo, E.P.; Bujak, A.L.; Wang, H.; Ford, R.J.; Collins, A.; Blümer, R.M.; Fullerton, M.D.; Yabut, J.M.; et al. Inhibiting peripheral serotonin synthesis reduces obesity and metabolic dysfunction by promoting brown adipose tissue thermogenesis. *Nat. Med.* **2015**, *21*, 166–172. [CrossRef]
25. Martin, A.M.; Young, R.L.; Leong, L.; Rogers, G.B.; Spencer, N.J.; Jessup, C.F.; Keating, D.J. The Diverse Metabolic Roles of Peripheral Serotonin. *Endocrinology* **2017**, *158*, 1049–1063. [CrossRef] [PubMed]
26. Chang, S.H.; Stoll, C.R.; Song, J.; Varela, J.E.; Eagon, C.J.; Colditz, G.A. The effectiveness and risks of bariatric surgery: An updated systematic review and meta-analysis, 2003–2012. *JAMA Surg.* **2014**, *149*, 275–287. [CrossRef]

27. Parrott, J.; Frank, L.; Rabena, R.; Craggs-Dino, L.; Isom, K.A.; Greiman, L. American Society for Metabolic and Bariatric Surgery integrated health nutritional guidelines for the surgical weight loss patient 2016 update: Micronutrients. *Surg. Obes. Relat. Dis.* **2017**, *13*, 727–741. [CrossRef]
28. Borg, G.A. Psychophysical bases of perceived exertion. *Med. Sci. Sports Exerc.* **1982**, *14*, 377–381. [CrossRef]
29. Shaham, O.; Wei, R.; Wang, T.J.; Ricciardi, C.; Lewis, G.D.; Vasan, R.S.; Carr, S.A.; Thadhani, R.; Gerszten, R.E.; Mootha, V.K. Metabolic profiling of the human response to a glucose challenge reveals distinct axes of insulin sensitivity. *Mol. Syst. Biol.* **2008**, *4*, 214. [CrossRef]
30. Huffman, K.M.; Shah, S.H.; Stevens, R.D.; Bain, J.R.; Muehlbauer, M.; Slentz, C.A.; Tanner, C.J.; Kuchibhatla, M.; Houmard, J.A.; Newgard, C.B.; et al. Relationships between circulating metabolic intermediates and insulin action in overweight to obese, inactive men and women. *Diabetes Care* **2009**, *32*, 1678–1683. [CrossRef]
31. Liu, R.; Hong, J.; Xu, X.; Feng, Q.; Zhang, D.; Gu, Y.; Shi, J.; Zhao, S.; Liu, W.; Wang, X.; et al. Gut microbiome and serum metabolome alterations in obesity and after weight-loss intervention. *Nat. Med.* **2017**, *23*, 859–868. [CrossRef] [PubMed]
32. Gralka, E.; Luchinat, C.; Tenori, L.; Ernst, B.; Thurnheer, M.; Schultes, B. Metabolomic fingerprint of severe obesity is dynamically affected by bariatric surgery in a procedure-dependent manner. *Am. J. Clin. Nutr.* **2015**, *102*, 1313–1322. [CrossRef] [PubMed]
33. Modesitt, S.C.; Hallowell, P.T.; Slack-Davis, J.K.; Michalek, R.D.; Atkins, K.A.; Kelley, S.L.; Arapovic, S.; Shupnik, M.A.; Hoehn, K. Women at extreme risk for obesity-related carcinogenesis: Baseline endometrial pathology and impact of bariatric surgery on weight, metabolic profiles and quality of life. *Gynecol. Oncol.* **2015**, *138*, 238–245. [CrossRef] [PubMed]
34. Doi, M.; Yamaoka, I.; Nakayama, M.; Mochizuki, S.; Sugahara, K.; Yoshizawa, F. Isoleucine, a blood glucose-lowering amino acid, increases glucose uptake in rat skeletal muscle in the absence of increases in AMP-activated protein kinase activity. *J. Nutr.* **2005**, *135*, 2103–2108. [CrossRef] [PubMed]
35. Nishimura, J.; Masaki, T.; Arakawa, M.; Seike, M.; Yoshimatsu, H. Isoleucine prevents the accumulation of tissue triglycerides and upregulates the expression of PPARα and uncoupling protein in diet-induced obese mice. *J. Nutr.* **2010**, *140*, 496–500. [CrossRef]
36. Bertrand, R.L.; Senadheera, S.; Markus, I.; Liu, L.; Howitt, L.; Chen, H.; Murphy, T.V.; Sandow, S.L.; Bertrand, P.P. A Western diet increases serotonin availability in rat small intestine. *Endocrinology* **2011**, *152*, 36–47. [CrossRef]
37. Young, R.L.; Lumsden, A.L.; Martin, A.M.; Schober, G.; Pezos, N.; Thazhath, S.S.; Isaacs, N.J.; Cvijanovic, N.; Sun, E.W.L.; Wu, T.; et al. Augmented capacity for peripheral serotonin release in human obesity. *Int. J. Obes.* **2018**, *42*, 1880–1889. [CrossRef]
38. Kwak, S.H.; Park, B.L.; Kim, H.; German, M.S.; Go, M.J.; Jung, H.S.; Koo, B.K.; Cho, Y.M.; Choi, S.H.; Cho, Y.S.; et al. Association of variations in TPH1 and HTR2B with gestational weight gain and measures of obesity. *Obesity* **2012**, *20*, 233–238. [CrossRef]
39. Sumara, G.; Sumara, O.; Kim, J.K.; Karsenty, G. Gut-derived serotonin is a multifunctional determinant to fasting adaptation. *Cell Metab.* **2012**, *16*, 588–600. [CrossRef]
40. Yabut, J.M.; Crane, J.D.; Green, A.E.; Keating, D.J.; Khan, W.I.; Steinberg, G.R. Emerging Roles for Serotonin in Regulating Metabolism: New Implications for an Ancient Molecule. *Endocr. Rev.* **2019**, *40*, 1092–1107. [CrossRef]
41. Cummings, N.E.; Williams, E.M.; Kasza, I.; Konon, E.N.; Schaid, M.D.; Schmidt, B.A.; Poudel, C.; Sherman, D.S.; Yu, D.; Arriola Apelo, S.I.; et al. Restoration of metabolic health by decreased consumption of branched-chain amino acids. *J. Physiol.* **2018**, *596*, 623–645. [CrossRef] [PubMed]
42. Qin, L.Q.; Xun, P.; Bujnowski, D.; Daviglus, M.L.; Van Horn, L.; Stamler, J.; He, K. Higher branched-chain amino acid intake is associated with a lower prevalence of being overweight or obese in middle-aged East Asian and Western adults. *J. Nutr.* **2011**, *141*, 249–254. [CrossRef] [PubMed]

Journal of
Clinical Medicine

MDPI

Article

Additional Metabolic Effects of Bariatric Surgery in Patients with a Poor Mid-Term Weight Loss Response: A 5-Year Follow-Up Study

David Benaiges [1,2,3,4,*], Maria Bisbe [1], Juan Pedro-Botet [1,2,3], Aleix de Vargas-Machuca [1], Jose M. Ramon [5], Manuel Pera [5], Montserrat Villatoro [3], Laia Fontané [3,4], Helena Julià [1,3], Elisenda Climent [1,2,3], Olga Castañer [2,6], Juana A. Flores-Le Roux [1,2,3] and Alberto Goday [1,2,3,6]

1 Departament de Medicina, Universitat Autònoma de Barcelona, 08139 Barcelona, Spain; mbisbe01@gmail.com (M.B.); 86620@parcdesalutmar.cat (J.P.-B.); aleixdevargasmachuca@gmail.com (A.d.V.-M.); 62257@parcdesalutmar.cat (H.J.); 61063@parcdesalutmar.cat (E.C.); 94066@parcdesalutmar.cat (J.A.F.-L.R.); Agoday@parcdesalutmar.cat (A.G.)
2 Cardiovascular Risk and Nutrition Research Group (CARIN-ULEC), IMIM-Hospital del Mar, Barcelona, Biomedical Research Park (Parc de Recerca Biomèdica de Barcelona-PRBB), 08003 Barcelona, Spain; ocastaner@imim.es
3 Department of Endocrinology and Nutrition, Hospital del Mar, 08003 Barcelona, Spain; 93954@parcdesalutmar.cat (M.V.); lfontane@parcdesalutmar.cat (L.F.)
4 Consorci Sanitari de l'Alt Penedès i Garraf, 08720 Vilafranca del Pendès, Spain
5 Unit of Gastrointestinal Surgery, Hospital del Mar, Institut de Recerca IMIM-Hospital del Mar, 08003 Barcelona, Spain; 16350@parcdesalutmar.cat (J.M.R.); 95405@parcdesalutmar.cat (M.P.)
6 Centro de Investigaciones Biomédicas en Red de Obesidad y Nutrición, CIBERobn, 28029 Madrid, Spain
* Correspondence: 96002@parcdesalutmar.cat; Tel.: +34-932483902; Fax: +34-932483254

Received: 3 August 2020; Accepted: 28 September 2020; Published: 1 October 2020

Abstract: To ascertain the 5-year metabolic effects of bariatric surgery in poor weight loss (WL) responders and establish associated factors. Methods: Retrospective analysis of a non-randomised prospective cohort of bariatric surgery patients completing a 5-year follow-up. Mid-term poor WL was considered when 5-year excess weight loss was <50%. Results: Forty-three (20.3%) of the 212 included patients were mid-term poor WL responders. They showed an improvement in all metabolic markers at 2 years, except for total cholesterol. This improvement with respect to baseline was maintained at 5 years for plasma glucose, HbA1c, HOMA, HDL and diastolic blood pressure; however, LDL cholesterol, triglycerides and systolic blood pressure were similar to presurgical values. Comorbidity remission rates were comparable to those obtained in the good WL group except for hypercholesterolaemia (45.8% vs. poor WL, $p = 0.005$). On multivariate analysis, lower baseline HDL cholesterol levels, advanced age and lower preoperative weight loss were independently associated with poor mid-term WL. Conclusions: Although that 1 in 5 patients presented suboptimal WL 5 years after bariatric surgery, other important metabolic benefits were maintained.

Keywords: bariatric surgery; obesity; severe obesity; weight loss; weight regain; sleeve gastrectomy; gastric bypass

1. Introduction

Undoubtedly, bariatric surgery (BS) has proved to be the most effective treatment for morbidly-obese patients when conventional therapy has failed. Its health benefits have been shown to extend beyond weight loss, with improvement in or even remission of obesity-related comorbidities such as type 2 diabetes, hypertension or dyslipidaemia [1,2].

Several studies have shown that post-surgical weight loss varies widely among patients and a notable percentage can be qualified as poor weight loss (WL) responders [3–6]. They are more frequently identified at mid-term follow-up taking into account that most patients experience a slight weight regain from the first year post-surgery [3,7,8]. Despite being a widely recognised group, no previous studies focused on the evolution of metabolic parameters and comorbidity remission rates 5 years after BS. To our knowledge, the Farias et al. study is the only work comparing good and poor WL responders. Those authors only reported results on the remission rates of obesity-related comorbidities with a shorter follow-up (2 years) [6].

We can hypothesise that patients with poor WL at 5 years will also benefit from BS considering two aspects: firstly, weight loss is not the only factor responsible for the improvement in comorbidities in BS; other phenomena, such as hormonal mechanisms, have been established [9–12]. Secondly, patients considered as poor WL responders have been defined by a percentage excess weight loss (%EWL) < 50%. However, despite not achieving an optimal WL at 5 years, patient weight remained lower than that at baseline. Thus, the primary aim of the present study was to determine the benefits of BS in poor WL responders at 5 years, compare them with good WL responders and identify the pre-surgical factors associated with a poor WL response to BS.

2. Experimental Section

2.1. Study Protocol

A retrospective analysis was conducted of a non-randomised prospective cohort study of severely-obese patients undergoing BS at the Hospital del Mar, Barcelona from January 2004 to December 2014. Patients were between 18 and 60 years of age and met the 1991 BS criteria of the National Institutes of Health [13]. Patients with a body mass index (BMI) of 35–39 kg/m^2 and metabolic abnormalities as well as patients with BMI > 40 kg/m^2 were included. The indication for the type of surgical procedure (laparoscopic sleeve gastrectomy [LSG] and laparoscopic Roux-en-Y gastric bypass [LRYGB]) was based on clinical criteria and the consensus of the BS Unit. In this respect, LSG was preferred in younger patients, in those with a BMI 35–40 kg/m^2, as a first-step treatment in cases with BMI > 50 kg/m^2 (although given the positive LSG outcomes none of these patients had to further undergo LRYGB), and when drug malabsorption was to be avoided. Patients who did not complete a minimum of 5 years of follow-up were excluded. In accordance with the study protocol, all patients were evaluated preoperatively and at 3, 6, 12, 18 and 24 months post-surgery and annually thereafter by the same surgeon, endocrinologist and nutritionist. Protocol visits included measurements of weight, waist, hip circumferences, blood pressure, assessment of comorbidity status and laboratory tests for glucose, insulin, glycated haemoglobin (HbA1c), total cholesterol, high-density lipoprotein (HDL) cholesterol and triglyceride levels. All subjects provided their informed consent for the procedure and the study. The Ethics Committee of Parc de Salut Mar (2017/7722) approved the protocol in accordance with the ethical guidelines of the 1975 Declaration of Helsinki.

2.2. Anthropometric and Biochemical Measurements

BMI was calculated as weight in kilograms divided by the square of height in metres and the %EWL was based on weight in excess of that corresponding to a BMI of 25 kg/m^2 for each patient. Poor WL responders were defined as those whose EWL did not reach 50% during post-surgical follow-up [3]. Patients whose %EWL at 5 years was under 50% were considered poor mid-term WL responders. Glucose was determined by the oxidase method. HbA1c was quantified by chromatography (Biosystem, Barcelona, Spain). Insulin was measured by radioimmunoassay (Insulin kit, DPC, Los Angeles, CA, USA). Homeostasis model assessment for insulin-resistance (HOMA-IR) indices was estimated using the following formula [14]: HOMA-IR = insulin (U/mL) fasting glucose (mmol/L)/22.5. Total cholesterol and triglycerides were determined using enzymatic methods in a Cobas Mira automatic analyser (Baxter Diagnostics AG, Düdingen, Switzerland). HDL cholesterol was measured using separation by precipitation with phosphotungstic acid and magnesium chloride and low-density lipoprotein (LDL) cholesterol concentration was calculated with the Friedewald formula [15]. In accordance with data from our population, the cut-off level for the HOMA-IR index to define insulin resistance was ≥3.29 [16]. Diabetes was considered when at least one of the following criteria was met: plasma glucose determination > 126 mg/dL, HbA1c > 6.5% or current treatment with antidiabetic medication or insulin. By contrast, diabetes remission was considered when plasma glucose < 100 mg/dL, HbA1c < 6.0% and no anti-diabetic medication was needed. Hypercholesterolaemia was defined as total cholesterol > 200 mg/dL or use of statin treatment. Remission was considered when total cholesterol was < 200 mg/dL in the absence of statin treatment. Hypertriglyceridaemia implied triglyceride levels > 150 mg/dL or fibrate treatment. Remission was considered when triglyceridaemia <150 mg/dL and no fibrate treatment was needed. Hypertension was defined as systolic blood pressure > 140 mmHg and/or diastolic blood pressure > 90 mmHg or need for antihypertensive treatment. Remission was considered when systolic < 140 mmHg and diastolic blood pressure < 90 mmHg and no antihypertensive treatment was needed.

2.3. Surgical Techniques

The LRYGB technique consisted of a 150 cm antecolic Roux limb with a 25-mm circular pouch-jejunostomy and exclusion of 50 cm of the proximal jejunum. In LSG, a longitudinal resection of the stomach from the angle of His to approximately 5 cm proximal to the pylorus was made using a 36 French bougie inserted along the lesser curvature. The same team of surgeons performed all operations [12].

2.4. Study Power Calculation

Accepting an alpha risk of 0.05 and a beta risk of 0.2 in a two-sided test, 135 subjects were necessary in the first group and 33 in the second to recognize as statistically significant a difference greater than or equal to 20 mg/dL in 5 years total cholesterol change. The common standard deviation for total cholesterol change was assumed to be 37 [17].

2.5. Statistical Analysis

Statistical analysis was calculated with IBM SPSS Statistics for Windows, Version 25.0 (Armonk, NY, USA: IBM Corp.). Data were expressed as percentages and frequencies for categorical variables, as mean ± standard deviation for continuous variables with a normal distribution and as median with interquartile range for continuous variables with a non-normal distribution. Normality was evaluated using the Kolmogorov-Smirnov test. For skewed variables, a logarithmic transformation was used to achieve normality. Fisher exact test or ×2 test was applied to determine the association between qualitative variables and Student t test to compare mean and standard deviations of quantitative variables Two-factor mixed ANOVA models were used to evaluate the evolution of continuous variables in each group and analyse differences between groups at each time point from baseline. Logistic regression analysiswas applied to evaluate factors independently associated with poor mid-term WL. All variables associated on univariate analysis ($p < 0.1$) with poor weight loss responders were included in the regression model. A p value < 0.05 was considered statistically significant.

3. Results

One hundred and forty-four (40.4%) of the 356 patients who underwent BS between January 2004 and December 2014 were excluded due to lack of follow-up beyond 5 years. Therefore, 212 patients completed 5 years of follow-up and were included in this study. Baseline characteristics of the included patients are shown in Table 1.

As shown in Figure 1, the maximum proportion of good WL was present at 18 months post-surgery with a progressive decline thereafter. At 5 years, 43 patients (20.3%) presented EWL <50% and were considered poor mid-term WL responders. Baseline characteristics of poor WL responders at 5 years were comparable to good WL responders except for age, HDL cholesterol and type of surgery (Table 1). The %EWL and BMI trajectories of the two groups of subjects are depicted in Figures 2 and 3, respectively. Differences between groups, in %EWL and BMI, were already apparent 6 months after surgery ($p < 0.001$) and remained significant throughout follow-up.

Table 1. Baseline characteristics of all included patients, good and poor mid-term weight loss responders.

	Included Patients ($n = 212$)	Good Mid-Term WL Responders ($n = 169$)	Poor Mid-Term WL Responders ($n = 43$)	p Value *
Age (years)	45.4 ± 8.9	44.7 ± 8.9	48.4 ± 8.4	0.015
Female (%)	176 (83.0)	140 (82.8)	36 (83.7)	0.548
BMI (kg/m^2)	44.2 ± 5.0	44.1 ± 4.9	44.7 ± 5.5	0.482
LRYGB (%)	131 (61.8)	110 (65.1)	21 (48.8)	0.038
Preoperative %EWL (%)	12.1 ± 13.0	12.9 ± 12.7	8.7 ± 13.5	0.064
Abdominal waist (cm)	126.3 ± 11.9	125.9 ± 12	127.7 ± 11.6	0.468
Systolic BP (mmHg)	139 ± 19.5	138.6 ± 20.0	140.6 ± 17.8	0.538
Diastolic BP (mmHg)	85.9 ± 11.7	86.12 ± 11.9	85.1 ± 11.0	0.603
Glycaemia (mg/dL)	118.4 ± 40.4	116 ± 41.6	127.7 ± 33.9	0.089
Insulin (mU/mL)	16.8 ± 14.4	16.8 ± 15.5	16.9 ± 9.0	0.959
HOMA-IR	5.5 ± 7.7	5.5 ± 8.4	5.5 ± 3.5	0.999
HbA1c (%)	5.97 ± 3.42	5.98 ± 3.8	5.93 ± 0.79	0.944
Total cholesterol (mg/dL)	194.8 ± 34.1	195.5 ± 34.5	191.72 ± 32.7	0.512
HDL cholesterol (mg/dL)	50.7 ± 15.6	51.9 ± 16.3	45.9 ± 11.5	0.023
LDL cholesterol (mg/dL)	118.6 ± 33.0	118.4 ± 34.2	119.6 ± 28.4	0.828
Triglycerides (mg/dL)	106.5 (82.3–151.5)	119.0 (90.0–146.0)	104.0 (77.5–152.5)	0.583
Hypertension * (%)	93 (43.9)	77 (45.6)	16 (37.2)	0.209
Anti-hypertensive drugs	77 (36.3)	62 (36.7)	15 (34.9)	0.826
Diabetes (%)	53 (25)	38 (22.5)	15 (34.9)	0.072
Oral antidiabetic drugs	26 (12.3)	15 (8.9)	11 (25.6)	0.002
Insulin	5 (2.4)	5 (3.0)	0	0.253
Dyslipidaemia (%)	61 (28.8)	45 (26.6)	16 (37.2)	0.120
Statins	31 (14.6)	21 (12.4)	10 (23.3)	0.065
Fibrates	12 (5.7)	9 (5.3)	3 (7.0)	0.454
Cigarette smoking (%)	58 (27.5)	47 (28.0)	11 (25.6)	0.458

WL = weight loss; BMI = body mass index; LRYGB = laparoscopic Roux en Y gastric bypass; %EWL = percentage excess weight loss; BP = blood pressure; HbA1c = glycated haemoglobin; HDL = high-density lipoprotein; HOMA-IR = homeostasis model assessment for insulin resistance; LDL = low-density lipoprotein. * p values for comparisons between poor and good weight loss.

Changes in metabolic markers after BS in good and poor WL responders are shown in Table 2. Good mid-term WL responders showed a significant decrease in systolic and diastolic blood pressure, plasma glucose, HbA1c, HOMA-IR, total cholesterol, LDL cholesterol, and triglycerides and an increase in HDL cholesterol 2 years after BS. Improvement in these metabolic parameters was maintained at 5 years. Poor mid-term WL responders also showed an improvement in all metabolic markers at 2 years, except for total cholesterol. This improvement with respect to baseline was maintained at 5 years for plasma glucose, HbA1c, HOMA, HDL cholesterol and diastolic blood pressure; LDL cholesterol, triglycerides, systolic blood pressure became similar to pre-surgical values. When the 2- and 5-year evolution of these metabolic parameters was compared between good and poor WL responders, significant differences were found regarding 2- and 5-year total cholesterol changes and 5-year triglyceride variation.

When the remission rates of obesity-associated comorbidities were analysed, no significant differences were found between good and poor WL responders at 2 and 5 years post-surgery except for hypercholesterolaemia remission (Table 3).

On the multivariate analysis, lower baseline HDL cholesterol levels, advanced age and lower preoperative weight loss were independently associated with poor mid-term WL (Table 4).

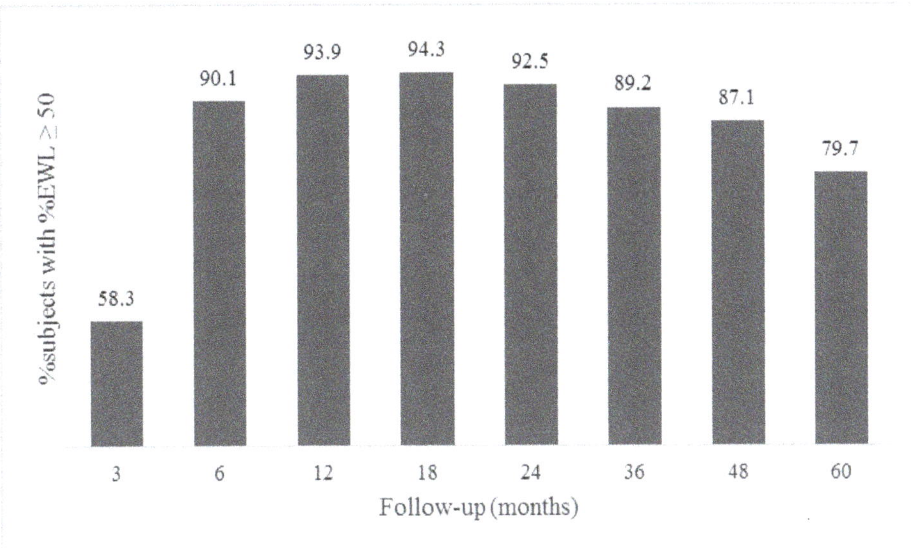

Figure 1. Percentage of good weight loss responders throughout follow-up. %EWL = percentage excess weight loss.

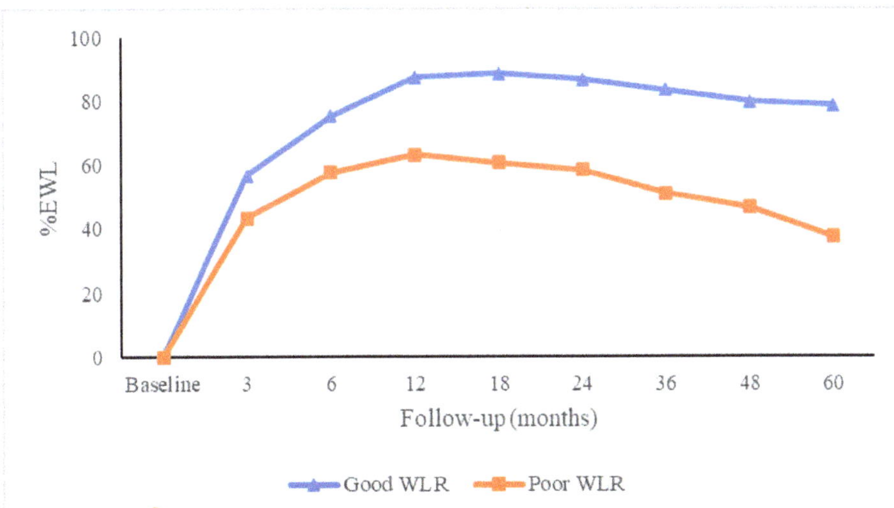

Figure 2. Changes in percentage of excess weight loss in good and poor weight loss responders during follow-up after the bariatric surgical procedure. %EWL = percentage excess weight loss; WLR = weight loss responders.

Table 2. Evolution of metabolic markers of good and poor WL at baseline, 2 and 5 years after bariatric surgery.

	Good Mid-Term WLR (n = 169)					Poor Mid-Term WLR (n = 43)					Good vs. Poor WLR 2 Years	Good vs. Poor WLR 5 Years
	Baseline	2 Years	* p Value	5 Years	† p Value	Baseline	2 Years	* p Value	5 Years	† p Value	p Value	p Value
Glucose (mg/dL)	116.8 ± 43.1	90.0 ± 11.5	<0.001	91.7 ± 11.1	<0.001	126.4 ± 33.5	93.8 ± 12.1	<0.001	98.4 ± 13.1	<0.001	0.244	0.379
HbA1c (%)	5.8 ± 1.1	5.3 ± 0.6	<0.001	5.5 ± 0.6	<0.001	6.0 ± 0.8	5.4 ± 0.4	<0.001	5.5 ± 0.4	0.018	0.496	0.261
HOMA	5.8 ± 10.0	1.0 ± 0.8	<0.001	1.1 ± 0.9	<0.001	5.6 ± 3.4	1.7 ± 1.7	<0.001	2.3 ± 1.9	<0.001	0.701	0.447
Cholesterol (mg/dL)	197.4 ± 34.1	182.2 ± 31.8	<0.001	190.4 ± 34.9	0.015	192.3 ± 33.5	187.5 ± 34.7	0.714	196.9 ± 35.7	0.107	0.018	0.027
HDL cholesterol (mg/dL)	52.5 ± 17.1	68.7 ± 16.4	<0.001	70.7 ± 17.4	<0.001	45.5 ± 11.6	61.7 ± 14.3	<0.001	60.7 ± 18.6	<0.001	0.926	0.382
LDL cholesterol (mg/dL)	118.8 ± 35.5	98.8 ± 28.9	<0.001	103.5 ± 29.1	<0.001	120.8 ± 28.2	109.9 ± 27.1	0.016	114.3 ± 30.5	0.114	0.073	0.130
Triglycerides (mg/dL)	104.0 (77.5–52.5)	66.0 (53.0–83.0)	<0.001	70.0 (58.0–96.5)	<0.001	119.0 (90.0–146.0)	84.0 (69.0–115.0)	<0.001	90.0 (73.0–140.0)	0.243	0.109	0.006
Systolic BP (mmHg)	141.2 ± 21.0	120.4 ± 17.6	<0.001	128.4 ± 17.4	<0.001	143.8 ± 16.9	122.3 ± 15.5	<0.001	134.4 ± 16.8	0.072	0.340	0.131
Diastolic BP (mmHg)	86.6 ± 12.5	72.5 ± 11.4	<0.001	75.4 ± 10.6	<0.001	87.2 ± 11.4	75.3 ± 8.6	<0.001	78.6 ± 11.5	0.001	0.074	0.085

WLR= weight loss responders; BP = blood pressure; HbA1c = glycated haemoglobin; HDL= high-density lipoprotein; HOMA-IR = homeostasis model assessment for insulin resistance; LDL = low-density lipoprotein. * p values for comparisons within study group between baseline and 2 years. † p values for comparisons within study group between baseline and 5 years.

Table 3. Remission rate of metabolic comorbidities in good and poor weight loss responders at 2 and 5 years post-surgery.

	Good WLR at 2 Years	Poor WLR at 2 Years	* p Value	Good WLR at 5 Years	Poor WLR at 5 Years	† p Value
Type 2 diabetes (%)	32/38 (84.2)	14/15 (93.3)	0.351	27/38 (71.1)	11/15 (73.3)	0.577
Hypertension (%)	40/77 (51.9)	7/16 (43.8)	0.374	37/77 (48.1)	7/16 (43.8)	0.486
Hypercholesterolaemia (%)	44/83 (53.0)	6/22 (27.3)	0.027	38/83 (45.8)	3/22 (13.6)	0.005
Hypertriglyceridaemia (%)	21/25 (84.0)	4/6 (66.7)	0.327	22/25 (88.0)	3/6 (50.0)	0.069

* p value for comparison between study groups at 2 years. † p value for comparison between study groups at 5 years.

Table 4. Multivariate analysis of factors associated with poor mid-term WL after bariatric surgery.

	Odds Ratio	95% CI	p Value
Age (for each 5 years)	1.429	1.100–1.857	0.007
Baseline HDL cholesterol (for each 5 mg/dL)	0.753	0.629–0.901	0.002
Type 2 diabetes mellitus	1.009	0.445–2.287	0.983
Sleeve gastrectomy	1.643	0.798–3.383	0.178
Preoperative %EWL (for each 5%)	0.832	0.720–0.963	0.014

CI = confidence interval; HDL = high-density lipoproteins; %EWL = percentage excess weight loss.

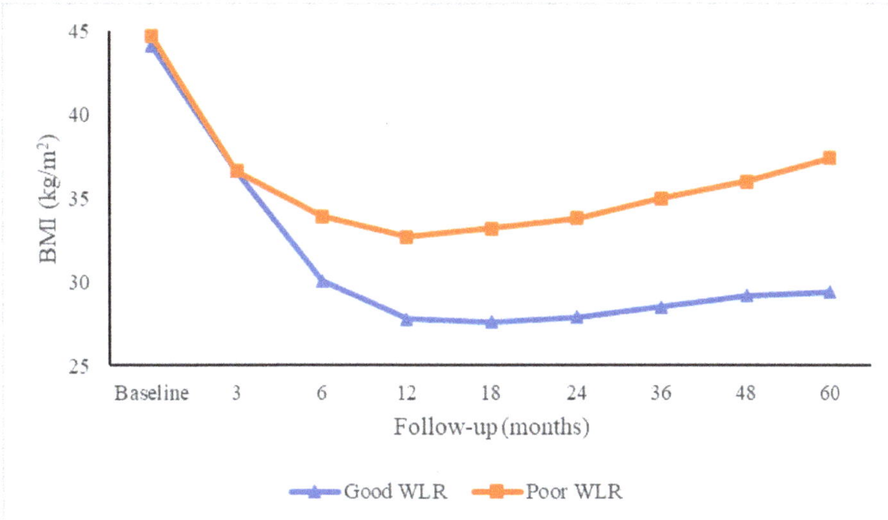

Figure 3. Changes in BMI of good and poor weight loss responders during follow-up after the bariatric surgical procedure. BMI = body mass index; WLR = weight loss responders.

4. Discussion

Different weight loss patterns were observed following BS. Although most participants maintained their weight loss over time, 20.3% had an EWL < 50% at 5 years. Interestingly, the present study found that, despite remaining in obesity range, improvements in several metabolic markers persisted at 5 years after surgery. Moreover, remission rates of several comorbidities associated with obesity showed no significant differences between good and poor mid-term WL. Predictors associated with a poor WL pattern were also identified in this study.

Despite the lack of uniform criteria to determine unsuccessful outcomes after BS, poor WL has been extensively defined as EWL < 50%. Most studies had short-term follow-up periods (1–2 years) and yielded highly variable poor WL rates, varying from 15 to 35% [4,5]. A study by de Hollanda et al., which included the same surgical techniques as the present study and a similar follow-up period, revealed a 24.3% rate of non-responsive patients [3].

Both groups presented clearly different weight loss trajectories. Of note, good WL responders reached on average a %EWL of approximately 80% between 1 and 2 years of follow-up and were subsequently able to remain within overweight range (BMI 25–30 kg/m^2) until 5 years of follow-up. By contrast, poor WL responders achieved a lower maximum weight loss of around 60% and also had a greater weight regain so that mean BMI in poor mid-term WL responders was in class I obesity range (BMI 30–35 kg/m^2) from 6 months to 2 years and worsened to class II obesity range (BMI 35–40 kg/m^2) from 3 to 5 years of follow-up.

As expected, good mid-term WL in our cohort showed an improvement in all metabolic parameters and similar results to other study cohorts in which no distinction regarding weight response was taken into account [7,18,19]. Interestingly, poor WL also showed an improvement in all metabolic parameters at 2 years, except for total cholesterol. These results can be explained by the fact that the maximum weight loss in this group of patients was observed around this follow-up timepoint. In contrast, at 5 years, two different patterns emerged with some of these parameters worsening to levels similar to those at baseline and others maintaining the improvement at 5 years.

The fact that glucose, HbA1c and HOMA-IR did not worsen with weight gain suggests that the improvement in these metabolic parameters after BS was partially independent of weight. In this respect, amelioration in insulin resistance and glucose metabolism occurred soon after the procedure, when significant weight loss had not yet been achieved, suggesting the involvement of gut hormonal mechanisms such as increased secretion of incretins that enhance insulin sensitivity [9–12]. The other parameter that remained greater at 5 years compared with baseline despite weight recovery was HDL cholesterol. In this case, it seems that a reduction in insulin resistance and systemic inflammation favoured the production of large HDL particles which in turn improves cholesterol efflux [20].

In contrast, other parameters such as triglycerides, LDL cholesterol or systolic blood pressure showed worsening between 2 and 5 years after surgery in poor WL responders in line with the weight increase. For triglyceridaemia, the close relationship between triglyceride decrease and weight reduction after surgery is well known [21]. As for LDL cholesterol, no significant differences were found between good and poor WL responders. However, while LDL cholesterol levels at 2 and 5 years post-surgery remained lower than those at baseline in good responders, LDL in poor responders rose to levels similar to those at baseline from 2 to 5 years. These findings can be explained by the fact that the poor responder group did not as frequently undergo the LRYGB technique and the malabsorptive component seems to be the most significant factor in LDL cholesterol reduction following BS [22]. Finally, differences in total cholesterol were justified by the changes in LDL and HDL levels. While total cholesterol dropped in good responders owing to a notable decrease in LDL, total cholesterol in poor responders increased due to a rise in HDL cholesterol.

With regard to the clinical evolution of systolic and diastolic blood pressure, no differences were found between study groups at either 2 or 5 years. Despite that, systolic blood pressure increased after surgery in poor WL responders from 2 to 5 years, showing no significant differences with baseline values at 5 years. These results are in line with epidemiological studies that had reported a close relationship between weight loss and blood pressure reduction [23,24]. In a previous study of 197 patients who underwent RYGB or SG, relapse of hypertension at 3 years was observed in >20% of patients who had achieved apparent hypertension remission at 12 months [24]. The only independent predictor of relapse was the greater use of preoperative antihypertensive medication. This suggested a waning effect of BS on blood pressure control over time, although further high-quality data regarding the mid- and long-term effects on hypertension remission are required. In this respect, in the present study, diastolic blood pressure remained lower than baseline throughout follow-up, suggesting that systolic blood pressure appears to be more sensitive to weight regain than diastolic blood pressure [23]. The worsening of systolic blood pressure from 2 to 5 years in poor WL responders would especially harm subjects over 50 years of age, since above this age systolic blood pressure would be a greater predictor of cardiovascular events and in subjects <50 years old it would be diastolic blood pressure [25].

When comorbidity remission rates were compared, results pointed in the same direction as those obtained on analysing the evolution of metabolic parameters. Hence, no significant differences were found between the remission rates of good and poor WL responders, except for hypercholesterolaemia. Of note, hypertriglyceridaemia showed a greater tendency towards poor WL (p = 0.069), which concurs with the differences observed in the change in triglyceride levels at 5 years. However, these results contrast with those reported by Farias et al. [6] who compared good and poor responders after a 2-year period post-LRYGB. Significant differences in remission rates of type 2 diabetes, hypertension and hyperlipidaemia were found between good and poor responders. The distinct findings of both studies can be attributed to a shorter follow-up period, differences in sample size, LRYGB as the only surgical technique studied and a different proportion of poor responders.

Various predictors of weight change after BS were suggested in previous studies with variable magnitudes of effects [26–28]. A negative correlation has been reported between EWL and age, tobacco consumption, pre-operative BMI, female sex, diabetes and LSG, among others. In the present study, the only pre-surgical parameters showing a significant association were age, pre-surgical weight loss and baseline HDL cholesterol. These findings could be explained by the fact that ageing is associated with a progressive decline in the quantity and quality of muscle tissue, the basal metabolic rate and energy requirements. These metabolic changes could influence the response to BS [26]. Regarding pre-surgical weight loss, it seems reasonable to assume that patients who manage to lose more weight before surgery will be more efficient in maintaining weight loss over time. Other studies also favour this association [29,30]. On the other hand, HDL cholesterol has not been previously identified as a predictive factor of WL. However, some studies demonstrated a significant association between both moderate and vigorous physical activity and higher HDL concentration [31]. Hence, HDL could be interpreted as an exercise marker, thereby indicating that subjects with higher HDL concentrations and thus physically more active had a clear trend towards greater weight loss patterns. The differences between this study and others in identifying predictive factors could partially be explained by differences in baseline characteristics or how weight loss was defined (as a continuous variable or used as a cut-off point to define poor WL).

The present study had some limitations. There was a lack of follow-up of around 40%, which may have influenced the final results since the sample of patients used could not have been representative of the initial patient cohort. Nevertheless, the loss of a follow-up rate was similar to that of other studies with a 5-year follow-up conducted in other countries with a National Health Service such as ours. Unfortunately, no other factors that may have contributed to a poor WL, such as physical activity, eating behaviour, quality of life or interpersonal support were taken into account. Moreover, other comorbidities such as obstructive sleep apnea were not studied.

5. Conclusions

One out of 5 patients undergoing BS will fail to achieve and maintain an optimal WL 5 years after surgery. Despite what may be expected, these patients obtain and preserve clinical benefits, such as improvement in glucose and lipid metabolism, comparable to those achieved by good WL. In view of these data, it could reasonably be argued that in some patients BS, despite achieving slight weight loss, continues to provide other major metabolic benefits. These findings support the idea of changing the concept of bariatric surgery to metabolic surgery.

Author Contributions: D.B. contributed to the study design, data collection, data analysis and writing. M.B. contributed to the study design and writing; J.P.-B. contributed to the data analysis and writing; A.d.V.-M. contributed to the data collection; J.M.R. contributed to the study design; M.P. contributed to the study design; M.V. contributed to the data collection; L.F. contributed to the data collection; H.J. contributed to the study design; E.C. contributed to the study design; O.C. contributed to the study design and writing; J.A.F.-L.R. contributed to the study design and writing; A.G. contributed to the study design, data analysis and writing. All authors have read and agreed to the published version of the manuscript.

Funding: This research received no external funding.

Acknowledgments: We thank Christine O'Hara for review of the English version of the manuscript.

Conflicts of Interest: The authors declare no conflict of interest.

References

1. Sjöström, L.; Lindroos, A.-K.; Peltonen, M.; Torgerson, J.; Bouchard, C.; Carlsson, B.; Dahlgren, S.; Larsson, B.; Narbro, K.; Sjöström, C.D.; et al. Lifestyle, diabetes, and cardiovascular risk factors 10 years after bariatric surgery. *N. Engl. J. Med.* **2004**, *351*, 2683–2693. [CrossRef] [PubMed]
2. Buchwald, H.; Avidor, Y.; Braunwald, E.; Jensen, M.D.; Pories, W.; Fahrbach, K.; Schoelles, K. Bariatric surgery: A systematic review and meta-analysis. *JAMA* **2004**, *292*, 1724–1737. [CrossRef] [PubMed]
3. de Hollanda, A.; Ruiz, T.; Jiménez, A.; Flores, L.; Lacy, A.; Vidal, J. Patterns of weight loss response following gastric bypass and sleeve gastrectomy. *Obes. Surg.* **2015**, *25*, 1177–1183. [CrossRef] [PubMed]
4. Rawlins, M.L.; Teel, D.; Hedgcorth, K.; Maguire, J.P. Revision of Roux-en-Y gastric bypass to distal bypass for failed weight loss. *Surg. Obes. Relat. Dis.* **2011**, *7*, 45–49. [CrossRef]
5. Brolin, R.E.; Cody, R.P. Adding malabsorption for weight loss failure after gastric bypass. *Surg. Endosc.* **2007**, *21*, 1924–1926. [CrossRef]

6. Farias, G.; Thieme, R.D.; Teixeira, L.M.; Heyde, M.E.V.D.; Bettini, S.C.; Radominski, R.B. Good weight loss responders and poor weight loss responders after Roux-en-Y gastric bypass: Clinical and nutritional profiles. *Nutr. Hosp.* **2016**, *33*, 574. [CrossRef]
7. Courcoulas, A.P.; King, W.C.; Belle, S.H.; Berk, P.; Flum, D.R.; Garcia, L.; Gourash, W.; Horlick, M.; Mitchell, J.E.; Pomp, A.; et al. Seven-year weight trajectories and health outcomes in the Longitudinal Assessment of Bariatric Surgery (LABS) study. *JAMA Surg.* **2018**, *153*, 427–434. [CrossRef]
8. Sjöström, L. Review of the key results from the Swedish Obese Subjects (SOS) trial—A prospective controlled intervention study of bariatric surgery. *J. Intern. Med.* **2013**, *273*, 219–234. [CrossRef]
9. Rao, R.S.; Yanagisawa, R.; Kini, S. Insulin resistance and bariatric surgery. *Obes. Rev.* **2012**, *13*, 316–328. [CrossRef]
10. Laferrère, B.; Heshka, S.; Wang, K.; Khan, Y.; McGinty, J.; Teixeira, J.; Hart, A.B.; Olivan, B. Incretin levels and effect are markedly enhanced 1 month after Roux-en-Y gastric bypass surgery in obese patients with type 2 diabetes. *Diabetes Care* **2007**, *30*, 1709–1716. [CrossRef]
11. Benaiges Boix, D.; Goday Arno, A.; Pedro-Botet, J. La cirugía bariátrica como tratamiento de la diabetes tipo 2. *Med. Clin. (Barc.)* **2012**, *138*, 391–396. [CrossRef] [PubMed]
12. Benaiges, D.; Flores Le-Roux, J.A.; Pedro-Botet, J.; Chillarón, J.J.; Renard, M.; Parri, A.; Ramón, J.M.; Pera, M.; Goday, A. Sleeve gastrectomy and Roux-en-Y gastric bypass are equally effective in correcting insulin resistance. *Int. J. Surg.* **2013**, *11*, 309–313. [CrossRef] [PubMed]
13. Gastrointestinal surgery for severe obesity: National Institutes of Health Consensus Development Conference Statement. *Am. J. Clin. Nutr.* **1992**, *55*, 615S–619S. [CrossRef] [PubMed]
14. Matthews, D.R.; Hosker, J.P.; Rudenski, A.S.; Naylor, B.A.; Treacher, D.F.; Turner, R.C. Homeostasis model assessment: Insulin resistance and β-cell function from fasting plasma glucose and insulin concentrations in man. *Diabetologia* **1985**, *28*, 412–419. [CrossRef]
15. Friedewald, W.T.; Levy, R.I.; Fredrickson, D.S. Estimation of the concentration of low-density lipoprotein cholesterol in plasma, without use of the preparative ultracentrifuge. *Clin. Chem.* **1972**, *18*, 499–502. [CrossRef]
16. Goday, A.; Gabriel, R.; Ascaso, J.F.; Franch, J.; Ortega, R.; Martinez, O.; Lerones, N. Cardiovascular risk in subjects with high probability of metabolic syndrome and insulin resistance. DESIRE study. *Rev. Clin. Esp.* **2008**, *208*, 377–385. [CrossRef]
17. Benaiges, D.; Flores-Le-Roux, J.A.; Pedro-Botet, J.; Ramon, J.M.; Parri, A.; Villatoro, M.; Carrera, M.J.; Pera, M.; Sagarra, E.; Grande, L.; et al. Impact of restrictive (sleeve gastrectomy) vs hybrid bariatric surgery (Roux-en-Y gastric bypass) on lipid profile. *Obes Surg.* **2012**, *22*, 1268–1275. [CrossRef]
18. Helmiö, M.; Victorzon, M.; Ovaska, J.; Leivonen, M.; Juuti, A.; Jaser, N.; Peromaa, P.; Tolonen, P.; Hurme, S.; Salminen, P. SLEEVEPASS: A randomized prospective multicenter study comparing laparoscopic sleeve gastrectomy and gastric bypass in the treatment of morbid obesity: Preliminary results. *Surg. Endosc.* **2012**, *26*, 2521–2526. [CrossRef]
19. Salminen, P.; Helmiö, M.; Ovaska, J.; Juuti, A.; Leivonen, M.; Peromaa-Haavisto, P.; Hurme, S.; Soinio, M.; Nuutila, P.; Victorzon, M. Effect of laparoscopic sleeve gastrectomy vs laparoscopic Roux-en-Y gastric bypass on weight loss at 5 years among patients with morbid obesity: The SLEEVEPASS randomized clinical trial. *JAMA* **2018**, *319*, 241–254. [CrossRef]
20. Osto, E.; Doytcheva, P.; Corteville, C.; Bueter, M.; Dörig, C.; Stivala, S.; Buhmann, H.; Colin, S.; Rohrer, L.; Hasballa, R.; et al. Rapid and body weight-independent improvement of endothelial and high-density lipoprotein function after Roux-en-Y gastric bypass role of glucagon-like peptide-1. *Circulation* **2015**, *131*, 871–881. [CrossRef]
21. Cunha, F.M.; Oliveira, J.; Preto, J.; Saavedra, A.; Costa, M.M.; Magalhães, D.; Lau, E.; Bettencourt-Silva, R.; Freitas, P.; Varela, A.; et al. The effect of bariatric surgery type on lipid profile: An age, sex, body mass index and excess weight loss matched study. *Obes. Surg.* **2016**, *26*, 1041–1047. [CrossRef] [PubMed]
22. Pihlajamäki, J.; Grönlund, S.; Simonen, M.; Käkelä, N.P.; Moilanen, L.; Pääkkönen, M.; Pirinen, E.; Kolehmainen, M.; Kärjä, V.; Kainulainen, S.; et al. Cholesterol absorption decreases after Roux-en-Y gastric bypass but not after gastric banding. *Metabolism* **2010**, *59*, 866–872. [CrossRef] [PubMed]
23. Aucott, L.; Rothnie, H.; McIntyre, L.; Thapa, M.; Waweru, C.; Gray, D. Long-term weight loss from lifestyle intervention benefits blood pressure?: A systematic review. *Hypertension* **2009**, *54*, 756–762. [CrossRef] [PubMed]

24. Benaiges, D.; Saguéa, M.; Flores-Le Roux, J.A.; Pedro-Botet, J.; Ramón, J.M.; Villatoro, M.; Chillarón, J.J.; Pera, M.; Más, A.; Grande, L.; et al. Predictors of hypertension remission and recurrence after bariatric surgery. *Am. J. Hypertens.* **2016**, *29*, 653–659. [CrossRef] [PubMed]
25. Vishram, J.K.; Borglykke, A.; Andreasen, A.H.; Jeppesen, J.; Ibsen, H.; Jorgensen, T.; Broda, G.; Palmieri, L.; Giampaoli, S.; Donfrancesco, C.; et al. MORGAM Project. Impact of age on the importance of systolic and diastolic blood pressures for stroke risk: The MOnica, Risk, Genetics, Archiving, and Monograph (MORGAM) project. *Hypertension* **2012**, *60*, 1117–1123. [CrossRef] [PubMed]
26. Parri, A.; Benaiges, D.; Schröder, H.; Izquierdo-Pulido, M.; Ramón, J.; Villatoro, M.; Flores-Le Roux, J.; Goday, A. Preoperative predictors of weight loss at 4 years following bariatric surgery. *Nutr. Clin. Pract.* **2015**, *30*, 420–424. [CrossRef] [PubMed]
27. Courcoulas, A.P.; Christian, N.J.; O'Rourke, R.W.; Dakin, G.; Patchen Dellinger, E.; Flum, D.R.; Melissa Kalarchian, P.D.; Mitchell, J.E.; Patterson, E.; Pomp, A.; et al. Preoperative factors and 3-year weight change in the Longitudinal Assessment of Bariatric Surgery (LABS) consortium. *Surg. Obes. Relat. Dis.* **2015**, *11*, 1109–1118. [CrossRef]
28. Campos, G.M.; Rabl, C.; Mulligan, K.; Posselt, A.; Rogers, S.J.; Westphalen, A.C.; Lin, F.; Vittinghoff, E. Factors associated with weight loss after gastric bypass. *Arch. Surg.* **2008**, *143*, 877–883. [CrossRef]
29. Livhits, M.; Mercado, C.; Yermilov, I.; Parikh, J.A.; Dutson, E.; Mehran, A.; Ko, C.Y.; Gibbons, M.M. Preoperative predictors of weight loss following bariatric surgery: Systematic review. *Obes. Surg.* **2012**, *22*, 70–89. [CrossRef]
30. Alvarado, R.; Alami, R.S.; Hsu, G.; Safadi, B.Y.; Sanchez, B.R.; Morton, J.M.; Curet, M.J. The impact of preoperative weight loss in patients undergoing laparoscopic Roux-en-Y gastric bypass. *Obes. Surg.* **2005**, *15*, 1282–1286. [CrossRef]
31. Da Silva, R.C.; de Fátima Haueisen Sander Diniz, M.; Alvim, S.; Vidigal, P.G.; Fedeli, L.M.G.; Barreto, S.M. Physical activity and lipid profile in the ELSA-Brasil study. *Arq. Bras. Cardiol.* **2016**, *107*, 10–19. [CrossRef] [PubMed]

Journal of
Clinical Medicine

MDPI

Review

The Metabolic Rearrangements of Bariatric Surgery: Focus on Orexin-A and the Adiponectin System

Anna Valenzano [1,†], Nicola Tartaglia [2,†], Antonio Ambrosi [2], Domenico Tafuri [3], Marcellino Monda [4], Antonietta Messina [4], Francesco Sessa [1], Angelo Campanozzi [5], Vincenzo Monda [4], Giuseppe Cibelli [1], Giovanni Messina [1,*] and Rita Polito [1,*]

1. Department of Clinical and Experimental Medicine, University of Foggia, 71100 Foggia, Italy; anna.valenzano@unifg.it (A.V.); francesco.sessa@unifg.it (F.S.); giuseppe.cibelli@unifg.it (G.C.)
2. General Surgery, Department of Medical and Surgical Sciences, University of Foggia, 71100 Foggia, Italy; nicola.tartaglia@unifg.it (N.T.); antonio.ambrosi@unifg.it (A.A.)
3. Department of Motor Sciences and Wellness, University of Naples "Parthenope", 80133 Naples, Italy; domenico.tafuri@uniparthenope.it
4. Department of Experimental Medicine, Section of Human Physiology and Unit of Dietetic and Sport Medicine, Università degli Studi della Campania Luigi Vanvitelli, 80138 Naples, Italy; marcellino.monda@unicampania.it (M.M.); Antonietta.messina@unicampania.it (A.M.); vincenzo.monda@unicampania.it (V.M.)
5. Pediatrics, Department of Medical and Surgical Sciences, University of Foggia, 71100 Foggia, Italy; angelo.campanozzi@unifg.it

* Correspondence: giovanni.messina@unifg.it (G.M.); rita.polito@unifg.it (R.P.); Tel.: +39-0881588095 (G.M.)
† These authors equally contributed.

Received: 9 September 2020; Accepted: 10 October 2020; Published: 16 October 2020

Abstract: The accumulation of adipose tissue represents one of the characteristics of obesity, increasing the risk of developing correlated obesity diseases such as cardiovascular disease, type 2 diabetes, cancer, and immune diseases. Visceral adipose tissue accumulation leads to chronic low inflammation inducing an imbalanced adipokine secretion. Among these adipokines, Adiponectin is an important metabolic and inflammatory mediator. It is also known that adipose tissue is influenced by Orexin-A levels, a neuropeptide produced in the lateral hypothalamus. Adiponectin and Orexin-A are strongly decreased in obesity and are associated with metabolic and inflammatory pathways. The aim of this review was to investigate the involvement of the autonomic nervous system focusing on Adiponectin and Orexin-A after bariatric surgery. After bariatric surgery, Adiponectin and Orexin-A levels are strongly increased independently of weight loss showing that hormone increases are also attributable to a rearrangement of metabolic and inflammatory mediators. The restriction of food intake and malabsorption are not sufficient to clarify the clinical effects of bariatric surgery suggesting the involvement of neuro-hormonal feedback loops and also of mediators such as Adiponectin and Orexin-A.

Keywords: obesity; adipose tissue; adiponectin; central nervous system; Orexin-A; bariatric surgery

1. Introduction

Obesity is characterized by an altered metabolic and inflammatory profile leading to various metabolic, inflammatory, and immune diseases [1]. The accumulation of visceral adipose tissue is a principal characteristic of obesity. It accumulates in the abdominal area of the body and is dangerous for health. Indeed, the endocrine function of adipose tissue is strongly influenced by the presence of visceral adipose tissue. As reported by Xin et al., 2020, in obesity, adipocytes are dysfunctional with an excessive secretion of multiple pro-inflammatory adipokines, contributing to a chronic inflammatory reaction and promoting the progression of metabolic and cardiovascular complications [2]. It is well known that white adipocytes of visceral fat are particularly active in the release of adipokines. Although adipocytes secrete a large variety of bioactive molecules with widespread systemic effects contributing to numerous physiological and pathological processes, the autocrine and paracrine actions of these molecules are highly complex, and our understanding of these processes is likely rudimentary [3]. The complexity of obesity consists of adipose tissue recognized as an endocrine organ producing adipokines, the active protein with pleiotropic functions in the regulation of energy metabolism, insulin sensitivity, inflammation, atherosclerosis, and proliferation. Among these, Adiponectin is the most abundant product of white adipose tissue (WAT). It is produced in various oligomers of different molecular weight and it is negatively correlated with obesity [4].

During obesity development there is also an involvement of the sympathetic system. The central nervous system, through the production of hypotalamic mediators, acts on adipose tissue (AT) regulating its function, both physiologically and patho-physiologically. In particular, through the production of Orexin-A, a hypothalamic peptide, the central nervous system increases the sympathetic stimulation of WAT and thereby increasing lipolysis [5–7]. Bariatric surgery is necessary when there is severe obesity and this technique is able to induce an improvement or resolution of many obese related conditions and to improve quality of life, inducing weight loss and a rearrangement of metabolic and hormone pathways. From data in the literature, it is clear that bariatric surgery is capable not only of acting from a mechanical-anatomical point of view, reducing the size of the stomach and therefore the intake of food, but also improving some metabolic parameters such as the production of adipocytokines and hypothalamic peptides. There is a strong metabolic interconnection between the central nervous system, the digestive system and adipose tissue. In light of this evidence, in this review, the functional metabolic changes in the sympathetic and para-sympathetic nervous systems through the production of Adiponectin and Orexin-A induced by bariatric surgery are elucidate.

2. Adipose Tissue: General Characteristics

AT is an endocrine organ, composed of adipocytes and pervaded by many innate and adaptative immune cells [8–10]. In obesity, the excessive expansion of AT mass induces the recruitment of numerous immune cells leading to an imbalance in adipokine production. AT exerts its metabolic function through the production of adipokines, among these is Adiponectin [11–13]. Literature data demonstrated that obesity strongly correlates to immune and autoimmune disease development [11]. The immune system monitors and responds to specific metabolic cues in both pathologic and non-pathologic settings. The immune system continuously communicates with AT. These systems influence each other. In addition, it is well known that the immune system is influenced by environmental changes as well as nutritional factors [11,12]. Imbalanced nutrition strongly influences the function and development of the immune system, depressing it and/or reducing immune competence. As previously reported, AT is pervaded by immune system cells leading to an alteration of pro-inflammatory cytokines such as leptin, TNF-α, L-6, IL8 and anti-inflammatory cytokines such as Adiponectin and IL-10 [11–15].

3. Adiponectin: General Characteristics

Adiponectin is an abundant adipokine produced by AT, representing about 0.1% of total serum proteins. This adipokine is present as oligomers of different molecular weight: low molecular weight (LMW), medium molecular weight (MMW) and high molecular weight (HMW) that are the most biologically active [8]. Adiponectin has pleiotropic functions on different target tissues through the presence of its receptors: AdipoR1, AdipoR2 and T-cadherin. The main metabolic functions of Adiponectin are exerted on the liver, muscle, and AT; in fact, the metabolites of Adiponectin affect glucose homeostasis and the metabolism of fatty acids through a primary action at the level of muscles and the liver [9]. It increases insulin sensitivity and reduces hepatic neoglucogenesis, increases glucose uptake by adipocytes and myocytes, increasing the oxidation of free fatty acids in muscles and preventing the increase of free fatty acids and triglycerides as a result of a high fat diet. Numerous studies, both in vitro and in vivo, have also characterized the anti-inflammatory, anti-atherogenic and anti-angiogenic effects of this protein. The anti-inflammatory effects of Adiponectin include the suppression of pro-inflammatory cytokine production, such as TNF-α and IL-6, C-reactive protein and growth factors, and the modulation of the expression of the anti-inflammatory cytokine IL-10 in monocytes and macrophages. On the contrary, TNF-α and other inflammatory markers (IL-6, C-reactive protein, SAA, tPA, MCP-1) and glucocorticoids suppress and regulate Adiponectin production [10] (Figure 1). The anti-atherogenic effects include the modulation of the inflammatory response inhibiting monocyte adhesion and macrophage polarization. In addition, Adiponectin is able to inhibit endothelial cell proliferation and promote apoptosis with a consequent antitumor effect [1]. On the contrary, in cases of vascular damage, Adiponectin regulates the endothelial response to damage by suppressing apoptosis acting on the regulation of proliferation and differentiation of osteoblasts. This adipokine has a pleiotropic function, it is not only a metabolic mediator, but also an inflammatory and immune mediator [11]. As regards its metabolic effects, Adiponectin is involved in glucose and lipid metabolism. It is involved in glucose homeostasis and in the metabolism of fatty acids through a primary action in muscles and the liver by means of AMPK phosphorilation [12]. Furthermore, Adiponectin increases insulin sensitivity and glucose uptake increasing GLUT-4 translocation by adipocytes and myocytes. In the muscle, it increases the oxidation of free fatty acids and prevents the increase of free fatty acids and triglycerides as a result of a high fat diet [12]. Many data in the literature report that Adiponectin negatively correlates with anthropometric parameters such as body mass index (BMI) and body weight, and also with metabolic parameters such as glycemia, total cholesterol, and LDL cholesterol. On the contrary, it is positively correlated with HDL-cholesterol [13]. In addition, several studies report that Adiponectin serum levels are strongly decreased in obese subjects compared to healthy subjects; however, Adiponectin serum levels negatively correlate with the risk of developing obesity related diseases [14] (Figure 1A).

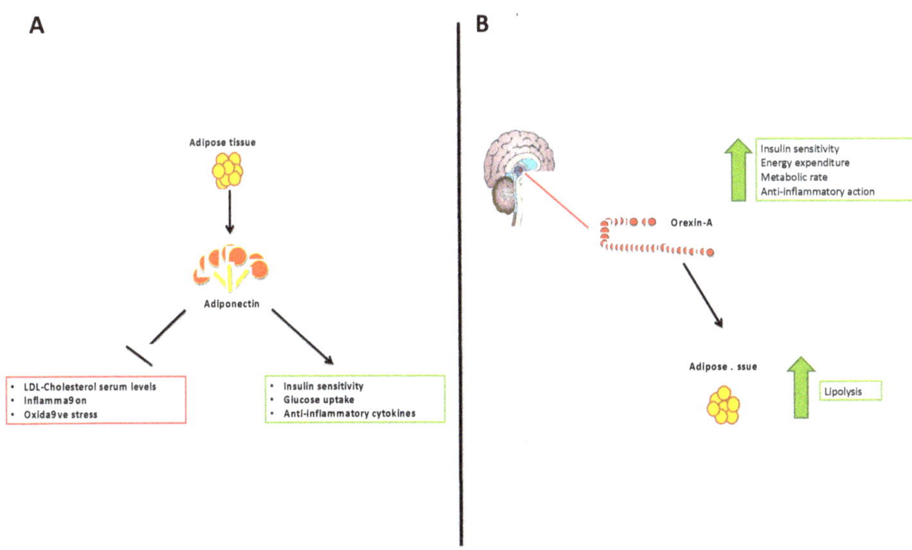

Figure 1. The principal beneficial effects of Adiponectin (panel (**A**)) and of Orexin-A (panel (**B**)).

4. Orexin-A: General Characteristics

The lateral hypothalamus produces an important neuropeptide; Orexin-A (hypocretin-1) [16]. It plays an important role in peripheral energy balance, suggesting the involvement of central nervous system (CNS) mechanisms, and coordinates sleep-wakefulness and food-seeking, especially in the physiological state of fasting stress [17]. Orexin-A exerts its functions by binding its receptors, Orexin-1 receptor (Ox1) and Orexin-2 receptor (Ox2), two G-protein coupled receptors [18–20]. The Orexin system is involved in physiological and pathophysiological processes [21–23] (Figure 1B). Many metabolic molecules influence Orexin-A activity; in particular, glucose, leptin, and amino acids and also some environmental factors increase Orexin-A levels during the waking phase of the circadian cycles and fasting or periods of caloric restriction. This neuropeptide is able to regulate physiological and behavioral processes impacting on energy balance and metabolic status, physical activity, blood glucose levels, and food intake [20–22]. Overall, it is well known that Orexin-A is involved in the regulation of insulin sensitivity, energy expenditure and metabolic rate. In addition, it regulates immune processes and inflammatory response, in particular, it has an anti-inflammatory action [21,24,25]. Orexin-A exerts its metabolic effects acting on MAPK pathways, through PGC-1α. Data in the literature report that PGC-1α is able to act on neuronal metabolism involving the orexinergic system [20]. It is involved in metabolic pathways and also in different pathologies such as obesity, diabetes, and chronic neurodegenerative diseases [20]. In vitro studies report that Orexin-A, through PGC-1α, activates HIF-1a that may be a link between Orexin and cellular metabolic signaling pathways relevant to obesity [22]. In addition, it is well known that Orexin-A regulates various physiological functions activating phospholipase C/protein kinase C and AC/cAMP/PKA pathways [5,26]. In addition, this neuropeptide exerts its metabolic functions on energy metabolism regulating feeding behavior and energy expenditure [26–29]. Orexin-A directly acts on AT inducing lipolysis, independently of food intake. As reported by Perez-Leighton et al., the injection of Orexin-A into the lateral thalamus of SD rats for 10 consecutive days reduced diet-induced obesity without affecting food intake [30] (Figure 1B). Previous studies demonstrated that Orexin-A reduces adipogenesis in human intra-abdominal, but not subcutaneous, adipocytes [31,32].

Orexin-A is involved in inflammatory responses as an anti-inflammatory mediator [15]. In obesity, Orexin-A serum levels are strongly reduced and inversely correlate with BMI and with pro-inflammatory mediators such as C-reactive protein and TNF-a. On the contrary, Orexin-A levels positively correlate with Adiponectin serum levels and HDL-cholesterol [33].

5. Bariatric Surgery: Why Is It Done and Who Is It for?

The prevalence of overweight and obese people is increasing globally. Recently, many young people (20–30 years old) have been reported to be overweight or obese. Being overweight and obesity are associated with an increased risk of morbidity and mortality [34].

Bariatric surgery is a valid strategy for weight loss. Gastric bypass and other weight loss surgeries are characteristics of bariatric surgery. It is used when diet and physical activity are insufficient for weight loss and/or various serious health problems have caused excessive weight.

The current indications for bariatric surgery refer to the severity of obesity and the potential reversibility of the clinical conditions. The evaluation of BMI is considered a marker for the indication for surgery. In particular, this surgery is performed in subjects with a BMI > 40 kg/m^2, in the absence of any other comorbidities and with BMI > 35 kg/m^2 with obesity-associated comorbidities [35–37].

Bariatric surgery consists of some procedures limiting food intake and other procedures reducing the body's ability to absorb nutrients. Malabsorptive bariatric procedures divert the flow of bile and pancreatic enzymes from food and therefore limit the digestion and absorption of nutrients, resulting in reduced calorie intake and subsequent weight loss. Essential micronutrients such as vitamins and trace elements are also absorbed to a lesser extent, potentially leading to severe side effects [35]. In addition, various bariatric surgery techniques use both procedures. Among these, gastric bypass is a reversible technique, decreasing the amount of food intake and also the absorption of nutrients. The most common performed bariatric surgery worldwide is sleeve gastrectomy as reported by Angrisani et al., 2014 [38]. This procedure consists of removing about 80% of the stomach, leaving a long, tube-like pouch. Generally, sleeve gastrectomy induces notable weight loss, because it reduces stomach size and limits food intake. It also produces less of the appetite-regulating hormone ghrelin, which may lessen the desire to eat. In addition, ghrelin reduction is induced by both gastric bypass and sleeve gastrectomy [39]. In addition, an adjustable gastric band (AGB) is another surgery technique. It has advantages including significant weight loss. It is an inflatable silicone device placed around the top portion of the stomach to treat obesity, intended to decrease food consumption [38]. Another procedure is a biliopancreatic diversion with duodenal switch (BPD/DS). It is a complex procedure that tackles weight loss in three different ways. First, a sleeve gastrectomy is performed. For this, a large portion of the stomach is removed with a stapling instrument, leaving a narrow tube, or sleeve, from the top to near the bottom of the stomach. The second part of the procedure reroutes food away from the upper part of the small intestine, which is the natural path of digestion. This cuts back on how many calories and nutrients the body is able to absorb. The small intestine is divided and a connection is made near the end of the small intestine. The third part of the BPD/DS procedure changes the normal way that bile and digestive juices break down food. This cuts back on how many calories are absorbed, causing still more weight loss. One end of the small intestine is connected to the duodenum, near the bottom of the stomach [40]. Bariatric surgery has many beneficial effects, but it has many serious risks and side effects [41]. Moreover, after bariatric surgery, a lifestyle change is necessary through healthy diet and regular physical activity making the beneficial effects of bariatric surgery last longer [36]. Among the beneficial effects of bariatric surgery is knowing that it increases weight loss and reduces the risk of obesity and its associated diseases. In addition, before bariatric surgery, obese subjects are put on a healthy diet with physical activity to induce weight loss. This surgical intervention is carried out on subjects with severe obesity. The current indications for bariatric surgery state that the surgery is necessary when there is severe obesity and the potential reversibility of the clinical conditions. Classically, starting from the Consensus Conference of the American National Institute of Health (1991), BMI is considered to be decisive, but it must be kept in mind that it has important limits; not being in able to highlight the distribution and breakdown of lipid accumulation in the form of somatic or visceral fat, a key factor in determining the metabolic syndrome; and also the different distribution of fat in relation to age, sex and race. For this reason, BMI is considered an important benchmark, but not the only one for establishing the indication for surgery. At the same time, BMI, also considered in its historical dimension as the maximum value reached by the patient, makes it possible to give indications for bariatric surgery. Finally, BMI is evaluated, together with metabolic, functional and psychological parameters, always in an overall balance between risks and benefits, in patients with a BMI > 40 kg/m^2, in the absence of any other comorbidities; or with a BMI > 35 kg/m^2, in the presence of comorbidities among those classically considered to be associated with obesity, including type 2 diabetes mellitus (T2DM) resistant to medical treatment [36,37].

As reported by Chang et al., bariatric surgery has substantial and sustained effects on weight and significantly ameliorates obesity-attributable comorbidities in the majority of bariatric surgery patients [35]. The reoperation rate of an adjustable gastric band is higher than that of gastric bypass and sleeve gastrectomy, and the weight loss outcomes of an adjustable gastric band are less substantial than sleeve gastrectomy or gastric bypass [41]. Bariatric surgery is able to induce an improvement or resolution of many obese related conditions and to improve quality of life, also inducing a rearrangement of metabolic and hormone pathways [42]. As reported by Zsombok, there is an improvement in metabolic profile and the remission of type 2 diabetes after bariatric surgery well before weight loss [38]. The author reported that bariatric surgery could alter the neural communication between the gastrointestinal system and the brain, interfering with the autonomic output to the visceral organs, including the liver. In addition, incretins, among these is glucagon-like peptide 1 (GLP-1), are able to influence the central nervous system. Data in the literature reported that the level of GLP-1 is significantly increased after bariatric surgery and could have a key anti-diabetic effect, regardless of weight loss [42]. Moreover, bariatric surgery, the central nervous system and AT influence each other through the production of neuropeptide such as Orexin-A and adipocytokines such as Adiponectin, as suggested by several studies [6].

6. Effects of Bariatric Surgery on Adiponectin and Orexin-A

It is well known that the beneficial effects of bariatric surgery have shifted from the contribution of simple gastric diversion and restriction to an energetic pursuit of the contribution of gastrointestinal hormones, secretions, and the microbiome [43]. There is an involvement of sympathetic and parasympathetic nervous systems in bariatric surgery. Several studies reported that the automatic nervous system and parasympathetic tone are involved in the regulation of inflammation. In addition, it is associated with hypothalamus-pituitary-adrenal axis (HPA) function, glucose regulation and autoimmune disorders through the production of many mediators, among which is Orexin-A [44]. The main effects of bariatric surgery on the nervous system are attributable to the vagus nerve that is involved during bariatric surgery. Geronikolou et al. reported that bariatric surgery has a greater effect on both branches of the cardiac automatic nervous system, making it more beneficial for severe cardiovascular patients. Furthermore, bariatric surgery has positive effects on insulin resistance by decreasing it. Moreover, this intervention is able to increase vagal tone, improving cardiac function. Heinonen et al. reported that gastric banding and/or gastric bypass are effective for weight loss, but among the beneficial effects of bariatric surgery there are many other factors such as neurohormonal feedback loops. Data in the literature report that peptide hormones such as Adiponectin, orexins, and leptin might play a part in this regulation [44,45].

Heinonen et al. reported that in the stomach and intestine enterochromaffin-like cells display Orexin immunoreactivity. Kirchgessner and Liu reported that Orexins play a role in the gastric and intestinal phase of secretion [46]. In addition, many literature data report the role of Orexin-A and B in appetite control [47,48]. Furthermore, it is known that Orexin inhibited responses to CCK suggesting its role in modulating gut-to-brain signaling. Several studies report that Orexin-A levels are influenced by bariatric surgery independent of weight loss. As reported by Gupta et al., in the acute post-operative phase (after 1 day) and prior to any weight loss, some subjects demonstrate an increase in Orexin while others have decreased plasma Orexin levels. This raises the question as to what factors regulate these acute changes in Orexin during the acute post-operative phase [49]. On the contrary, Federico et al. reported that Orexin-A serum levels were comparable in obese patients before and after bariatric surgery [50]. Moreover, Cigdem et al. showed that laparoscopic gastric band application resulted not only in significant weight loss but also in decreased Orexin-A serum levels [51]. Amin et al. demonstrated a rise in Orexin and a decrease in leptin in a cohort of obese subjects affected by obstructive sleep apnea, after bariatric surgery, showing that metabolic changes were also occurring in the same time span and thus it was plausible that physiologic rather than anatomic changes may underlie the clinically significant improvement in obstructive sleep apnea as early as 11 days following bariatric surgery [52]. The regulation of Orexin and the involvement of the nervous system both depend on mechanical factors but also on chemical mediators and hormones that are in circulation after the intervention. It is also reported that bariatric surgery has an impact on AT. Sams et al. reported that bariatric surgery has numerous beneficial effects on glucose homeostasis through the regulation and modulation of insulin sensitivity. The inflammatory mechanism of insulin resistance involves an early phase of improved insulin sensitivity and a late phase of decreased inflammatory mediators. The authors reported that gastric bypass induces a rearrangement of gastrointestinal anatomy and an amelioration in glucose homeostasis [53,54]. Regarding the rearrangement of gastrointestinal anatomy, bariatric surgery induces significant changes in gut hormone production that contribute to ameliorate general health [51]. It is well known that obesity induces not only an alteration of many metabolic mediators alerting glucose and lipid profiles, but also induces an imbalance in the expression of pro- and anti-inflammatory adipokines such as Adiponectin. As reported by Salman et al. bariatric surgery induces a significant increase in serum Adiponectin levels and a significant decline in serum levels of leptin, resisitin, and pre-B cell enhancing factor/Nampt/visfatin, confirming the role of this technique in hormonal rearrangement [55].

Moreover, recent studies have reported that bariatric surgery is associated with a reduction in specific adipokines including leptin, chemerin, and PAI-1, whereas Adiponectin is raised;

adaptations that could be indicative of improved fat mass and function [56,57]. After bariatric surgery, obese subjects have an increase in Adiponectin serum levels. This increase is associated not only with weight loss, but also with a decrease of inflammation reducing insulin resistance (Table 1 and Figure 2).

Table 1. The main effects of bariatric surgery on adipose tissue and the central nervous system.

Bariatric Surgery	
Adipose Tissue	**Central Nervous System**
Increased Adiponectin	Increased Orexin-A
Decreased Leptin	Increased Vagal Tone
Decreased Insulin Resistance	Orexin-A Controls Appetite

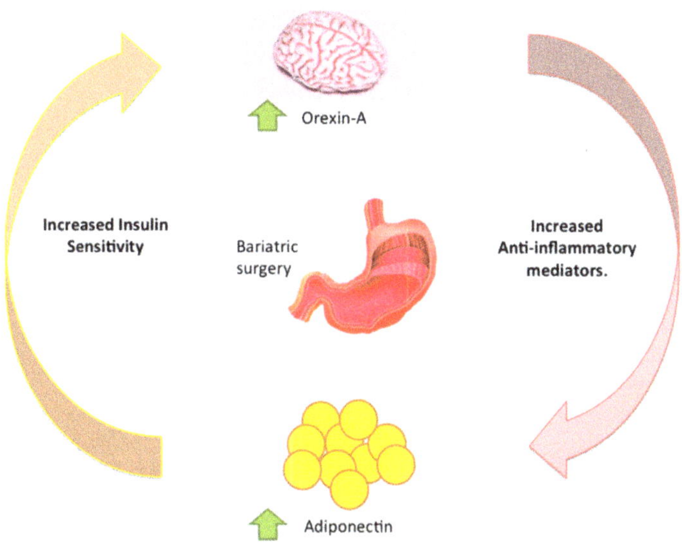

Figure 2. Adiponectin and Orexin-A levels are increased after bariatric surgery independently of weight loss showing the involvement of neuro-hormonal feedback loops.

7. Conclusions

Adiponectin and Orexin-A are both involved in obesity and its correlated diseases. These proteins are strongly reduced in obese patients. Both Adiponectin and Orexin-A have beneficial metabolic effects, increasing glucose uptake and insulin sensitivity; on the other hand, they are anti-inflammatory mediators. After bariatric surgery, Adiponectin and Orexin-A levels are increased and this is attributable not only to weight loss, but also to a rearrangement of metabolic and inflammatory mediators. The restriction of food intake or a combination of a restriction and malabsorption induced by bariatric surgery are, however, not sufficient to explain the profound clinical effects of bariatric surgery, suggesting the involvement of neuro-hormonal feedback loops and also of mediators such as Adiponectin and Orexin-A. Further studies are needed to clarify the molecular mechanism underlying this regulation.

Author Contributions: Conceptualization A.V., G.M. and R.P.; writing-original draft preparation A.V., N.T., A.A., D.T. and R.P.; writing review and editing A.M., F.S., A.C. and V.M.; visualization M.M., G.C. and G.M. All authors have read and agreed to the published version of the manuscript.

Funding: This research received no external funding.

Acknowledgments: The authors thank the Scientific Bureau of the University of Catania for language support.

Conflicts of Interest: The authors declare no conflict of interest.

References

1. Nigro, E.; Scudiero, O.; Monaco, M.L.; Palmieri, A.; Mazzarella, G.; Costagliola, C.; Bianco, A.; Daniele, A. New Insight into Acrp30 Role in Obesity and Obesity-Related Diseases. *BioMed Res. Int.* **2014**, *2014*, 658913. [CrossRef] [PubMed]
2. Xin, S.; Daoquan, P. Adipokines as novel biomarkers of cardio-metabolic disorders. *Clin. Chim. Acta* **2020**, *507*, 31–38.
3. Richard, A.J.; White, U.; Elks, C.M.; Stephens, J.M. *Adipose Tissue: Physiology to Metabolic Dysfunction*; Endotext. MDText.com, Inc.: South Dartmouth, MA, USA, 2020.
4. Messina, A.; Monda, M.; Valenzano, A.; Messina, G.; Villano, I.; Moscatelli, F.; Cibelli, G.; Marsala, G.; Polito, R.; Ruberto, M.; et al. Functional Changes Induced by Orexin A and Adiponectinon the Sympathetic/Parasympathetic Balance. *Front. Physiol.* **2018**, *9*, 259. [CrossRef] [PubMed]
5. Liu, L.; Wang, Q.; Liu, A.; Lan, X.; Huang, Y.; Zhao, Z.; Jie, H.; Chen, J.; Zhao, Y.-J. Physiological Implications of Orexins/Hypocretins on Energy Metabolism and Adipose Tissue Development. *ACS Omega* **2020**, *5*, 547–555. [CrossRef]
6. Sams, V.G.; Blackledge, C.; Wijayatunga, N.; Barlow, P.; Mancini, M.; Mancini, G.; Moustaid-Moussa, N. Effect of bariatric surgery on systemic and adipose tissue inflammation. *Surg. Endosc.* **2016**, *30*, 3499–3504. [CrossRef]
7. Colquitt, J.L.; Pickett, K.; Loveman, E.; Frampton, G. Surgery for weight loss in adults. *Cochrane Database Syst. Rev.* **2014**, *8*, CD003641. [CrossRef]
8. Kadowaki, T.; Yamauchi, T. Acrp30 and Acrp30 receptors. *Endocr. Rev.* **2005**, *26*, 439–451. [CrossRef]
9. Yamauchi, T.; Kamon, J.; Ito, Y.; Tsuchida, A.; Yokomizo, T.; Kita, S.; Sugiyama, T.; Miyagishi, M.; Hara, K.; Tsunoda, M.; et al. Cloning of Acrp30 receptors that mediate antidiabetic metabolic effects. *Nature* **2003**, *423*, 762–769. [CrossRef]
10. Di Gregorio, P.A.; Lu, G.B.; Rassuoli, N.; Ranganathan, G. Acrp30 expression from human adipose tissue: Relation to obesity, insulin resistance, and tumor necrosis factor-alpha expression. *Diabetes* **2003**, *52*, 1779–1785.
11. Pecoraro, A.; Nigro, E.; Polito, R.; Monaco, M.L.; Scudiero, O.; Mormile, I.; Marcelli, A.C.; Capasso, M.; Habetswallner, F.; Genovese, A.; et al. Total and High Molecular Weight Acrp30 Expression Is Decreased in Patients with Common Variable Immunodeficiency: Correlation with Ig Replacement Therapy. *Front. Immunol.* **2017**, *8*, 895. [CrossRef]
12. De Rosa, A.; Monaco, M.L.; Capasso, M.; Forestieri, P.; Pilone, V.; Nardelli, C.; Buono, P.; Daniele, A. Acrp30 oligomers as potential indicators of adipose tissue improvement in obese subjects. *Eur. J. Endocrinol.* **2013**, *169*, 37–43. [CrossRef] [PubMed]
13. Lacedonia, D.; Nigro, E.; Matera, M.G.; Scudiero, O.; Monaco, M.L.; Polito, R.; Carpagnano, G.E.; Barbaro, M.P.F.; Mazzarella, G.; Bianco, A.; et al. Evaluation of Acrp30 profile in Italian patients affected by obstructive sleep apnea syndrome. *Pulm. Pharmacol. Ther.* **2016**, *40*, 104–108. [CrossRef] [PubMed]
14. Corbi, G.; Polito, R.; Monaco, M.L.; Cacciatore, F.; Scioli, M.; Ferrara, N.; Daniele, A.; Nigro, E. Adiponectin Expression and Genotypes in Italian People with Severe Obesity Undergone a Hypocaloric Diet and Physical Exercise Program. *Nutrients* **2019**, *11*, 2195. [CrossRef] [PubMed]
15. Polito, R.; Nigro, E.; Messina, A.; Monaco, M.L.; Monda, V.; Scudiero, O.; Cibelli, G.; Valenzano, A.; Picciocchi, E.; Zammit, C.; et al. Adiponectin and Orexin-A as a Potential Immunity Link between Adipose Tissue and Central Nervous System. *Front. Physiol.* **2018**, *9*, 982. [CrossRef]
16. Kotz, C.M.; Teske, J.A.; Levine, J.A.; Wang, C. Feeding and activity induced by Orexin A in the lateral hypothalamus in rats. *Regul. Pept.* **2002**, *104*, 27–32. [CrossRef]
17. Kotz, C.M.; Wang, C.; Teske, J.A.; Thorpe, A.; Novak, C.; Kiwaki, K.; Levine, J. Orexin A mediation of time spent moving in rats: Neural mechanisms. *Neuroscience* **2006**, *142*, 29–36. [CrossRef]
18. Boss, C.; Roch, C. Recent trends in Orexin research—2010 to 2015. *Bioorg. Med. Chem. Lett.* **2015**, *25*, 2875–2887. [CrossRef]

19. Salerno, M.; Villano, I.; Nicolosi, D.; Longhitano, L.; Loreto, C.; Lovino, A.; Sessa, F.; Polito, A.N.; Monda, V.; Chieffi, S.; et al. Modafinil and Orexin system: Interactions and medico-legal considerations. *Front. Biosci. Landmark.* **2019**, *24*, 564–575. [CrossRef]
20. Inutsuka, A.; Yamanaka, A. The physiological role of Orexin/hypocretin neurons in the regulation of sleep/wakefulness and neuroendocrine functions. *Front. Endocrinol.* **2013**, *4*, 18. [CrossRef]
21. Chieffi, S.; Carotenuto, M.; Monda, V.; Valenzano, A.; Villano, I.; Precenzano, F.; Tafuri, D.; Salerno, M.; Filippi, N.; Nuccio, F.; et al. Orexin system: The key for a healthy life. *Front. Neurol.* **2017**, *8*, 357. [CrossRef]
22. Milasta, S.; Evans, N.A.; Ormiston, L.; Wilson, S.; Lefkowitz, R.J.; Milligan, G. The sustainability of interactions between the Orexin-1 receptor and b-arrestin-2 is defined by a single C-terminal cluster of hydroxy amino acids and modulates the kinetics of ERK MAPK regulation. *Biochem. J.* **2005**, *387*, 573–584. [CrossRef] [PubMed]
23. Messina, A.; Bitetti, I.; Precenzano, F.; Iacono, D.; Messina, G.; Roccella, M.; Parisi, L.; Salerno, M.; Valenzano, A.; Maltese, A.; et al. Non-rapid eye movement sleep paras- omnias and migraine: A role of Orexinergic projections. *Front. Neurol.* **2018**, *9*, 95. [CrossRef] [PubMed]
24. Messina, G.; Dalia, C.; Tafuri, D.; Monda, V.; Palmieri, F.; Dato, A.; Russo, A.; De Blasio, S.; Messina, G.; De Luca, V.; et al. Orexin-A controls sympathetic activity and eating behavior. *Front. Psychol.* **2014**, *5*, 997. [CrossRef] [PubMed]
25. Messina, A.; De Fusco, C.; Monda, V.; Esposito, M.; Moscatelli, F.; Valenzano, A.; Carotenuto, M.; Viggiano, E.; Chieffi, S.; De Luca, V.; et al. Role of the Orexin system on the hypothalamus-pituitary-thyroid axis. *Front. Neural Circuits* **2016**, *10*, 66. [CrossRef] [PubMed]
26. Monda, M.; Viggiano, A.; Viggiano, A.; Viggiano, E.; Messina, G.; Tafuri, D.; De Luca, V. Sympathetic and hyperthermic reactions by Orexin A: Role of cerebral catecholaminergic neurons. *Regul. Pept.* **2007**, *139*, 39–44. [CrossRef] [PubMed]
27. Messina, G.; Monda, V.; Moscatelli, F.; Valenzano, A.A.; Monda, G.; Esposito, T.; De Blasio, S.; Messina, A.; Tafuri, D.; Barillari, M.R.; et al. Role of Orexin system in obesity. *Biol. Med.* **2015**, *7*, 4. [CrossRef]
28. Monda, V.; Salerno, M.; Sessa, F.; Bernardini, R.; Valenzano, A.; Marsala, G.; Zammit, C.; Avola, R.; Carotenuto, M.; Messina, G.; et al. Functional Changes of Orexinergic Reaction to Psychoactive Substances. *Mol. Neurobiol.* **2018**, *55*, 6362–6368. [CrossRef] [PubMed]
29. Santacroce, R.; Santoro, R.; Sessa, F.; Iannaccaro, P.; Sarno, M.; Longo, V.; Gallone, A.; Vecchione, G.; Muleo, G.; Margaglione, M. Screening of mutations of hemophilia A in 40 Italian patients: A novel G-to-A mutation in intron 10 of the F8 gene as a putative cause of mild hemophilia a in southern Italy. *Blood Coagul. Fibrinolysis* **2008**, *19*, 197–202. [CrossRef] [PubMed]
30. Perez-Leighton, C.E.; Boland, K.; Teske, J.A.; Billington, C.; Kotz, C.M. Behavioral responses to Orexin, Orexin receptor gene expression, and spontaneous physical activity contribute to individual sensitivity to obesity. *Am. J. Physiol. Endocrinol. Metab.* **2012**, *303*, E865–E874. [CrossRef] [PubMed]
31. Digby, J.E.; Chen, J.; Tang, J.Y.; Lehnert, H.; Matthews, R.N.; Randeva, H.S. Orexin receptor expression inhuman adipose tissue: Effects of Orexin-A and Orexin-B.J. *Endocrinology* **2006**, *191*, 129–136. [CrossRef] [PubMed]
32. Valenzano, A.; Polito, R.; Trimigno, V.; Di Palma, A.; Moscatelli, F.; Corso, G.; Sessa, F.; Salerno, M.; Montana, A.; Di Nunno, N.; et al. Effects of Very Low Calorie Ketogenic Diet on the Orexinergic System, Visceral Adipose Tissue, and ROS Production. *Antioxidants* **2019**, *13*, 643. [CrossRef] [PubMed]
33. Odgen, C.L.; Carroll, M.D.; Kit, B.K.; Flegal, K.M. Prevalence of obesity among adults: United States, 2011–2012. *NCHS Data Brief* **2013**, *131*, 1–8.
34. Buchwald, H.; Estok, R.; Fahrbach, K.; Banel, D.; Jensen, M.D.; Pories, W.J.; Bantle, J.P.; Sledge, I. Weightand type 2 diabetes after bariatric surgery: Systematic review and meta-analysis. *Am. J. Med.* **2009**, *122*, 248–256. [CrossRef]
35. Chang, S.H.; Stoll, C.R.; Song, J.; Varela, J.E.; Eagon, C.J.; Colditz, G.A. The effectiveness and risks of bariatric surgery: An updated systematic review and meta-analysis, 2003–2012. *JAMA Surg.* **2014**, *149*, 275–287. [CrossRef] [PubMed]
36. Zsombok, A. Automic control and bariatric procedures. *Review* **2013**, *177*, 81–86.

37. Foschi, D.; de Luca, M.; Sarro, G.; Bernante, P.; Zappa, M.A.; Moroni, R.; Navarra, G.; Foletto, M.; Ceriani, V.; Piazza, L.; et al. *Linea Guida di Chirurgia Dell'obesita-Linee Guida Di Buona Pratica Clinica Nella Selezione, Nella Preparazione, Nel Trattamento Perioperatorio e a Lungo Termine Del Paziente Obeso Sottoposto a Chirurgia Bariatrica*; Edizione: Treviso, Italy, 2016.
38. Angrisani, L.; Santonicola, A.; Iovino, P.; Vitiello, A.; Zundel, N.; Buchwald, H.; Scopinaro, N. Bariatric surgery and endoluminal procedures: IFSO Worldwide Survery 2014. *Obes. Surg.* **2017**, *27*, 2279–2289. [CrossRef]
39. Svane, M.S.; Bojsen-Møller, K.N.; Martinussen, C.; van Hall, G.; Holst, J.J.; Madsbad, S. Postprandial Nutrient Handling and Gastrointestinal Hormone Secretion After Roux-en-Y Gastric Bypass vs Sleeve Gastrectomy. *Orig. Res. Full Rep. Clin. Aliment. Tract* **2019**, *156*, 1627–1641. [CrossRef]
40. Saverio, F.; Elghadban, H.; Parodi, C.; Pagliardi, F.; Weiss, A. BPD and BPD-DS Concerns and Results. In *Advanced Bariatric and Metabolic Surgery*; IntechOpen: London, UK, 2012. [CrossRef]
41. Poirier, P.; Cornier, M.A.; Mazzone, T.; Stiles, S.; Cummings, S.; Klein, S.; McCullough, P.A.; Fielding, C.R.; Franklin, B.A. American Heart Association Obesity Committee of the Council on Nutrition, Physical Activity, and Metabolism. Bariatricsurgery and cardiovascular risk factors: A scientific statement from the AmericanHeart Association. *Circulation* **2011**, *123*, 1683–1701. [CrossRef]
42. O'Brien, P.E.; McPhail, T.; Chaston, T.B.; Dixon, J.B. Systematic review ofmedium-term weight loss after bariatric operations. *Obes. Surg.* **2006**, *16*, 1032–1040. [CrossRef]
43. Ganjavi, H.; Shapiro, C.M. Hypocretin/Orexin: A molecular link betweensleep, energy regulation, and pleasure. *J. Neuropsychiatry Clin. Neurosci.* **2007**, *19*, 413–419. [CrossRef]
44. Heinonen, M.V.; Purhonen, A.K.; Miettinen, P.; Pääkkönen, M.; Pirinen, E.; Alhava, E.; Akerman, K.; Herzig, K.H. Apelin, Orexin-A and leptin plasma levels in morbid obesity and effect of gastric banding. *Regul. Pept.* **2005**, *130*, 7–13. [CrossRef] [PubMed]
45. Kirchgessner, A.L.; Liu, M. Orexin synthesis and response in the gut. *Neuron* **1999**, *24*, 941–951. [CrossRef]
46. Edwards, C.M.; Abusnana, S.; Sunter, D.; Murphy, K.G.; Ghatei, M.A.; Bloom, S.R. The effect of the Orexins on food intake: Comparison with neuropeptide Y, melanin-concentrating hormone and galanin. *J. Endocrinol.* **1999**, *160*, R7–R12. [CrossRef] [PubMed]
47. Burdyga, G.; Lal, S.; Spiller, D.; Jiang, W.; Thompson, D.; Attwood, S.; Saeed, S.; Grundy, D.; Varro, A.; Dimaline, R.; et al. Localization of Orexin-1 receptors to vagal afferent neurons in the rat and humans. *Gastroenterology* **2003**, *124*, 129–139. [CrossRef] [PubMed]
48. Gupta, A.; Miegueu, P.; Lapointe, M.; Poirier, P.; Martin, J.; Bastien, M.; Tiwari, S.; Cianflone, K. Acute Post-Bariatric Surgery Increase in Orexin Levels Associates with Preferential Lipid Profile Improvement. *PLoS ONE* **2014**, *9*, e84803. [CrossRef] [PubMed]
49. Luo, N.; Liu, J.; Chung, B.H.; Yang, Q.; Klein, R.L.; Garvey, W.T.; Fu, Y. Macrophage Adiponectinexpression improves insulin sensitivity and protects against inflammation and atherosclerosis. *Diabetes* **2010**, *59*, 791–799. [CrossRef]
50. Federico, A.; Dallio, M.; Tolone, S.; Gravina, A.G.; Patrone, V.; Romano, M.; Tuccillo, C.; Mozzillo, A.L.; Amoroso, V.; Misso, G.; et al. Gastrointestinal Hormones, Intestinal Microbiota and Metabolic Homeostasis in Obese Patients: Effect of Bariatric Surgery. *In Vivo* **2016**, *30*, 21–30.
51. Cigdem, A.P.; Kocael, A.; Tabak, O.; Taskin, M.; Zengin, K.; Uzun, H. Plasma ghrelin, leptin, and Orexin-A levels and insulin resistance after laparoscopic gastric band applications in morbidly obese patients. *Minerva Med.* **2013**, *104*, 309–316.
52. Amin, R.; Simakajornboon, N.; Szczesniak, R.; Inge, T. Early improvement in obstructive sleep apnea and increase in Orexin levels after bariatric surgery in adolescents and young adults. *Surg. Obes. Relat. Dis.* **2017**, *13*, 95–100. [CrossRef]
53. Rubino, F.; Schauer, P.R.; Lee, K.M.; Cummings, D.E. Metabolic surgery to treat type 2 diabetes: Clinical outcomes and mecha- nisms of action. *Annu. Rev. Med.* **2010**, *61*, 393–411. [CrossRef] [PubMed]
54. Pournaras, D.J.; Aasheim, E.T.; Bueter, M.; Ahmed, A.R.; Welbourn, R.; Olbers, T.; le Roux, C.W. Effect of bypassing the proximal gut on gut hormones involved with gly-cemic control and weight loss. *Surg. Obes. Relat. Dis.* **2012**, *8*, 371–374. [CrossRef] [PubMed]
55. Salman, A.A.; Sultan, A.A.E.A.; Abdallah, A.; Abdelsalam, A.; Mikhail, H.M.S.; Tourky, M. Effect of weight loss induced by laparoscopic sleeve gastrectomy on liver histology and serum adipokine levels. *J. Gastroenterol. Hepatol.* **2020**, *35*, 1769–1773. [CrossRef]

56. Askarpour, M.; Alizadeh, S.; Hadi, A.; Symonds, M.E.; Miraghajani, M.; Sheikhi, A.; Ghaedi, E. Effect of Bariatric Surgery on the Circulating Level of Adiponectin, Chemerin, Plasminogen Activator Inhibitor-1, Leptin, Resistin, and Visfatin: A Systematic Review and Meta-Analysis. *Horm. Metab. Res.* **2020**, *52*, 207–215. [CrossRef] [PubMed]
57. Cavaliere, G.; Viggiano, E.; Trinchese, G.; De Filippo, C.; Messina, A.; Monda, V.; Valenzano, A.; Cincione, R.I.; Zammit, C.; Cimmino, F.; et al. Long feeding high-fat diet induces hypothalamic oxidative stress and inflammation, and prolonged hypothalamic AMPK activation in rat animal model. *Front. Physiol.* **2018**, *9*, 818. [CrossRef]

Journal of
Clinical Medicine

MDPI

Article

Variables Associated with Short-Term Weight Loss in a Cohort of Patients with Morbid Obesity According to Age and Three Types of Bariatric Surgery

Maria D. Alvarez-Bermudez [1,2,†], Flores Martin-Reyes [3,4,†], Luis Ocaña-Wilhelmi [5,6], Francisco J. Moreno-Ruiz [5,7], Juan Alcaide Torres [2,3], Diego Fernandez-Garcia [1,2], Sergio Valdes [3,8,9], Noelia Moreno-Morales [10], Eduardo Garcia-Fuentes [3,4,*], Francisco J. Tinahones [1,2,3,11,*] and Lourdes Garrido-Sanchez [1,2,3]

1 CIBER Fisiopatología Obesidad y Nutrición (CIBERObn), Instituto Salud Carlos III, Km., 228220 Madrid, Spain; mar17alv@gmail.com (M.D.A.-B.); diegofernandezgarcia@hotmail.com (D.F.-G.); lourdes.garrido@ibima.eu (L.G.-S.)
2 Unidad de Gestión Clínica de Endocrinología y Nutrición, Hospital Universitario Virgen de la Victoria, 29010 Málaga, Spain; juan.alcaidetorres@gmail.com
3 Instituto de Investigación Biomédica de Málaga-IBIMA, 29010 Málaga, Spain; floresmarey@hotmail.com (F.M.-R.); sergio.valdes@hotmail.es (S.V.)
4 Unidad de Gestión Clínica de Aparato Digestivo, Hospital Universitario Virgen de la Victoria, 29010 Málaga, Spain
5 Departamento de Especialidades Quirúrgicas, Bioquímica e Inmunología, Universidad de Málaga, 29010 Málaga, Spain; luisowilhelmi@hotmail.com (L.O.-W.); javier.morenoruiz@gmail.com (F.J.M.-R.)
6 Unidad de Gestión Clínica de Cirugía General, Digestiva y Trasplantes, Hospital Universitario Virgen de la Victoria, 29010 Malaga, Spain
7 Unidad de Gestión Clínica de Cirugía General, Digestiva y Trasplantes, Hospital Regional Universitario, 29010 Málaga, Spain
8 CIBER Diabetes y Enfermedades Metabolicas Asociadas (CIBERDEM), Instituto Salud Carlos III, Km. 228220, Madrid, Spain
9 Unidad de Gestión Clínica de Endocrinología y Nutrición, Hospital Regional Universitario, 29010 Málaga, Spain
10 Departamento Fisioterapia. Facultad Ciencias de la Salud, Universidad de Malaga, 29010 Malaga, Spain; nmm@uma.es
11 Departamento de Medicina y Dermatología, Universidad de Málaga, 29010 Málaga, Spain
* Correspondence: edugfl@gmail.com (E.G.-F.); fjtinahones@uma.es (F.J.T.)
† These authors contributed equally to this work.

Received: 21 October 2020; Accepted: 29 October 2020; Published: 2 November 2020

Abstract: Background The percentage of excess weight lost (%EWL) after bariatric surgery (BS) shows great discrepancies from one individual to another. **Objective** To evaluate the %EWL one year after BS and to determine the existence of baseline biomarkers associated with weight loss. **Methods** We studied 329 patients with morbid obesity undergoing three types of BS (biliopancreatic diversion (BPD), Roux-en-Y gastric bypass (RYGB) and sleeve gastrectomy (SG)), depending on the %EWL one year after surgery: good responders (GR) (%EWL ≥ 50%) and non-responders (NR) (%EWL < 50%). **Results** The GR presented a higher percentage of change in anthropometric and biochemical variables compared to the NR group, even within each type of BS. There was a greater percentage of GR among those who underwent RYGB. The patients who underwent SG showed the lowest decrease in biochemical variables, both in GR and NR. Within the GR group, those with a lower age showed greater improvement compared to the other age groups. A %EWL ≥50% was negatively associated with the age and atherogenic index of plasma (AIP), and positively with the type of BS (RYGB). **Conclusions** The GR group was associated with lower age and AIP and undergoing RYGB. Additionally, those patients who underwent SG showed a lower metabolic improvement.

Keywords: morbid obesity; bariatric surgery; excess weight loss

1. Introduction

Obesity and related comorbidities are health problems worldwide. In 2016, about 13% of the world's adult population was shown to be obese [1]. Bariatric surgery (BS) is a therapeutic approach to obesity and its comorbidities, and results in huge benefits in comparison with pharmacological actions [2]. It has been demonstrated that weight loss due to surgery was greater than other conservative therapy effects, and produced better glucose control than medical therapy did [3]. That reduction reaches its maximum between 6 months and 3 years post-surgery [2–4].

Several studies suggest that weight loss is an important contributor to the health outcomes associated with BS [5]. It was considered favourable to lose at least 50% of excess weight after surgery [6]. However, the weight reduction after BS shows great discrepancies from one individual to another [7], with a minority of patients (5–20%) who do not achieve successful long-term weight loss [7]. Considering post-operative weight loss and subsequent recovery, a classification that stratifies the patients into good responders and non-responders was established [8].

Several studies have compared the percentage of excess weight loss (%EWL) between different types of BS [9] or even different techniques of the same type of surgery [10], while others have analyzed several preoperative predictors with discordant results [11,12]. However, the surgery response, even performed with the same technique, is variable among different subjects. This fact could be explained due to metabolic differences before undergoing BS which can be reflected in anthropometric measurements or baseline serum markers [13]. Therefore, these biomarkers may be able to predict the weight loss response rate. However, it is unclear which factors are associated with the amount of excess weight loss after BS [14,15]. A more profound study of pre-surgical factors that are able to predict treatment success would be very useful in clinical practice in order to select the best candidates for each intervention. Some preoperative factors are a predictor of weight loss after Roux-en-Y gastric bypass (RYGB), such as body mass index (BMI) and waist circumference, and age [16]. There is evidence that increased age is associated with a lower %EWL [17]. However, other studies suggest that for patients older than 50 and 60 years, age does not influence the outcome after BS [18].

According to this background, the aim of this retrospective observational study was the evaluation of the response regarding weight loss in the short term (1 year after BS) on all patients with morbid obesity who underwent different BS techniques, as well as to determine the existence of baseline biomarker associated to weight loss.

2. Experimental Section

2.1. Subjects of Study

Patients with morbid obesity (BMI > 40 kg/m^2) in our retrospective observational study were selected among the 582 subjects that underwent BS at the Virgen de la Victoria University Hospital and at the Regional University Hospital of Malaga between 2008–2017 and consented to participate in the study. From those, only those patients that attended at baseline and at the follow-up one year after BS, and with data in all the variables analyzed were included (n = 329). There are no significant differences in biochemical and anthropometric variables and comorbidities between patients included and not included in this study (data not shown). Three types of surgical techniques (sleeve gastrectomy (SG), biliopancreatic diversion (BPD) and RYGB) were performed. The surgical technique used depended on the multidisciplinary team that followed the patient. RYGB and SG were performed at the Regional University Hospital, and BPD and SG were performed at the Virgen de la Victoria University Hospital. The characteristics of these techniques have been shown in previous studies [19,20]. RYGB consists of a small longitudinal gastric pouch (20 mL) created along the lesser curvature that is totally separated from the main stomach. The jejunum is divided 40 cm distal to the ligament of Treitz and advanced in an antecolic/antegastric position to create a 125 cm Roux-en-Y limb, which is anastomosed to the gastric pouch [20]. BPD consists of a distal gastrectomy with a long Roux-en-Y reconstruction with the enteroenteric anastomosis performed 50 cm proximal to the ileocecal valve and the gastroenteric anastomosis performed 250 cm proximal to the ileocecal valve, with 200 mL of gastric volume [19]. SG is a technique that involves a longitudinal section parallel to the gastric lesser curvature supervised by the Fouche probe. The vascularization of the stomach is not compromised as the arterial supply of the celiac trunk remains intact [19]. The SG technique was similar in these two hospitals. The study was conducted in accordance with the guidelines laid down in the Declaration of Helsinki. All participants gave their informed consent to participate in this study prior to BS, and the study was reviewed and approved by the Ethics Committee of the Provincial Research of Malaga. The patients with morbid obesity were evaluated at baseline (prior to BS) and were followed up one year after the intervention by a multidisciplinary team (surgeons, endocrinologists and researchers), during which different anthropometric and biochemical data were prospectively collected. When the patients gave their consent, they were also informed that the data to be collected would be used for studies other than this one.

2.2. Clinical and Anthropometric Variables

Data were prospectively collected prior to BS and at 12 months in the postsurgical period. Anthropometric variables, both before BS and one year after, were measured in all the patients with morbid obesity included in the study. These included measurements of weight, height, waist and hip circumferences, and blood pressure. BMI was calculated as weight in kilograms divided by height in square metres. The %EWL was based on the excess weight compared to the weight corresponding to a BMI of 25 kg/m^2 for each patient.

2.3. Assessment of Weight Change

We assessed %EWL as 100 × (preoperative weight—weight at the time of evaluation)/(preoperative weight—weight corresponding to BMI = 25 Kg/m^2) [21]. The different patterns of weight loss were defined based on the EWL Reinhold criteria. Weight loss was considered insufficient when %EWL <50% in analogy with the Reinhold criteria [22]. The Reinhold criteria were modified by Christou et al. [23]. The patients with %EWL >50% of the weight at the beginning and throughout follow-up were considered as good responders (GR). On the other hand, patients with %EWL <50% of the weight at the beginning and up to the follow-up were considered as non-responders (NR).

2.4. Biochemical Variables

Blood samples were collected after a 12-h fast. The serum was separated and immediately frozen at −80 °C [19]. Serum glucose, cholesterol, triglycerides and HDL were analysed using an Advia Chemistry XPT autoanalyzer (Siemens Healthcare Diagnostics). Coefficients of variation for glucose, cholesterol, triglycerides and HDL were 1.8%, 2.5%, 3.9% and 4.5% respectively. The LDL was calculated from the Friedewald equation. Serum insulin levels were measured by immunoassay using an ADVIA Centaur autoanalyzer (Siemens Healthcare Diagnostics). Insulin resistance was calculated by the following formula: HOMA-IR = fasting insulin (μIU/mL) × fasting glucose (mmol/L)/22.5. The determination of leptin and adiponectin was performed by commercial enzyme-linked immunosorbent assay (ELISA) (Mediagnost, Germany, BLK Diagnostics, Spain, respectively). C-reactive protein (CRP) was performed by commercial ELISA (DRG Instruments GmbH, Marburg, Germany). Atherogenic index of plasma (AIP) was calculated as log (triglycerides/HDL) [24]. Total cholesterol/HDL cholesterol (TC/HDL) and triglycerides/HDL cholesterol (TG/HDL) index were also calculated [25]. The percentages of change (Δ) of the different anthropometric and biochemical variables at one year after BS were calculated using the following formula: (baseline variable—one-year variable) × 100/baseline variable [19].

Alterations in hydrocarbon metabolism were defined according to the criteria proposed by the American Diabetes Association (ADA) [26]. Type 2 diabetes mellitus (T2DM) was defined as two fasting plasma glucose values >125 mg/dl or glycated haemoglobin ≥6.5% or treatment with non-insulin hypoglycaemic agents or insulin. Criteria for hypertension diagnosis were current treatment with antihypertensive agents and/or systolic blood pressure >140 mmHg and/or diastolic blood pressure >90 mmHg [27]. Hypercholesterolemia was defined as total cholesterol >200 mg/dl or the use of cholesterol-lowering drugs [28].

2.5. Statistical Analysis

The statistical analysis was performed with SPSS (Windows 15.0; SPSS, Chicago, IL, USA). Data were expressed as mean ± standard deviation for continuous variables and as percentages for categorical variables. Student's *t*-test was performed to assess differences between two means. The differences in the variables within the same group, before and after BS, were compared with the Student's t-test for paired samples. Comparison between the results of the different groups was made with the one-way ANOVA and the post hoc analysis with the Bonferroni test. A Chi-square test was used to evaluate the degree of association between categorical variables. Pearson correlation coefficients were calculated to estimate the lineal associations between variables. The strength of association between variables was analysed by multivariate logistic regression models controlled for potential confounders such as age, sex, BMI at baseline, among others. Values were considered to be statistically significant when $p \leq 0.05$.

3. Results

We followed 329 patients with morbid obesity during the first year after BS. Table 1 shows the characteristic of patients included in this study according to the type of BS. Patients underwent BPD were slightly more obese (higher weight (p = 0.001), BMI (p = 0.001), and waist (p = 0.045) and hip circumferences (p = 0.018)), and those underwent SG had lower glucose levels (p = 0.004). Patients lost the same total weight regardless of the type of BS (BPD: 44.2 ± 15.5 kg; RYGB: 48.4 ± 16.8 kg; SG: 44.8 ± 17.7 kg; p = 0.230). However, there was a lower percentage of total weight-loss (Δ-Weight) after BPD (29.7 ± 8.9%) than after RYGB (35.2 ± 8.1%) and SG (32.6 ± 9.3%) (p = 0.002).

Table 1. Characteristics of patients with morbid obesity at baseline classified according to the type of bariatric surgery.

	Pre-Surgery		
	BPD	**RYGB**	**SG**
N (%)	66	83	180
Sex (men/women)	24/42	20/63	59/121
Age (years)	42.9 ± 9.6	43.9 ± 9.4	44.1 ± 10.1
Weight (Kg)	147.4 ± 22.8 [a]	135.3 ± 23.7 [b]	135.1 ± 23.7 [b]
BMI (kg/m^2)	53.8 ± 6.5 [a]	49.7 ± 8.0 [b]	50.2 ± 7.7 [b]
Waist (cm)	141.4 ± 16.7 [a]	135.8 ± 15.4 [b]	134.4 ± 13.4 [b]
Hip (cm)	152.6 ± 13.3 [a]	147.6 ± 17.2 [b]	146.1 ± 14.9 [b]
SBP (mmHg)	138.5 ± 20.9	137.9 ± 18.3	137.5 ± 19.1
DBP (mmHg)	84.9 ± 14.5	81.7 ± 12.5	83.0 ± 10.4
Glucose (mg/dL)	117.1 ± 40.6 [a]	119.8 ± 51.9 [a]	104.8 ± 49.9 [b]
Total cholesterol (mg/dL)	193.3 ± 44.9	197.8 ± 37.0	187.5 ± 33.7
Triglycerides (mg/dL) *	151.3 (101.2–208.0)	127.0 (99.0–184.0)	122.0 (77.1–145.5)
HDL (mg/dL)	44.6 ± 10.4	47.1 ± 11.5	44.4 ± 11.3
LDL (mg/dL)	119.9 ± 36.3	121.6 ± 31.6	109.8 ± 31.7
Insulin (µIU/mL) *	19.2 (16.2–24.3)	15.3 (13.2–21.9)	13.1 (11.1–20.4)
HOMA-IR *	5.03 (4.2–7.7)	4.01 (3.3–6.2)	3.6 (2.6–4.9)
Leptin (ng/mL) *	58.8 (52.3–84.6)	62.3 (49.0–81.5)	41.9 (33.4–57.4)
Adiponectin (µg/mL)	8.8 ± 4.5	7.9 ± 3.8	8.2 ± 3.5
CRP (mg/L) *	5.3 (3.9–9.3)	9.7 (7.8–16.4)	3.3 (1.5–8.1)
TG/HDL *	3.7 (1.9–5.6)	2.7 (2.1–3.5)	2.1 (1.7–3.2)
TC/HDL	4.3 ± 1.2	4.3 ± 1.1	4.3 ± 1.2
AIP	0.46 ± 0.26	0.45 ± 0.27	0.47 ± 0.27

Table 1. *Cont.*

	Pre-Surgery		
	BPD	**RYGB**	**SG**
Comorbidities			
%Patients with T2DM (n)	39.4 (26)	44.6 (37)	32.7 (59)
%Patients with hypertension (n)	74.3 (49)	82.0 (68)	72.7 (131)
%Patients with hypercholesterolemia (n)	47.0 (31)	67.5 (56)	41.7 (75)

The results are given as the mean ± SD. * These results are given as median (interquartile range). BMI: Body mass index. SBP: Systolic blood pressure; DBP: Diastolic blood pressure; HOMA-IR: homeostasis model assessment of insulin resistance index. CRP: C-reactive protein. TG: triglycerides; TC: total cholesterol. AIP: atherogenic index of plasma. Different letters show significant differences between the means of the three types of bariatric surgery: $p < 0.05$.

The characteristics of patients classified according to the %EWL are presented in Table 2. Those patients with %EWL <50% presented a higher age (p = 0.031), baseline BMI (p = 0.005) and hip circumference (p = 0.037) than those with %EWL ≥50%. There was a decrease in the percentage of comorbidities after BS, both in the group of patients with %EWL <50% and with %EWL ≥50% (Table 2). However, these changes were more significant in those with %EWL ≥50%.

Table 2. Characteristics of patients with morbid obesity at baseline and one year after bariatric surgery, classified according to the percentage of excess weight loss (%EWL).

	Pre-Surgery		Post-Surgery	
	%EWL <50%	**%EWL ≥50%**	**%EWL <50%**	**%EWL ≥50%**
N (%)	64 (19.4%)	265 (80.6%)	64 (19.4%)	265 (80.6%)
Sex (men/women)	18/46	85/180		
Age (years)	46.6 ± 10.2	43.9 ±9.7 ^{1}		
Weight (Kg)	142.2 ± 24.9	137.1 ± 23.7	111.9 ± 17.6 ‡	87.9 ± 14.1 ^{2,‡}
BMI (kg/m^2)	53.4 ± 8.6	50.1 ± 7.4 ^{1}	42.0 ± 5.8 ‡	32.1 ± 4.5 ^{2,‡}
Waist (cm)	140.9 ± 14.3	136.6 ± 15.8	120.0 ± 12.5 ‡	102.4 ± 12.2 ^{2,‡}
Hip (cm)	152.5 ± 14.5	147.1 ± 15.4 ^{1}	132.1 ± 12.1 ‡	113.5 ± 12.8 ^{2,‡}
SBP (mmHg)	142.8 ± 19.9	137.8 ± 18.6	131.6 ± 19.6 ‡	127.9 ± 20.4 ‡
DBP (mmHg)	84.5 ± 10.7	82.7 ± 11.9	81.4 ± 13.0 ‡	76.7 ± 12.3 ^{1,‡}
Glucose (mg/dL)	115.3 ± 34.1	110.7 ± 41.9	91.6 ± 12.2 ‡	83.9 ± 15.5 ^{2,‡}
Total cholesterol (mg/dL)	196.7 ± 39.1	188.1 ± 36.7	182.3 ± 50.6	173.7 ± 38.2 ‡
Triglycerides (mg/dL) *	183.0 (123.2–234.5)	122.1 (92.9–168.0)	147.0 (106.5–168.0) †	82.0 (60.5–114.0) ^{2,‡}
HDL (mg/dL)	44.9 ± 10.9	45.5 ± 11.3	50.7 ± 15.5 †	53.7 ± 13.3 ‡
LDL (mg/dL)	120.8 ± 34.0	113.9 ± 32.2	108.8 ± 40.0	103.5 ± 32.8 ‡
Insulin (μIU/mL) *	15.3 (13.4–20.6)	17.1 (12.9–23.6)	9.1 (7.4–11.4) ‡	7.5 (5.2–9.1) ^{2,‡}
HOMA-IR *	4.3 (3.5–5.5)	4.4 (3.3–6.7)	2.1 (1.5–2.4) ‡	1.5 (1.1–1.9) ^{2,‡}
Leptin (ng/mL) *	78.4 (45.8–88.1)	58.2 (43.7–75.0)	25.4 (15.1–39.2) ‡	12.0 (8.8–16.0) ^{2,‡}
Adiponectin (μg/mL)	9.1 ± 4.0	7.9 ± 4.1	11.1 ± 5.3	13.8 ± 6.7 ‡
CRP (mg/L) *	7.5 (5.7–11.7)	8.1 (3.9–11.4)	0.3 (0.2–1.7) †	0.7 (0.3–2.3) ‡
TG/HDL *	4.0 (2.7–5.9)	2.6 (1.9–3.6)	3.1 (2.9–4.0) ‡	1.6 (1.0–2.4) ^{2,‡}
TC/HDL	4.6 ± 1.2	4.3 ± 1.1	3.7 ± 1.1 ‡	3.3 ± 0.9 ^{1,‡}
AIP	0.50 ± 0.26	0.45 ± 0.27	0.36 ± 0.25 ‡	0.19 ± 0.21 ^{2,‡}
Comorbidities				
%Patients with T2DM (n)	45.3 (29)	35.4 (94)	3.2 (2) †	0.8 (2) ‡
%Patients with hypertension (n)	82.8 (53)	73.5 (195)	60.9 (39) †	49.1 (130) ‡
%Patients with hypercholesterolemia (n)	56.2 (36)	48.3 (128)	39.0 (25) †	28.3 (75) ‡

The results are given as the mean ± SD. * These results are given as median (interquartile range). BMI: Body mass index. SBP: Systolic blood pressure; DBP: Diastolic blood pressure; HOMA-IR: homeostasis model assessment of insulin resistance index. CRP: C-reactive protein. TG: triglycerides; TC: total cholesterol. AIP: atherogenic index of plasma. Significant differences between patients with morbid obesity with %EWL < 50 and those with %EWL ≥50%, both baseline and one year after bariatric surgery: ^{1} $p < 0.05$; ^{2} $p < 0.001$. Significant differences in patients with morbid obesity between before and after bariatric surgery, both in those with %EWL <50% and in those with %EWL ≥ 50%: † $p < 0.05$; ‡ $p < 0.001$.

3.1. Association Between %EWL and the Variables Studied

The next step was to analyse the linear association between %EWL and anthropometric and biochemical variables through correlation analysis. There was a significant linear association between

%EWL and age ($r = -0.302$, $p < 0.001$), weight ($r = 0.280$, $p < 0.001$), BMI ($r = 0.259$, $p < 0.001$), waist ($r = 0.215$, $p < 0.001$) and hip circumference ($r = 0.287$, $p < 0.001$) and AIP ($r = -0.211$, $p < 0.001$). No other significant associations were found (data not shown).

The variables associated with a %EWL ≥50% in a logistic regression model were the age, AIP and the type of BS (RYGB) (Table 3). This regression was adjusted for sex, BMI, HOMA-IR, CRP and hypertension (yes/no), which are related to the metabolic alterations most frequently associated with the presence and development of obesity: insulin resistance (HOMA-IR) [29], inflammation (CRP) [30] and hypertension [31].

Table 3. Variables associated with a %EWL ≥50% (%EWL <50% (0) and %EWL ≥50% (1)) obtained from a logistic regression model.

	B Coefficient	*p*	OR	(95% Confidence Interval)
Sex (women = 0/men = 1)	−0.462	0.449	0.630	0.191–2.081
Age	−0.066	0.050	0.936	0.876–0.999
BMI	−0.001	0.977	0.999	0.913–1.092
Hypertension (yes = 0/no = 1)	−0.673	0.416	0.510	0.101–2.579
AIP	−3.188	0.019	0.041	0.003–0.591
Type of surgery		0.045		
Type of surgery (SG)	0.958	0.196	2.607	0.610–11.147
Type of surgery (RYGB)	1.850	0.014	6.360	1.465–27.606
HOMA-IR	0.106	0.227	1.112	0.936–1.320
CRP	−0.015	0.692	0.985	0.914–1.062

3.2. %EWL According to the Type of BS

One year after BS, 80.5% of patients reached %EWL ≥50%. When analysed according to the type of BS, 86.7% of patients who underwent RYGB were GR. For SG, 82.2% were GR and of those undergoing BPD, 68.2% were GR. There was a greater percentage of patients who underwent RYGB who reached %EWL ≥50% compared to the other types of BS ($p = 0.012$).

Table 4 shows the characteristics of patients classified according to %EWL and the surgical technique used. A worse metabolic profile was found in those patients with %EWL <50%, both within BPD and SG groups. Within RYGB, we did not find significant differences.

3.3. %EWL and Comorbidities According the Type of BS

We analysed whether there were significant differences in these comorbidities within each type of BS, according to %EWL (Table 4). Within the SG group, we found a higher percentage of patients with T2DM ($p = 0.034$) and hypertension ($p = 0.017$) in the group of patients with %EWL <50%. No significant differences were observed within the BPD and RYGB groups.

3.4. %EWL According to Sex

Regarding sex, there were no significant differences in the percentage of women and men between the group of patients with %EWL ≥50% or with %EWL <50%.

3.5. %EWL According to Age

When the age was classified in quartiles (≤37 years, >37 and ≤44 (37–44) years, >44 and ≤52 (45–52) years and >52 years), we did not find significant differences in the percentage of GR, although a tendency was observed: the age ≤37 years group: 85.5%; the 37–44 years group: 82.7%; the 45–52 years group: 78.7%; the >52 years group: 75.3%.

Subsequently, we analysed whether there were significant differences according to the %EWL within each age group (Table 5). The main differences were within the 37–44 years group, with higher levels in the group of patients with %EWL <50%.

Table 4. Baseline characteristics of patients with morbid obesity classified according to %EWL and the type of bariatric surgery.

	%EWL <50%			%EWL ≥50%		
	BPD	**RYGB**	**SG**	**BPD**	**RYGB**	**SG**
N (% within each type of BS)	21 (31.8%)	11 (13.3%)	32 (17.8%)	45 (68.2%)	72 (86.7%)	148 (82.2%)
Sex (men/women)	8/13	2/9	8/24	16/29	18/54	51/97
Age (years)	42.0 ± 8.9	46.6 ± 11.8	48.1 ± 9.9	41.6 ± 10.1	43.5 ± 9.1	44.4 ± 9.9
Weight (Kg)	148.9 ± 24.6	137.8 ± 23.5	137.5 ± 26.6	146.6 ± 21.6 [a]	134.8 ± 23.1 [b]	134.7 ± 23.8 [b]
BMI (kg/m2)	54.4 ± 7.8	52.4 ± 8.2	52.3 ± 9.8	53.5 ± 5.9 [a]	49.9 ± 7.6 [b]	49.2 ± 7.4 [b]
Waist (cm)	143.8 ± 14.7	135.0 ± 13.2	139.5 ± 13.8	140.3 ± 15.8	137.1 ± 16.2	135.1 ± 15.6
Hip (cm)	153.6 ± 10.4	147.5 ± 20.3	150.6 ± 14.7	152.2 ± 13.3 [a]	147.6 ± 16.9 [a,b]	145.2 ± 14.8 [b]
SBP (mmHg)	138.0 ± 23.5	134.6 ± 5.5	145.1 ± 17.4	138.7 ± 20.2	137.6 ± 18.2	136.7 ± 18.2 [1]
DBP (mmHg)	84.4 ± 15.1	77.0 ± 3.4	85.7 ± 8.8	85.1 ± 14.9	82.1 ± 12.8	82.5 ± 10.8
Glucose (mg/dL)	120.2 ± 31.6	116.2 ± 52.9	105.7 ± 20.1	115.4 ± 44.9 [a,b]	120.2 ± 52.2 [a]	103.4 ± 32.9 [b,1]
Total cholesterol (mg/dL)	200.0 ± 42.9	207.6 ± 45.8	183.4 ± 31.6	189.6 ± 46.1 [a,b]	196.5 ± 35.9 [a]	182.3 ± 34.2 [b]
Triglycerides (mg/dL) *	165.5 (130.0–210.0)	175.0 (96.0–183.0)	179.0 (143.0–222.0)	105.0 (87.0–169.0) [b,1]	138.5 (100.0–202.0) [a]	110.0 (75.5–128.4) [a,b]
HDL (mg/dL)	40.6 ± 10.4 [b]	50.0 ± 9.3 [a]	45.4 ± 11.7 [a,b]	46.7 ± 9.8 [1]	46.7 ± 11.8	44.2 ± 11.2
LDL (mg/dL)	125.7 ± 39.6	129.0 ± 40.7	109.3 ± 25.3	117.2 ± 34.5	118.3 ± 32.7	109.9 ± 33.0
Insulin (μIU/mL) *	17.9 (13.3–22.2)	17.0 (13.7–25.8)	12.5 (11.9–15.4)	22.2 (16.7–28.6)	16.9 (13.5–24.1)	17.3 (11.0–22.5)
HOMA-IR *	5.4 (4.2–6.4)	4.1 (3.4–9.9)	3.5 (2.9–4.3)	6.9 (4.2–9.2)	4.3 (3.3–6.8)	3.8 (2.7–5.5)
Leptin (ng/mL) *	88.1 (57.7–91.2)	78.7 (42.0–122.3)	39.8 (39.5–106.0)	56.8 (51.0–67.0) [1]	63.2 (46.0–94.0)	43.8 (35.5–68.8)
Adiponectin (μg/mL)	8.6 ± 4.2	9.1 ± 4.4	9.8 ± 2.3	8.8 ± 4.7	7.1 ± 3.7	7.9 ± 3.6
CRP (mg/L) *	5.9 (3.4–9.4)	7.9 (2.4–15.6)	9.4 (4.8–10.8)	4.3 (3.0–9.8) [a,b]	8.5 (3.8–12.7) [a]	3.3 (1.4–9.2) [b]
TG/HDL *	3.7 (2.9–5.8)	3.1 (2.5–3.5)	2.8 (2.5–5.0)	2.5 (1.7–3.9) [2]	3.0 (2.0–4.0)	2.2 (1.5–3.1)
TC/HDL	5.2 ± 1.2 [a]	4.2 ± 0.8 [b]	4.2 ± 1.2 [b]	4.1 ± 1.1 [2]	4.4 ± 1.2	4.3 ± 1.2
AIP	0.60 ± 0.27	0.43 ± 0.19	0.47 ± 0.27	0.38 ± 0.23 [2]	0.47 ± 0.28	0.47 ± 0.27
Comorbilities						
%Patients with T2DM (n)	42.9 (9)	36.7 (4)	46.8 (15)	37.8 (17)	45.8 (33)	29.1 (43) [1]
%Patients with hypertension (n)	66.7 (14)	100.0 (11)	87.5 (28)	80.0 (36)	80.5 (58)	69.6 (103) [1]
%Patients with hypercholesterolemia (n)	57.1 (12)	81.8 (9)	40.6 (13)	42.2 (19)	65.3 (47)	41.9 (62)

The results are given as the mean ± SD. * These results are given as median (interquartile range). BMI: Body mass index. SBP: Systolic blood pressure; DBP: Diastolic blood pressure; HOMA-IR: homeostasis model assessment of insulin resistance index. CRP: C-reactive protein. TG: triglycerides; TC: total cholesterol; AIP: atherogenic index of plasma. Different letters show significant differences between the means of the three types of bariatric surgery: $p < 0.05$. Significant differences between patients with morbid obesity with %EWL <50 and those with %EWL ≥50% according to the type of bariatric surgery: [1] $p < 0.05$; [2] $p < 0.01$ and [3] $p < 0.001$ (to simplify these data, significant differences are marked in bold).

Table 5. Baseline characteristics of patients with morbid obesity classified according to the percentage of excess weight loss (%EWL) and age.

	%EWL <50%				%EWL ≥50%			
	≤37 Years	**37–44 Years**	**45–52 Years**	**>52 Years**	**≤37 Years**	**37–44 Years**	**45–52 Years**	**>52 Years**
N (% within each group of age)	12 (14.5%)	14 (17.3%)	17 (21.3%)	21 (24.7%)	71 (85.5%)	67 (82.7%)	63 (78.7%)	64 (75.3%)
Sex (men/women)	4/8	5/9	5/12	4/17	23/48	16/51	23/40	23/41
Age (years)	31.2 ± 4.6 ^{d}	40.6 ± 1.9 ^{c}	48.7 ± 2.1 ^{b}	57.9 ± 2.4 ^{a}	31.4 ± 4.7 ^{d}	41.4 ± 1.8 ^{c}	47.8 ± 2.1 ^{b}	56.4 ± 3.4 ^{a,1}
Weight (Kg)	146.2 ± 28.1 ^{a,b}	159.9 ± 24.5 ^{a}	137.7 ± 20.9 ^{b,c}	128.2 ± 21.4 ^{c}	144.9 ± 24.9 ^{a}	133.3 ± 21.0 ^{b,2}	137.0 ± 22.8 ^{b}	131.8 ± 23.2 ^{b}
BMI (kg/m2)	52.6 ± 10.5 ^{a,b}	58.6 ± 7.8 ^{a}	51.2 ± 8.9 ^{b}	51.3 ± 7.0 ^{b}	51.8 ± 8.1 ^{a}	49.7 ± 7.6 ^{a,b,2}	49.4 ± 6.4 ^{a,b}	49.1 ± 7.0 ^{b}
Waist (cm)	148.6 ± 16.6 ^{a}	146.4 ± 16.7 ^{a,b}	134.7 ± 11.2 ^{c}	136.9 ± 13.3 ^{b,c}	137.3 ± 16.9 ^{a,b}	132.6 ± 15.4 ^{b,2}	136.9 ± 14.2 ^{a,b}	139.1 ± 15.6 ^{a}
Hip (cm)	152.9 ± 18.8	156.8 ± 15.4	149.3 ± 13.1	149.8 ± 14.9	151.0 ± 16.4 ^{a}	146.2 ± 14.2 ^{a,b,2}	144.7 ± 16.3 ^{b}	145.7 ± 13.6 ^{ab}
SBP (mmHg)	127.8 ± 9.8 ^{b}	135.2 ± 12.4 ^{b}	138.7 ± 22.2 ^{b}	156.7 ± 15.8 ^{a}	135.6 ± 15.5 ^{b}	135.3 ± 18.2 ^{b}	136.1 ± 20.6 ^{b}	143.2 ± 20.1 ^{a,1}
DBP (mmHg)	83.8 ± 8.9	83.5 ± 9.3	83.6 ± 13.8	86.6 ± 9.3	82.0 ± 11.2	83.8 ± 12.1	81.3 ± 12.0	83.8 ± 12.2
Glucose (mg/dL)	111.7 ± 40.6	127.0 ± 38.3	107.1 ± 25.6	114.3 ± 33.6	97.0 ± 31.0 ^{c}	107.1 ± 31.3 ^{b,c,2}	111.6 ± 46.6 ^{b}	126.2 ± 50.2 ^{a}
Total cholesterol (mg/dL)	189.7 ± 35.2	198.2 ± 45.3	185.1 ± 39.9	206.4 ± 36.5	184.7 ± 36.6	185.4 ± 37.2	190.2 ± 37.3	190.7 ± 36.5
Triglycerides (mg/dL) *	194.5 (127.5–351.4)	1710 (150.5–216.0)	149.9 (112.7–185.4)	179.0 (122.5–193.0)	117.5 (71.0–147.0) ^{b}	120.0 (89.5–187.5) ^{ab,1}	105.0 (88.0–157.0) ^{b}	138.8 (121.0–209.0) ^{a}
HDL (mg/dL)	40.1 ± 8.1 ^{b}	43.0 ± 11.2 ^{b}	40.9 ± 9.4 ^{b}	52.8 ± 10.8 ^{a}	43.6 ± 11.7	45.4 ± 12.1	45.9 ± 9.4 ^{1}	46.7 ± 11.9 ^{1}
LDL (mg/dL)	114.5 ± 23.9	119.1 ± 39.1	118.0 ± 37.1	125.0 ± 33.4	114.2 ± 28.0	114.3 ± 34.1	114.3 ± 35.0	112.2 ± 33.0
Insulin (μIU/mL) *	15.2 (12.1–23.4)	25.8 (20.3–33.6)	13.1 (11.9–16.3)	15.4 (13.1–18.8)	18.4 (12.8–29.4)	18.1 (12.8–24.5)	20.1 (15.1–24.0)	16.8 (13.1–23.5)
HOMA-IR *	5.6 (4.1–6.1)	9.4 (5.9–14.2)	4.0 (3.0–4.3)	3.9 (3.3–4.7)	4.1 (2.7–7.5)	4.7 (3.5–6.9) ^{1}	5.1 (3.8–7.5)	4.3 (3.3–7.1)
Leptin (ng/mL) *	67.0 (37.1–98.7)	90.7 (83.6–93.5)	60.8 (34.0–91.2)	68.3 (39.6–109.0)	59.1 (49.0–83.3)	53.4 (41.0–85.4)	62.3 (35.9–82.9)	53.0 (38.0–64.2)
Adiponectin (μg/mL)	5.4 ± 2.6 ^{b}	7.9 ± 5.8 ^{a,b}	9.8 ± 2.4 ^{a}	10.8 ± 3.2 ^{a}	7.5 ± 3.7	8.5 ± 4.7	8.6 ± 3.8	8.9 ± 3.9
CRP (mg/L) *	7.8 (4.3–28.9)	8.3 (4.1–17.7)	4.9 (3.4–5.7)	8.5 (5.5–13.2)	8.3 (3.4–11.3)	4.2 (1.8–8.9)	7.3 (1.7–11.8)	7.3 (3.8–9.8)
TG/HDL *	4.6 (3.3–11.5)	4.2 (2.8–5.8)	3.0 (2.9–4.0)	2.8 (2.5–4.2)	2.6 (1.5–3.1)	2.6 (1.7–3.9) ^{1}	2.2 (2.0–3.5)	3.1 (2.1–5.6)
TC/HDL	4.8 ± 1.3	4.8 ± 1.4	4.6 ± 1.1	4.1 ± 0.9	4.4 ± 1.3	4.4 ± 1.2	4.2 ± 1.0	4.2 ± 1.2
AIP	0.55 ± 0.29	0.59 ± 0.27	0.51 ± 0.24	0.41 ± 0.26	0.43 ± 0.26	0.41 ± 0.27 ^{1}	0.45 ± 0.25	0.51 ± 0.29
Comorbidities								
%Patients with T2DM (n)	25.0 (3)	57.1 (8)	47.0 (8)	47.6 (10)	18.3 (13)	26.8 (18) ^{1}	34.9 (22)	62.5 (40)
%Patients with hypertension (n)	58.3 (7)	64.2 (9)	82.4 (14)	100.0 (21)	59.1 (42)	74.6 (50)	77.8 (49)	84.3 (54) ^{1}
%Patients with hypercholesterolemia (n)	41.7 (5)	71.4 (10)	35.3 (6)	71.4 (15)	35.2 (25)	43.2 (29) ^{1}	50.8 (32)	68.8 (44)

The results are given as the mean ± SD or * as median (interquartile range). BMI: Body mass index. SBP: Systolic blood pressure; DBP: Diastolic blood pressure; HOMA-IR: homeostasis model assessment of insulin resistance index. CRP: C-reactive protein. TG: triglycerides; TC: total cholesterol. AIP: atherogenic index of plasma. Different letters show significant differences between the means of the four groups of age: $p < 0.05$. Significant differences between patients with morbid obesity with %EWL <50 and those with %EWL ≥50% according to age: ^{1} $p < 0.05$; ^{2} $p < 0.01$ and ^{3} $p < 0.001$ (to simplify these data, significant differences are marked in bold).

3.6. %EWL and Comorbidities According to Age

We also analysed whether there were significant differences in the comorbidities within each age group according to %EWL (Table 5). No significant differences were observed in the group of patients age ≤37 years and 45–52 years. Within the 37–44 years group, we observed a higher percentage of patients with T2DM ($p = 0.035$) and hypercholesterolemia ($p = 0.048$) in the group of patients with %EWL <50%. Finally, within the >52 years group, we observed a higher percentage of hypertensive patients ($p = 0.049$) in the group of patients with %EWL <50%.

3.7. %EWL and Percentage Change (Δ) of Anthropometric and Biochemical Variables

We analysed the Δ-anthropometric and Δ-biochemical variables according to the %EWL. Those patients with %EWL ≥ 50% presented a significant higher percentage of change compared to the group with %EWL < 50% in Δ-weight ($p < 0.001$), Δ-IMC ($p < 0.001$), Δ-waist ($p < 0.001$), Δ-hip ($p < 0.001$), Δ-triglycerides ($p = 0.002$), Δ-leptin ($p < 0.001$), Δ-HOMA-IR ($p < 0.001$), Δ-adiponectin ($p = 0.024$) and Δ-TG/HDL index ($p = 0.009$). No other significant differences were found.

3.8. %EWL and Δ-Anthropometric and Δ-Biochemical Variables According to Type of BS

We also analysed the Δ-anthropometric and Δ-biochemical variables according to %EWL and type of BS (Table 6). Higher Δ-anthropometric and Δ-biochemical variables were found in those patients with %EWL ≥50% within the three types of BS.

Within the %EWL <50% group (Table 6), the patients underwent SG showed the lowest decrease in glucose ($p = 0.035$) and CRP levels ($p = 0.015$), and the greatest increase in cholesterol ($p < 0.001$), HDL ($p = 0.017$) and LDL ($p < 0.001$) levels. The patients underwent RYGB showed the lowest decrease in waist circumference ($p = 0.019$).

Within the %EWL ≥50% group (Table 6), the patients underwent SG showed the lowest decrease in glucose ($p = 0.023$) and TC/HDL ($p = 0.006$) levels, and the greatest increase in cholesterol ($p < 0.001$), HDL ($p < 0.001$), LDL ($p < 0.001$) and adiponectin ($p = 0.004$) levels. The patients underwent BPD showed the lowest decrease in weight ($p = 0.042$), BMI ($p = 0.042$), waist circumference ($p = 0.045$), triglycerides ($p < 0.001$), TG/HDL ($p < 0.001$) and AIP ($p = 0.038$).

3.9. %EWL and Δ-Anthropometric and Δ-Biochemical Variables According to Age

We also analysed the Δ-anthropometric and Δ-biochemical variables according to %EWL and age (Table 7). Higher Δ-anthropometric and Δ-biochemical variables were found in those patients with %EWL ≥50% within the four groups of age.

Within the %EWL <50% group (Table 7), there was no age group that was clearly different compared to the other groups.

Within the %EWL ≥50% group (Table 7), the ≤37 years group showed the greatest decreases compared to the other groups (in weight ($p < 0.001$), BMI ($p < 0.001$), waist ($p = 0.001$) and hip circumference ($p = 0.002$), systolic ($p = 0.012$) and diastolic blood pressure ($p = 0.025$) and HOMA-IR ($p = 0.035$)). The >52 years group showed the greatest decrease in glucose ($p = 0.016$). The 45–52 years group showed the greatest increase in adiponectin ($p = 0.014$).

Table 6. Percentage change (Δ) of anthropometric and biochemical variables of patients with morbid obesity classified according to the percentage of excess weight loss (%EWL) and the type of bariatric surgery.

	%EWL <50%			%EWL ≥50%		
	BPD	**RYGB**	**SG**	**BPD**	**RYGB**	**SG**
Δ-Weight	20.9 ± 7.5	22.1 ± 7.3	20.0 ± 5.2	34.3 ± 5.8 [b,3]	36.0 ± 6.6 [a,3]	35.2 ± 7.6 [a,b,3]
Δ-BMI	20.9 ± 7.5	22.1 ± 7.3	20.0 ± 5.2	34.3 ± 5.8 [b,3]	36.0 ± 6.6 [a,3]	35.2 ± 7.6 [a,b,3]
Δ-Waist	17.7 ± 5.5 [a]	12.6 ± 7.1 [b]	14.2 ± 5.5 [a,b]	22.4 ± 6.1 [b,1]	25.4 ± 8.1 [a,3]	24.9 ± 7.7 [a,b,3]
Δ-Hip	14.2 ± 3.7	11.0 ± 9.2	12.6 ± 3.9	21.2 ± 5.6 [3]	23.2 ± 14.1 [3]	22.3 ± 6.6 [3]
Δ-SBP	9.9 ± 10.5	7.1 ± 20.1	6.6 ± 12.0	9.7 ± 13.6	8.1 ± 13.8	6.2 ± 15.2
Δ-DBP	11.3 ± 12.9	2.6 ± 16.9	0.7 ± 16.0	8.4 ± 16.7	4.7 ± 22.5	5.1 ± 17.3
Δ-Glucose	20.5 ± 16.4 [a]	22.4 ± 19.8 [a]	9.0 ± 14.3 [b]	20.7 ± 17.8 [a,b]	24.6 ± 21.9 [a]	14.6 ± 16.4 [b]
Δ-Cholesterol	31.6 ± 14.8 [a]	−0.5 ± 15.6 [b]	−10.7 ± 24.2 [b]	24.9 ± 18.0 [a]	11.2 ± 22.6 [b,1]	−6.0 ± 21.9 [c]
Δ-Triglycerides *	24.9 (2.9–58.9)	18.9 (8.6–41.2)	5.46 (−10.9–26.2)	12.8 (−12.9–30.3) [b]	34.6 (13.1–51.1) [a]	41.0 (4.3–50.3) [a,2]
Δ-HDL	0.8 ± 29.0 [a]	−8.8 ± 25.1 [a,b]	−30.5 ± 44.2 [b]	−3.7 ± 26.5 [a]	−20.2 ± 27.8 [b]	−30.2 ± 31.1 [b]
Δ-LDL	38.4 ± 14.0 [a]	−5.5 ± 30.9 [b]	−11.3 ± 36.2 [b]	35.2 ± 21.2 [a]	11.2 ± 34.2 [a,b]	−2.3 ± 103.0 [c]
Δ-Insulin *	47.4 (40.9–60.7)	20.1 (13.2–35.1)	16.3 (13.2–29.3)	62.9 (55.3–70.9) [2]	54.6 (37.9–67.2)	58.4 (44.1–70.6) [3]
Δ-HOMA-IR *	55.5 (46.2–77.6)	26.8 (21.6–39.8)	32.3 (29.1–42.4)	73.5 (64.1–76.8) [1]	67.4 (52.3–77.7)	60.6 (51.7–77.2) [3]
Δ-Leptin *	53.2 (47.8–69.6)	52.3 (48.5–61.2)	51.9 (50.8–56.5)	85.4 (77.9–88.3) [2]	76.9 (70.7–85.1) [2]	76.6 (64.0–79.9) [1]
Δ-Adiponectin	−12.0 ± 37.0	−82.7 ± 59.5	−55.9 ± 60.1	−33.5 ± 56.0 [a]	−119.1 ± 150.4 [b]	−156.0 ± 124.3 [b]
Δ-CRP *	95.8 (87.7–97.2) [a]	71.7 (65.4–82.2) [a,b]	65.2 (54.9–71.8) [b]	84.8 (72.1–93.2)	83.8 (66.6–94.2)	89.2 (60.2–91.9) [3]
Δ-TG/HDL *	31.4 (11.0–45.5)	35.7 (15.6–49.7)	8.8 (−17.4–34.6)	0.23 (−12.9–24.7) [b]	47.5 (26.1–61.1) [a]	52.6 (7.7–62.7) [a,1]
Δ-TC/HDL	28.1 ± 17.9 [a]	2.6 ± 29.7 [b]	9.2 ± 25.6 [b]	25.0 ± 16.4 [a]	23.4 ± 19.8 [a,1]	15.2 ± 22.0 [b]
Δ-AIP	53.1 ± 154.0	19.9 ± 98.1	53.1 ± 77.6	21.2 ± 213.1 [b]	49.6 ± 72.2 [a,b]	70.0 ± 87.9 [a,1]

The results are given as the mean ± SD or * as median (interquartile range). BMI: Body mass index. SBP: Systolic blood pressure; DBP: Diastolic blood pressure; HOMA-IR: homeostasis model assessment of insulin resistance index. CRP: C-reactive protein. TC: total cholesterol. TG: triglycerides; AIP: atherogenic index of plasma. Different letters show significant differences between the means of the three types of bariatric surgery: $p < 0.05$. Significant differences between patients with morbid obesity with %EWL <50 and those with %EWL ≥50% according to the type of bariatric surgery: [1] $p < 0.05$; [2] $p < 0.01$ and [3] $p < 0.001$ (to simplify these data, significant differences are marked in bold).

Table 7. Percentage change (Δ) of anthropometric and biochemical variables of patients with morbid obesity classified according to the percentage of excess weight loss (%EWL) and age.

	%EWL <50%				%EWL ≥50%			
	≤37 Years	37–44 Years	45–52 Years	>52 Years	≤37 Years	37–44 Years	45–52 Years	>52 Years
Δ-Weight	20.4 ± 6.3	23.5 ± 5.9	19.3 ± 7.1	19.5 ± 5.5	39.6 ± 7.3 [a,3]	34.8 ± 6.6 [b,3]	33.8 ± 6.0 [b,3]	32.9 ± 5.8 [b,3]
Δ-BMI	20.4 ± 6.3	23.5 ± 5.9	19.3 ± 7.1	19.5 ± 5.5	39.6 ± 7.3 [a,3]	34.8 ± 6.6 [b,3]	33.8 ± 6.0 [b,3]	32.9 ± 5.8 [b,3]
Δ-Waist	15.1 ± 5.2	15.8 ± 6.3	14.5 ± 5.1	14.8 ± 6.9	27.8 ± 6.8 [a,3]	23.7 ± 9.1 [b,2]	23.1 ± 5.2 [b,3]	23.1 ± 7.5 [b,3]
Δ-Hip	12.9 ± 4.7	13.7 ± 6.4	13.4 ± 4.0	11.8 ± 4.9	25.2 ± 6.7 [a,3]	23.2 ± 10.3 [a,b,3]	19.8 ± 10.8 [c,3]	20.6 ± 5.6 [b,c,3]
Δ-SBP	3.6 ± 9.8	4.9 ± 9.8	5.7 ± 16.2	13.1 ± 8.3	12.0 ± 12.2 [a,1]	6.3 ± 14.4 [b]	4.3 ± 15.1 [b]	5.4 ± 15.9 [b]
Δ-DBP	7.1 ± 14.4	0.5 ± 11.6	0.4 ± 21.0	6.4 ± 14.8	11.4 ± 15.6 [a]	6.3 ± 17.8 [a,b]	−0.6 ± 17.5 [b]	3.8 ± 19.9 [b]
Δ-Glucose	14.7 ± 19.1 [a,b]	25.1 ± 16.5 [a]	9.7 ± 17.5 [b]	12.9 ± 12.2 [a,b]	12.8 ± 19.1 [c]	16.1 ± 15.4 [b,c]	19.5 ± 17.5 [a,b]	24.5 ± 18.7 [a,1]
Δ-Cholesterol	18.2 ± 20.2 [a]	11.3 ± 27.4 [a,b]	−1.6 ± 32.7 [a,b]	−3.1 ± 24.0 [b]	9.4 ± 21.6	3.4 ± 25.7	4.6 ± 23.8	−1.2 ± 26.8
Δ-Triglycerides *	66.7 (58.3–75.2)	22.4 (−2.5–40.9)	−15.6 (−23.5–2.9)	27.5 (16.5–37.2)	25.0 (10.5–50.1)	23.9 (−3.4–55.5)	32.8 (15.8–45.2) [1]	35.5 (−1.1–53.8) [1]
Δ-HDL	−1.2 ± 15.4 [a]	−0.6 ± 23.8 [a]	−45.5 ± 55.8 [b]	−12.0 ± 29.1 [a]	−22.3 ± 30.7 [1]	−24.7 ± 34.8 [1]	−24.5 ± 28.0	−22.5 ± 31.9
Δ-LDL	14.7 ± 21.1	6.8 ± 38.0	4.5 ± 42.7	−10.6 ± 36.8	9.7 ± 30.2	0.9 ± 40.0	24.7 ± 145.6	−7.0 ± 45.7
Δ-Insulin *	46.8 (43.2–50.5)	70.8 (40.5–78.7)	44.3 (41.4–47.5)	32.6 (24.5–37.4)	58.3 (50.1–63.3) [2]	58.8 (38.6–68.3)	53.4 (40.7–68.7) [3]	58.8 (24.7–72.9) [2]
Δ-HOMA-IR *	62.5 (47.5–77.6)	77.7 (54.9–84.9)	53.2 (49.0–55.4)	43.0 (34.5–47.8)	66.6 (56.3–73.1) [a,1]	71.0 (50.1–77.1) [b]	67.7 (52.6–79.1) [a,b,3]	72.0 (51.7–78.5) [a,b,2]
Δ-Leptin *	53.2 (50.8–55.6)	49.7 (49.2–70.8)	47.0 (40.3–59.6)	61.1 (56.5–64.1)	82.1 (73.3–88.2) [1]	75.7 (65.9–81.5)	77.6 (71.0–85.0) [2]	79.9 (62.3–83.8) [1]
Δ-Adiponectin	−54.1 ± 25.6	−10.8 ± 43.9	−1.7 ± 39.4	−50.1 ± 58.6	−91.6 ± 92.2 [a]	−81.2 ± 101.0 [a]	−213.7 ± 193.9 [b,1]	−105.1 ± 82.3 [a]
Δ-CRP *	96.8 (95.9–97.8)	93.3 (85.9–96.2)	82.1 (78.7–88.9)	65.2 (54.9–80.9)	91.7 (80.7–96.1)	79.1 (50.4–87.8)	81.1 (69.4–91.3)	85.5 (54.4–95.4)
Δ-TG/HDL *	62.2 (50.1–74.2)	20.1 (−11.7–30.5)	1.9 (−27.5–15.0)	34.6 (21.7–47.5)	29.4 (7.7–58.3)	50.3 (−5.5–53.4)	48.3 (19.3–60.8)	46.2 (−9.6–58.1) [1]
Δ-TC/HDL	17.5 ± 24.9 [a,b]	9.9 ± 27.2 [a,b]	24.8 ± 24.6 [a]	3.1 ± 24.1 [b]	22.8 ± 20.1	18.8 ± 20.1	21.5 ± 22.6	14.8 ± 20.8 [1]
Δ-AIP	18.7 ± 39.0 [a,b]	9.4 ± 73.4 [b]	95.4 ± 175.0 [a]	46.9 ± 58.7 [a,b]	43.2 ± 77.0 [1]	37.4 ± 150.0 [1]	79.2 ± 121.2	64.2 ± 92.8

The results are given as the mean ± SD. * These results are given as median (interquartile range). BMI: Body mass index. SBP: Systolic blood pressure; DBP: Diastolic blood pressure; HOMA-IR: homeostasis model assessment of insulin resistance index. CRP: C-reactive protein. TG: triglycerides; TC: total cholesterol. AIP: aterogenic index of plasma. Different letters show significant differences between the means of the four groups of age: $p < 0.05$. Significant differences between patients with morbid obesity with %EWL <50 and those with %EWL ≥50% according to age: [1] $p < 0.05$; [2] $p < 0.01$ and [3] $p < 0.001$.

4. Discussion

The main finding of our study is that the main variables associated with a higher chance of a good weight loss response were age and the type of BS (RYGB), with the weight loss and AIP improvement being associated with each other; those patients with less age (≤37 years) are those that show a greater improvement in the variables analysed, mainly in the group with %EWL ≥50%. Additionally, those patients who underwent SG were those who showed a lower metabolic improvement (triglycerides, insulin, HOMA-IR, leptin and CRP), mainly in the group with %EWL <50%.

We found that BS achieves successful results in most of the variables studied in the short term, with an adequate percentage of post-surgery success 12 months after BS. Moreover, we observed significant improvements both in the non-responders group and in the good responder group. However, there are slight differences. The good responder group presents a greater improvement, and not only in anthropometric variables. However, the effects of all types of BS are not equal [32]. We also found slight differences between the effects of three types of BS. RYGP produced a higher %EWL than SG and, mainly, BPD. However, these patients had worse anthropometric characteristics. This could be conditioning that the %EWL was slightly lower in these patients. Other variables not considered in this study, such as the metabolic state of adipose tissue, could affect %EWL. The worse anthropometric characteristics of patients underwent BPD could alter the metabolism of adipose tissue: higher adipocyte hypertrophy is closely associated with a metabolic dysregulation [33], which could be associated with the evolution of these patients after BS [34]. On the other hand, and according to our results, there are studies showing a similar %EWL with RYGB [13,23]. We found that the percentage of patients with morbid obesity who do not achieve the desired weight loss depends on the type of surgery. Ma et al. [17] found that 85% of the patients who underwent gastric bypass achieved ≥50% EWL [17]. With regard to patients undergoing SG, and according to our results, other studies showed %EWL between 43 to 86% [35]. However, SG was the type of BS that produced the least improvement in the metabolic profile, mainly in the group with %EWL < 50%. This agrees with previous studies in which techniques with an important malabsorptive component were more effective than SG for weight outcomes and improvement of obesity-related comorbidities [36].

In addition to the effect of the type of bariatric surgery on %EWL, we observed that the weight loss is influenced by the age of the patient. Our study shows a tendency, with a higher %EWL in younger patients, as in other studies [16–18]. Different studies suggested that patients older than 50 years lost 40% less weight 2 years after BS than younger patients [18,37], with morbidity and mortality rates higher in older patients [11,38]. In addition to the influence of age on %EWL, we also found that there are differences between good responders and non-responders within each group of age. In general, good responder patients have a better baseline biochemical and anthropometric profile than those non-responders, mainly in the 37–44 years group. However, this better profile disappears as age increases. We observed that patients with a lower age showed some predictive factors of a %EWL ≥50%, mainly the group with 37–44 years; a better anthropometric (weight, BMI, waist and hip circumference), glycaemic (glucose, insulin and HOMA-IR) and atherosclerotic (triglycerides, TG/HDL index and AIP) profile. Overall, these patients have a better metabolic profile. These results suggest that there is a group of young patients with morbid obesity with a better metabolic profile, who are more favourable to adequate weight loss.

The last variable that we found to be associated with %EWL is AIP. It is a strong risk factor for atherosclerosis and a predictive factor for emergency cardiovascular events [39]. This index significantly improved after BS in all patients. Additionally, baseline AIP is lower in the group of BPD with %EWL ≥50%. As is known, and as we also found, BPD produces a significant improvement of the lipidic profile, which is closely linked to cardiovascular risk. Immediate post-surgical results showed a greater improvement in the lipid profile in patients who underwent BPD than in those who underwent SG [40].

We also found a significant decrease in the percentage of patients with T2DM, hypertension and hypercholesterolemia after BS regardless of %EWL (Table 2). In addition to weight loss, other metabolic factors related to surgical technique may determine the evolution of these comorbidities.

There are numerous studies that support the results obtained in our study regarding weight reduction and control of cardiovascular risk factors in the short term. Piché et al. showed a reduction in comorbidities such as hypertension, T2DM and dyslipidemia [41]. Other studies found similar results in patients who underwent RYGB and SG after a 17-month follow-up [42]. Although the comorbidities decrease after BS, weight loss (%EWL <50% or ≥50%) in those patients undergoing BPD and RYGB was not associated with a higher or lower pre-surgical presence of T2DM, hypertension and hypercholesterolemia. However, a lower presence of T2DM and hypertension in those patients undergoing SG was associated with a %EWL ≥50%. This suggests that baseline characteristics of patients may be associated with weight loss [4].

The present study is not exempt from limitations. We only analysed a few variables that can potentially influence the results that are measured. Additionally, although potential post-surgery features that could be determinants of the final effects were not considered, it is a strength that all patients followed homogeneous therapeutic recommendations after each type of BS. We also used 50% as a cut-off for the EWL, although other cut-offs could have been used. Studies for short- and long-term weight-loss show different results. While some reviews show similar %EWL with SG and RYGB at short and long-term [43], other reviews show better results with RYGB [44], with a greater treatment failure after six years for SG [44]. Most of the studies demonstrated and maintained weight loss through follow-up at five years and even for longer intervals (up to 11 years) [43]. However, a slow weight gain between the second and third years of postsurgery follow-up is found, increasing up to 5 years postsurgery [45]. Although, based on previous reviews, our results could be generalized to long-term weight loss, we cannot confirm this hypothesis without data. A long-term follow-up time would be necessary to compare the different surgical techniques and to determine the true variables associated with weight loss after BS, because many patients recover weight, as well as the associated comorbidities after the first years [3,4]. Another limitation that should be mentioned is that two hospitals contributed patients and shared only one surgery. However, this is performed with the same technical characteristics, so it would hardly affect the results obtained.

In conclusion, we show that the relevant variables associated with a %EWL ≥50% after 12 months of follow-up after BS were the type of surgery, mainly RYGB, and age, which is also associated with AIP. Our study confirms that BS, and mainly RYGB, is an effective procedure to metabolically the patients with morbid obesity, even in those non-responders. SG seems to be the one that showed a lower metabolic improvement, mainly in the non-responders group. More extensive knowledge would serve to predict the response to surgery.

Author Contributions: Design and coordination of the study: F.J.T., E.G.-F. and L.G.-S. Selection of subject: D.F.-G., S.V., L.O.-W. and F.J.M.-R. Sample collection and processing: M.D.A.-B., J.A.T. and N.M.-M. Performed the experiments: F.M.-R. Analyzed the data: E.G.-F. and L.G.-S. Contributed reagents/materials/analysis tools: F.J.T., E.G.-F. and L.G.-S. Wrote the paper: E.G.-F. and L.G.-S. All authors have read and agreed to the published version of the manuscript.

Funding: This work was supported in part by grants from the Instituto de Salud Carlos III ((PI17/01407) (Spain) and de la Consejería de Salud de la Junta de Andalucía (PI-0194-2017) (Spain). This study has been co-funded by FEDER funds.

Acknowledgments: LGS is supported by the Miguel Servet program from the ISCIII (Spain) ("Miguel Servet II" program, CPII18/00030) and Nicolas Monardes program from the Consejería de Salud de Andalucía (Spain) (C-0028-2018). FMR and JA are supported by a grant from the ISCIII (Spain) ("PFIS" program, FI19/00189 and FI19/00177, respectively). EGF is supported by the Nicolas Monardes program from the Consejería de Salud de Andalucía (Spain) (C-0031-2016). CIBER Fisiopatología de la Obesidad y Nutrición (CIBEROBN) and CIBER Diabetes y Enfermedades Metabólicas Asociadas are ISCIII projects (Spain).

Conflicts of Interest: The authors declare no conflict of interest.

References

1. World Health Organization. Obesity and Overweight. 2017. Available online: https://www.who.int/news-room/fact-sheets/detail/obesity-and-overweight (accessed on 30 September 2020).
2. Sjöström, L.; Narbro, K.; Sjöström, D.; Karason, K.; Larsson, B.; Wedel, H. Effects of bariatric surgery on mortality in swedish obese subjects. *N. Engl. J. Med.* **2007**, *357*, 741–752. [CrossRef] [PubMed]
3. Sjöström, L. Review of the key results from the Swedish Obese Subjects (SOS) trial-a prospective controlled intervention study of bariatric surgery. *J. Intern. Med.* **2013**, *273*, 219–234. [CrossRef] [PubMed]
4. Still, C.D.; Wood, G.C.; Chu, X.; Manney, C.; Strodel, W.; Petrick, A.; Gabrielsen, J.; Mirshahi, T.; Argyropoulos, G.; Seiler, J.; et al. Clinical factors associated with weight loss outcomes after Roux-en-Y gastric bypass surgery. *Obesity* **2014**, *22*, 888–894. [CrossRef] [PubMed]
5. Camastra, S.; Muscelli, E.; Gastaldelli, A.; Holst, J.J.; Astiarraga, B.D.; Baldi, S.; Nannipieri, M.; Ciociaro, D.; Anselmino, M.; Mari, A.; et al. Long-Term Effects of Bariatric Surgery on Meal Disposal and β-Cell Function in Diabetic and Nondiabetic Patients. *Diabetes* **2013**, *62*, 3709–3717. [CrossRef] [PubMed]
6. MacLean, L.D.; Rhode, B.M.; Sampalis, J.; Forse, R.A. Results of the surgical treatment of obesity. *Am. J. Surg.* **1993**, *165*, 155–162. [CrossRef]
7. Maggard, M.A.; Shugarman, L.R.; Suttorp, M.; Maglione, M.; Sugerman, H.J.; Livingston, E.H.; Nguyen, N.T.; Li, Z.; Mojica, W.A.; Hilton, L.; et al. Meta-Analysis: Surgical Treatment of Obesity. *Ann. Intern. Med.* **2005**, *142*, 547. [CrossRef]
8. Sarzynski, M.; Jacobson, P.; Rankinen, T.; Carlsson, B.; Sjöström, L.; Bouchard, C.; Carlsson, L.M.S. Associations of markers in 11 obesity candidate genes with maximal weight loss and weight regain in the SOS bariatric surgery cases. *Int. J. Obes.* **2010**, *35*, 676–683. [CrossRef]
9. Sugerman, H.J.; Londrey, G.L.; Kellum, J.M.; Wolf, L.; Liszka, T.; Engle, K.M.; Birkenhauer, R.; Starkey, J.V. Weight loss with vertical banded gastroplasty and Roux-Y gastric bypass for morbid obesity with selective versus random assignment. *Am. J. Surg.* **1989**, *157*, 93–102. [CrossRef]
10. Stefanidis, D.; Kuwada, T.S.; Gersin, K.S. The Importance of the Length of the Limbs for Gastric Bypass Patients—An Evidence-based Review. *Obes. Surg.* **2010**, *21*, 119–124. [CrossRef]
11. Nguyen, N.T.; Rivers, R.; Wolfe, B.M. Factors associated with operative outcomes in laparoscopic gastric bypass. *J. Am. Coll. Surg.* **2003**, *197*, 548–555. [CrossRef]
12. Melton, G.B.; Steele, K.E.; Schweitzer, M.A.; Lidor, A.O.; Magnuson, T.H. Suboptimal Weight Loss after Gastric Bypass Surgery: Correlation of Demographics, Comorbidities, and Insurance Status with Outcomes. *J. Gastrointest. Surg.* **2007**, *12*, 250–255. [CrossRef]
13. Sans, A.; Bailly, L.; Anty, R.; Sielezenef, I.; Gugenheim, J.; Tran, A.; Gual, P.; Iannelli, A. Baseline Anthropometric and Metabolic Parameters Correlate with Weight Loss in Women 1-Year After Laparoscopic Roux-En-Y Gastric Bypass. *Obes. Surg.* **2017**, *27*, 2940–2949. [CrossRef] [PubMed]
14. Campos, G.M. Factors Associated With Weight Loss After Gastric Bypass. *Arch. Surg.* **2008**, *143*, 877–884. [CrossRef]
15. Coupaye, M.; Sabate, J.M.; Castel, B.; Jouët, P.; Clerici, C.; Msika, S.; LeDoux, S. Predictive Factors of Weight Loss 1 Year after Laparoscopic Gastric Bypass in Obese Patients. *Obes. Surg.* **2010**, *20*, 1671–1677. [CrossRef]
16. Barhouch, A.S.; Padoin, A.V.; Casagrande, D.S.; Chatkin, R.; Süssenbach, S.P.; Pufal, M.A.; Rossoni, C.; Mottin, C.C. Predictors of Excess Weight Loss in Obese Patients After Gastric Bypass: A 60-Month Follow-up. *Obes. Surg.* **2015**, *26*, 1178–1185. [CrossRef]
17. Ma, Y.; Pagoto, S.L.; Olendzki, B.C.; Hafner, A.R.; Perugini, R.A.; Mason, R.; Kelly, J.J. Predictors of Weight Status following Laparoscopic Gastric Bypass. *Obes. Surg.* **2006**, *16*, 1227–1231. [CrossRef]
18. Contreras, J.E.; Santander, C.; Court, I.; Bravo, J. Correlation Between Age and Weight Loss after Bariatric Surgery. *Obes. Surg.* **2013**, *23*, 1286–1289. [CrossRef]
19. Garrido-Sanchez, L.; Murri, M.; Rivas-Becerra, J.; Ocaña-Wilhelmi, L.; Cohen, R.; Garcia-Fuentes, E.; Tinahones, F. Bypass of the duodenum improves insulin resistance much more rapidly than sleeve gastrectomy. *Surg. Obes. Relat. Dis.* **2012**, *8*, 145–150. [CrossRef] [PubMed]
20. García-Fuentes, E.; Garrido-Sanchez, L.; Garcia-Almeida, J.M.; Garcia-Arnes, J.; Gallego-Perales, J.L.; Rivas-Marin, J.; Morcillo, S.; Cardona, I.; Soriguer, F. Different Effect of Laparoscopic Roux-en-Y Gastric Bypass and Open Biliopancreatic Diversion of Scopinaro on Serum PYY and Ghrelin Levels. *Obes. Surg.* **2008**, *18*, 1424–1429. [CrossRef] [PubMed]

21. De Hollanda, A.; Ruiz, T.; Jiménez, A.; Flores, L.; Lacy, A.; Vidal, J. Patterns of Weight Loss Response Following Gastric Bypass and Sleeve Gastrectomy. *Obes. Surg.* **2014**, *25*, 1177–1183. [CrossRef]
22. Reinhold, R.B. Critical analysis of long term weight loss following gastric bypass. *Surg. Gynecol. Obstet.* **1982**, *155*, 385–394.
23. Christou, N.V.; Look, D.; MacLean, L.D. Weight Gain After Short- and Long-Limb Gastric Bypass in Patients Followed for Longer Than 10 Years. *Ann. Surg.* **2006**, *244*, 734–740. [CrossRef]
24. Shen, S.-W.; Lu, Y.; Li, F.; Yang, C.-J.; Feng, Y.-B.; Li, H.-W.; Yao, W.-F.; Shen, Z.-H. Atherogenic index of plasma is an effective index for estimating abdominal obesity. *Lipids Health Dis.* **2018**, *17*, 1–6. [CrossRef]
25. Lemieux, I.; Lamarche, B.; Couillard, C.; Pascot, A.; Cantin, B.; Bergeron, J.; Dagenais, G.R.; Després, J.-P. Total Cholesterol/HDL Cholesterol Ratio vs LDL Cholesterol/HDL Cholesterol Ratio as Indices of Ischemic Heart Disease Risk in Men. *Arch. Intern. Med.* **2001**, *161*, 2685–2692. [CrossRef]
26. Statements, P. Standards of medical care in diabetes—2012. *Diabetes Care* **2012**, *35* (Suppl. 1), S11–S63.
27. Chobanian, A.V.; Bakris, G.L.; Black, H.R.; Cushman, W.C.; Green, L.A.; Izzo, J.L.; Jones, D.W.; Materson, B.J.; Oparil, S.; Wright, J.T., Jr.; et al. The Seventh Report of the Joint National Committee on Prevention, Detection, Evaluation, and Treatment of High Blood Pressure: The JNC 7 Report. *JAMA* **2003**, *289*, 2560–2571. [CrossRef] [PubMed]
28. Brethauer, S.A.; Kim, J.; Chaar, M.E.; Papasavas, P.; Eisenberg, D.; Rogers, A. Standardized outcomes reporting in metabolic and bariatric surgery. *Obes. Surg.* **2015**, *25*, 587–606. [CrossRef]
29. Villarreal-Calderón, J.R.; Cuéllar, R.X.; Ramos-González, M.R.; Rubio-Infante, N.; Castillo, E.C.; Elizondo-Montemayor, L. Interplay between the Adaptive Immune System and Insulin Resistance in Weight Loss Induced by Bariatric Surgery. *Oxid. Med. Cell Longev.* **2019**, *2019*, 3940739. [CrossRef]
30. Cottam, D.R.; Mattar, S.G.; Barinas-Mitchell, E.; Eid, G.; Kuller, L.; Kelley, D.E.; Schauer, P.R. The Chronic Inflammatory Hypothesis for the Morbidity Associated with Morbid Obesity: Implications and Effects of Weight Loss. *Obes. Surg.* **2004**, *14*, 589–600. [CrossRef]
31. Leggio, M.; Lombardi, M.; Caldarone, E.; Severi, P.; D'Emidio, S.; Armeni, M.; Bravi, V.; Bendini, M.G.; Mazza, A. The relationship between obesity and hypertension: An updated comprehensive overview on vicious twins. *Hypertens. Res.* **2017**, *40*, 947–963. [CrossRef] [PubMed]
32. Park, C.H.; Korean Research Group for Endoscopic Management of Metabolic Disorder and Obesity; Nam, S.-J.; Choi, H.S.; Kim, K.O.; Kim, D.H.; Kim, J.-W.; Sohn, W.; Yoon, J.H.; Jung, S.H.; et al. Comparative Efficacy of Bariatric Surgery in the Treatment of Morbid Obesity and Diabetes Mellitus: A Systematic Review and Network Meta-Analysis. *Obes. Surg.* **2019**, *29*, 2180–2190. [CrossRef] [PubMed]
33. Liu, F.; He, J.; Wang, H.; Zhu, D.; Bi, Y. Adipose Morphology: A Critical Factor in Regulation of Human Metabolic Diseases and Adipose Tissue Dysfunction. *Obes. Surg.* **2020**, 1–15. [CrossRef] [PubMed]
34. Garrido-Sánchez, L.; Tomé, M.; Santiago-Fernández, C.; García-Serrano, S.; García-Fuentes, E.; Tinahones, F.J. Adipose tissue biomarkers involved in early resolution of type 2 diabetes after bariatric surgery. *Surg. Obes. Relat. Dis.* **2017**, *13*, 70–77. [CrossRef] [PubMed]
35. Diamantis, T.; Apostolou, K.G.; Alexandrou, A.; Griniatsos, J.; Felekouras, E.; Tsigris, C. Review of long-term weight loss results after laparoscopic sleeve gastrectomy. *Surg. Obes. Relat. Dis.* **2014**, *10*, 177–183. [CrossRef] [PubMed]
36. Yu, J.; Zhou, X.; Li, L.; Li, S.; Tan, J.; Li, Y.; Sun, X. The Long-Term Effects of Bariatric Surgery for Type 2 Diabetes: Systematic Review and Meta-analysis of Randomized and Non-randomized Evidence. *Obes. Surg.* **2014**, *25*, 143–158. [CrossRef]
37. Printen, K.J.; Mason, E.E. Gastric bypass for morbid obesity in patients more than fifty years of age. *Surg. Gynecol. Obstet.* **1977**, *144*, 192–194.
38. Livingston, E.H.; Huerta, S.; Arthur, D.; Lee, S.; De Shields, S.; Heber, D. Male Gender is a Predictor of Morbidity and Age a Predictor of Mortality for Patients Undergoing Gastric Bypass Surgery. *Ann. Surg.* **2002**, *236*, 576–582. [CrossRef]
39. Dobiášová, M. Atherogenic Index of Plasma [Log(Triglycerides/HDL-Cholesterol)]: Theoretical and Practical Implications. *Clin. Chem.* **2004**, *50*, 1113–1115. [CrossRef]
40. Murri, M.; García-Fuentes, E.; García-Almeida, J.M.; Garrido-Sanchez, L.; Mayas, M.D.; Bernal, R.; Tinahones, F.J. Changes in Oxidative Stress and Insulin Resistance in Morbidly Obese Patients After Bariatric Surgery. *Obes. Surg.* **2009**, *20*, 363–368. [CrossRef]

41. Piché, M.-È.; Martin, J.; Cianflone, K.; Bastien, M.; Marceau, S.; Biron, S.; Hould, F.-S.; Poirier, P. Changes in predicted cardiovascular disease risk after biliopancreatic diversion surgery in severely obese patients. *Metabolism* **2014**, *63*, 79–86. [CrossRef]
42. Perathoner, A.; Weißenbacher, A.; Sucher, R.; Laimer, E.; Pratschke, J.; Mittermair, R. Significant Weight Loss and Rapid Resolution of Diabetes and Dyslipidemia During Short-Term Follow-Up After Laparoscopic Sleeve Gastrectomy. *Obes. Surg.* **2013**, *23*, 1966–1972. [CrossRef] [PubMed]
43. Khaitan, L.; Shea, B.J. Laparoscopic vertical sleeve gastrectomy, long and short-term impact on weight loss and associated co-morbidities. *Ann. Transl. Med.* **2020**, *8*, S5. [CrossRef]
44. Bhandari, M.; Reddy, M.; Kosta, S.; Mathur, W.; Fobi, M.; Mohit, B.; Manoj, R.; Susmit, K.; Winni, M.; Mathias, F. Laparoscopic sleeve gastrectomy versus laparoscopic gastric bypass: A retrospective cohort study. *Int. J. Surg.* **2019**, *67*, 47–53. [CrossRef] [PubMed]
45. Osland, E.; Yunus, R.M.; Khan, S.; Memon, B.; Memon, M.A. Weight Loss Outcomes in Laparoscopic Vertical Sleeve Gastrectomy (LVSG) Versus Laparoscopic Roux-en-Y Gastric Bypass (LRYGB) Procedures. *Surg. Laparosc. Endosc. Percutaneous Tech.* **2017**, *27*, 8–18. [CrossRef]

Journal of
Clinical Medicine

MDPI

Article

Metabolomic Profiles Predict Diabetes Remission after Bariatric Surgery

Jane Ha [1,†], Mi Jang [2,†], Yeong-Keun Kwon [3,†], Young-Suk Park [4], Do-Joong Park [5], Joo-Ho Lee [6], Hyuk-Joon Lee [5], Tae-Kyung Ha [7], Yong-Jin Kim [8], Sang-Moon Han [9], Sang-Uk Han [10], Yoon-Seok Heo [11] and Sung-Soo Park [3,*]

1 Department of Medicine, Korea University College of Medicine, Seoul 02841, Korea; janehapti@korea.ac.kr
2 Department of Biotechnology and Food Science, Norwegian University of Science and Technology, 7491 Trondheim, Norway; kia3111@gmail.com
3 Division of Foregut Surgery, Korea University College of Medicine, Seoul 02841, Korea; kukwon@korea.ac.kr
4 Department of Surgery, Seoul National University Bundang Hospital, Seongnam 13620, Korea; youngsukmd@gmail.com
5 Department of Surgery, Seoul National University Hospital, Seoul 03080, Korea; dojoongpark@gmail.com (D.-J.P.); appe98@snu.ac.kr (H.-J.L.)
6 Department of Surgery, Nowon Eulji Medical Center, Seoul 01830, Korea; gsljh7@gmail.com
7 Department of Surgery, Hanyang University College of Medicine, Seoul 04763, Korea; missurgeon@hanyang.ac.kr
8 Department of Surgery, H+ Yangji Hospital, Seoul 08779, Korea; yjgs1997@gmail.com
9 Department of Surgery, Cheil General Hospital, Seoul 04619, Korea; surgeryhan@gmail.com
10 Department of Surgery, Ajou University Hospital, Suwon 16499, Korea; hansu@ajou.ac.kr
11 Department of Surgery, Inha University Hospital, Incheon 22332, Korea; gshur@inha.ac.kr
* Correspondence: kugspss@korea.ac.kr; Tel.: +82-2-920-6772
† J.H., M.J. and Y.K. (Co-first authors) contributed equally to this work.

Received: 22 October 2020; Accepted: 23 November 2020; Published: 1 December 2020

Abstract: Background: Amino acid metabolites (AAMs) have been linked to glucose homeostasis and type 2 diabetes (T2D). We investigated whether (1) baseline AAMs predict T2D remission 12 months after bariatric surgery and (2) whether AAMs are superior for predicting T2D remission postoperatively compared with existing prediction models. Methods: Among 24 participants undergoing bariatric surgery, 16 diabetes-related AAMs were quantified at baseline and postoperative 3 and 12 months. Existing prediction models included the ABCD, DiaRem, and IMS models. Results: Baseline L-dihydroxyphenylalanine (L-DOPA) (areas under receiver operating characteristic curves (AUROC), 0.92; 95% confidence interval (CI), 0.75 to 1.00) and 3-hydroxyanthranilic acid (3-HAA) (AUROC, 0.85; 95% CI, 0.67 to 1.00) better predicted T2D remission 12 months postoperatively than the ABCD model (AUROC, 0.81; 95% CI, 0.54 to 1.00), which presented the highest AUROC value among the three models. The superior prognostic performance of L-DOPA (AUROC at 3 months, 0.97; 95% CI, 0.91 to 1.00) and 3-HAA (AUROC at 3 months, 0.86; 95% CI, 0.63 to 1.00) continued until 3 months postoperatively. Conclusions: The AAM profile predicts T2D remission after bariatric surgery more effectively than the existing prediction models.

Keywords: bariatric surgery; metabolic surgery; diabetes; amino acid; metabolomics

1. Introduction

In recent years, it has become apparent that bariatric surgery not only promotes dramatic weight loss, but also induces the improvement or remission of type 2 diabetes (T2D) [1,2]. Current clinical guidelines recommend that bariatric surgery be considered to treat inadequately controlled T2D in people with a body mass index (BMI) as low as 30 kg/m^2 or as low as 27.5 kg/m^2 in Asian patients [3,4].

However, previous studies showed that 25% to 65% of T2D patients did not experience postoperative T2D remission [1,2] and that over 20% of patients with T2D remission experienced T2D recurrence during long-term follow-up [5,6]. Given that T2D remission or improvement is a major benefit of bariatric surgery, the ability to preoperatively predict T2D prognosis is crucial for patients and healthcare providers.

Interestingly, a number of studies have highlighted that the circulating concentrations of branched-chain amino acids (BCAAs) and aromatic amino acids, including leucine, isoleucine, valine, phenylalanine, tyrosine, and tryptophan, are closely correlated to insulin resistance and future diabetes [7–10]. Tryptophan derivatives, especially those from the kynurenine pathway (KynP) and serotonin pathway (SerP), are also highly associated with glucose homeostasis and energy expenditure [11–14]. Metabolites from the tyrosine pathway (TyrP), such as L-dihydroxyphenylalanine (L-DOPA) and dopamine, have been also suggested to contribute to the interplay between insulin signaling and glucose homeostasis [15,16]. Nonetheless, whether these amino acid metabolites (AAMs) mediate or predict the prognosis of T2D after bariatric surgery remains unclear.

The Korean Obesity Surgical Treatment Study (KOBESS) is based on a nationwide prospective multicenter cohort, the results of which led to the coverage of bariatric surgery by the National Health Insurance for the first time in Korea [17]. In this preplanned substudy of the KOBESS trial conducted to elucidate the role of AAMs as potential predictors of T2D prognosis after bariatric surgery, we investigated whether preoperative AAMs could predict T2D remission after bariatric surgery and compared the prognostic performance of AAMs with that of existing prediction models.

2. Methods

2.1. Study Participants

This substudy included 24 individuals with type 2 diabetes who participated in the main KOBESS trial (Supplemental Figure S1). The rationale and design of the KOBESS has been previously reported [17]. It was a prospective, multicenter, single-arm, longitudinal study in which 100 patients (including 54 patients with T2D) were enrolled to assess the effect of bariatric surgery on obese patients in Korea. Patients who provided written informed consent were screened for study eligibility and underwent physical and laboratory evaluations to confirm their eligibility (Institutional Review Board approval number: 2019AN0294).

2.2. Surgical Procedures

Study participants selected surgical procedures among sleeve gastrectomy (SG) and Roux-en-Y gastric bypass (RYGB) after being fully informed as to the strengths and weaknesses of both. For SG, a sleeve was fashioned starting 4–6 cm proximal to the pylorus using serial applications of linear staplers over a 36–40 Fr orogastric bougie. The last firing was 1–2 cm away from the angle of His. For RYGB, a lesser curve-based gastric pouch (approximately 30 mL in volume) was created using linear staplers. The length of the Roux and biliopancreatic limbs was 100 cm.

2.3. Management of Nutrition and Blood Glucose

After study enrollment, all patients were provided with American Diabetes Association dietary and lifestyle recommendations to optimize their glucose control. A bariatric physician and registered dietitian provided patient education and nutrition guidelines, including dietary principles such as carbohydrate counting, advice to engage in regular aerobic exercise (if medically fit to do so according to the physician providing their medical care), technical and interpretive skills of blood glucose monitoring, and education about managing hypoglycemia. All patients started guideline-based micronutrient supplementation after study enrollment and baseline assessment [18]. During the postoperative period, patients received education about a protocol-derived staged meal progression. A protein intake of 50 g/day and up to 1.5 g/kg ideal body weight per day was recommended. All patients were followed up every 4 to 12 weeks via outpatient clinic visit to check on glucose control and ensure compliance with the nutritional recommendations.

2.4. Measurements of Serum AAMs

Serum samples were collected before and at 3 and 12 months after bariatric surgery. Preoperative sampling was performed before the patients started the calorie-restricted diet and micronutrient supplementation. Patients fasted for 8 hours before the sampling. AAM profiling was performed using liquid chromatography–mass spectrometry. We selected 16 diabetes-related AAMs such as BCAAs (leucine, isoleucine, and valine), AAAs (phenylalanine, tyrosine, and tryptophan), KynP metabolites (kynurenine, anthranilic acid (AA), 3-hydroxykynurenine (3-HK), 3-hydroxyanthranilic acid (3-HAA), kynurenic acid (KA), xanthurenic acid (XA)), SerP metabolites (5-hydroxytryptophan (5-HTP), serotonin, 5-hydroxyindoleacetic acid (5-HIAA)), and TyrP metabolites (L-dihydroxyphenylalanine (L-DOPA)) based on previous studies on AAMs and glucose homeostasis or T2D (Supplemental Figure S2). The detailed protocol for measuring serum metabolites is presented in Supplemental Tables S1 and S2.

2.5. Outcome Measures

We assessed whether serum AAMs could predict T2D remission 12 months after bariatric surgery. T2D remission was defined as a normal glucose level (glycated hemoglobin < 6%, fasting plasma glucose < 100 mg/dL) in the absence of antidiabetic medications at 12 months postoperatively. Non-remission was defined when the criteria for remission were not met. In addition, the prognostic performances of AAMs were compared with scores from the following three prediction models: the ABCD [19], DiaRem [20], and IMS [21] models. Based on a systematic review of the relevant literature, we selected the prediction models that (1) provided scores implying T2D prognosis after bariatric surgery and (2) underwent external validation.

2.6. Statistical Analysis

Summary data are presented as percentages for categorical variables and as means with standard deviations (SDs) for continuous variables. Patients' characteristics were compared between the remission and non-remission groups using the Student's t-test or Mann–Whitney test for continuous variables and the Pearson chi square test or Fisher's exact test for categorical variables. Areas under receiver operating characteristic curves (AUROCs) were calculated to analyze the performances of the individual AAMs in predicting T2D remission at 12 months postoperatively. Based on the AUROC values, we selected the superior prognostic metabolites, defined as AUROC $\geq$ 0.80. Statistical analyses were performed using Stata12 (Stata Corp., College Station, TX, USA), and two-sided values of $p < 0.05$ were considered statistically significant.

3. Results

3.1. Patients' Baseline Characteristics

The mean age of the study participants was 45.4 years (SD, 10.2 years), and 17 (70.8%) participants were women (Table 1). Among the participants, 14 (58.3%) experienced T2D remission and 10 (41.7%) did not experience T2D remission at 12 months postoperatively. Baseline BMIs were 39.6 kg/m^2 (SD, 7.9 kg/m^2) in the remission group and 33.9 kg/m^2 (SD, 4.5 kg/m^2) in the non-remission group, respectively. Among the participants, 2 (14.3%) in the remission group and 3 (30.0%) in the non-remission group used insulin for glycemic control preoperatively; 9 (64.3%) in the remission group and 5 (50.0%) in the non-remission group received SG, and the rest of patients received RYGB. The remission and non-remission groups were similar for all observed characteristics, except for age (remission group, 41.0 years (SD, 8.7 years); non-remission group, 54.8 years (SD, 8.0 years); $p = 0.004$) and T2D duration (remission group, 2.2 years (SD, 1.4 years); non-remission group, 8.9 years (SD, 8.6 years); $p = 0.009$).

Scores calculated by the three existing prediction models showed significant differences between groups, indicating a higher probability of glycemic control in the remission group.

Table 1. Baseline characteristics.

Variables	Diabetes Status 1 Year after Bariatric Surgery		p Value
	Remission (n = 14)	Non-Remission (n = 10)	
Age, y	41.0 ± 8.7	54.8 ± 8.0	0.004
Female sex, no. (%)	12 (85.7)	5 (50.0)	0.058
Body mass index, kg/m^2	39.6 ± 7.9	33.9 ± 4.5	0.116
Body weight, kg	106.1 ± 31.2	89.7 ± 18.4	0.251
Waist circumference, cm	120.5 ± 19.9	112.1 ± 9.7	0.347
Waist-to-hip ratio	0.97 ± 0.05	1.03 ± 0.01	0.017
Duration of diabetes, y	2.2 ± 1.4	8.9 ± 8.6	0.009
Use of insulin, no. (%)	2 (14.3)	3 (30.0)	0.350
Current smoker, no. (%)	3 (21.4)	2 (20.0)	0.932
Hypertension, no. (%)	5 (35.7)	5 (50.0)	0.484
Dyslipidemia, no. (%)	9 (64.2)	6 (60.0)	0.831
Surgical methods (RYGB/SG), no. (%)	5/9 (35.7/64.3)	5/5 (50.0/50.0)	0.484
ABCD score	6.2 ± 2.0	3.3 ± 2.7	0.015
DiaRem score	4.7 ± 5.4	12.0 ± 5.3	0.013
IMS score	39.3 ± 22.9	88.2 ± 30.6	0.001

Plus–minus values are mean ± standard deviation. Remission was defined as normal glucose level (glycated hemoglobin < 6%, fasting plasma glucose < 100 mg/dL) in the absence of antidiabetic medications at 1 year postoperatively. Non-remission was defined when the criteria for remission were not met. Body mass index is the weight in kilograms divided by the square of the height in meters. Refer to the Methods section for details of the ABCD, DiaRem, and IMS scores. Abbreviations: RYGB, Roux-en-Y gastric bypass; SG, sleeve gastrectomy.

3.2. Patients' Characteristics at 3 and 12 Months Postoperatively

While the levels of glycated hemoglobin and fasting plasma glucose (FPG) at 3 and 12 months postoperatively were significantly different (p value for 3 months, <0.001 (glycated hemoglobin) and <0.001 (FPG); p value for 12 months, <0.001 (glycated hemoglobin) and <0.001 (FPG)) between the remission and non-remission groups, both groups were similar in terms of all other observed characteristics at baseline and 3 and 12 months postoperatively (Table 2). The mean glycated hemoglobin levels at baseline and 12 months postoperatively were 7.2% (SD, 2.0%) and 5.4% (SD, 0.2%) in the remission group and 8.9% (SD, 1.1%) and 7.6% (SD, 1.0%) in the non-remission group, respectively. Patients in the remission group presented 62.9% excess weight loss (EWL) (SD, 31.5%) and 90.6% EWL (SD, 38.3%) at 3 and 12 months, respectively, while patients in the non-remission group presented 59.4% EWL (SD, 24.7%) and 68.8% EWL (SD, 32.4%) at 3 and 12 months, respectively. There were no significant differences in blood pressure (systolic and diastolic), HDL cholesterol level, or triglyceride level between the remission and non-remission groups at baseline and 3 and 12 months postoperatively.

Table 2. Average values and percentage changes at 3 and 12 months after bariatric surgery.

Variables	Remission			Non-Remission			p Value for Baseline	p Value for 3 Months	p Value for 12 Months
	Baseline (n = 14)	3 Months (n = 14)	12 Months (n = 14)	Baseline (n = 10)	3 Months (n = 10)	12 Months (n = 10)			
Glycated hemoglobin, %	7.2 ± 2.0	5.6 ± 0.3	5.4 ± 0.2	8.9 ± 1.1	7.3 ± 1.1	7.6 ± 1.0	0.067	<0.001	<0.001
Fasting plasma glucose, mg/dL	151.1 ± 65.3	98.3 ± 9.8	97.2 ± 7.8	146.1 ± 51.9	129 ± 22.9	131 ± 26.6	0.871	<0.001	<0.001
Body mass index, kg/m^2	39.6 ± 7.9	32.3 ± 7.7	28.8 ± 6.6	33.9 ± 4.5	29.4 ± 4.5	28.9 ± 5.6	0.116	0.409	0.974
Body weight, kg	106.1 ± 31.2	87.7 ± 29.8	77.0 ± 24.9	89.7 ± 18.4	77.9 ± 17.6	76.7 ± 20.1	0.251	0.471	0.977
% Excess weight loss	-	62.9 ± 31.5	90.6 ± 38.3	-	59.4 ± 24.7	68.8 ± 32.4	-	0.818	0.240
% Weight loss	-	18.2 ± 4.1	27.6 ± 5.2	-	13.4 ± 2.7	15.1 ± 5.8	-	0.019	<0.001
Waist circumference, cm	120.5 ± 19.9	104.6 ± 21.0	93.8 ± 16.5	112.1 ± 9.7	98.4 ± 12.4	98.1 ± 12.5	0.347	0.515	0.573
Systolic blood pressure, mmHg	135.7 ± 9.8	125.1 ± 12.1	120.1 ± 13.1	136.8 ± 8.4	124.1 ± 11.5	130 ± 10.2	0.812	0.870	0.120
Diastolic blood pressure, mmHg	84.5 ± 9.8	77.6 ± 10.9	74.5 ± 9.1	85.0 ± 4.9	73.6 ± 12.7	77.1 ± 11.40	0.908	0.496	0.585
High-density lipoprotein cholesterol, mg/dL	49.5 ± 9.8	48.6 ± 10.7	60.1 ± 12.2	46.6 ± 8.5	46.1 ± 13.1	52.5 ± 11.2	0.549	0.671	0.208
Triglycerides, mg/dL	204.4 ± 232.3	110.6 ± 38.7	94.5 ± 36.0	174.6 ± 140.6	149.5 ± 88.6	139 ± 77.5	0.776	0.193	0.091

Plus–minus values are mean ± standard deviation. Body mass index is the weight in kilograms divided by the square of the height in meters. % Excess weight loss was calculated by dividing the number of kilograms lost by the number of kilograms of the patient's excess body weight. % Weight loss was calculated by dividing the number of kilograms by the number of kilograms of the patient's baseline body weight.

3.3. Prediction of T2D Remission after Bariatric Surgery

Levels of baseline AAMs were presented in Supplemental Table S3. No significant differences in AAMs were identified with respect to hypertension and dyslipidemia. Based on the receiver operating characteristic (ROC) curves of AAMs, L-DOPA (AUROC, 0.92; 95% CI, 0.75 to 1.00) and 3-HAA (AUROC, 0.85; 95% CI, 0.67 to 1.00) at baseline showed a superior performance in the prediction of T2D remission 12 months after bariatric surgery (Figure 1) (Supplemental Table S4). The ABCD model (AUROC, 0.81; 95% CI, 0.54 to 1.00) showed the highest AUROC among the three existing prediction models, which was lower than those of L-DOPA and 3-HAA (Supplemental Table S5). Given that we found significant differences in age and diabetes duration between the remission and non-remission groups (Table 1), additional analyses were performed on the subgroups therein. The prognostic performance of 3-HAA and L-DOPA for T2D remission was represented by an AUROC ≥ 0.75 (Supplemental Table S6).

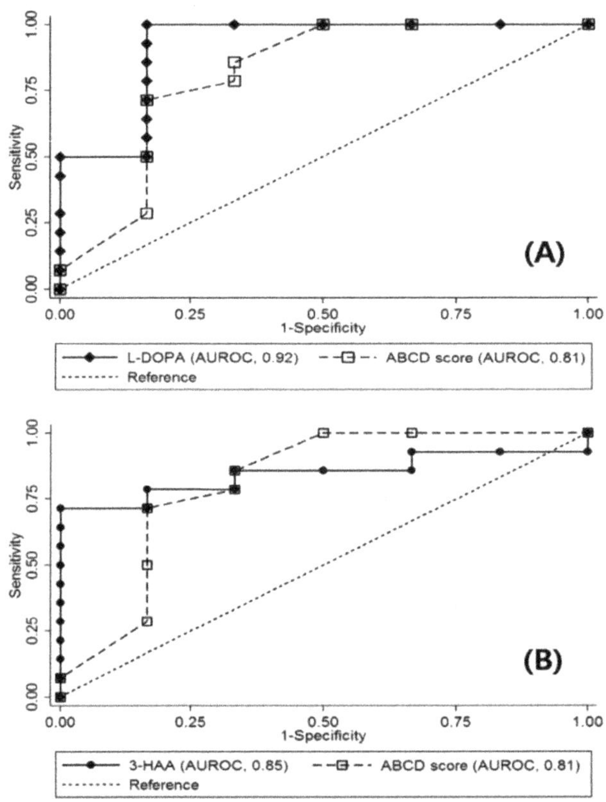

Figure 1. Prognostic performance of L-dihydroxyphenylalanine (L-DOPA), 3-hydroxyanthranilic acid (3-HAA), and the ABCD prediction model. Using 16 diabetes-related amino acid metabolites, receiver operating characteristic (ROC) curves were generated. Among the test serum metabolites, L-DOPA and 3-HAA showed superior prognostic performances with the best discrimination ability in the prediction of type 2 diabetes (T2D) remission 12 months after bariatric surgery. Figure (**A**,**B**) represent the different prognostic outcomes of L-DOPA and 3-HAA, respectively. AUROC, area under receiver operating characteristic curve.

3.4. Postoperative Changes in L-DOPA and 3-HAA

Serum levels of L-DOPA and 3-HAA at 3 and 12 months were measured to characterize the postoperative changes between groups (Figure 2) (Supplemental Table S7). The remission group showed higher levels of L-DOPA (remission group, 0.042 μmol/L (SE, 0.004 μmol/L); non-remission group, 0.022 μmol/L (SE, 0.002 μmol/L); $p = 0.014$) and 3-HAA (remission group, 0.059 μmol/L (SE, 0.006 μmol/L); non-remission group, 0.027 μmol/L (SE, 0.003 μmol/L); $p = 0.005$) at baseline. The statistical significance of the higher baseline levels of L-DOPA and 3-HAA was sustained up to 3 months postoperatively (p values for 3 months, 0.004 (L-DOPA) and 0.303 (3-HAA)). The superior prognostic performance of baseline L-DOPA and 3-HAA in the prediction of T2D remission was also sustained up to 3 months postoperatively (L-DOPA at 3 months (AUROC, 0.97; 95% CI, 0.91 to 1.00); 3-HAA at 3 months (AUROC, 0.86; 95% CI, 0.63 to 1.00)) (Figure 3). At 12 months, no differences in the levels of L-DOPA and 3-HAA were observed between the groups.

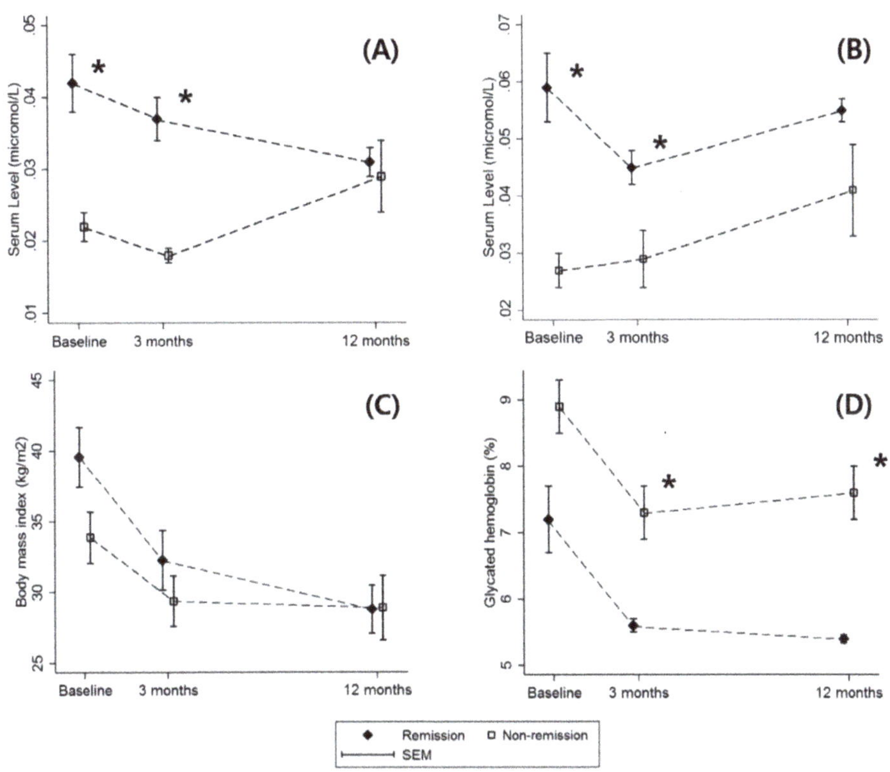

Figure 2. Longitudinal changes of four parameters after bariatric surgery. Figure (**A–D**) represent the postoperative changes in L-dihydroxyphenylalanine (L-DOPA), 3-hydroxyanthranilic acid (3-HAA), body mass index, and glycated hemoglobin, respectively. Measurements were obtained at baseline and 3 and 12 months postoperatively. While the serum levels of L-DOPA and 3-HAA at baseline and 3 months were higher in the type 2 diabetes (T2D) remission group, no significant differences between the remission and non-remission groups were identified 12 months postoperatively. * represent $p < 0.05$ in the comparison of the remission and non-remission groups.

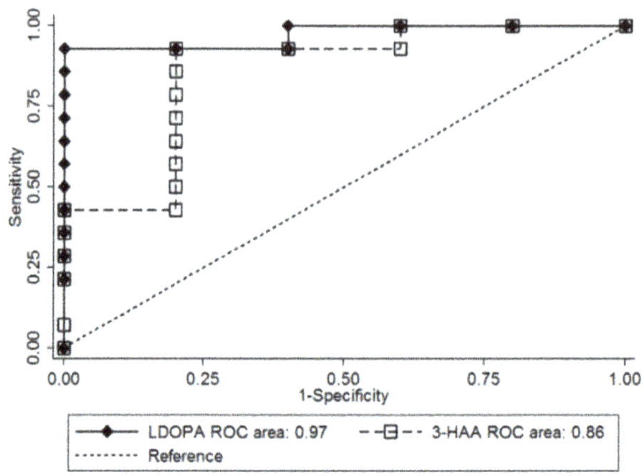

Figure 3. Prognostic performance of L-dihydroxyphenylalanine (L-DOPA) and 3-hydroxyanthranilic acid (3-HAA) measured at 3 months after bariatric surgery. Using L-DOPA and 3-HAA measured at 3 months after surgery, receiver operating characteristic (ROC) curves were generated. The superior prognostic performance of L-DOPA and 3-HAA continued until 3 months postoperatively, and they showed the best discrimination ability in predicting type 2 diabetes (T2D) remission 12 months after bariatric surgery.

4. Discussion

We showed that the profiles of diabetes-related AAMs before bariatric surgery could predict T2D remission 12 months postoperatively. In particular, serum levels of L-DOPA and 3-HAA showed superior prognostic performance with the best discrimination ability at 12 months postoperatively compared with the existing prediction models. We also showed that the superior prognostic performance of L-DOPA and 3-HAA continued for up to 3 months postoperatively.

Our results underscore the importance of KynP metabolites for predicting T2D prognosis after bariatric surgery and must be considered in the context of previous studies suggesting that KynP metabolites were potential biological mediators in T2D pathogenesis [7,9]. The majority of free tryptophan in humans is metabolized via KynP [22], which shifts in favor of the breakdown of tryptophan into downstream products in inflammatory states such as diabetes or obesity [23,24]. Consequently, levels of downstream metabolites such as 3-HAA [25], kynurenine [13], XA [26], and 3-HK [27] are higher in T2D patients than in non-diabetics. In particular, XA was found to contribute to diabetes development by chelating complexes with insulin and exerting pathological apoptosis effects on pancreatic beta cells; furthermore, 3-HAA plays a key role in anti-inflammation and neuroprotection, demonstrating strong antioxidative properties [28].

In patients who underwent bariatric surgery, plasma levels of KynP metabolites decreased 1 year after surgery along with metabolic improvements, implying that KynP metabolites should be assessed as potential biomarkers of metabolic improvement in bariatric patients [27]. According to our results, the baseline level of 3-HAA among the KynP metabolites showed superior performance in predicting T2D remission 1 year after bariatric surgery. Given that no significant differences in the 3-HAA level between the remission and non-remission groups were observed at 12 months postoperatively (Figure 2), our results imply that lower levels of 3-HAA may represent an early manifestation of postoperative T2D remission. Our results are the first to suggest that KynP metabolites predict T2D remission after bariatric surgery and are in line with those of recent studies indicating that KynP metabolites are biological mediators in T2D pathophysiology.

Our findings highlighting the TyrP are noteworthy in the context of experimental and clinical data that suggest that TyrP metabolites may contribute to energy expenditure and glucose homeostasis.

Dopamine is synthesized in the beta-cells from circulating L-DOPA, and exogenous dopamine inhibits insulin secretion from pancreatic beta-cells [29–31]. In this negative feedback loop, dopamine serves as an autocrine signal that is co-secreted with insulin and causes a tonic inhibition on glucose-stimulated insulin secretion [29–31]. Beta-cells co-secrete dopamine as well as insulin in response to glucose stimulus and express dopamine 2-like receptors (D2R), which are responsible for the import of L-DOPA [32]. Experiments with dopamine antagonists suggest that the co-secreted dopamine binds to D2R to downregulate beta-cell insulin secretion [32].

In the present study, the T2D remission group showed higher levels of serum L-DOPA at baseline and 3 months postoperatively than the non-remission group. Recently, it has been suggested that dopamine and glucagon-like peptide-1 exert opposing effects on the glucose-stimulated insulin secretion regulatory system and the anti-incretin effect of dopamine have been indicated as a potential mechanism of diabetes remission after bariatric surgery [16,33]. Given that the proximal gastrointestinal tract is the major source of peripheral circulating dopamine and L-DOPA [34], bariatric surgeries such as SG and RYGB might reduce the secretion and anti-incretin effect of dopamine and L-DOPA. This hypothesis regarding the decrease in dopaminergic action after bariatric surgery is in line with our findings; while the serum level of L-DOPA decreased continuously until 12 months after surgery in the remission group, no significant difference between baseline and 12 months was identified in the non-remission group (Figure 2).

For the preoperative prediction of T2D remission, several prediction models have been proposed. However, these prediction models have been challenged by insufficient validation studies and discordance between models [35]. We calculated the AUROCs of the three existing prediction models (the ABCD, DiaRem, and IMS models) and clinical parameters, according to existing prediction models for the prediction of T2D remission after bariatric surgery (Supplemental Table S5). However, the prognostic performances of the AAMs (especially L-DOPA and 3-HAA) were superior to those of the existing prediction models and other clinical parameters. Hence, AAMs should be further evaluated and considered as potential biomarkers for T2D remission.

This study had some limitations. First, our results did not exclude the possibility that other AAMs may also predict T2D remission after bariatric surgery. Further analysis of downstream KynP metabolites, such as quinolinic acid and nicotinamide adenine dinucleotide, and BCAA metabolites, such as alanine, glutamine, and glutamate, is necessary. Second, the postoperative individual diet pattern may affect the prognosis of T2D postoperatively. In animal studies, a low-BCAA diet improved glycemic control independent of energy balance [36], whereas leucine enriched the diet and improved glucose homeostasis [37]. Further studies to investigate the effect of postoperative diet pattern on the predictive performance of AAMs in bariatric patients are warranted. Third, the subjects were not randomized to the surgical procedures. In light of the high prevalence of gastric cancer in Korea, allocation to RYGB could raise ethical issues, because postoperative esophagogastroduodenoscopy for gastric cancer screening is not allowed in patients undergoing RYGB [17]. Although no significant difference in the surgical methods between the remission and non-remission groups was identified, further investigation of the effect of surgical methods on the prognostic performance of AAMs is warranted. Fourth, our study was conducted on a small number of Asian patients with relatively low BMIs. Caution is advised in applying our results to patients of other ethnicities, or patients with higher BMIs. Our results should be further validated in studies with more patients.

In conclusion, our data provide new insights into preoperative AAMs and the prediction of T2D remission after bariatric surgery. In our comprehensive metabolomics study targeting diabetes-related AAMs, preoperative levels of L-DOPA and 3-HAA more effectively predicted T2D remission 1 year after bariatric surgery compared with the existing prediction models. In addition, the predictive performance of these two metabolites persisted until 3 months postoperatively. The higher levels of L-DOPA and 3-HAA in the T2D remission group have significant clinical implications for the further development and application of surgical indications for the treatment of obesity and T2D.

Supplementary Materials: The following are available online at http://www.mdpi.com/2077-0383/9/12/3897/s1, Table S1: Protocol for measurement of serum amino acids metabolites; Table S2: Chromatographic retention time (RT), selected MRM parameters, DP, EP, CE, and CXP for each analyte measured; Table S3: Levels of baseline amino acid metabolites according to comorbidities; Table S4: Prognostic performance of amino acid metabolites to predict diabetes remission 12 months after bariatric surgery; Table S5: Prognostic performance of existing prediction models and clinical parameters to predict diabetes remission 12 months after bariatric surgery; Table S6, Subgroup analyses; Table S7, Longitudinal changes of serum metabolites after bariatric surgery; Figure S1: Study participants; Figure S2: Diabetes-related amino acid metabolites.

Author Contributions: Conceptualization, Y.-K.K., M.J. and J.H.; methodology, Y.-K.K., Y.-S.P., D.-J.P., J.-H.L., H.-J.L., T.-K.H., Y.-J.K., S.-M.H., S.-U.H. and Y.-S.H.; formal analysis, Y.-K.K. and M.J.; investigation, Y.-K.K. and M.J.; writing—original draft preparation, Y.-K.K. and J.H.; writing—review and editing, Y.-K.K., J.H. and S.-S.P.; visualization, Y.-K.K. and S.-S.P. All authors have read and agreed to the published version of the manuscript.

Funding: This work was supported by grants from the Korean Health Technology R&D Project (HC15C1322), Ministry of Health and Welfare, Republic of Korea (for Y.H.), the Health Fellowship Foundation (for J.H.), and Basic Science Research Program through the National Research Foundation of Korea funded by the Ministry of Education (2020R1I1A1A01070106) (for Y.K.).

Acknowledgments: We thank the College of Life Sciences and Biotechnology, Korea University for technical support; the Korea Basic Science Institute for technical support; and STARDOM Biobank for the storage of the study samples.

Conflicts of Interest: The authors declare no conflict of interest.

References

1. Mingrone, G.; Panunzi, S.; De Gaetano, A.; Guidone, C.; Iaconelli, A.; Leccesi, L.; Nanni, G.; Pomp, A.; Castagneto, M.; Ghirlanda, G.; et al. Bariatric surgery versus conventional medical therapy for type 2 diabetes. *N. Engl. J. Med.* **2012**, *366*, 1577–1585. [CrossRef] [PubMed]
2. Schauer, P.R.; Kashyap, S.R.; Wolski, K.; Brethauer, S.A.; Kirwan, J.P.; Pothier, C.E.; Thomas, S.; Abood, B.; Nissen, S.E.; Bhatt, D.L. Bariatric surgery versus intensive medical therapy in obese patients with diabetes. *N. Engl. J. Med.* **2012**, *366*, 1567–1576. [CrossRef] [PubMed]
3. American Diabetes Association. 8. Obesity Management for the Treatment of Type 2 Diabetes: Standards of Medical Care in Diabetes-2019. *Diabetes Care* **2019**, *42*, S81–S89. [CrossRef] [PubMed]
4. Rubino, F.; Nathan, D.M.; Eckel, R.H.; Schauer, P.R.; Alberti, K.G.; Zimmet, P.Z.; Del Prato, S.; Ji, L.; Sadikot, S.M.; Herman, W.H.; et al. Metabolic Surgery in the Treatment Algorithm for Type 2 Diabetes: A Joint Statement by International Diabetes Organizations. *Diabetes Care* **2016**, *39*, 861–877. [CrossRef]
5. Schauer, P.R.; Bhatt, D.L.; Kirwan, J.P.; Wolski, K.; Aminian, A.; Brethauer, S.A.; Navaneethan, S.D.; Singh, R.P.; Pothier, C.E.; Nissen, S.E.; et al. Bariatric Surgery versus Intensive Medical Therapy for Diabetes—5-Year Outcomes. *N. Engl. J. Med.* **2017**, *376*, 641–651. [CrossRef]
6. Sjostrom, L.; Peltonen, M.; Jacobson, P.; Ahlin, S.; Andersson-Assarsson, J.; Anveden, A.; Bouchard, C.; Carlsson, B.; Karason, K.; Lonroth, H.; et al. Association of bariatric surgery with long-term remission of type 2 diabetes and with microvascular and macrovascular complications. *JAMA* **2014**, *311*, 2297–2304. [CrossRef]
7. Floegel, A.; Stefan, N.; Yu, Z.; Muhlenbruch, K.; Drogan, D.; Joost, H.G.; Fritsche, A.; Haring, H.U.; Hrabe de Angelis, M.; Peters, A.; et al. Identification of serum metabolites associated with risk of type 2 diabetes using a targeted metabolomic approach. *Diabetes* **2013**, *62*, 639–648. [CrossRef]
8. Roberts, L.D.; Koulman, A.; Griffin, J.L. Towards metabolic biomarkers of insulin resistance and type 2 diabetes: Progress from the metabolome. *Lancet Diabetes Endocrinol.* **2014**, *2*, 65–75. [CrossRef]
9. Wang, T.J.; Larson, M.G.; Vasan, R.S.; Cheng, S.; Rhee, E.P.; McCabe, E.; Lewis, G.D.; Fox, C.S.; Jacques, P.F.; Fernandez, C.; et al. Metabolite profiles and the risk of developing diabetes. *Nat. Med.* **2011**, *17*, 448–453. [CrossRef]
10. Wurtz, P.; Soininen, P.; Kangas, A.J.; Ronnemaa, T.; Lehtimaki, T.; Kahonen, M.; Viikari, J.S.; Raitakari, O.T.; Ala-Korpela, M. Branched-chain and aromatic amino acids are predictors of insulin resistance in young adults. *Diabetes Care* **2013**, *36*, 648–655. [CrossRef]
11. Le Floc'h, N.; Otten, W.; Merlot, E. Tryptophan metabolism, from nutrition to potential therapeutic applications. *Amino Acids* **2011**, *41*, 1195–1205. [CrossRef] [PubMed]
12. Oxenkrug, G. Insulin resistance and dysregulation of tryptophan-kynurenine and kynurenine-nicotinamide adenine dinucleotide metabolic pathways. *Mol. Neurobiol.* **2013**, *48*, 294–301. [CrossRef] [PubMed]

13. Pedersen, E.R.; Tuseth, N.; Eussen, S.J.; Ueland, P.M.; Strand, E.; Svingen, G.F.; Midttun, O.; Meyer, K.; Mellgren, G.; Ulvik, A.; et al. Associations of plasma kynurenines with risk of acute myocardial infarction in patients with stable angina pectoris. *Arterioscler. Thromb. Vasc. Biol.* **2015**, *35*, 455–462. [CrossRef] [PubMed]
14. Yabut, J.M.; Crane, J.D.; Green, A.E.; Keating, D.J.; Khan, W.I.; Steinberg, G.R. Emerging Roles for Serotonin in Regulating Metabolism: New Implications for an Ancient Molecule. *Endocr. Rev.* **2019**, *40*, 1092–1107. [CrossRef] [PubMed]
15. Nash, A.I. Crosstalk between insulin and dopamine signaling: A basis for the metabolic effects of antipsychotic drugs. *J. Chem. Neuroanat.* **2017**, *83–84*, 59–68. [CrossRef] [PubMed]
16. Ustione, A.; Piston, D.W.; Harris, P.E. Minireview: Dopaminergic regulation of insulin secretion from the pancreatic islet. *Mol. Endocrinol.* **2013**, *27*, 1198–1207. [CrossRef]
17. Park, Y.S.; Park, D.J.; Lee, J.H.; Lee, H.J.; Ha, T.K.; Kim, Y.J.; Ryu, S.W.; Han, S.M.; Yoo, M.W.; Park, S.; et al. Korean OBEsity Surgical Treatment Study (KOBESS): Protocol of a prospective multicentre cohort study on obese patients undergoing laparoscopic sleeve gastrectomy and Roux-en-Y gastric bypass. *BMJ Open* **2017**, *7*, e018044. [CrossRef]
18. Parrott, J.; Frank, L.; Rabena, R.; Craggs-Dino, L.; Isom, K.A.; Greiman, L. American Society for Metabolic and Bariatric Surgery Integrated Health Nutritional Guidelines for the Surgical Weight Loss Patient 2016 Update: Micronutrients. *Surg. Obes. Relat. Dis.* **2017**, *13*, 727–741. [CrossRef]
19. Lee, W.J.; Almulaifi, A.; Chong, K.; Chen, S.C.; Tsou, J.J.; Ser, K.H.; Lee, Y.C.; Chen, J.C. The Effect and Predictive Score of Gastric Bypass and Sleeve Gastrectomy on Type 2 Diabetes Mellitus Patients with BMI < 30 kg/m(2). *Obes. Surg.* **2015**, *25*, 1772–1778. [CrossRef]
20. Still, C.D.; Wood, G.C.; Benotti, P.; Petrick, A.T.; Gabrielsen, J.; Strodel, W.E.; Ibele, A.; Seiler, J.; Irving, B.A.; Celaya, M.P.; et al. Preoperative prediction of type 2 diabetes remission after Roux-en-Y gastric bypass surgery: A retrospective cohort study. *Lancet Diabetes Endocrinol.* **2014**, *2*, 38–45. [CrossRef]
21. Aminian, A.; Brethauer, S.A.; Andalib, A.; Nowacki, A.S.; Jimenez, A.; Corcelles, R.; Hanipah, Z.N.; Punchai, S.; Bhatt, D.L.; Kashyap, S.R.; et al. Individualized Metabolic Surgery Score: Procedure Selection Based on Diabetes Severity. *Ann. Surg.* **2017**, *266*, 650–657. [CrossRef] [PubMed]
22. Schwarcz, R. The kynurenine pathway of tryptophan degradation as a drug target. *Curr. Opin. Pharmacol.* **2004**, *4*, 12–17. [CrossRef] [PubMed]
23. Brandacher, G.; Hoeller, E.; Fuchs, D.; Weiss, H.G. Chronic immune activation underlies morbid obesity: Is IDO a key player? *Curr. Drug Metab.* **2007**, *8*, 289–295. [CrossRef] [PubMed]
24. Oxenkrug, G.; van der Hart, M.; Summergrad, P. Elevated anthranilic acid plasma concentrations in type 1 but not type 2 diabetes mellitus. *Integr. Mol. Med.* **2015**, *2*, 365–368. [CrossRef]
25. Muzik, O.; Burghardt, P.; Yi, Z.; Kumar, A.; Seyoum, B. Successful metformin treatment of insulin resistance is associated with down-regulation of the kynurenine pathway. *Biochem. Biophys. Res. Commun.* **2017**, *488*, 29–32. [CrossRef]
26. Oxenkrug, G.F. Increased Plasma Levels of Xanthurenic and Kynurenic Acids in Type 2 Diabetes. *Mol. Neurobiol.* **2015**, *52*, 805–810. [CrossRef]
27. Christensen, M.H.E.; Fadnes, D.J.; Rost, T.H.; Pedersen, E.R.; Andersen, J.R.; Vage, V.; Ulvik, A.; Midttun, O.; Ueland, P.M.; Nygard, O.K.; et al. Inflammatory markers, the tryptophan-kynurenine pathway, and vitamin B status after bariatric surgery. *PLoS ONE* **2018**, *13*, e0192169. [CrossRef]
28. Krause, D.; Suh, H.S.; Tarassishin, L.; Cui, Q.L.; Durafourt, B.A.; Choi, N.; Bauman, A.; Cosenza-Nashat, M.; Antel, J.P.; Zhao, M.L.; et al. The tryptophan metabolite 3-hydroxyanthranilic acid plays anti-inflammatory and neuroprotective roles during inflammation: Role of hemeoxygenase-1. *Am. J. Pathol.* **2011**, *179*, 1360–1372. [CrossRef]
29. Farino, Z.J.; Morgenstern, T.J.; Maffei, A.; Quick, M.; De Solis, A.J.; Wiriyasermkul, P.; Freyberg, R.J.; Aslanoglou, D.; Sorisio, D.; Inbar, B.P.; et al. New roles for dopamine D2 and D3 receptors in pancreatic beta cell insulin secretion. *Mol. Psychiatry* **2019**. [CrossRef]
30. Rubi, B.; Ljubicic, S.; Pournourmohammadi, S.; Carobbio, S.; Armanet, M.; Bartley, C.; Maechler, P. Dopamine D2-like receptors are expressed in pancreatic beta cells and mediate inhibition of insulin secretion. *J. Biol. Chem.* **2005**, *280*, 36824–36832. [CrossRef]
31. Shankar, E.; Santhosh, K.T.; Paulose, C.S. Dopaminergic regulation of glucose-induced insulin secretion through dopamine D2 receptors in the pancreatic islets in vitro. *IUBMB Life* **2006**, *58*, 157–163. [CrossRef] [PubMed]

32. Simpson, N.; Maffei, A.; Freeby, M.; Burroughs, S.; Freyberg, Z.; Javitch, J.; Leibel, R.L.; Harris, P.E. Dopamine-mediated autocrine inhibitory circuit regulating human insulin secretion in vitro. *Mol. Endocrinol.* **2012**, *26*, 1757–1772. [CrossRef] [PubMed]
33. Rubino, F.; R'Bibo, S.L.; del Genio, F.; Mazumdar, M.; McGraw, T.E. Metabolic surgery: The role of the gastrointestinal tract in diabetes mellitus. *Nat. Rev. Endocrinol.* **2010**, *6*, 102–109. [CrossRef] [PubMed]
34. Eisenhofer, G.; Aneman, A.; Friberg, P.; Hooper, D.; Fandriks, L.; Lonroth, H.; Hunyady, B.; Mezey, E. Substantial production of dopamine in the human gastrointestinal tract. *J. Clin. Endocrinol. Metab.* **1997**, *82*, 3864–3871. [CrossRef]
35. Ha, J.; Kwon, Y.; Kim, N.H.; Park, S.; Menzo, E.L.; Rosenthal, R.J. Discordance in prediction for prognosis of type 2 diabetes after metabolic surgery: Comparison of the ABCD, DiaRem, and individualized metabolic surgery models. *Ann. Surg. Treat. Res.* **2019**, *97*, 309–318. [CrossRef]
36. Fontana, L.; Cummings, N.E.; Arriola Apelo, S.I.; Neuman, J.C.; Kasza, I.; Schmidt, B.A.; Cava, E.; Spelta, F.; Tosti, V.; Syed, F.A.; et al. Decreased Consumption of Branched-Chain Amino Acids Improves Metabolic Health. *Cell Rep.* **2016**, *16*, 520–530. [CrossRef]
37. Zhang, Y.; Guo, K.; LeBlanc, R.E.; Loh, D.; Schwartz, G.J.; Yu, Y.H. Increasing dietary leucine intake reduces diet-induced obesity and improves glucose and cholesterol metabolism in mice via multimechanisms. *Diabetes* **2007**, *56*, 1647–1654. [CrossRef]

Journal of
Clinical Medicine

MDPI

Article

Anxiety and Depression Affect Early Postoperative Pain Dimensions after Bariatric Surgery

Sofia Gravani [1,*], Maria Matiatou [1], Pantelis T. Nikolaidis [2,*], Evangelos Menenakos [3], Constantinos G. Zografos [4], George Zografos [1] and Konstantinos Albanopoulos [1]

1 1st Propaedeutic Surgical Department, Medical School, National and Kapodistrian University of Athens, Hippocratio General Hospital of Athens, 11527 Athens, Greece; m.matiatou@gmail.com (M.M.); surg-clinic-uoa@hippocratio.gr (G.Z.); albanopoulos_Kostis@yahoo.gr (K.A.)
2 School of Health and Caring Sciences, University of West Attica, 12243 Athens, Greece
3 5th Propaedeutic Surgical Department, Medical School, National and Kapodistrian University of Athens, Eugenideio General Hospital of Athens, 11528 Athens, Greece; evmenenakos@hotmail.com
4 1st Propaedeutic Surgical Department, Medical School, National and Kapodistrian University of Athens, Laiko General Hospital of Athens, 11527 Athens, Greece; Koszogra92@hotmail.com
* Correspondence: sofgrav@yahoo.gr (S.G.); pademil@hotmail.com (P.T.N.)

Abstract: Uncontrolled postoperative pain and prolonged immobilization after bariatric surgery have been associated with increased postoperative complications and prolonged hospitalization. The aim of our study was to evaluate the postoperative pain that follows bariatric surgery and identify any psychological factors that may affect the early postoperative perception of pain. The study included 100 patients with obesity (women, $n = 61$; age 37.4 ± 9.9 years, mean ± standard deviation; Body Mass Index (BMI) 47.6 ± 6.5 kg/m^2) who underwent bariatric surgery. Preoperative anxiety and depression were evaluated by the Hospital Anxiety and Depression Scale (HADS), and the quantitative and qualitative dimension of early postoperative pain were evaluated by the McGill Pain Questionnaire Short Form (MPQ-SF). Furthermore, the postoperative analgesia protocol was recorded for each patient. Pain declined gradually during the first 24 h postoperative. Although preoperative anxiety had no correlation with the overall pain of postoperative Day 0, patients with a higher level of preoperative anxiety had significantly more intense and more unpleasant pain at 1 h post operation. In addition, depression influences both the intensity and unpleasantness of pain at different time points (1 h, 4 h and 24 h postoperative). Preoperative pain correlated with educational level, but not with age, BMI, gender, marital status, smoking and surgery type. In conclusion, preoperative anxiety and depression influence the early postoperative pain after bariatric surgery, and their preoperative identification is of major importance to enhance the implementation of fast-track postoperative protocols to prevent complications and prolonged hospitalization.

Keywords: obesity; bariatric surgery; pain dimensions; postoperative pain; preoperative anxiety; preoperative depression

Citation: Gravani, S.; Matiatou, M.; Nikolaidis, P.T.; Menenakos, E.; Zografos, C.G.; Zografos, G.; Albanopoulos, K. Anxiety and Depression Affect Early Postoperative Pain Dimensions after Bariatric Surgery. *J. Clin. Med.* **2021**, *10*, 53. https://doi.org/10.3390/jcm10010053

Received: 20 November 2020
Accepted: 22 December 2020
Published: 25 December 2020

Publisher's Note: MDPI stays neutral with regard to jurisdictional claims in published maps and institutional affiliations.

1. Introduction

The prevalence of severe obesity, i.e., body mass index (BMI) higher than 35 kg/m^2, is increasing rapidly in the developing world [1] and has become a global problem [2]. Obesity relates to an increased prevalence of comorbidities [3,4], including type 2 diabetes, cardiovascular diseases, respiratory diseases, back and lower extremity weight-bearing degenerative problems, several forms of cancer, and mental health problems leading to increased mortality [2,4,5]. When conservative methods of obesity treatment fail, bariatric surgery remains the only effective method of weight loss [6–8]. Bariatric surgery is gaining more and more popularity since it offers efficient weight loss with proven long-term effects, contributing to improved physical and mental quality of life [9]. The obese population [2,3,10] and the number of bariatric surgeries performed are increasing worldwide [11,12]. Technological advances and progress in surgical techniques have resulted in the adoption of new surgical procedures, classified as restrictive and/or malabsorptive based on the presumed weight loss mechanism [10].

Currently, the most common bariatric procedures worldwide are the laparoscopic Roux-en-Y gastric bypass (LRYGB) and the laparoscopic sleeve gastrectomy (LSG) [11,13]. The one anastomosis gastric bypass (OAGB), also known as single anastomosis gastric bypass or mini gastric bypass, is an effective, safe and simple alternative of LRYGB. Moreover, it has a significant reduction of technical complexity, shorter operative time and a potential reduction in morbidity and mortality [14,15]. Although the laparoscopic surgical approach has the advantage of less postoperative pain [16], patients undergoing laparoscopic bariatric surgery still require efficient analgesia to prevent postoperative complications. Effective pain control reduces the risk of postoperative complications such as pneumonia or atelectasis by enhancing deep breathing, deep vein thrombosis and pulmonary embolism, by encouraging early mobilization [17]. Furthermore, the effective control of perioperative pain helps prevent its transition to chronic pain [14]. A restriction concerning the efficient postoperative analgesia of obese patients is that these patients frequently suffer from comorbidities such as obstructive sleep apnea and other forms of sleep-disordered breathing, making the use of systemic opioids at the early postoperative period very challenging [18]. Postoperative pain management strategies for obesity surgery focuses on ensuring adequate pain relief and mitigating the risk of complications in analgesic use.

Pain is a subjective experience that is characterized by its intensity and its quality characteristics. The quality characteristics of pain are described by words that reflect (a) the sensory qualities of pain in terms of temporal, spatial, pressure, thermal and other properties; and (b) the affective qualities of pain in terms of tension, fear and autonomic properties that are part of the pain experience [19]. The sensory and affective dimensions are considered to be separate and differentially modifiable [20]. A variety of factors are associated with postoperative pain such as patients' demographic and psychological parameters, different types of surgery and surgical characteristics [21,22]. The correlation between psychological parameters and perception of pain is well established [21], and so is the association between morbid obesity and psychopathological conditions [23]. Preoperative depression and anxiety are two identified psychological factors influencing the experience of postoperative pain in many types of surgeries [24–26], but little is known about how they could affect the early postoperative pain following bariatric surgery.

Identifying the psychological factors affecting the postoperative perception of pain for this group of patients may lead to more efficient pain protocols, thus enhancing the implementation of fast-track bariatric protocols [27–29]. Therefore, the aim of the present study is to evaluate the early postoperative pain of patients undergoing bariatric surgery and investigate the relationship between pain and the preoperative feeling of anxiety and depression.

2. Material and Methods

The study was approved by the Institutional Human Subjects Review Board of our hospital. During a 2-year period (2016–2018), 250 patients with obesity underwent bariatric surgery at our Laparoscopic Bariatric Unit. Our inclusion criteria were as follows: age 18–65 years, BMI $\geq$ 30 kg/m^2, laparoscopic bariatric procedure of LSG or OAGB, and patients with I and II physical status according to the classification system of the American Society of Anesthesiologists. The exclusion criteria were history of bariatric or other upper abdominal surgery, diagnosis of a psychiatric disorder, diagnosis of chronic pain, intraoperative placement of a drain, simultaneous cholecystectomy, and postoperative complication and reoperation. In total, 100 patients (women, n = 61; age 37.4 $\pm$ 9.9 years, mean $\pm$ standard deviation; BMI, 47.6 $\pm$ 6.5 kg/m^2) were eligible to participate in our study. The sample size (n = 100) of the study was determined using the statistical software G*Power 3.1.9.6 for macOS (https://www.psychologie.hhu.de/arbeitsgruppen/allgemeine-psychologie-und-arbeitspsychologie/gpower.html, Heinrich Heine University Düsseldorf, Düsseldorf,

Germany) considering tail one, effect size 0.3, error probability alpha 0.05 and power (1-error probability beta) 0.93 for correlational analysis.

Prior to the experimental procedures, the patients were informed in writing and orally about the surgical procedure and the survey protocol. After signed written consent was obtained, all patients were asked to complete a questionnaire about their medical history, socioeconomic status and the Hospital Anxiety and Depression Scale (HADS). In the intraoperative period, the researcher provided a questionnaire about the surgery and analgesia protocol. All patients were asked to complete the Greek version of the McGill Pain Questionnaire Short Form (MPQ-SF) [30,31] during the postoperative Day 0 (POD #0) at 1, 4, 8, 12 and 24 h after the completion of the operation.

The research protocol predetermined the intraoperative and postoperative analgesia consisting of a bolus intravenous infusion of 1gr paracetamol plus 2 mcg/kg fentanyl 30 min before the animation. Postoperatively, the protocol consisted of an intravenous infusion (IV) of 1gr paracetamol every 6 h, in addition to a fentanyl solution (10 mcg/mL) infusion through a patient-controlled analgesia (PCA) pump, with a stable rate of 2.5 mL/h. Furthermore, the PCA pump allowed patients to self-administer small IV doses of fentanyl (2 mL) with a lockout interval of 10 min. The self-administrated fentanyl volume during the first 24 h was recorded for each patient.

2.1. Assessment of Preoperative Psychological Status

HADS is a tool to measure the feeling of anxiety (HADS-A) and depression (HADS-D) [32]. It is used to identify patients in the general hospital who require more systematic psychiatric assessment and care. This tool consists of seven questions that evaluate anxiety and seven questions that evaluate depression. Respondents can answer every question on a four-stage Likert scale scoring from 0 to 3. The scores attributed to the questions are summed up separately for the questions assessing depression and those evaluating anxiety, leading to two scores that range between 0 and 21. High score values indicate high levels of anxiety or depression. Scores between 0–7 points indicate normal levels, scores between 8–10 points indicate border-line abnormal levels and scores between 11–21 points indicate abnormal levels.

2.2. Evaluation of Postoperative Pain

Postoperative pain was evaluated by using the validated Greek version of MPQ-SF [30,31]. The questionnaire consists of 15 descriptive adjectives for the pain sensation, 11 sensory and 4 affective, each one assessed by four levels of intensity (none, mild, moderate, severe). Each level scores different points (none = 0, mild = 1, moderate = 2 and severe = 3 points). A sensory and an affective score are calculated by adding the points attributed to the selected adjectives. In addition, a total score (SFMPQ-total) obtained by adding the sensory and the affective score is also calculated. Furthermore, the questionnaire includes a Numeric Rating Scale (NRS), which is a visual horizontal 10 cm analogue scale (VAS) to describe the intensity of pain (0 = no pain, 10 = pain as bad as it could possibly be). A 6-point verbal rating scale pain (Present Pain Index—PPI) is also a component of the MPQ-SF that uses adjectives to describe the feeling of pain at the time of completion of the questionnaire (no pain = 0, mild = 1, discomforting = 2, distressing = 3, horrible = 4 and excruciating = 5). In addition to the use of MPQ-SF, postoperative pain was evaluated by recording the self-administration of small IV doses of fentanyl (2 mL) through the PCA pump during the first 24 h.

2.3. Statistical Analysis

Parametric (mean $\pm$ SD) and non-parametric statistics (median and interquartile range) described variables. Despite the use of variables described by ordinal scales, we presented data with both parametric and non-parametric statistics to have comparable data with the literature [29,30]. The Spearman correlation coefficient (r) was used to explore the association between two quantitative variables. The correlation is considered low when rho ranges from 0.1 to 0.3, moderate when rho ranges from 0.31 to 0.5 and high when rho is greater than 0.5. Linear regression analysis was used to find independent factors related to the pain scales from which dependence factors (b) and their standard errors (standard errors = SE) were derived. Age, gender, BMI, marital status, smoking, educational level and type of surgery were considered as potential prognostic factors of postoperative pain. The validity of the models, i.e., normality of the residuals, homoscedasticity and multicollinearity, were checked. Statistical significance was set at $p < 0.05$. Analyses were conducted using SPSS statistical software (version 22.0, IBM, Armonk, NY, USA).

3. Results

3.1. Sample Characteristics

The operations performed were LSG on 58 patients (58%) and laparoscopic OAGB on 42 patients (42%). Table 1 outlines patients' characteristics and surgical procedures.

Table 1. Information about the surgical procedure and descriptions of general and demographic features of the study sample.

Variable		*n* (%)
Gender, *n* (%)	Female	61 (61%)
	Male	39 (39%)
Educational level, *n* (%)	Primary	5 (5%)
	Secondary	53 (53%)
	Two-year degree	18 (18%)
	University	23 (23%)
	Postgraduate university education	1 (1%)
Smoking, *n* (%)	No	52 (52%)
	Yes	35 (35%)
	In the past	13 (13%)
Operation, *n* (%)	LSG	58 (58%)
	OAGB	42 (42%)

BMI, body mass index; LSG, laparoscopic sleeve gastrectomy; OAGB, one anastomosis gastric by-pass.

3.2. Preoperative Psychological Characteristics

The preoperative feeling of anxiety and depression was evaluated using the HADS. With respect to the preoperative level of anxiety, 76% of patients were assessed as having a normal level, 15% as having a border-line level and 9% as having an abnormal level. As for the preoperative depression level, 89% were assessed as having a normal level, 7% as having a border-line level and 4% as abnormal. The mean values of the sample's preoperative anxiety and depression levels were both normal (0–7 points). The mean preoperative anxiety score was at 4.24 (out of 21), and the mean preoperative depression score at 5.78 (out of 21) (Table 2).

Table 2. Sample's level of preoperative anxiety and depression.

Preoperative Level	Normal (%)	Border-Line (%)	Abnormal (%)	Mean ± SD	Median (IQR)
Anxiety	76	15	9	4.24 ± 3.09	4 (2–6)
Depression	89	7	4	5.78 ± 3.55	5 (3–7)

SD, standard deviation; IQR = 25th–75th interquartile range.

3.3. Early Postoperative Pain

At POD #0, the NRS was 4.61 (out of 10), the PPI was 1.79 (out of 5), the sensory score was 6.32 (out of 33), the affective score was 2.81 (out of 12) and the SFMPQ total was 9.16 (out of 45) (Table 3). Although the pain measurements at different time points showed a gradual decrease of pain during the first 24 postoperative hours, distressing (PPI = 3) and severe pain (NRS $\geq$ 7) was present in the 1st postoperative hour that remained moderate ($4 \leq$ NRS ≤ 6) until the 8th postoperative hour.

Table 3. McGill Pain Questionnaire Short Form (MPQ-SF) parameters for every predetermined time point and during the first 24 postoperative hours.

	1 h	4 h	8 h	12 h	24 h	Overall Day 0
	Mean ± SD (Median, IQR)	Mean ± SD (Median, IQR)	Mean ± SD (Median, IQR)	Mean ± SD (Median, IQR)	Mean ± SD (Median, IQR)	Mean ± SD (Median, IQR)
NRS	7.4 ± 2.1 (8, 6–9)	5.4 ± 2.5 (5, 3–7)	4.3 ± 2.5 (4, 2–6)	3.6 ± 2.4 (3, 1–5)	2.3 ± 2.1 (2, 1–4)	4.61 ± 1.71 (4.8, 3.2–6.0)
PPI	3.00 ± 1.27 (3, 2–4)	2.01 ± 0.98 (2, 1–2)	1.58 ± 0.96 (1, 1–2)	1.31 ± 0.79 (1, 1–2)	1.02 ± 0.76 (1, 0.5–1.5)	1.79 ± 0.62 (1.8, 1.4–2.2)
Sensory	11.9 ± 6.2 (11, 7–16)	8.1 ± 5.5 (7, 4–11)	4.8 ± 4.8 (4, 2–6)	3.4 ± 3.7 (2, 1.3–4)	3.0 ± 3.4 (2, 0–4)	6.32 ± 3.67 (5.4, 3.8–8.0)
Affective	5.4 ± 2.9 (5, 3–8)	3.4 ± 2.5 (3, 2–4)	2.3 ± 2.2 (2, 1–3)	1.6 ± 1.6 (1, 0–2)	1.2 ± 1.6 (1, 0–2)	2.81 ± 1.53 (2.4, 1.8–3.8)
SFMPQ Total	17.3 ± 8.5 (16, 10.5–25)	11.5 ± 7.2 (10, 7–15)	7.1 ± 6.4 (6, 3–9)	5.1 ± 5.0 (4, 2–6)	4.1 ± 4.7 (3.5, 1–5)	9.16 ± 4.88 (7.8, 5.6–11.6)

SD, standard deviation; IQR = 25th–5th interquartile range; NRS, Numeric Rating Scale; PPI, Present Pain Index; SFMPQ—total score, Short Form McGill Pain Questionnaire—total score; Day 0, First 24 postoperative hours.

The need for extra bolus infusions of the analgesic drug through the Patient Controlled Analgesia (PCA) pump during the POD #0 was recorded; patients' attempts were 19.0 ± 14.7, while the amount of analgesic drug delivered from the attempts was 0.4 ± 0.3 mg. Table 4 shows Spearman correlation between the average pain scores for each pain scale NRS, PPI, Sensory, Affective and SFMPQ total with data from PCA such as patient attempts, bolus provided by attempts, bolus provided by continues rate and the total bolus. The amount provided by patients' attempts was found to be significantly positively correlated with the average intensity score NRS (p = 0.042) and the average score on the Sensory (p = 0.048), affective (p = 0.049) and total emotional score SFMPQ (p = 0.043), with patients in more pain seeking extra analgesic drugs by using the PCA pump.

Table 4. Correlations between PCA pump amounts and average pain scores for each pain scale during the first 24 postoperative hours.

		NRS	PPI	Sensory	Affective	SFMPQ Total
Patient attempts	r	0.20	0.15	0.19	0.19	0.19
	p	0.062	0.152	0.075	0.073	0.066
Patient bolus given from attempts (mg)	r	0.21	0.17	0.21	0.21	0.21
	p	0.042	0.117	0.048	0.049	0.043
Patient bolus given from continuous rate (mg)	r	−0.01	0.10	0.06	−0.03	0.04
	p	0.962	0.330	0.599	0.780	0.725
Total bolus given(mg)	r	0.10	0.16	0.15	0.12	0.15
	p	0.347	0.132	0.157	0.240	0.163

PCA: Patient Controlled Analgesia, NRS: Numerical Rating Scale, PPI: Present Pain Index, SFMPQ—total score: Short Form McGill Pain Questionnaire—total score.

3.4. Early Postoperative Pain and Sociodemographic Characteristics/Type of Surgery

The multiple linear regression showed that age, gender, BMI, marital status, smoking and type of surgery did not have any association (positive or negative) with pain ratings for the first 24 postoperative hours. The educational level had a positive association ($p \leq 0.05$) with all pain parameters' ratings (NRS, PPI, sensory score, affective score and SFMPQ—total score). Patients with a higher educational level experienced more severe pain both in terms of quality and intensity during the first 24 hours. Furthermore, the multiple linear regression analysis between the bolus infusions of the analgesic drug through the PCA attempts showed no association with all the above characteristics (Table 5).

Table 5. Correlations between all pain scales with educational level of participants.

Pain Scale	Educational Level	b +	SE ++	*p*
NRS	Primary Secondary	0.142	0.046	0.003
PPI	Primary Secondary	0.125	0.045	0.007
Sensory	Primary Secondary	0.117	0.057	0.043
Affective	Primary Secondary	0.125	0.065	0.050
SFMPQ total	Primary Secondary	0.110	0.055	0.047

+ Dependency factor, ++ standard factor error. NRS: Numeric Rating Scale, PPI: Present Pain Index, SFMPQ—total score: Short Form McGill Pain Questionnaire—total score.

3.5. Early Postoperative Pain and Preoperative Psychological Status

The investigation of the influence of preoperative anxiety or depression on the experience of pain in every predetermined time point revealed an association between psychological factors and pain at different postoperative time points during POD #0. An important positive correlation was observed between the preoperative feeling of anxiety and the pain of the 1st postoperative hour, with most of the questionnaire's parameters being affected. Patients reporting a higher level of preoperative anxiety experienced severe pain at the 1st preoperative hour in terms of both pain intensity and unpleasantness. In contrast, preoperative feelings of depression seem to influence only the perception of the quality of postoperative pain at the 1st hour (affective score) but extract an important influence on severity and unpleasantness of pain (NRS, PPI, affective score) at the 4th postoperative hour. Furthermore, patients with higher levels of preoperative depression report less severe unpleasantness (affective and SF-MPQ score) at the 24th postoperative pain measurement (Table 6).

Table 6. Spearman's correlation coefficients of the preoperative anxiety and depression scores with the MPQ-SF parameters for every predetermined time point.

	Postoperative Hour	NRS		PPI		Sensory Score		Affective Score		SFMPQ Total Score	
		r	*p*	r	*p*	r	*p*	r	*p*	r	*p*
Preoperative Anxiety	1st hour	0.22	0.030	0,.04	0.676	0.28	0.005	0.29	0.004	0.31	0.002
	4th hour	0.04	0.731	−0.02	0.850	0.12	0.257	0.07	0.514	0.13	0.215
	8th hour	0.04	0.675	0.00	0.987	0.06	0.550	−0.06	0.540	0.02	0.844
	12th hour	−0.03	0.744	−0.07	0.508	−0.02	0.868	−0.05	0.653	−0.02	0.812
	24th hour	−0.07	0.516	−0.08	0.424	−0.02	0.857	−0.10	0.340	−0.07	0.494
Preoperative Depression	1st hour	0.14	0.158	0.04	0.662	0.14	0.181	0.22	0.034	0.17	0.096
	4th hour	0.21	0.038	0.20	0.046	0.14	0.185	0.22	0.029	0.16	0.110
	8th hour	0.10	0.303	0.01	0.906	0.05	0.625	0.10	0.319	0.06	0.531
	12th hour	−0.02	0.871	−0.03	0.755	0.04	0.710	0.04	0.690	0.06	0.569
	24th hour	0.05	0.644	0.00	0.994	−0.09	0.395	−0.28	0.004	−0.23	0.038

NRS: Numeric Rating Scale, PPI: Present Pain Index, SFMPQ—total score: Short Form McGill Pain Questionnaire—total score.

4. Discussion

Many studies have demonstrated a higher prevalence of psychological disorders among obese patients who are candidates for bariatric surgery [33–35]. In our hospital, the preoperative assessment of patients planning to undergo bariatric surgery includes a professional psychiatric evaluation, and for patients with proven pathology, the operation is postponed. A reevaluation is performed after psychiatric treatment, and if the patient is proven to be psychologically stabilized, the operation is performed. This strategy could explain why the preoperative assessment of the feelings of anxiety and depression using HADS classifies most of our patients in the normal range. Nonetheless, 24% and 11% of our patients were assessed as having border-line or abnormal anxiety or depression levels, respectively.

It is well known that psychological factors play a role in the perception of postoperative pain [21,25,36]. This is the first study demonstrating the influence of preoperative anxiety and depression on postoperative pain at different time points of POD #0 after a bariatric surgery. Furthermore, the assessment of pain using a well-structured questionnaire (MPQ-SF) that evaluates both the quantitative and qualitative dimensions of pain permits a detailed description of the perception of postoperative pain.

In this study, pain control during the first eight postoperative hours was insufficient, with patients experiencing severe and distressing pain at the 1st postoperative hour decreasing to moderate pain 4 h after the surgery and persisting until the 8th postoperative hour. Furthermore, anxiety seemed to play a role on pain perception at the 1st postoperative hour, with patients with higher levels of preoperative anxiety experiencing more severe pain in terms of intensity and quality. This finding confirmed the results of previous studies showing that anxiety is a significant positive predictor of severe pain shortly after the operation [37,38]. Moreover, this study extended this knowledge by being the first to evaluate the impact of the preoperative level of anxiety on the qualitative dimension of pain after bariatric surgery. Depression, on the other hand, had a statistically significant positive correlation only with the affective dimension of pain at the 1st postoperative hour. However, depression influenced both quantity and quality characteristics of pain at the 4th postoperative hour, with patients with a higher preoperative level of depression experiencing an intense and unpleasant pain. This finding is also in line with a previous study describing the positive correlation of depression with the intensity of postoperative pain after a bariatric surgery [21]. Our study is the first to show a positive correlation with the intensity of quality characteristics of pain at different time points during POD #0.

An unexpected finding of our study was the impact of preoperative depression on the affective dimension of pain at the 24th postoperative hour measurement. Patients with higher levels of preoperative depression experienced less unpleasantness (affective component) of pain 24 h after the surgery. Moreover, it also influenced the total perception of pain in terms of pain sensation at this time point (SFMPQ—total score). Studies evaluating the experimental pain in depressive patients have reported equivocal results, with some describing increased or decreased pain thresholds [39] depending on the underlying mode of pain application [40] or type of surgery [41,42] and only one examining the affective dimension of experimental pain [43]. At this time point (24th postoperative hour), pain is mild, with the score of the affective component being 1.2 (out of 12) and the score of the SFMPQ-total being 4.1 (out of 45). We can assume that this finding has no clinical significance.

Another interesting finding is that patients' educational level is an independent factor influencing the perception of quantitative and qualitative characteristics of pain, with patients with higher educational levels reporting more severe pain during the POD #0 after a bariatric surgery. This positive correlation was significant with all the MPQ-SF parameters. On the other hand, age, gender, BMI, marital status, smoking and type of surgery had no influence on postoperative pain. Our findings are supported by the results of other studies about bariatric surgery, which reported that gender, age, surgical technique and smoking are not related to postoperative pain [44–46]. However, these results are in contrast with the positive correlations observed in another investigation between age and postoperative pain, at the first 24 h after Laparoscopic gastric by-pass surgery [46]. In terms of educational status, there is no study in bariatric surgery (except in general surgery) demonstrating the impact of educational status on the perception of pain [47]. An informative discussion with patients before surgery may have helped patients with a high or low educational level to have lower pain scores.

5. Conclusions

In conclusion, preoperative anxiety and depression and a high educational level are factors influencing the qualitative and quantitative dimension of early postoperative pain during the first postoperative day (POD #0). The preoperative identification of these factors may be useful for designing personalized and time-dependent postoperative analgesic protocols to improve clinical outcomes. Furthermore, regular and systematic pain assessment during different time points at the POD #0 after bariatric surgery is essential for the efficient control of early postoperative pain. The efficient control of early postoperative pain enhances early mobilization and promotes the implementation of fast-track bariatric protocols. This strategy is of major importance due to the susceptibility of bariatric patients to postoperative complications.

Author Contributions: Conceptualization, S.G.; methodology, S.G. and M.M.; software, S.G.; validation, S.G.; formal analysis, S.G.; investigation, S.G.; resources K.A.; data curation, S.G., C.G.Z. and E.M.; writing—original draft preparation, S.G.; writing—review and editing, S.G., M.M. and P.T.N.; visualization, S.G. and M.M.; supervision, G.Z. and K.A.; project administration, S.G. All authors have read and agreed to the published version of the manuscript.

Funding: This research received no external funding.

Institutional Review Board Statement: The study was conducted according to the guidelines of the Declaration of Helsinki, and approved by the Scientific-Ethics Committee of the Hospital with protocol number 10262 and date 19/07/2016.

Informed Consent Statement: Informed consent was obtained from all subjects involved in the study.

Data Availability Statement: All data are available by the corresponding author (S.G.) upon reasonable request.

Acknowledgments: The authors would like to acknowledge the support of patients who have generously given their time to complete the questionnaires of the research protocol.

Conflicts of Interest: The authors declare no conflict of interest.

References

1. Wang, M.; Xu, S.; Liu, W.; Zhang, C.; Zhang, X.; Wang, L.; Liu, J.; Zhu, Z.; Hu, J.; Luo, X.; et al. Prevalence and changes of BMI categories in China and related chronic diseases: Cross-sectional National Health Service Surveys (NHSSs) from 2013 to 2018. *EClinicalMedicine* **2020**, *26*, 100521. [CrossRef] [PubMed]
2. Di Angelantonio, E.; Bhupathiraju, S.N.; Wormser, D.; Gao, P.; Kaptoge, S.; de Gonzalez, A.B.; Cairns, B.J.; Huxley, R.; Jackson, C.L.; Joshy, G.; et al. Body-mass index and all-cause mortality: Individual-participant-data meta-analysis of 239 prospective studies in four continents. *Lancet* **2016**, *388*, 776–786. [CrossRef]
3. Residori, L.; García-Lorda, P.; Flancbaum, L.; Pi-Sunyer, F.X.; Laferrére, B. Prevalence of co-morbidities in obese patients before bariatric surgery: Effect of race. *Obes. Surg.* **2003**, *13*, 333–340. [CrossRef] [PubMed]
4. Buchwald, H.; Avidor, Y.; Braunwald, E.; Jensen, M.D.; Pories, W.; Fahrbach, K.; Schoelles, K. Bariatric surgery: A systematic review and meta-analysis. *J. Am. Med. Assoc.* **2004**, *292*, 1724–1737. [CrossRef]
5. Pantalone, K.M.; Hobbs, T.M.; Chagin, K.M.; Kong, S.X.; Wells, B.J.; Kattan, M.W.; Bouchard, J.; Sakurada, B.; Milinovich, A.; Weng, W.; et al. Prevalence and recognition of obesity and its associated comorbidities: Cross-sectional analysis of electronic health record data from a large US integrated health system. *BMJ Open* **2017**, *7*. [CrossRef]
6. Noria, S.F.; Grantcharov, T. Biological effects of bariatric surgery on obesity-related comorbidities. *Can. J. Surg.* **2013**, *56*, 47–57. [CrossRef]
7. Picot, J.; Jones, J.; Colquitt, J.L.; Gospodarevskaya, E.; Loveman, E.; Baxter, L.; Clegg, A.J. The clinical effectiveness and cost-effectiveness of bariatric (weight loss) surgery for obesity: A systematic review and economic evaluation. *Health Technol. Assess.* **2009**, *13*. [CrossRef]
8. Douglas, I.J.; Bhaskaran, K.; Batterham, R.L.; Smeeth, L. Bariatric Surgery in the United Kingdom: A Cohort Study of Weight Loss and Clinical Outcomes in Routine Clinical Care. *PLoS Med.* **2015**, *12*, e1001925. [CrossRef]
9. Raaijmakers, L.C.H.; Pouwels, S.; Thomassen, S.E.M.; Nienhuijs, S.W. Quality of life and bariatric surgery: A systematic review of short- and long-term results and comparison with community norms. *Eur. J. Clin. Nutr.* **2017**, *71*, 441–449. [CrossRef]
10. NCD Risk Factor Collaboration (NCD-RisC). Trends in adult body-mass index in 200 countries from 1975 to 2014: A pooled analysis of 1698 population-based measurement studies with 19.2 million participants. *Lancet* **2016**, *387*, 1377–1396. [CrossRef]
11. Angrisani, L.; Santonicola, A.; Iovino, P.; Formisano, G.; Buchwald, H.; Scopinaro, N. Bariatric Surgery Worldwide 2013. *Obes. Surg.* **2015**, *25*, 1822–1832. [CrossRef] [PubMed]
12. Parker, M.; Loewen, M.; Sullivan, T.; Yatco, E.; Cerabona, T.; Savino, J.A.; Kaul, A. Predictors of outcome after obesity surgery in New York state from 1991 to 2003. *Surg. Endosc.* **2007**, *21*, 1482–1486. [CrossRef] [PubMed]
13. Kozlowski, T.; Kozakiewicz, K.; Dadan, J.; Mysliwiec, P. Innovative solutions in bariatric surgery. *Gland Surg.* **2016**, *5*, 529–536. [CrossRef] [PubMed]
14. Chaim, E.A.; Ramos, A.C.; Cazzo, E. Mini-Gastric Bypass: Description of the Technique and Preliminary Results. *Arq. Bras. Cir. Dig.* **2017**, *30*, 264–266. [CrossRef] [PubMed]
15. Carbajo, M.A.; Luque-de-León, E.; Jiménez, J.M.; Ortiz-de-Solórzano, J.; Pérez-Miranda, M.; Castro-Alija, M.J. Laparoscopic One-Anastomosis Gastric Bypass: Technique, Results, and Long-Term Follow-Up in 1200 Patients. *Obes. Surg.* **2017**, *27*, 1153–1167. [CrossRef]
16. El Shobary, H.; Christou, N.; Backman, S.B.; Gvocdic, B.; Schricker, T. Effect of laparoscopic versus open gastric bypass surgery on postoperative pain and bowel function. *Obes. Surg.* **2006**, *16*, 437–442. [CrossRef]
17. Gan, T.J. Poorly controlled postoperative pain: Prevalence, consequences, and prevention. *J. Pain Res.* **2017**, *10*, 2287–2298. [CrossRef]
18. Adams, J.P.; Murphy, P.G. Obesity in anaesthesia and intensive care. *Br. J. Anaesth.* **2000**, *85*, 91–108. [CrossRef]
19. Melzack, R.; Katz, J. The McGill pain questionnaire: Development, psychometric properties, and usefulness of the long form, short form, and short form-2. In *Handbook of Pain Assessment*, 3rd ed.; The Guilford Press: New York, NY, USA, 2011; pp. 45–66.
20. Auvray, M.; Myin, E.; Spence, C. The sensory-discriminative and affective-motivational aspects of pain. *Neurosci. Biobehav. Rev.* **2010**, *34*, 214–223. [CrossRef]
21. Ip, H.Y.V.; Abrishami, A.; Peng, P.W.H.; Wong, J.; Chung, F. Predictors of postoperative pain and analgesic consumption: A qualitative systematic review. *Anesthesiology* **2009**, *111*, 657–677. [CrossRef]
22. Yang, M.M.; Hartley, R.L.; Leung, A.A.; Ronksley, P.E.; Jetté, N.; Casha, S.; Riva-Cambrin, J. Preoperative predictors of poor acute postoperative pain control: A systematic review and meta-analysis. *BMJ Open* **2019**, *9*. [CrossRef] [PubMed]
23. Malik, S.; Mitchell, J.E.; Engel, S.; Crosby, R.; Wonderlich, S. Psychopathology in bariatric surgery candidates: A review of studies using structured diagnostic interviews. *Compr. Psychiatry* **2014**, *55*, 248–259. [CrossRef] [PubMed]
24. Kavaki, O.; Altuntas, E.; Muderris, S. Effects of the preoperative anxiety and depression on the postoperative pain in ear, nose, and throat surgery. *Indian J. Otol.* **2012**, *18*, 82–87. [CrossRef]
25. Sobol-Kwapinska, M.; Bąbel, P.; Plotek, W.; Stelcer, B. Psychological correlates of acute postsurgical pain: A systematic review and meta-analysis. *Eur. J. Pain.* **2016**, *20*, 1573–1586. [CrossRef]
26. C.A.H.; Diaz, M.A.C.; Bonisson, P.L.V.; Simino, G.P.R.; Barbosa, M.H.; de Mattia, A.L. Relationship of anxiety and preoperative depression with post-operative pain. *Texto Contexto Enferm.* **2020**, *29*, 1–13. [CrossRef]

27. Elliott, J.A.; Patel, V.M.; Kirresh, A.; Ashrafian, H.; Le Roux, C.W.; Olbers, T.; Athanasiou, T.; Zacharakis, E. Fast-track laparoscopic bariatric surgery: A systematic review. *Updates Surg.* **2013**, *65*, 85–94. [CrossRef]
28. Bamgbade, O.A.; Oluwole, O.; Khaw, R.R. Perioperative Analgesia for Fast-Track Laparoscopic Bariatric Surgery. *Obes. Surg.* **2017**, *27*, 1828–1834. [CrossRef]
29. Nijland, L.M.G.; de Castro, S.M.M.; van Veen, R.N. Risk Factors Associated with Prolonged Hospital Stay and Readmission in Patients After Primary Bariatric Surgery. *Obes. Surg.* **2020**, *30*, 2395–2402. [CrossRef]
30. Georgoudis, G.; Watson, P.J.; Oldham, J.A. The development and validation of a Greek version of the short-form McGill Pain Questionnaire. *Eur. J. Pain* **2000**, *4*, 275–281. [CrossRef]
31. Georgoudis, G.; Oldham, J.A.; Watson, P.J. Reliability and sensitivity measures of the greek version of the short form of the McGill Pain Questionnaire. *Eur. J. Pain* **2001**, *5*, 109–118. [CrossRef]
32. Zigmond, A.S.; Snaith, R.P. The Hospital Anxiety and Depression Scale. *Acta Psychiatr. Scand.* **1983**, *67*, 361–370. [CrossRef]
33. Van Hout, G.C.M.; Van Oudheusden, I.; Van Heck, G.L. Psychological profile of the morbidly obese. *Obes. Surg.* **2004**, *14*, 579–588. [CrossRef]
34. Marzocchi, R.; Moscatiello, S.; Villanova, N.; Suppini, A.; Marchesini, G. Psychological Profile and Quality of Life of Morbid Obese Patients Attending a Cognitive Behavioural Program. *Psihol. Teme* **2008**, *17*, 349–360.
35. McGarrity, L.A.; Perry, N.S.; Derbidge, C.M.; Trapp, S.K.; Terrill, A.L.; Smith, T.W.; Ibele, A.R.; MacKenzie, J.J. Associations Between Approach and Avoidance Coping, Psychological Distress, and Disordered Eating Among Candidates for Bariatric Surgery. *Obes. Surg.* **2019**, *29*, 3596–3604. [CrossRef] [PubMed]
36. Hah, J.M.; Hilmoe, H.; Schmidt, P.; McCue, R.; Trafton, J.; Clay, D.; Sharifzadeh, Y.; Ruchelli, G.; Boussard, T.H.; Goodman, S.; et al. Preoperative factors associated with remote postoperative pain resolution and opioid cessation in a mixed surgical cohort: Post hoc analysis of a perioperative gabapentin trial. *J. Pain Res.* **2020**, *13*, 2959–2970. [CrossRef] [PubMed]
37. Kalkman, C.J.; Visser, K.; Moen, J.; Bonsel, G.J.; Grobbee, D.E.; Moons, K.G.M. Preoperative prediction of severe postoperative pain. *Pain* **2003**, *105*, 415–423. [CrossRef]
38. Kain, Z.N.; Sevarino, F.; Alexander, G.M.; Pincus, S.; Mayes, L.C. Preoperative anxiety and postoperative pain in women undergoing hysterectomy: A repeated-measures design. *J. Psychosom. Res.* **2000**, *49*, 417–422. [CrossRef]
39. Dickens, C.; McGowan, L.; Dale, S. Impact of depression on experimental pain perception: A systematic review of the literature with meta-analysis. *Psychosom. Med.* **2003**, *65*, 369–375. [CrossRef]
40. Bär, K.J.; Brehm, S.; Boettger, M.K.; Boettger, S.; Wagner, G.; Sauer, H. Pain perception in major depression depends on pain modality. *Pain* **2005**, *117*, 97–103. [CrossRef]
41. Caumo, W.; Schmidt, A.P.; Schneider, C.N.; Bergmann, J.; Iwamoto, C.W.; Adamatti, L.C.; Bandeira, D.; Ferreira, M.B.C. Preoperative predictors of moderate to intense acute postoperative pain in patients undergoing abdominal surgery. *Acta Anaesthesiol. Scand.* **2002**, *46*, 1265–1271. [CrossRef]
42. Pinto, P.R.; McIntyre, T.; Araújo-Soares, V.; Costa, P.; Almeida, A. Differential Predictors of Acute Post-Surgical Pain Intensity After Abdominal Hysterectomy and Major Joint Arthroplasty. *Ann. Behav. Med.* **2015**, *49*, 384–397. [CrossRef] [PubMed]
43. Dworkin, R.H.; Clark, W.C.; Lipsitz, J.D. Pain responsivity in major depression and bipolar disorder. *Psychiatry Res.* **1995**, *56*, 173–181. [CrossRef]
44. Ferreira, A.T.; Duarte, N.M.; Caetano, A.M.; Albuquerque, K.A.; Buenos Aires, V.; Brainer-Lima, J.P.; Hinrichsen, E.A.; Santa-Cruz, F.; Campos, J.M. Postoperative pain following bariatric surgery: Correlation between intensity and clinical-surgical variables. *Bariatr. Surg. Pract. Patient Care* **2019**, *14*, 57–61. [CrossRef]
45. Karlnoski, R.A.; Puri, S.; Chen, R.; Mangar, D.; Murr, M.M.; Camporesi, E.M. Reduced postoperative pain and complications after a modified multidisciplinary approach for bariatric surgery. *Open Obes. J.* **2013**, *5*, 60–64. [CrossRef]
46. Hartwig, M.; Allvin, R.; Bäckström, R.; Stenberg, E. Factors Associated with Increased Experience of Postoperative Pain after Laparoscopic Gastric Bypass Surgery. *Obes. Surg.* **2017**, *27*, 1854–1858. [CrossRef]
47. Lanitis, S.; Mimigianni, C.; Raptis, D.; Sourtse, G.; Sgourakis, G.; Karaliotas, C. The impact of educational status on the postoperative perception of pain. *Korean J. Pain* **2015**, *28*, 265–274. [CrossRef]

Journal of
Clinical Medicine

MDPI

Article

Improvement of Arterial Stiffness One Month after Bariatric Surgery and Potential Mechanisms

Anna Oliveras [1,2,3,4,*], Isabel Galceran [1,2], Albert Goday [2,5,6], Susana Vázquez [1,2], Laia Sans [1,2,4], Marta Riera [2,4], David Benaiges [2,5] and Julio Pascual [1,2]

1 Nephrology Department, Hospital Universitari del Mar, 08003 Barcelona, Spain; igalceran@hospitaldelmar.cat (I.G.); svazquez@hospitaldelmar.cat (S.V.); lsans@hospitaldelmar.cat (L.S.); JPascualSantos@hospitaldelmar.cat (J.P.)
2 IMIM (Hospital del Mar Medical Research Institute), 08003 Barcelona, Spain; agoday@hospitaldelmar.cat (A.G.); mriera1@imim.es (M.R.); dbenaiges@hospitaldelmar.cat (D.B.)
3 Department of Experimental and Health Sciences, Area of Medicine, Universitat Pompeu Fabra, 08002 Barcelona, Spain
4 Red de Investigación Renal (REDINREN), Instituto Carlos III-FEDER, 28029 Madrid, Spain
5 Endocrinology Department, Hospital Universitari del Mar, 08003 Barcelona, Spain
6 Medicine Department, Universitat Autònoma de Barcelona, 08193 Barcelona, Spain
* Correspondence: aoliveras@hospitaldelmar.cat; Tel.: +34-932-483-483

Abstract: Arterial stiffness (AS) is an independent predictor of cardiovascular risk. We aimed to analyze changes (Δ) in AS 1-month post-bariatric surgery (BS) and search for possible pathophysiological mechanisms. Patients with severe obesity (43% hypertensives) were prospectively evaluated before and 1-month post-BS, with AS assessed by pulse-wave velocity (PWV), augmentation index (AIx@75) and pulse pressure (PP). Ambulatory 24 h blood pressure (BP), anthropometric data, renin-angiotensin-aldosterone system (RAAS) components and several adipokines and inflammatory markers were also analyzed. Overall reduction in body weight was mean (interquartile range (IQR)) = 11.0% (9.6–13.1). A decrease in PWV, AIx@75 and PP was observed 1-month post-BS (all, $p < 0.01$). There were also significant Δ in BP, RAAS components, adipokines and inflammatory biomarkers. Multiple linear regression adjusted models showed that Δaldosterone was an independent variable (B coeff.95%CI) for final PWV (B = −0.003, −0.005 to 0.000; $p = 0.022$). Angiotensin-converting enzyme (ACE)/ACE2 and ACE were independent variables for final AIx@75 (B = 0.036, 0.005 to 0.066; $p = 0.024$) and PP (B = 0.010, 0.003 to 0.017; $p = 0.01$), respectively. There was no correlation between ΔAS and anthropometric changes nor with Δ of adipokines or inflammatory markers except high-sensitivity C-reactive protein (hs-CRP). Patients with PWV below median decreased PWV (mean, 95%CI = −0.18, −0.25 to −0.10; $p < 0.001$) and both AIx@75 and PP at 1-month, but not those with PWV above median. In conclusion, there is an improvement in AS 1-month post-BS that correlates with ΔBP and Δrenin-angiotensin-aldosterone components. The benefit is reduced in those with higher PWV.

Keywords: bariatric surgery; arterial stiffness; renin-angiotensin axis

Citation: Oliveras, A.; Galceran, I.; Goday, A.; Vázquez, S.; Sans, L.; Riera, M.; Benaiges, D.; Pascual, J. Improvement of Arterial Stiffness One Month after Bariatric Surgery and Potential Mechanisms. *J. Clin. Med.* **2021**, *10*, 691. https://doi.org/10.3390/jcm10040691

Academic Editor: Tomoaki Morioka
Received: 23 December 2020
Accepted: 4 February 2021
Published: 10 February 2021

1. Introduction

The World Health Organization reported that more than 1.9 billion adults were overweight and, of these, over 650 million were obese [1]. Obesity is a well-established contributor to cardiac and all-cause mortality, independently of other associated cardiovascular risk factors [2,3]. Bariatric surgery (BS) consistently has shown to reduce cardiovascular morbidity and overall mortality [4,5], although the underlying mechanisms continue to be investigated.

Arterial stiffness (AS), considered as an independent cardiovascular risk factor [6], is a decrease in the ability of an artery to expand and contract in response to a given pressure change [7]. AS can be measured in many different ways [8]: pulse pressure (PP), pulse wave velocity (PWV), given that one of the fundamental principles of vascular pathophysiology is that pulse waves travel faster in stiffer arteries, and augmentation index (AIx), that expresses the degree of "augmentation" of central systolic blood pressure (SBP) as a consequence of systolic pressure waves travelling back to the heart and being received in late systole. Although these three indices are frequently used as AS markers, the most reliable seems to be PWV. It has been shown that PWV predicts mortality and cardiovascular outcomes [9], even independently of the Framingham Risk Score, showing better survival of individuals whose PWV responded to antihypertensive treatment independently of SBP reduction [10]. Moreover, high PWV is associated with increased cardiovascular disease risk regardless of hypertension status [11].

Excess body weight is associated with higher aortic stiffness in young and older adults [12]. Therefore, increased AS may be one of the mechanisms by which obesity increases cardiovascular risk independently of traditional risk factors. It is generally accepted that body weight decrease either by lifestyle intervention or by BS results in a reduction in AS. Some studies have reported a significant decrease In PWV or AIx at 3 months [13], 6 months [14,15], or beyond two years [16] after the intervention. There is no evidence or negative results regarding changes in PWV after weight loss in earlier stages [13,17].

The previously published BARIHTA (Hemodynamic Changes and Vascular Tone Control after Bariatric Surgery. Prognostic Value Regarding Hyper Tension and Target Organ Damage) study [18] analyses haemodynamic changes after BS. Here, changes in AS markers are analyzed, mainly as early as one month after BS. Additionally, we explore the role of different mechanisms potentially responsible for such changes.

2. Materials and Methods

2.1. Methods

2.1.1. Study Design and Patients

The BARIHTA study is a prospective observational trial in a cohort of consecutively recruited patients with severe obesity scheduled to undergo BS (clinicaltrials.gov identifier: NCT03115502). Details about BARIHTA trial have been published elsewhere [18]. In brief, the BARIHTA study enrolled outpatients attending consults in the Hospital del Mar (Barcelona, Catalonia, Spain), because of severe obesity and looking for surgical treatment. All participants of both sexes aged 18–60 years with medical indication for treatment with BS and who agreed to undergo the surgical intervention, were invited to participate. Both normotensive and hypertensive patients were included. The exclusion criteria comprised the exclusion of the BS program for any reason or the refusal to give informed consent. The trial was approved by the local institutional Ethic Committee in accordance with the Declaration of Helsinki.

Here, we report additional analysis focused on the effect of BS on AS and its relationship with several renin-angiotensin-aldosterone system (RAAS) components, as well as with inflammatory markers and adipokines, according to pre-specified secondary endpoints.

Demographic and clinical data were recorded from all participants in the inclusion visit. Anthropometric characteristics, pharmacological treatment and 24 h blood pressure (BP) recordings, including data on PWV and AIx, and laboratory tests were obtained at baseline and 1, 3, 6 and 12 months after surgery. Hypertension was considered if patient received antihypertensive drugs and/or if the baseline 24 h-BP was $\geq$130/80 mmHg. Diabetes mellitus (DM) was diagnosed if the patient was under antidiabetic treatment or had $\geq$2 fasting plasma glucose determinations $\geq$7.0 mmol/L or if glycosylated haemoglobin A1c was >6.5%.

2.1.2. Procedures

Mobil-O-Graph® Device and Measurements

A Mobil-O-Graph® NG-ambulatory blood pressure (NG-ABPM) by IEM, Stolberg, Germany device was used to measure brachial-BP and indirectly calculate aortic-BP and other arterial parameters through the oscillometric method (ARCSolver algorithm). Several studies have validated this device for estimating PWV and AIx [19,20]. Using suitable sized cuffs, the monitor was placed at 08:00–10:00 h A.M., and brachial artery waveforms were automatically recorded at 20-min intervals. Then, a generalized transfer function is applied to the averaged waveform to generate a corresponding aortic waveform. AIx was calculated as the ratio of the difference between the second systolic peak and the diastolic pressure and the difference between the first systolic peak and the diastolic pressure × 100. AIx was corrected for heart rate at 75 beats/min (AIx@75), as is standard [19,21,22]. The device also provided an indirect estimation of cardiac output.

All patients had recordings of good technical quality (≥70% valid readings). Otherwise, a new ambulatory-BP-monitoring (ABPM) was repeated within 1-week and used as the valid one.

Renin-Angiotensin-Aldosterone System (RAAS) Components

Plasma renin activity (PRA) and plasma aldosterone concentration, as well as angiotensin-converting enzyme (ACE) and angiotensin-converting enzyme-2 (ACE2) activities, were measured by validated laboratory methods [23]. Details on assay performance are reported in Appendix A.

Adipokines and Inflammatory Parameters

Leptin, adiponectin, and some cytokines and inflammatory markers, i.e., resistin, angiopoietin-2, MCP-1 and high-sensitivity C-reactive protein (hs-CRP) were also determined. See Appendix B.

Surgical Techniques

Either laparoscopic Roux-en-Y gastric bypass (LRYGB) or laparoscopic sleeve gastrectomy (LSG) were chosen for each patient based on clinical criteria and the consensus of the Bariatric Surgery Unit. Thus, LSG was preferred in younger patients, in those with BMI ranged 35–40 kg/m^2, as a first-step treatment in cases with a body mass index (BMI) > 50 kg/m^2 and when drug malabsorption was to be avoided [24]. The LRYGB technique involved a 150-cm antecolic Roux limb with 25-mm circular pouch–jejunostomy and exclusion of 50 cm of the proximal jejunum. In LSG, the longitudinal resection of the stomach from the angle of His to approximately 5 cm proximal to the pylorus was performed using a 36-French bougie inserted along the lesser curvature.

2.1.3. Statistical Analyses

Descriptive data are presented as mean ± standard deviation (S.D.) for those normally distributed variables or summarized as median (interquartile range, IQR) in case of a non-normal distribution according to the Kolmogorov–Smirnov test. Categorical and dichotomous variables are presented as frequencies and percentages. Comparisons of variables between two periods were carried out by paired *t*-tests in continuous normally distributed data or by Wilcoxon-test in non-normally distributed continuous data. Multiple linear regression models were constructed for the resulting 1-month value of each AS parameter (dependent variable) adjusting for age, sex, variation (Δ) of body weight, Δ 24 h-systolic BP, Δ cardiac output, the baseline value of the correspondent AS marker and Δ of each assessed RAAS components (independent variables). Results are shown by the B coefficient and corresponding 95% confidence intervals (95%CI). Pearson's or Spearman's correlation coefficients, when appropriate, were obtained to measure the association between AS indexes and BP estimates, RAAS components, adipokines, inflammatory markers and glucose homeostasis parameters.

A sample size calculation was initially calculated and 61 subjects were assumed as needed to answer the primary outcome [18]. A post-hoc power calculation was performed regarding the paired *t*-test for the variable Δ 24 h-PWV (1-month after BS vs. baseline), the secondary endpoint analyzed here, having a sample size of 47 patients. Since we have a mean difference of −0.26 and a standard deviation of 0.40 (effect size = −0.65), for an $\alpha = 0.05$, a power of 99.4% was found.

Statistical package SPSS for Windows version 25.0 (Cary, NC, USA) was used. A change was considered significant if the two-side alpha level was ≤0.05.

A quarter of the study population received treatment with one or more drugs that interfered with RAAS, being modified within the first month post-BS. For this reason, the main analyses, especially those which include BP and/or RAAS parameters, were performed separately in both the whole cohort and in the normotensive patients.

3. Results

Sixty-two patients completed the BARIHTA study. Complete data on AS were available for 47 subjects, and these comprise the cohort reported here (a flowchart is supplied in Supplementary Figure S1). Main baseline clinical characteristics are described in Table 1.

Table 1. Baseline clinical characteristics.

Age, year (mean ± SD)	42.7 ± 9.4
Sex, women, *n* (%)	34 (72.3)
Body weight, kg (mean ± SD)	118.1 ± 19.5
Waist circumference, cm (mean ± SD)	131.6 ± 10.7
Body mas index, kg/m^2 (mean ± SD)	42.2 ± 5.4
Race, Caucasian, *n* (%)	45 (95.7)
Current smokers, *n* (%)	10 (21.3)
Surgical procedure, *n* (%): Sleeve gastrectomy Roux-en-Y gastric bypass	 20 (42.6) 27 (57.4)
Hypertension, *n* (%)	20 * (42.6)
T2-Diabetes Mellitus, *n* (%)	4 (8.5)
Dyslipidemia, *n* (%)	12 (25.5)
Previous major vascular event **, *n* (%)	3 (6.4)
Sleep apnea syndrome, *n* (%) CPAP, *n* (%)	11 (23.4) 9 (81.8)

T2 = type 2; CPAP = continuous positive airway pressure. * Three of them, never-treated hypertensives. ** Coronary artery disease, heart failure, ictus or peripheral vascular disease.

There was a higher prevalence of female patients, and 43% of individuals were hypertensives. None of the patients died in the follow-up period. Of note, no patient in this study was treated with a sodium-glucose transport protein 2-inhibitor or a glucagon-like peptide-1 receptor agonist.

3.1. Changes in Anthropometric and Hemodynamic Parameters

As regards the primary outcome of the BARIHTA study, there was a 12-month decrease in both 24 h-central and 24 h-peripheral SBP (mean, 95% CI) of −4.4 mmHg (−8.3 to −0.5) and −4.0 mmHg (−7.8 to −0.2) respectively.

Changes (Δ) in AS were statistically significant 1-month post-BS (Table 2).

Table 2. Changes 1-month after bariatric surgery.

Parameter	All Patients (n = 47)			Patients without Antihypertensive Treatment at Baseline ** (n = 30)		
	Baseline Mean ± SD	1-Month Mean ± SD	p	Baseline Mean ± SD	1-Month Mean ± SD	p
Anthropometric parameters						
Body weight, kg	118.1 ± 19.5	104.5 ± 17.5	<0.001	116.1 ± 17.7	102.5 ± 15.2	<0.001
Waist circumference, cm	132.0 ± 12.0	122.4 ± 10.2	<0.001	130.2 ± 10.6	120.2 ± 9.3	<0.001
Arterial stiffness						
24 h-PP, mmHg	46.4 ± 7.5	44.2 ± 7.1	0.001	45.8 ± 6.9	43.1 ± 6.6	0.010
24 h-PWV, m/s	6.64 ± 1.03	6.24 ± 0.97	<0.001	6.2 ± 1.0	6.11 ± 0.99	0.001
AIx@75, %	26.4 ± 7.5	22.7 ± 7.1	<0.001	24.8 ± 5.9	22.2 ± 6.0	0.028
Blood pressure, heart rate and cardiac output						
24 h-SBP, mmHg	120.0 ± 11.7	114.3 ± 9.9	<0.001	118.6 ± 10.7	113.5 ± 9.7	<0.001
24 h-DBP, mmHg	73.7 ± 9.0	70.2 ± 6.9	<0.001	72.1 ± 7.7	69.4 ± 6.8	<0.001
24 h-HR, bpm	73.2 ± 10.1	66.7 ± 8.8	<0.001	75.2 ± 9.2	68.7 ± 7.6	<0.001
Cardiac output	4.6 ± 0.6	4.5 ± 0.5	<0.001	4.7 ± 0.5	4.5 ± 0.4	0.004
Glucose metabolism parameters						
Fasting glucose, mg/dL	99.6 ± 19.1	86.5 ± 10.1	<0.001	95.9 ± 12.9	85.7 ± 9.2	<0.001
Glycosylated hemoglobin, %	5.7 ± 0.8	5.3 ± 0.6	<0.001	5.7 ± 1.0	5.3 ± 0.6	0.001
Fasting insulin *, mcU/mL	12.0 [8.3; 17.3]	6.8 [3.9; 9.4]	<0.001	11.7 [7.1; 17.3]	6.3 [2.9; 9.2]	<0.001
Insulin resistance (HOMA-IR) *	54.5 [37.2; 87.1]	23.8 [13.8; 39.3]	<0.001	50.4 [28.3; 82.2]	23.3 [10.3; 39.3]	<0.001
RAAS components						
PRA *, ng/mL/h	0.8 [0.3; 1.3]	0.8 [0.5; 1.2]	0.726	0.8 [0.4; 1.2]	0.9 [0.5; 1.5]	0.411
Aldosterone *, ng/dL	87.8 [56.8; 134.5]	82.0 [61.4; 139.5]	0.747	76.7 [59.3; 108.3]	86.0 [65.8; 128.5]	0.210
ACE activity, RFU/µL	1320.2 ± 385.8	1099.0 ± 293.7	<0.001	1307.9 ± 337.4	1126.6 ± 258.0	<0.001
ACE2 activity *, RFU/µL/h	7.9 [5.8; 10.8]	6.0 [4.7; 7.8]	<0.001	7.6 [5.5; 9.4]	5.8 [4.2; 7.8]	0.001
ACE act./ACE2 act.	170.0 ± 82.0	194.1 ± 108.7	0.009	183.0 ± 93.3	207.4 ± 118.1	0.072
Adipokines & Inflammatory Markers						
Leptin *, ng/mL	56.5 [28.8; 73.7]	21.4 [12.1; 37.3]	<0.001	45.1 [24.3; 67.1]	15.9 [9.5; 31.5]	<0.001
Adiponectine *, µg/mL	19.0 [12.5; 33.3]	23.6 [12.9; 40.5]	0.050	22.5 [16.0; 35.5]	27.1 [16.8; 45.6]	0.043
Resistin, ng/mL	36.8 ± 13.3	37.3 ± 14.9	0.822	35.9 ± 11.2	39.4 ± 12.7	0.106
MCP-1, pg/mL	544.9 ± 197.5	601.5 ± 249.4	0.041	530.0 ± 199.5	632.6 ± 274.7	0.014
Angiopoietin2 *, pg/mL	2676.2 [1815.4; 4067.0]	4039.6 [2076.8; 5380.9]	0.042	2721.4 [1815.4; 4655.1]	4366.8 [2011.9; 5293.3]	0.046
hs-CRP *, mg/dL	0.77 [0.43; 1.41]	0.45 [0.24; 0.74]	0.001	0.57 [0.32; 0.93]	0.56 [0.25; 0.74]	0.249

* Data shown as median [interquartile range]. ** normotensive patients (n = 27) plus mild hypertensive patients without antihypertensive treatment (n = 3). ACE = angiotensin converting enzyme; ACE2 = angiotensin converting enzyme 2; AIx@75 = augmentation index at 75 beats/minute; DBP = diastolic blood pressure; HOMA = homeostasis model assessment; HR = heart rate; hs-CRP = C-reactive protein; MCP-1 = monocyte chemoattractant protein-1; PP = pulse pressure; PRA = plasma renin activity; PWV = pulse-wave velocity; RAAS = renin-angiotensin aldosterone system; RFU = relative fluorescence units; SBP = systolic blood pressure; ACE = angiotensin converting enzyme; ACE2 = angiotensin converting enzyme 2; AIx@75 = augmentation index at 75 beats/min.

Although there was a trend towards a decrease in all AS markers from baseline to 3, 6 and 12 months [25], only the decrease of 24 h PP at 12 months was statistically significant: mean (95%CI) = −2.1 mmHg (−4.1 to −0.1), p = 0.042. Since our goal was to analyze changes in AS and their potential mechanisms, most of the analyses shown from now on are referred to the evaluation 1-month post-BS. Thus, 1-month changes in anthropometric and hemodynamic parameters and arterial stiffness estimates are shown in Table 2, both in the whole cohort and after excluding patients with any antihypertensive treatment, and for all these variables there was a statistically significant decrease ($p < 0.01$ for all).

Statistically significant decreases in body weight and waist circumference are also shown in Table 2. The overall reduction in body weight was mean (IQR) = 11.0% (9.6–13.1).

3.2. Changes in Glucose Metabolism, RAAS Components, Adipokines and Inflammatory Markers

There was a statistically significant decrease in all glucose metabolism parameters ($p < 0.001$) (Table 2).

Table 2 also describes the baseline and 1-month post-BS values of the RAAS components, showing statistically significant decreases in both ACE and ACE2 activities. However, none change was observed in either PRA or plasma aldosterone concentration values. Figure S2 (Supplementary Figure S2) shows that decreases in PRA and plasma aldosterone concentration occur from 3-months on. As regards adipokines and inflammatory markers, there was a statistically significant decrease in leptin and a trend towards a decrease in hs-CRP, as well as increases in other adipokines (adiponectine, MCP-1 and angiopoietin-2).

When analyzing anthropometrics, arterial stiffness and hemodynamic changes according to the surgical technique (Supplementary Table S1), to having or not sleep-apnea or to sex [25], no between-groups remarkable differences were observed.

Multiple linear regression models were built for each of the statistically significant change in AS markers (Table 3).

In all tested models for final (1-month post-BS) 24 h PP and final PWV, Δ 24 h systolic BP and baseline values of each correspondent AS marker were statistically significant independent variables. Another independent variable for 24 h PP post-BS was Δ ACE. On the other hand, Δ aldosterone was an independent variable for the final PWV value. As regards final AIx@75, age and baseline AIx@75 value were statistically significant independent variables in all models. In addition, the ratio ACE/ACE2 was also an independent variable for the final AIx@75 value in this cohort. Neither Δ body weight nor Δ cardiac output influenced the final value of any AS marker. Equivalent results were found when the same models were tested including Δ waist circumference instead of Δ body weight [25].

In addition, Pearson's or Spearman's correlation coefficients, as appropriate, were obtained to measure the association between the observed changes.

Table 3. Role of several factors, including RAAS components, on changes in arterial stiffness markers in patients without antihypertensive treatment.

	Dep. Variable	B Coefficient	95% (CI)	p
	1-month 24 h PP			
Model 1	Age			
	Sex			
	Δ 24 h-SBP	0.481	0.272–0.689	0.001
	Δ body weight			
	Δ cardiac output			
	Baseline 24 h-PP	0.996	0.771–1.220	< 0.001
	Δ ACE			

Table 3. *Cont.*

	Dep. Variable	B Coefficient	95% (CI)	*p*
		1-month PWV		
Model 2	Age			
	Sex			
	Δ 24 h-SBP	0.032	0.008–0.056	0.014
	Δ body weight			
	Δ cardiac output			
	Baseline PWV	0.651	0.416–0.886	< 0.001
	Δ aldosterone	−0.003	−0.005–0.000	0.022
		1-month AI@75		
Model 3	Age			
	Sex			
	Δ 24 h-SBP			
	Δ body weight			
	Δ cardiac output			
	Baseline AI@75	0.326	0.013–0.639	0.043
	Δ ACE/ACE2	0.036	0.005–0.006	0.024

Δ = change; ACE = angiotensin converting enzyme; ACE2 = angiotensin converting enzyme 2; AIx@75 = augmentation index at 75 beats/minute; PP = pulse pressure; PWV = pulse-wave velocity; SBP = systolic blood pressure. Adjusted squared R = 0.863 (Model 1), 0.900 (Model 2) and 0.689 (Model 3).

3.3. Correlations

3.3.1. Correlations of Changes in Arterial Stiffness (AS) with Changes in Anthropometric Parameters, Glucose Metabolism, Adipokines and Inflammatory Markers

At 1-month, there was no statistically significant correlation between changes in PWV, AIx@75 or PP with changes in body weight or waist circumference. When the correlations between the variation of each of these three AS markers with changes in fasting glucose, fasting insulin or the HOMA-IR index were explored, again no correlation was found.

In addition, none of the changes in any of the analyzed adipokines or inflammatory markers showed a statistically significant correlation with changes in PWV, AIx@75 or PP. except between variation of 24 h PP and variation of hs-CRP: Rho = 0.382; $p = 0.041$ [25].

3.3.2. Correlations of Changes in AS with Changes in BP Estimates

Variation of 24 h-PWV (Figure 1A) correlated with Δ 24 h-SBP (Pearson's coefficient = 0.384; $p = 0.036$. No statistically significant correlation was observed between ΔAIx@75 and any BP estimate.

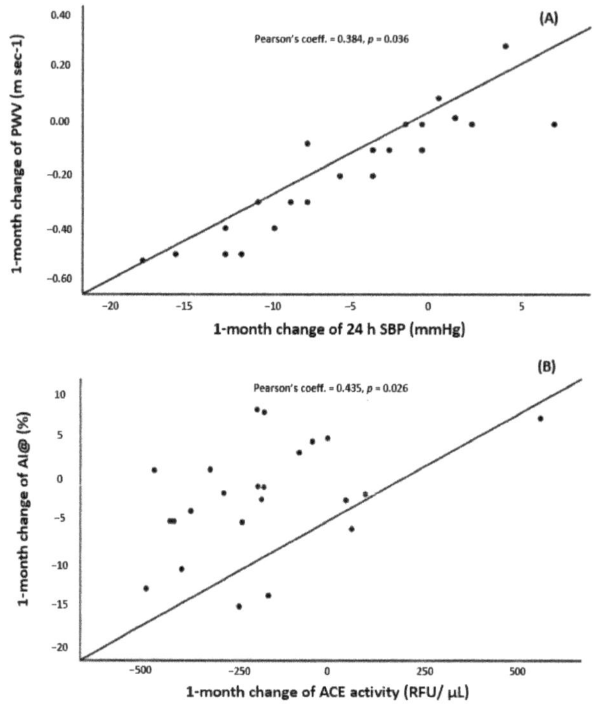

Figure 1. (**A**) Scatter plot for the correlation between change of PWV and change of 24 h SBP one-month after bariatric surgery. (**B**) Scatter plot for the correlation between change of AIx@75 and change of ACE one month after bariatric surgery. ACE = angiotensin converting enzyme; AIx@75 = augmentation index at 75 beats/minute; PWV = pulse-wave velocity; SBP = systolic blood pressure.

3.3.3. Correlations of Changes in AS with Changes in the RAAS Components

Variation of 24 h PWV correlated with Δ ACE/ACE2 ratio (Pearson's coefficient = −0.488; p = 0.013). There was also a direct correlation between Δ AIx@75 and Δ ACE (Pearson's coefficient = 0.435; p = 0.026) (Figure 1B). At 1-month there was no correlation between changes in PRA or aldosterone levels and changes in any AS marker. On the other hand, there was no correlation between changes in aldosterone levels and changes in ACE activity.

Finally, given the fact that some authors [12] reported significant improvement of AS after BS only in those with pathological preoperative PWV, we explored three quantile regression models for changes in AS markers. Therefore, we segmented the sample into two subsets above and below the median of baseline 24 h PWV, AIx@75 and 24 h-PP, respectively (Table 4).

Table 4. Changes in AS markers according to the segmented population into two subsets above and below the median of baseline PWV, baseline AIx@75 and baseline 24 h PP, respectively.

	Below Median Baseline 24 h-PWV (*n* = 21)		**Above Median Baseline 24 h-PWV (*n* = 15)**		**Below Median Baseline 24 h AIx@75 (*n* = 18)**		**Above Median Baseline 24 h-AIx@75 (*n* = 18)**		**Below Median Baseline 24 h-PP (*n* = 18)**		**Above Median Baseline 24 h-PP (*n* = 18)**	
	Mean (95%CI)	***p***	**Mean (95%CI)**	***p***	**Mean (95%CI)**	***p***	**Mean (95%CI)**	***p***	**Mean (95%CI)**	***p***	**Mean (95%CI)**	***p***
						Δ 24 h-PWV						
1 month	−0.18 (−0.25 to −0.10)	**<0.001**	−0.31 (−0.64 to 0.02)	0.060	−0.18 (−0.28 to −0.08)	**0.002**	−0.29 (−0.55 to −0.03)	**0.034**	−0.16 (−0.28 to −0.04)	0.013	−0.31 (−0.56 to −0.05)	**0.020**
						Δ 24 h-AIx@75						
1 month	−3.8 (−6.7 to −0.9)	**0.014**	−1.6 (−4.6 to 1.3)	0.261	−0.0 (−2.8 to 2.7)	0.990	−5.7 (−8.3 to −3.2)	**<0.001**	−1.9 (−4.3 to 0.4)	0.106	−4.3 (−6.7 to −1.9)	**0.001**
						Δ 24 h-PP						
1 month	−3.4 (−5.5 to −1.3)	**0.003**	−2.3 (−5.1 to 0.4)	0.563	−2.0 (−5.0 to 1.0)	0.177	−2.7 (−4.8 to −0.6)	**0.015**	−2.1 (−5.1 to 0.8)	0.149	−3.6 (−6.7 to −0.6)	**0.023**

Δ = change; AIx@75 = augmentation index at 75 beats/minute; PP = pulse pressure; PWV = pulse-wave velocity. Significant results are highlighted in bold format.

Patients with higher baseline 24 h PWV only showed a statistically significant decrease in PWV and AIx@75 1-month post-BS, but not in the PP. In contrast, those with 24 h-PWV below the median showed a decrease in all AS markers at 1-month. Conversely, patients with lower AIx@75 and lower PP only showed an improvement in 24 h PWV at 1-month. Remarkably, for patients with AIx@75 or PP above the median, statistically significant decreases were observed in all AS markers at 1-month.

4. Discussion

Arterial stiffness, assessed by three different methods, i.e., PWV, AIx@75 and PP, improved significantly as early as 1-month after BS in this cohort of patients with severe obesity. These changes were confirmed in the subset of patients strictly normotensives, as confirmed by the 24 h -ABPM, or who did not experience changes in their antihypertensive treatment regimen. In fact, it has been suggested that AS may precede elevations in systolic BP and incident hypertension in obese individuals [26]. Moreover, although there are several reports observing an improvement in AS after losing weight, these changes have demonstrated to be significant only from 3 months after BS, as summarized by Petersen [7] et al. In this systematic review and meta-analysis, where all studies had a follow-up time of more than 1-month, it is shown that although some AS measures improved 3 months after weight loss, these changes were not observed according to AIx or PP, while PWV was not evaluated. Even in a very recent study on this issue [12], no significant decrease in AS was observed 1-month post-BS except in patients with preoperative pathologic PWV. And another group reported very recently significant changes in PWV at 8 months after BS [27]. Along these lines, the second important point is that we have demonstrated that main changes in the different markers of AS occur in patients with lowest PWV, suggesting that perhaps PWV is a stronger marker of organ damage than AIx@75 or PP, and thus less susceptible to modification even after losing weight. On the contrary, for patients with AIx@75 or PP above the median, statistically significant decreases were observed in all AS markers. The set of these findings suggests that PWV is a more powerful marker of AS and less likely to change, whereas elevated AS based on AIx@75 or PP is more likely to improve after BS, and we believe that it adds knowledge to what is reported until now on relationships between obesity, AS and changes after BS. Thus, although PWV is the gold standard for AS measurement [21], perhaps AIx and PP should receive more attention as modifiable therapeutic targets, at least in the obese population. It is known that PWV closely relates to arterial wall stiffness whereas AIx is related to both arterial wall stiffness and wave reflection, which is dependent on peripheral resistance and affected by heart rate variation. This finding is in accordance with that reported by Rossi et al. [28] in primary aldosteronism, where it was suggested that vascular damage may be partially reversible and that both forward and backward pulse wave amplitudes might be more accurate than PWV to detect subtle changes of function in large arteries. It is probable that this difference between the two AS markers would justify the fact that AIx is a more modifiable parameter than PWV, given the changes in heart rate and peripheral resistances are associated with weight loss. We must also highlight the novelty of assessing AS parameters by an oscillometric device providing 24 h measurements. In fact, the vast majority of reports regarding changes in AS after BS use "office" methods, such as applanation tonometry. Here we have shown changes in 24 h ambulatory measurements, which add value to the findings, although confirmation in further studies would be desirable. Thirdly, there were significant changes in anthropometric parameters, glucose metabolism components and adipokines and inflammatory markers. However, none of them showed a statistically significant role in the observed AS improvement. Otherwise, and as expected, BP determined final PWV, while the main independent variable for final AIx@75 was age. Regarding the potential mechanisms responsible for the reduction of AS after weight loss, some authors [13] have found a correlation between weight loss and reduction of PWV independently of changes in established hemodynamic and cardiometabolic risk factors. Other groups [15], but not all [12], suggest that this correlation is mediated by the decrease in BP. Aside from conflicting reports on the role of BP in AS, elevated cardiac volume and output in obese individuals have also been noted as possible mediators of AS, more important than elevated BP [29]. Given the non-significant changes in PWV at 3, 6, and 12 months, also reported by Cooper et al. [14], we must keep in mind that AS is influenced by both functional and structural factors. We hypothesize that hemodynamic changes occur primarily in the first few weeks after BS, from which they are likely to stabilize, while surely the deepest structural changes remain. This could justify the lack of a permanent decrease of the PWV. In relation to carbohydrate metabolism, there are contrasting results regarding changes in glucose metabolism and insulin sensitivity parameters and AS modification: while some studies show a relationship with AIx [14], others suggest that there is no correlation [16].

What is relevant is the finding that changes in several RAAS components were also independent variables for the final values of each AS markers, after adjusting for confounding factors, relationships that were confirmed in correlation analyses. Some studies have previously suggested that the RAAS is an important determinant of AS, in addition to BP and other factors. Multiple mechanisms are responsible for the RAAS activation in obesity, including adipose tissue-derived RAAS components that might be involved in regulation of BP and AS through local production of angiotensin (Ang) II and aldosterone, conversion of adipocyte-derived angiotensinogen by systemic renin and ACE-activity, or forming Ang via alternative routes due to the presence of cathepsins and chymase in human adipose tissue [27,30]. The main changes in this BARIHTA study were observed in ACE and ACE2, but no significant change was found in PRA or plasma aldosterone concentration 1-month post-BS, nor were there any correlations between their changes and improvement on any AS marker. Surprisingly, aldosterone concentration did not change, but its variation was shown to determine PWV changes at 1 month, although, as mentioned, the decrease in aldosterone levels began at 3 months. Perhaps this relationship is statistically significant due to its inclusion in a model with other variables, but from our point of view, what is really important is that the RAAS components have an overall impact on AS, as can be deduced from the three models. There is a predominant role of adipose-tissue-derived RAAS components in the development of AS in obese individuals and its consequent improvement after BS. All components of RAAS, except renin, are known to be found in aortic and mesenteric perivascular adipose tissue, including angiotensinogen, ACE, ACE2, chymase, Ang I, Ang II, AT1, and AT2 receptors [31]. Other authors [32] have also suggested that the generation of some RAAS components through a non-renin-dependent pathway is likely. Taking together, this may explain why changes in AS are related to certain components of RAAS, but not to PRA or aldosterone, at least one month after BS. Moreover, it justifies why there is no correlation between changes at 1-month in ACE activity and changes in aldosterone concentration since, as described, the decrease in the latter occurred from 3 months. Another point to address is the finding that ACE2 activity is elevated at baseline and decreases after BS, considering that its metabolite Ang (1–7) exerts inhibitory effects on inflammation and on vascular and cell growth mechanisms. Recent studies have shown that increased activation of ACE2/Ang-(1–7)/MasR axis can revert and prevent local and systemic dysfunctions improving lipid profile and insulin resistance by modulating insulin actions, and reducing inflammation [32,33]. Therefore, the increased ACE2 would counterbalance the adverse effects of raised Ang II in obesity by increasing levels of the vasodilator Ang-(1–7), as has been shown in other pathological conditions, although it is only speculation. In addition, the increase in the ACE/ACE2 ratio suggests that the decrease in ACE2—probably overexpressed before surgery—is greater than the decrease in ACE, perhaps due to the faster normalization of a compensatory mechanism than that of a pathological one.

Our study has some limitations and several strengths. First, there is some debate about the reliability or not of the Mobile-O-Graph device for measuring AS in the general population and in patients with obesity or with Marfan's syndrome [34]. Recently, a couple of studies have concluded that the oscillometric PWV of Mobil-O-Graph is explained almost entirely by age and SBP compared to carotid-femoral PWV [35] or to the invasive aortic PWV measurement [36], since their relationship is explained by shared associations with age and SBP. However, it has been established that estimated PWV can be used to improve risk prediction in addition to traditional risk classification in conditions under which measuring carotid-femoral PWV is not feasible [8]. Anyway, we have used this same method at different time points for each individual, which is why we truly believe that the modification over time of this parameter has value. On the other hand, due to an otherwise common underrepresentation of male patients in the analyzed cohort, it is not possible to explore the influence of gender on the relationships between RAAS components and AS in this setting. Anyway, we discarded any between-sex differences in 1-month changes in anthropometric and AS measurements and, on the other hand, sex was included in the regression analyses. Otherwise, although we have not explored other possible mechanisms for AS, such as the overproduction of reactive oxygen species or the role of the sympathetic nervous system, we have analyzed the most important mechanisms of its overactivation in obesity, i.e., hyperinsulinemia, hyperleptinemia, RAAS activation and the presence of obstructive sleep-apnea [29]. Finally, it is said that other central obesity indices, such as the waist-to-hip ratio, may be a superior predictor of obesity-related cardiometabolic risk than BMI. However, using the waist circumference we obtained results similar to those obtained with body weight. There are several relevant strengths. Most of the results reported here refer to patients with confirmed normal 24 h BP, except for a small proportion of never-treated hypertensives or patients who did not change antihypertensive treatment throughout the study. This is of high relevance because it emphasizes that in patients with severe obesity there are subtle structural alterations, even below the cutoff values accepted as normality, which improve after BS, indicating a possible higher cardiovascular risk for to this otherwise normotensive population. Moreover, we want to highlight the relative youth of this cohort, which makes the structural changes in the arteries even more relevant. Finally, the inclusion of ACE and ACE2 in this study may contribute to deepen the exploration of pathophysiological mechanisms on the topic we are dealing with, although our study does not allow to establish causal relationships. These data support the need for broader studies questioning the link of AS with RAAS to determine how sustained weight loss reduces cardiovascular morbidity and whether treatment with RAAS inhibitors could have an equivalent benefit.

5. Conclusions

Severely obese patients, including normotensives, have some degree of AS that improves one-month post-BS. Patients with the highest baseline PWV are less likely to improve, but improvement of AS in those with higher baseline AIx@75 maintains over time. AS changes are probably related to modifications in the RAAS, specifically to ACE and ACE2 activities, although this possibility deserves further investigation.

Supplementary Materials: The following are available online at https://www.mdpi.com/2077-0383/10/4/691/s1. Figure S1: Flowchart for participants in the BARIHTA Study, Figure S2A. Variation of plasma renin activity (log-transformed) levels at follow-up. B. Variation of plasma aldosterone (log-transformed) concentration at follow-up, Table S1. Changes in anthropometric, blood pressure and arterial stiffness parameters one-month after bariatric surgery according to the type of surgery.

Author Contributions: Conceptualization, A.O., L.S. and A.G.; validation, S.V., D.B., M.R. and J.P.; formal analysis, M.R.; investigation, I.G., L.S.; resources, I.G., S.V.; data curation, A.G., D.B.; writing—original draft preparation, A.O.; writing—review and editing, A.O., M.R., A.G., D.B. and J.P.; supervision, D.B. and J.P.; project administration, A.O.; funding acquisition, A.O. and J.P. All authors have read and agreed to the published version of the manuscript.

Funding: Research reported in this publication was supported by the Spanish Society of Nephrology and by the Spanish Ministry of Health ISCIII RedinRen RD16/0009/0013. The funders of the study had no role in study design, data collection, data analysis, data interpretation, or writing of the report.

Institutional Review Board Statement: The study was conducted according to the guidelines of the Declaration of Helsinki, and approved by the Ethics Committee of Parc de Salut MAR, Barcelona, Spain (protocol code 2013/5248/I; date of approval 26 September 2013).

Informed Consent Statement: Informed consent was obtained from all subjects involved in the study.

Acknowledgments: We are indebted to Sara Alvarez, Maria Vera, Berta Xargay, Anna Faura and Tai Mooi Ho (Nephrology Dpt. Hospital del Mar and Hospital del Mar Medical Research Institute, Barcelona, Spain), for their effort and implication in the study. We are also indebted to David Benito (Hospital del Mar Medical Research Institute, Barcelona, Spain) for his valuable laboratory support and to Xavier Duran (Hospital del Mar Medical Research Institute) for his aid in performing the statistical analyses.

Conflicts of Interest: The authors declare no conflict of interest.

Appendix A

A.1. Angiotensin-Converting Enzyme (ACE2) Enzymatic Assay

The ACE2 fluorescent enzymatic assay protocol was performed as previously described [17,18], using an ACE2-quenched fluorescent substrate (Mca-Ala-Pro-Lys(Dnp)-OH, BioMol, Hamburg, Germany; Enzo, Life Sciences, Farmingdale, NY, USA). Serum samples (2 μL) were incubated with ACE2 assay buffer [100 mM Tris·HCl, 600 mM NaCl, 10 μM ZnCl2, pH 7.5 in presence of protease inhibitors 100 μM captopril, 5 μM amastatin, 5 μM bestatin, and 10 μM Z-Pro-prolinal (from Sigma-Aldrich, St. Louis, MO, USA and Enzo Life Sciences, Farmingdale, NY, USA)] and 10 μM fluorogenic substrate in a final volume of 100 μL at 37 °C for 16 h. Serum ACE2 cleaves the substrate proportionally to the enzyme activity. Results were obtained after subtracting the background when an ACE2-especific inhibitor was added (0.6 μM DX600). Experiments were carried out in duplicate for each data point. Plates were read using a fluorescence plate reader (Tecan Infinite 200; Germany) at λex320 nm and λem400 nm. Results were expressed as RFU (relative fluorescent units)/μL serum/h.

A.2. ACE Enzymatic Assay

The ACE fluorescent enzymatic assay was performed as previously described [19,20]. For this determination, 2 L of serum were incubated in duplicate with 73 L of reaction buffer (0.5 M borate buffer and 5.45 M N-hippuryl-His-Leu) for 25 min at 37 °C. Finally, 20 mM of o-phthalaldehyde was added to the samples and formed a fluorescent adduct with the enzyme-catalysed product L-histidyl-L-leucine. Fluorescence was measured at λex360 nm and λem485 nm. Results were expressed as RFU/μL serum.

Appendix B

Adipokines and Inflammatory Parameters

Cytokine and chemokine assays with Luminex kits were used. Three Milliplex MAP®kits from Millipore (Merck Millipore, Billerica, MA, USA) were used to test analytes: a 2-plex human adipokine magnetic bead panel 1 for Adiponectin and Resistin (#HADK1MAG-61K), a 3-plex human angiogenesis/growth factor magnetic bead panel 1 for Leptin (#HAGP1MAG-12K), and a 3-plex human cytokine/chemokine magnetic bead panel for MCP-1 (#HCYTOMAG-60K). According to manufacturers' instructions, all methods were performed by the same operator. All kits supplied lyophilized standards that were reconstituted and diluted at 7 serial concentrations (standard curves). Standards included all recombinant analytes tested and were considered as positive controls for the procedure. When indicated by the manufacturer, samples were diluted in assay buffer. Twenty-five μL of sample were used to capture an analyte on analyte-specific color-coded magnetic beads coated with capture antibodies. After the final wash, the beads were resuspended in sheath fluid and the median fluorescent intensity (MFI) data of 50 beads per bead set were analysed on a Luminex 200TM (Luminex Corp., Austin, TX, USA) and Bio-Plex Manager MP software (Bio-Rad, Hercules, CA, USA). Analyte concentrations were calculated by reference to an eight-point five-parameter logistic standard curve for each analyte.

References

1. World Health Organization. Obesity and Overweight. 2018. Available online: https://www.who.int/en/news-room/fact-sheets/detail/obesity-and-overweight (accessed on 10 August 2020).
2. Murphy, N.F.; MacIntyre, K.; Stewart, S.; Hart, C.L.; Hole, D.; McMurray, J.J. Long-term cardiovascular consequences of obesity: 20-year follow-up of more than 15 000 middle-aged men and women (the Renfrew-Paisley study). *Eur. Heart J.* **2006**, *27*, 96–106. [CrossRef]
3. Khan, S.S.; Ning, H.; Wilkins, J.T.; Allen, N.; Carnethon, M.; Berry, J.D.; Sweis, R.N.; Lloyd-Jones, D.M. Association of Body Mass Index with Lifetime Risk of Cardiovascular Disease and Compression of Morbidity. *JAMA Cardiol.* **2018**, *3*, 280–287. [CrossRef] [PubMed]
4. Sjöström, L.; Gummesson, A.; Sjöström, C.D.; Narbro, K.; Peltonen, M.; Wedel, H.; Bengtsson, C.; Bouchard, C.; Carlsson, B.; Dahlgren, S.; et al. Swedish Obese Subjects Study. Effects of bariatric surgery on mortality in Swedish obese subjects. *N. Engl. J. Med.* **2007**, *357*, 741–752. [CrossRef] [PubMed]
5. Adams, T.D.; Gress, R.E.; Smith, S.C.; Halverson, R.C.; Simper, S.C.; Rosamond, W.D.; LaMonte, M.J.; Stroup, A.M.; Hunt, S.C. Long-term mortality after gastric bypass surgery. *N. Engl. J. Med.* **2007**, *357*, 753–761. [CrossRef]
6. Safar, M.E. Arterial stiffness as a risk factor for clinical hypertension. *Nat. Rev. Cardiol.* **2018**, *15*, 97–105. [CrossRef] [PubMed]
7. Cecelja, M.; Chowienczyk, P. Role of arterial stiffness in cardiovascular disease. *JRSM Cardiovasc. Dis.* **2012**, *1*, 1–10. [CrossRef]
8. Petersen, K.S.; Clifton, P.M.; Lister, N.; Keogh, J.B. Effect of weight loss induced by energy restriction on measures of arterial compliance: A systematic review and meta-analysis. *Atherosclerosis* **2016**, *247*, 7–20. [CrossRef]
9. Vlachopoulos, C.; Aznaouridis, K.; Stefanadis, C. Prediction of cardiovascular events and all-cause mortality with arterial stiffness: A systematic review and meta-analysis. *J. Am. Coll. Cardiol.* **2010**, *55*, 1318–1327. [CrossRef] [PubMed]
10. Ben-Shlomo, Y.; Spears, M.; Boustred, C.; May, M.; Anderson, S.G.; Benjamin, E.J.; Boutouyrie, P.; Cameron, J.; Chen, C.H.; Cruickshank, J.K.; et al. Aortic pulse wave velocity improves cardiovascular event prediction: An individual participant meta-analysis of prospective observational data from 17,635 subjects. *J. Am. Coll. Cardiol.* **2014**, *63*, 636–646. [CrossRef]
11. Niiranen, T.J.; Kalesan, B.; Hamburg, N.M.; Benjamin, E.J.; Mitchell, G.F.; Vasan, R.S. Relative Contributions of Arterial Stiffness and Hypertension to Cardiovascular Disease: The Framingham Heart Study. *J. Am. Heart Assoc.* **2016**, *5*, e004271. [CrossRef]
12. Wildman, R.P.; Mackey, R.H.; Bostom, A.; Thompson, T.; Sutton-Tyrrell, K. Measures of obesity are associated with vascular stiffness in young and older adults. *Hypertension* **2003**, *42*, 468–473. [CrossRef]
13. Frey, S.; Jacobi, D.; Pichelin, M.; Cariou, B.; Mirallié, E.; Blanchard, C. Improvement in arterial stiffness (pOpmètre®) after bariatric surgery. Results from a prospective study. *Ann. Endocrinol.* **2020**, *81*, 44–50. [CrossRef]
14. Cooper, J.N.; Buchanich, J.M.; Youk, A.; Brooks, M.M.; Barinas-Mitchell, E.; Conroy, M.B.; Sutton-Tyrrell, K. Reductions in arterial stiffness with weight loss in overweight and obese young adults: Potential mechanisms. *Atherosclerosis* **2012**, *223*, 485–490. [CrossRef] [PubMed]

15. Samaras, K.; Viardot, A.; Lee, P.N.; Jenkins, A.; Botelho, N.K.; Bakopanos, A.; Lord, R.V.; Hayward, C.S. Reduced arterial stiffness after weight loss in obese type 2 diabetes and impaired glucose tolerance: The role of immune cell activation and insulin resistance. *Diab. Vasc. Dis. Res.* **2013**, *10*, 40–48. [CrossRef]
16. Petersen, K.S.; Blanch, N.; Keogh, J.B.; Clifton, P.M. Effect of weight loss on pulse wave velocity: Systematic review and meta-analysis. *Arterioscler. Thromb. Vasc. Biol.* **2015**, *35*, 243–252. [CrossRef] [PubMed]
17. Nordstrand, N.; Gjevestad, E.; Hertel, J.K.; Johnson, L.K.; Saltvedt, E.; Røislien, J.; Hjelmesaeth, J. Arterial stiffness, lifestyle intervention and a low-calorie diet in morbidly obese patients-a nonrandomized clinical trial. *Obesity (Silver Spring)* **2013**, *21*, 690–697. [CrossRef] [PubMed]
18. Oliveras, A.; Goday, A.; Sans, L.; Arias, C.E.; Vazquez, S.; Benaiges, D.; Ramon, J.M.; Pascual, J. Changes in Central 24-h Ambulatory Blood Pressure and Hemodynamics 12 Months After Bariatric Surgery: The Barihta Study. *Obes. Surg.* **2020**, *30*, 195–205. [CrossRef]
19. Papaioannou, T.G.; Argyris, A.; Protogerou, A.D.; Vrachatis, D.; Nasothimiou, E.G.; Sfikakis, P.P.; Stergiou, G.S.; Stefanadis, C.I. Non-invasive 24 h ambulatory monitoring of aortic wave reflection and arterial stiffness by a novel oscillometric device: The first feasibility and reproducibility study. *Int. J. Cardiol.* **2013**, *169*, 57–61. [CrossRef]
20. Hametner, B.; Wassertheurer, S.; Kropf, J.; Mayer, C.; Eber, B.; Weber, T. Oscillometric estimation of aortic pulse wave velocity: Comparison with intra-aortic catheter measurements. *Blood Press. Monit.* **2013**, *18*, 173–176. [CrossRef]
21. Laurent, S.; Cockcroft, J.; Van Bortel, L.; Boutouyrie, P.; Giannattasio, C.; Hayoz, D.; Pannier, B.; Vlachopoulos, C.; Wilkinson, I.; Struijker-Boudier, H. European Network for Non-invasive Investigation of Large Arteries. Expert consensus document on arterial stiffness: Methodological issues and clinical applications. *Eur. Heart J.* **2006**, *27*, 2588–2605. [CrossRef]
22. Laurent, S.; Marais, L.; Boutouyrie, P. The Noninvasive Assessment of Vascular Aging. *Can. J. Cardiol.* **2016**, *32*, 669–679. [CrossRef]
23. Soler, M.J.; Riera, M.; Crespo, M.; Mir, M.; Márquez, E.; Pascual, M.J.; Pascual, J. Circulating angiotensin-converting enzyme 2 activity in kidney transplantation: A longitudinal pilot study. *Nephron Clin. Pract.* **2012**, *121*, c144–c150. [CrossRef]
24. Tucker, O.N.; Szomstein, S.; Rosenthal, R.J. Indications for sleeve gastrectomy as a primary procedure for weight loss in the morbidly obese. *J. Gastrointest. Surg.* **2008**, *12*, 662–667. [CrossRef]
25. Oliveras, A. Barcelona, Spain. Unpublished work. 2021.
26. Weisbrod, R.M.; Shiang, T.; Al Sayah, L.; Fry, J.L.; Bajpai, S.; Reinhart-King, C.A.; Lob, H.E. Arterial stiffening precedes systolic hypertension in diet-induced obesity. *Hypertension* **2013**, *62*, 1105–1110. [CrossRef] [PubMed]
27. Giudici, A.; Palombo, C.; Kozakova, M.; Morizzo, C.; Losso, L.; Nannipieri, M.; Berta, R.; Hughes, A.D. Weight Loss after Bariatric Surgery Significantly Improves Carotid and Cardiac Function in Apparently Healthy People with Morbid Obesity. *Obes. Surg.* **2020**, *30*, 3776–3783. [CrossRef]
28. Rossi, G.P.; Maiolino, G. Excess Arterial Damage in Hyperaldosteronism. *Hypertension* **2019**, *74*, 502–504. [CrossRef] [PubMed]
29. Ikonomidis, I.; Mazarakis, A.; Papadopoulos, C.; Patsouras, N.; Kalfarentzos, F.; Lekakis, J.; Kremastinos, D.T.; Alexopoulos, D. Weight loss after bariatric surgery improves aortic elastic properties and left ventricular function in individuals with morbid obesity: A 3-year follow-up study. *J. Hypertens.* **2007**, *25*, 439–447. [CrossRef]
30. Schütten, M.T.; Houben, A.J.; de Leeuw, P.W.; Stehouwer, C.D. The Link Between Adipose Tissue Renin-Angiotensin-Aldosterone System Signaling and Obesity-Associated Hypertension. *Physiology (Bethesda)* **2017**, *32*, 197–209. [CrossRef] [PubMed]
31. Xia, N.; Li, H. The role of perivascular adipose tissue in obesity-induced vascular dysfunction. *Br. J. Pharmacol.* **2017**, *174*, 3425–3442. [CrossRef]
32. Chappell, M.C.; Marshall, A.C.; Alzayadneh, E.M.; Shaltout, H.A.; Diz, D.I. Update on the Angiotensin converting enzyme 2-Angiotensin (1-7)-MAS receptor axis: Fetal programing, sex differences, and intracellular pathways. *Front. Endocrinol.* **2014**, *4*, 201. [CrossRef]
33. Lelis, D.F.; Freitas, D.F.; Machado, A.S.; Crespo, T.S.; Santos, S.H.S. Angiotensin-(1-7), Adipokines and Inflammation. *Metabolism* **2019**, *95*, 36–45. [CrossRef] [PubMed]
34. Salvi, P.; Furlanis, G.; Grillo, A.; Pini, A.; Salvi, L.; Marelli, S.; Rovina, M.; Moretti, F.; Gaetano, R.; Pintassilgo, I.; et al. Unreliable Estimation of Aortic Pulse Wave Velocity Provided by the Mobil-O-Graph Algorithm-Based System in Marfan Syndrome. *J. Am. Heart Assoc.* **2019**, *8*, e04028. [CrossRef] [PubMed]
35. Schwartz, J.E.; Feig, P.U.; Izzo, J.L., Jr. Pulse Wave Velocities Derived From Cuff Ambulatory Pulse Wave Analysis. *Hypertension* **2019**, *74*, 111–116. [CrossRef] [PubMed]
36. Salvi, P.; Scalise, F.; Rovina, M.; Moretti, F.; Salvi, L.; Grillo, A.; Gao, L.; Baldi, C.; Faini, A.; Furlanis, G.; et al. Noninvasive Estimation of Aortic Stiffness Through Different Approaches. *Hypertension* **2019**, *74*, 117–129. [CrossRef] [PubMed]

Journal of
Clinical Medicine

MDPI

Review

Factors Affecting Metabolic Outcomes Post Bariatric Surgery: Role of Adipose Tissue

Sara H. Keshavjee [1], Katherine J. P. Schwenger [2], Jitender Yadav [3], Timothy D. Jackson [4], Allan Okrainec [4] and Johane P. Allard [2,*]

1 Vagelos College of Physicians & Surgeons, Columbia University, New York, NY 10032, USA; shk2176@cumc.columbia.edu
2 Division of Gastroenterology, Toronto General Hospital, University Health Network, Toronto, ON M5G 2N2, Canada; kschweng@uhnresearch.ca
3 Department of Immunology, University of Toronto, Toronto, ON M5S 1A8, Canada; jitu.yadav@mail.utoronto.ca
4 Division of General Surgery, University Health Network, University of Toronto, Toronto, ON M5T 2S8, Canada; timothy.jackson@uhn.ca (T.D.J.); allan.okrainec@uhn.ca (A.O.)
* Correspondence: dr.johane.allard@uhn.ca

Abstract: Obesity is an ever-growing public health crisis, and bariatric surgery (BS) has become a valuable tool in ameliorating obesity, along with comorbid conditions such as diabetes, dyslipidemia and hypertension. BS techniques have come a long way, leading to impressive improvements in the health of the majority of patients. Unfortunately, not every patient responds optimally to BS and there is no method that is sufficient to pre-operatively predict who will receive maximum benefit from this surgical intervention. This review focuses on the adipose tissue characteristics and related parameters that may affect outcomes, as well as the potential influences of insulin resistance, BMI, age, psychologic and genetic factors. Understanding the role of these factors may help predict who will benefit the most from BS.

Keywords: bariatric surgery; adipose tissue; metabolic outcomes

Citation: Keshavjee, S.H.; Schwenger, K.J.P.; Yadav, J.; Jackson, T.D.; Okrainec, A.; Allard, J.P. Factors Affecting Metabolic Outcomes Post Bariatric Surgery: Role of Adipose Tissue. *J. Clin. Med.* **2021**, *10*, 714. https://doi.org/10.3390/jcm10040714

Academic Editor: David Benaiges Boix

Received: 15 January 2021
Accepted: 9 February 2021
Published: 11 February 2021

1. Introduction

Obesity is an ever-growing problem and the World Health Organization estimated 650 million people to be obese in 2016 [1]. The main cause of obesity is the overconsumption of calories versus expenditure; however, other factors such as endocrine dysfunction, genetic makeup, and sleep debt can also contribute to obesity [2]. Along with obesity comes the burden of comorbidities, such as cardiovascular disease [3], diabetes [3], non-alcoholic fatty liver disease (NAFLD) [4], and hypertension (HTN) [5]. Specifically, obesity doubles the risk of HTN and triples the risk of type 2 diabetes mellitus (T2DM) in the 45–54 year old age category [6]. There is also a high prevalence of metabolic syndrome that accompanies obesity. Although criteria are controversial, someone is considered to have metabolic syndrome if they have three or more of the following: abdominal obesity, dyslipidemia, insulin resistance or hyperglycemia and HTN [7]. When compared to those of normal weight, individuals who are overweight have a 5.5-fold higher risk and individuals with obesity have a 32-fold higher risk of developing metabolic syndrome [8]. Despite this risk, not all individuals with obesity develop metabolic syndrome, and there is a stark contrast between those with "metabolically healthy" obesity verses "metabolically unhealthy" obesity. These relatively new categories of obesity came to light when noticing a subgroup of people with obesity, often early-onset, who have normal insulin sensitivity, and no signs of metabolic syndrome; "metabolically healthy" obesity [9]. Recently, the "metabolically healthy" obesity group has also been shown to have a decreased inflammatory state compared to similar-weight controls [10], and decreased liver fat content [11]. "Metabolically unhealthy" obesity is associated with a higher incidence of HTN, insulin resistance, and dyslipidemia, while "metabolically healthy" individuals with obesity have a lower risk of these comorbidities, along with a lesser degree of adipose tissue dysfunction [12].

One particularly effective treatment for obesity and its comorbidities is bariatric surgery (BS), which may be accomplished by various techniques such as Roux-en-Y gastric bypass (RYGB), sleeve gastrectomy (SG), and biliopancreatic diversion with duodenal switch (BPD) [13]. BS has been shown to be effective for achieving significant weight loss, with an average of 28.6% total body weight loss following RYGB and 25% following laparoscopic SG at five years post-surgery [14].

In addition to the direct benefits of weight loss, BS has been shown to decrease the magnitude of comorbidities such as HTN [15,16] and dyslipidemia, and even cause remission of T2DM [14,17,18]. The improvement on the three aforementioned comorbidities after RYGB surgery has been shown to be superior to medical and lifestyle management in a randomized controlled trial (RCT) of 120 patients [16]. Another RCT of 150 patients showed that an endpoint of HbA1c <6% without the use of diabetes medication was met by 29% of participants that received RYGB and by 23% who received SG, compared to only 5% for conventional medical therapy [19].

Despite huge successes in weight loss and comorbidity reduction from BS, not every patient achieves the significant weight loss and/or metabolic improvements. Approximately 10–20% of BS patients have insufficient weight loss one year after surgery, with excess body weight loss <40% or total weight loss <20% [20]. Additionally, even when patients initially achieve weight loss and improvements in T2DM, these problems can recur [21]. The challenge remains in predicting which patients will benefit most from BS. In this review, we will be summarizing the known predictors of BS outcomes, with a focus on the influence that adipose tissue characteristics may have.

2. Predictors of Bariatric Surgery Outcome

The success of bariatric surgery is generally evaluated based on percent total or percent excess body weight loss (EBWL) and reduction of comorbidities such as HTN, dyslipidemia, insulin resistance or T2DM. When attempting to predict the probability of BS success, studies often assess the severity of obesity (BMI, waist-to-hip ratio), age, and comorbidities at baseline. There are many other factors that are more recently being considered, such as social and psychological factors, as well as characteristics of the adipose tissue itself. This review focuses on adipose tissue characteristics and related parameters that may affect outcomes as well as the potential influence of insulin resistance, BMI, age, psychologic and genetic factors.

2.1. Adipose Tissue: Structure, Hypertrophy, Fibrosis

In obesity, as adipose tissue accommodates to caloric excess, it expands via hypertrophy or hyperplasia, to increase fatty acid storage [22]. This occurs in two maintain compartments: under the skin as the subcutaneous adipose tissue (SAT) or around abdominal organs as visceral adipose tissue (VAT). VAT includes the compartments of omental, retroperitoneal and mesenteric depots, each with varying metabolic properties [23]. Expansion of the visceral compartment is often associated with metabolically unhealthy obesity and development of comorbidities, whereas predominant SAT expansion is associated with metabolically healthy obesity [12]. Metabolic derangements and T2DM may be linked to VAT due to the fact that it is more metabolically active, and liver dysfunction can result from fatty acids, inflammatory cytokines and metabolites draining into portal circulation [24]. The visceral and subcutaneous fat is inherently different; subcutaneous fat confers fewer metabolic complications and may even be less harmful than VAT [25–27]. Adding to the complexity, even within one fat depot there are multiple subpopulations of adipocytes that have differing metabolic and physiological properties [28].

Clearly, expansion of adipose tissue is not benign in a patient with obesity. The depot of fat, along with method of expansion, has important effects on the development of comorbidities, including metabolic syndrome. Particularly, expansion of adipose tissue through hypertrophy can be indicative of dysfunctional adipocytes, inflammation, and risk for visceral adipose deposition [29]. Some studies have shown that the degree of adipocyte hypertrophy may predict increased risk of T2DM and a lower probability of T2DM remission after BS [30]. Hypertrophy, as opposed to hyperplasia, is also associated with worse metabolic derangements, such as dyslipidemia [31]. Thus, looking at adipocyte hypertrophy may provide important insight into the outcome of BS, especially in individuals with T2DM.

Additionally, during obesity, important changes occur in the extracellular matrix (ECM) of adipose tissue. As adipose tissue expands, the ECM is degraded; however, long-term inflammation, including macrophage infiltration [32], leads to a switch toward fibrosis, restricting adipose expansion [33]. This limitation in adipose expansion is thought to play a role in increasing visceral adipose deposition. Specifically, individuals with obesity show increased fibrosis [34] and expression of ECM component genes (such as various integrins, collagens, glycosaminoglycans and proteoglycans) in SAT compared to lean controls, along with a similar trend in liver fibrosis [35]. This may be mediated by a shift in adipocyte precursor population to a CD9+ phenotype, which has a pro-fibrotic effect [36]. There is, however, some evidence to show that fibrosis is not purely maladaptive, as VAT fibrosis may be protective against adipocyte hypertrophy and the consequent metabolic derangements, such as T2DM [37]. A study of 82 individuals undergoing BS found that SAT and VAT ECM deposition was decreased in both VAT and SAT of patients with T2DM, when observed by sirius red staining [37]. Consistent with the possible protective role of fibrosis, this study found that VAT fibrotic gene expression was decreased among diabetic patients, with a correlation to HbA1c levels [37]. Fibrosis may also be harmful, as another study of 65 patients found that those with increased SAT fibrosis had poorer fat mass loss percentage after RYGB surgery [31]. It is possible that despite fibrotic VAT's protective effect on T2DM, there remains a detriment to weight loss following BS due to dysfunctional ECM remodeling. Overall, the fibrotic response may be indicative of the degree of inflammation and metabolic dysregulation, helping to predict outcomes after BS.

Changes in the adipose tissue architecture and lipid composition do occur after BS. One month following RYGB, patients' VAT was found to have decreased fat fraction and increased T1 relaxation time on MRI in comparison to before surgery [38]. The T1 time is negatively correlated with fat content [39], showing that this may be a more nuanced measurement to take into account aside from adipose tissue mass, especially in regards to visceral adiposity. As soon as four weeks after BS, SAT adipocyte size has been shown to decrease significantly, along with a decrease in E2F1 expression, a marker of proliferation [40]. Interestingly, another study has shown that the number of adipocyte precursor cells is increased following BS and weight loss as compared to pre-BS, where numbers of precursors are often low in patients with obesity [41]. At two years post-RYGB, women's fat cell volume was more closely associated with improved insulin sensitivity than reduction in fat mass [42]. This shows that the remodeling of the adipose tissue through fat content and adipocyte size may be a useful indicator of underlying metabolic changes, possibly returning the tissue to a metabolically healthy state. Associated changes may also occur in the ECM, as there is decreased expression of ECM component genes and increased expression of ECM degradation pathways (such as via metallopeptidases) in patients three months post-BS when compared to pre-operative levels [35]. Although gene expression shows anti-fibrotic changes after weight loss, there is debate as to whether existing fibrosis is reversible or not [35].

2.2. Adipose Tissue: Inflammatory Response

Numerous metabolic and inflammatory changes occur within expanding adipose tissue in a patient with obesity, which may contribute to development of comorbidities, including metabolic syndrome. As a result of the stress-induced changes, obesity has come to be considered a form of chronic inflammatory disease, driven by the close interactions of adipocytes and adipose tissue macrophages (ATM) [43]. These changes in adipose tissue are significant, and it is of interest to find out whether the varying inflammatory phenotypes of adipose tissue correlate to the varying outcomes of BS procedures.

Expansion of adipose tissue can lead to tissue hypoperfusion and hypoxia [44]. This makes hypoxic markers a promising area of research for predicting adipose tissue dysfunction. This hypoxia and adipose tissue stress causes a change in released adipokines, becoming more pro-inflammatory via IL-1β, IL-6, TNF, IL-8, leptin, resistin and MCP-1 [45]. This causes the recruitment of monocytes and as obesity progresses, ATM have been shown to progress from predominantly M2 to M1 type, assuming a more pro-inflammatory phenotype [46]. Aside from M1 and M2, some macrophages may take on an entirely different phenotype in obesity, the metabolically activated macrophage, which contributes to both inflammation and clearance of dead adipocytes [47].

The overall increase of inflammatory cytokines, as mentioned above, contributes to insulin resistance through a variety of mechanisms [48]. Specifically, expression of IL-6 from adipose tissue is elevated in obesity, with a threefold higher expression in omental fat as opposed to subcutaneous fat [49]. IL-6 can induce expression of C reactive protein (CRP), which are together used as clinical markers of inflammation and risk of T2DM development, independent of obesity [50,51]. TNF-α, produced by macrophages, has also been targeted as a link between obesity and insulin resistance, as a TNF-α antagonist Etanercept causes improvements in fasting blood glucose levels in obese individuals with metabolic syndrome [52]. TNF-α has also been shown to be an antagonist of GLUT4, a key mechanism of glucose uptake in response to insulin [53]. Additionally, MCP-1 expression has been shown to be elevated in SAT in obese individuals [54], along with elevations in those with T2DM without obesity [55]. MCP-1 likely has a direct role in insulin resistance, as mouse models with MCP-1 deletions are protected from high-fat diet induced insulin resistance and have less macrophage infiltration in adipose tissue [56]. However, MCP-1 may have broad-reaching affects, as MCP-1 knockout mice also had protection from hepatic steatosis during high-fat diet induced obesity [56]. Taken together, markers of inflammation along with insulin resistance measurements may help to predict chance of T2DM remission and outcomes after BS.

Many changes have been seen to occur in the inflammatory response following BS. At the tissue level, there is a decrease in subcutaneous ATMs after BS and weight loss, with an increase in IL-10 cytokine expression, signaling a shift to an anti-inflammatory M2 phenotype [57]. Multiple studies have shown a decrease in M1 and increase in M2 macrophages [58] appearing within three months post-BS [59]. However, the omental adipose tissue macrophages are likely the most important to assess, as they may be largely responsible for metabolic derangements. Cancello et al. found twice the number of ATMs in omental versus subcutaneous fat, with only omental macrophage counts correlating to insulin resistance and hepatic fibroinflammatory lesions [60]. Another contributing factor to the inflammatory profile improvement after BS is that hypoxic dysfunction of adipose tissue was shown to be reduced, including a reduction in hypoxic marker HIF-1α, macrophage chemo-attractants (MCP-1, CSF-3, PLAUR), and macrophage numbers [57]. On a systemic level, a meta-analysis of 116 studies showed that circulating levels of inflammatory markers like IL-6, TNF-α, and CRP significantly decreased following BS, which is in line with other studies on traditional weight loss [57]. Therefore, the reduction in inflammation following BS may be a product of the weight loss rather than the surgery itself [61,62].

The change in adipose tissue mass and degree of inflammation post-BS may be predicted by pre-surgical systemic and adipose-specific markers. When looking at predicting BS outcome, higher pre-operative systemic CRP levels have been shown to be associated with increased weight loss post-BS [63]. Another study found that high hs-CRP in women is able to predict the degree of reduction in visceral fat area one year post-surgery [64]. In general, a study of 37 patients undergoing BS found that an increase in adipose tissue inflammatory response (as measured by CD11b and IL-10 mRNA expression in adipose tissue) was associated with lower BMI loss after BS [65]. When looking broadly at the level of the serum proteome, Wewer Albrechtsen et al. found that 88 proteins changed significantly from baseline when measured again one week after surgery [66]. Many of the implicated proteins are important in inflammatory processes (complement, acute phase proteins, CRP) or lipid homeostasis [66]. Some proteins showed changes up to two years later, which may illustrate the difference between rapid surgery-induced effects and long-term weight loss-induced effects. Although the changes of inflammatory markers in response to BS have been researched, the role for many of these markers in predicting BS outcomes remains to be studied. Certain markers, such as circulating hs-CRP and tissue IL-10, may be implicated in predicting BS response, but there remains large potential for research regarding the use of inflammatory markers.

2.3. Adipose Tissue: Adipokine Dysregulation

As adipose tissue expands in obesity, the cells experience hypertrophy, along with oxidative and inflammatory stressors. This leads many individuals with obesity to experience altered adipokine secretion from adipose tissue, which can have far-reaching effects on the body and metabolism. In Table 1, we will briefly review the function of the main adipokines and their relationship to metabolic syndrome, followed by the effect of BS.

Table 1. Adipokines implicated in obesity and changes noted post-bariatric surgery (BS).

Adipokine	Role in Obesity Pathogenesis	Changes after BS
Leptin	• ↑ with degree of adiposity [67], signals hypothalamus to ↑ energy expenditure, ↓ hunger [68]. • Pro-inflammatory effect on macrophages (increased TNF-α and IL-6), induces a Th1 cell inflammatory phenotype, releasing IL-2 and IFN-γ [50]. • Leptin resistance may occur in obesity, for a variety of reasons [69–71]. • Patients with increased circulating leptin pre-BS have increased weight loss post-BS [64]. However, other smaller studies have not found the same association [72].	↓ systemic leptin concentrations following various types of BS and weight loss [58,73].
Adiponectin	• Functions in anti-apoptotic signaling, ↓inflammation, ↓insulin sensitivity [74]. ↓macrophage activation, ↑IL-10 production [50]. • Levels are inversely correlated with adiposity [75] and degree of dysfunction in adipocytes [76]. • Serum adiponectin <4.0 μg/mL greatly increases the likelihood of metabolic syndrome [77], can also be correlated with probability of developing T2DM [78]. • Study of BS recipients (n = 1570) found that pre-BS adiponectin levels were not useful in predicting BS outcomes [79].	↑ circulating adiponectin within three months post-BS [80]. ↑ adiponectin adipose tissue expression with levels similar to normal weight controls within two years post-BS [81].
Resistin	• ↑IR, ↑hepatic glucose production, ↑inflammation (via monocyte secretion of IL6, TNF) [50]. • Role in IR due to its stimulation of SOC3 expression, which inhibits insulin signaling in the adipocyte [82] • Some studies show levels to be predictive of T2DM progression [83,84], where others have shown it to be associated with increased BMI rather than insulin resistance [85,86]. • Inflammatory role-correlates with circulating CRP, IL-6 and TNF-α levels in patients with inflammatory diseases or T2DM [87]. • Dyslipidemia—positive correlation with VLDL, and negative with HDL [87].	↓ in SAT expression 12 months post-BS [81]. However, results are conflicting [73].

Table 1. *Cont.*

Adipokine	Role in Obesity Pathogenesis	Changes after BS
Retinol Binding Protein 4 (RBP4)	• Main protein to which retinol (vitamin A) binds to in serum, produced by liver and adipose tissue. • ↑IR, which may be due to RBPP4's negative correlation with GLUT4, which is necessary to import glucose into cells to be metabolized [88] • ↑ Serum levels in obesity, associated with metabolic syndrome and T2DM [89]. • Adipose tissue expression levels associated with ↑ BMI, waist circumference, circulating RBP4 and HOMA IR [90]. • Dysregulated levels (high or low) are predictive of T2DM risk, independent of BMI [91].	↓ RBP4 in 12 months following BS, with a correlation to decreases in fasting glucose, serum triglycerides, and weight [92].

Along with the aforementioned adipokines in Table 1, many others have been studied and shown to have dysfunctional expression in obesity. These include visfatin [93], chemerin, lipocalin-2 [94], CXCL5, IL-18, and NAMPT [50], among others. Another area of interest regarding adipose tissue is that white adipose tissue, typically seen in obesity, [95] can change its phenotype into brown-like adipose tissue, called beige/brite adipose tissue, which is associated with improvements in IR, reduction in blood glucose and increased resting energy expenditure [96–98]. The increase in thermogenic capacity is mediated by UCP1 (uncoupling protein 1) [99,100], which is highly induced in brown-like adipocytes and expressed in the inner membrane of the mitochondria [95]. The transcription of UCP1 requires critical co-activators, specifically PCG1-α and PPARγ which commit the cells to thermogenesis [101,102]. This is of interest as recent research showed a decrease in functional brown adipose tissue in obesity [103].

In summary, analysis of adipokine levels pre-operatively may give insight into the degree of metabolic derangement and inflammation that is present in patients undergoing BS, while post-operative measures may track improvement in metabolic parameters. Although some adipokines have been shown to aid in BS outcome prediction as mentioned above, the role of others remains unclear.

2.4. Insulin Resistance and Type 2 Diabetes Mellitus

T2DM is a common phenomenon in individuals with obesity, as there is an association between obesity and insulin resistance in skeletal muscle, liver, and adipose tissue [104], along with pancreatic beta cell dysfunction [105]. T2DM remission often occurs after BS, especially from surgeries with a malabsorptive component; the highest remission rates occur after BPD (95%) and second-highest from RYGB (75%) [106]. However, remission after surgery is less likely in patients with poor glycemic control and increasing time since diabetes diagnosis, likely due to more extensive pancreatic beta cell damage and dysfunction [19,107].

A common clinical test for insulin resistance is the homeostatic model assessment for insulin resistance (HOMA-IR). HOMA-IR is generally increased in individuals with increased weight or obesity, and it is associated with T2DM and cardiometabolic complications [108]. In those with obesity, high HOMA-IR is also associated with steatosis and liver fibrosis [109]. Additionally, the probability of T2DM remission in the long and short term after RYGB surgery can be estimated with a DiaREM score, taking into account age, HbA1c and diabetes medication use [110,111]. Through predicting insulin resistance severity, these scores may help predict BS-related improvements in glycemic control.

Within one week after RYGB, before significant weight loss, patients experience improvements in glucose homeostasis [112]. This may be attributed to hepatic insulin sensitivity increase, as seen in one study measuring this via basal glucose and basal hepatic insulin sensitivity index [112]. Quick changes in insulin sensitivity following surgery may be due to calorie restriction after surgery, leading to reduced hepatic fat and subsequent insulin sensitivity increases [112,113]. Within one week, there are also increases in postprandial GLP-1 secretion, which enhances pancreatic beta cell function by stimulating insulin release [114]. One study using diet-induced obese rats found that the response to GLP-1 agonists has been shown to predict the efficacy of RYGB on glucose tolerance [115]. A recent study in T2DM individuals undergoing RYGB surgery found that those who experienced T2DM remission one year post-RYGB had significantly higher pre-RYGB GLP-1 concentrations [116]. However, research is limited and the degree in which GLP-1 predicts metabolic success post-RYGB is still contested [117]. In addition to GLP-1, HOMA_IR score has also been shown to decrease as soon as two weeks after surgery [118]. In the longer term, peripheral insulin resistance has been shown to improve by three months post-BS [119]. This may be mediated in part by continually decreasing intramyocellular fat [120], causing increased insulin sensitivity of skeletal muscle [121]. In another study, MRI analysis showed hepatic fat was reduced below the pathological range by six months and pancreatic fat 12 months post-BS, further explaining the long-term improvement in insulin resistance [122]. The beneficial effects of BS on the liver extend past insulin resistance, as a meta-analysis of 15 studies found that non-alcoholic steatohepatitis was resolved in 69.5% of cases and steatosis was improved in approximately 91.6% of cases [123]. There is evidence that surgeries with a malabsorptive component, such as RYGB, have better outcomes in terms of diabetes remission and improved HOMA-IR score than simply restrictive surgery in both short and long term [19,124–127]. In summary, there appears to be a role for using diabetes status and time since diagnosis to predict remission following BS, but its role in predicting weight loss and other metabolic parameters following BS remains to be studied.

2.5. BMI, Pre-Operative Weight Loss

Pre-operative BMI does seem to be an important predictor of BS results. Using a database of over seventy-thousand BS recipients, pre-operative weight has been shown to account for a large portion, approximately 18.5%, of the variation seen in weight loss post-BS [128]. Additionally, a meta-analysis has shown that many studies observed a lower EBWL percentage in those with a higher pre-operative BMI [129]. These results may be due to the fact that those with higher BMI are more likely to have the burden of comorbidities [130], including metabolic syndrome [8]. Along with BMI, surgery type is a major predictor of weight loss outcomes, explaining approximately 44.8% of the variability in a study of patients receiving RYGB, adjustable gastric band, or SG [128]. Evidently, BMI may be a major predictor in explaining BS outcome, and together with surgery type, these factors may explain a large portion of outcome variability.

The use of preoperative weight loss as a mandatory criterion before BS is a widely debated topic, with evidence for and against its utility. A study of the Swedish national registry for BS (n = 9570) found that there was a strong positive association between pre- and post-operative weight loss, especially in those in the highest BMI quartile [131]. Other studies saw similar data, such as a study of 884 patients undergoing RYGB that found those who achieved 10% EBWL preoperatively, were more likely to attain the goal of 70% EBWL post-BS [132]. A recent study of 355 RYGB or SG recipients asked patients to maintain a low calorie diet with the goal of 8% EBWL for four weeks before BS [133]. Those who achieved ≥8% EBWL had significantly greater EBWL at three, six and twelve months post-BS than those who did not achieve 8% EBWL pre-operatively [133]. Although many studies show a positive association between pre- and post-operative weight loss, it is difficult to tease out the impact of the pre-operative weight loss itself versus individual reactions to caloric restriction, along with the surgical candidate selection factors associated with mandatory preoperative EBWL.

2.6. Age

Along with the aforementioned factors, the age of the patient has been shown to have an effect on BS outcomes. In addition to having a negative impact on weight loss, higher age carries a higher risk of intraoperative and post-operative complications, which must be factored into the risk-benefit analysis of recommending BS. Some studies have reported significantly more complications in the older age group compared to those below 60 [134]. However, a recent study on more than three thousand patients undergoing RYGB or laparoscopic SG found no increase in intra-operative or post-operative complications for the 60+ age group [135]. Other studies have also found that EBWL is negatively affected by increasing age, including a study of more than thirteen-hundred patients aged 18–65 undergoing RYGB or SG [136].

2.7. Psychological Factors

Although many predictors of surgery outcome are not modifiable, some of the psychiatric conditions that correlate with poor outcome can be controlled and ameliorated before surgery. Patients with psychiatric disorders before SG surgery, such as personality disorders, adjustment disorders or depression, have been shown to have worse outcomes than those without mental illness [137]. Importantly, worse outcomes have been shown even in individuals with past mood disorders and no current episode, highlighting the possible role of additional treatment and social support before and after surgery in any patient with current or past mental health concerns [138].

2.8. Genetic Factors

Recently, studies have begun to look at how an individual's genotype may be able to predict their response to BS. Many genome wide association studies have shown that there are hundreds of heritable genes that correlate with phenotypes such as waist-to-hip ratio and BMI [139]. Some alleles are even associated with a more metabolically healthy obese picture, with decreased comorbidities such as HTN, T2DM and heart disease [140]. When trying to analyze whether single nucleotide polymorphisms (SNPs) are associated with weight loss after RYGB, a genome wide association study by Rinella et al. found that genetic variants clustering around the genes of PKHD1, HTR1A, GUCY1A2, NMBR, KCNK2 and IGF1R may be implicated [141]. These genes have previously been related to biological processes such as appetite, lipid and glucose homeostasis and early onset obesity [141]. Similar results were seen in a study by Aasbrenn et al. [142]. Paradoxically, Aasbrenn et al. also noticed that individuals genetically predisposed to "slimness" experienced significantly poorer weight loss after surgery, possibly signaling social rather than biological causes of obesity in these patients [142]. In the future, genetic testing for SNPs may be used to predict a portion of one's variable outcome after BS.

3. Conclusions

BS and the associated weight loss improve many metabolic and inflammatory parameters associated with changes in adipose tissue, adipokine expression, inflammatory profile and glucose/lipid homeostasis. The adipose tissue phenotype itself is very closely linked to the comorbidities that develop in individuals with obesity and their response to BS. Among pre-BS factors that may predict outcomes post-BS, those that have been found to be significant from the adipose tissue are VAT/SAT fibrosis, circulating CRP, Cd11b and IL10 adipose tissue mRNA levels, and possibly circulating leptin. In addition, other significant factors include diabetes status and time since diagnosis, pre-operative weight loss, age and psychological disorders. There may be other factors that can predict post-BS response, including a variety of adipokines and inflammatory markers (both circulating and expressed in adipose tissue), but further studies will be required in order to determine their significance. In the future, clinicians can use pre-operative data to better predict patient outcomes post-BS, as well as determine the optimal treatment plan for their patients.

Author Contributions: Writing—original draft preparation, S.H.K.; writing—review and editing, K.J.P.S., J.Y., T.D.J., A.O. and J.P.A.; supervision, K.J.P.S., J.Y., T.D.J., A.O. and J.P.A.; project administration, K.J.P.S. All authors have read and agreed to the published version of the manuscript.

Funding: This research received no external funding.

Institutional Review Board Statement: Not applicable.

Informed Consent Statement: Not applicable.

Conflicts of Interest: S.H.K., K.J.P.S., J.Y., T.D.J. and J.P.A. have no conflict of interest to declare. Author 5 (A.O.) has relevant financial activities outside of the submitted work. He is provided an honorarium for speaking and teaching from Ethicon, Medtronic and Merk. The funders had no role in the design of the study; in the collection, analyses, or interpretation of data; in the writing of the manuscript, or in the decision to publish the results.

References

1. WHO. Obesity and Overweight. 2020. Available online: https://www.who.int/news-room/fact-sheets/detail/obesity-and-overweight (accessed on 1 September 2020).
2. Keith, S.W.; Redden, D.T.; Katzmarzyk, P.T.; Boggiano, M.M.; Hanlon, E.C.; Benca, R.M.; Ruden, D.; Pietrobelli, A.; Barger, J.L.; Fontaine, K.R.; et al. Putative contributors to the secular increase in obesity: Exploring the roads less traveled. *Int. J. Obes.* **2006**, *30*, 1585–1594. [CrossRef]
3. Singh, G.M.; Danaei, G.; Farzadfar, F.; Stevens, G.A.; Woodward, M.; Wormser, D.; Kaptoge, S.; Whitlock, G.; Qiao, Q.; Lewington, S.; et al. The Age-Specific Quantitative Effects of Metabolic Risk Factors on Cardiovascular Diseases and Diabetes: A Pooled Analysis. *PLoS ONE* **2013**, *8*, e65174. [CrossRef] [PubMed]
4. Li, L.; Liu, D.W.; Yan, H.Y.; Wang, Z.Y.; Zhao, S.H.; Wang, B. Obesity is an independent risk factor for non-alcoholic fatty liver disease: Evidence from a meta-analysis of 21 cohort studies. *Obes. Rev.* **2016**, *17*, 510–519. [CrossRef] [PubMed]
5. Wang, Y.; Wang, Q.J. The prevalence of prehypertension and hypertension among US Adults According to the New Joint National Committee Guidelines: New challenges of the old problem. *Arch. Intern. Med.* **2004**, *164*, 2126–2134. [CrossRef] [PubMed]
6. Thompson, D.; Edelsberg, J.; Colditz, G.A.; Bird, A.P.; Oster, G. Lifetime health and economic consequences of obesity. *Arch. Intern. Med.* **1999**, *159*, 2177–2183. [CrossRef] [PubMed]
7. Grundy, S.M.; Brewer, H.B.; Cleeman, J.I.; Smith, S.C.; Lenfant, C. Definition of Metabolic Syndrome. *Arterioscler. Thromb. Vasc. Biol.* **2004**, *24*, 2. [CrossRef] [PubMed]
8. Johnson, W.D.; Kroon, J.J.M.; Greenway, F.L.; Bouchard, C.; Ryan, D.; Katzmarzyk, P.T. Prevalence of risk factors for metabolic syndrome in adolescents: National Health and Nutrition Examination Survey (NHANES), 2001–2006. *Arch. Pediatr. Adolesc. Med.* **2009**, *163*, 371–377. [CrossRef]
9. Sims, E.A.H. Are there persons who are obese, but metabolically healthy? *Metabolism* **2001**, *50*, 1499–1504. [CrossRef] [PubMed]
10. Shin, M.J.; Hyun, Y.J.; Kim, O.Y.; Kim, J.Y.; Jang, Y.; Lee, J.H. Weight loss effect on inflammation and LDL oxidation in metabolically healthy but obese (MHO) individuals: Low inflammation and LDL oxidation in MHO women. *Int. J. Obes.* **2006**, *30*, 1529–1534. [CrossRef]
11. Stefan, N.; Kantartzis, K.; Machann, J.; Schick, F.; Thamer, C.; Rittig, K.; Balletshofer, B.; Machicao, F.; Fritsche, A.; Häring, H.U. Identification and characterization of metabolically benign obesity in humans. *Arch. Intern. Med.* **2008**, *168*, 1609–1616. [CrossRef]
12. Iacobini, C.; Pugliese, G.; Blasetti Fantauzzi, C.; Federici, M.; Menini, S. Metabolically healthy versus metabolically unhealthy obesity. *Metabolism* **2019**, *92*, 51–60. [CrossRef] [PubMed]
13. Nguyen, N.T.; Varela, J.E. Bariatric surgery for obesity and metabolic disorders: State of the art. *Nat. Rev. Gastroenterol. Hepatol.* **2017**, *14*, 160–169. [CrossRef]
14. Peterli, R.; Wolnerhanssen, B.K.; Peters, T.; Vetter, D.; Kroll, D.; Borbely, Y.; Schultes, B.; Beglinger, C.; Drewe, J.; Schiesser, M.; et al. Effect of laparoscopic sleeve gastrectomy vs laparoscopic roux-en-y gastric bypass onweight loss in patients with morbid obesity the sm-boss randomized clinical trial. *JAMA J. Am. Med. Assoc.* **2018**, *319*, 255–265. [CrossRef]
15. Owen, J.G.; Yazdi, F.; Reisin, E. Bariatric Surgery and Hypertension. *Am. J. Hypertens.* **2018**, *31*, 11–17. [CrossRef]
16. Ikramuddin, S.; Korner, J.; Lee, W.-J.; Connett, J.E.; Inabnet III, W.B.; Billington, C.B.; Thomas, A.J.; Leslie, D.B.; Chong, K.; Jeffery, R.W.; et al. Roux-en-Y Gastric Bypass versus Intensive Medical Management for the Control of Type 2 Diabetes, Hypertension and Hyperlipidemia: An International, Multicenter, Randomized Trial. *JAMA* **2013**, *309*, 2240–2249. [CrossRef]
17. Mingrone, G.; Panunzi, S.; De Gaetano, A.; Guidone, C.; Iaconelli, A.; Nanni, G.; Castagneto, M.; Bornstein, S.; Rubino, F. Bariatric-metabolic surgery versus conventional medical treatment in obese patients with type 2 diabetes: 5 year follow-up of an open-label, single-centre, randomised controlled trial. *Lancet* **2015**, *386*, 964–973. [CrossRef]
18. Guidone, C.; Manco, M.; Valera-Mora, E.; Iaconelli, A.; Gniuli, D.; Mari, A.; Nanni, G.; Castagneto, M.; Calvani, M.; Mingrone, G. Mechanisms of Recovery From Type 2 Diabetes After Malabsorptive Bariatric Surgery. *Diabetes* **2006**, *55*, 2025–2031. [CrossRef] [PubMed]
19. Schauer, P.R.; Bhatt, D.L.; Kirwan, J.P.; Wolski, K.; Aminian, A.; Brethauer, S.A.; Navaneethan, S.D.; Singh, R.P.; Pothier, C.E.; Nissen, S.E.; et al. Bariatric surgery versus intensive medical therapy for diabetes—5-year outcomes. *N. Engl. J. Med.* **2017**, *376*, 641–651. [CrossRef]

20. Nielsen, M.S.; Christensen, B.J.; Schmidt, J.B.; Tækker, L.; Holm, L.; Lunn, S.; Ritz, C.; Wewer Albrechtsen, N.J.; Holst, J.J.; Schnurr, T.M.; et al. Predictors of weight loss after bariatric surgery—A cross-disciplinary approach combining physiological, social, and psychological measures. *Int. J. Obes.* **2020**, *44*, 2291–2302. [CrossRef]
21. Digiorgi, M.; Rosen, D.J.; Choi, J.J.; Milone, L.; Schrope, B.; Olivero-Rivera, L.; Restuccia, N.; Yuen, S.; Fisk, M.; Inabnet, W.B.; et al. Re-emergence of diabetes after gastric bypass in patients with mid- to long-term follow-up. *Surg. Obes. Relat. Dis.* **2010**, *6*, 249–253. [CrossRef] [PubMed]
22. Wang, Q.A.; Tao, C.; Gupta, R.K.; Scherer, P.E. Tracking adipogenesis during white adipose tissue development, expansion and regeneration. *Nat. Med.* **2013**, *19*, 1338–1344. [CrossRef] [PubMed]
23. Frikke-Schmidt, H.; O'Rourke, R.W.; Lumeng, C.N.; Sandoval, D.A.; Seeley, R.J. Does bariatric surgery improve adipose tissue function? *Obes. Rev.* **2016**, *17*, 795–809. [CrossRef] [PubMed]
24. Rytka, J.M.; Wueest, S.; Schoenle, E.J.; Konrad, D. The portal theory supported by venous drainage-selective fat transplantation. *Diabetes* **2011**, *60*, 56–63. [CrossRef] [PubMed]
25. Tran, T.T.; Yamamoto, Y.; Gesta, S.; Kahn, C.R. Beneficial Effects of Subcutaneous Fat Transplantation on Metabolism. *Cell Metab.* **2008**, *7*, 410–420. [CrossRef] [PubMed]
26. Vishvanath, L.; Gupta, R.K. Contribution of adipogenesis to healthy adipose tissue expansion in obesity. *J. Clin. Investig.* **2019**, *129*, 4022–4031. [CrossRef]
27. Fox, C.S.; Massaro, J.M.; Hoffmann, U.; Pou, K.M.; Maurovich-Horvat, P.; Liu, C.-Y.; Vasan, R.S.; Murabito, J.M.; Meigs, J.B.; Cupples, L.A.; et al. Abdominal Visceral and Subcutaneous Adipose Tissue Compartments. *Circulation* **2007**, *116*, 39–48. [CrossRef] [PubMed]
28. Lee, K.Y.; Luong, Q.; Sharma, R.; Dreyfuss, J.M.; Ussar, S.; Kahn, C.R. Developmental and functional heterogeneity of white adipocytes within a single fat depot. *EMBO J.* **2019**, *38*, e99291. [CrossRef]
29. Gustafson, B.; Hammarstedt, A.; Hedjazifar, S.; Smith, U. Restricted adipogenesis in hypertrophic obesity: The role of WISP2, WNT, and BMP4. *Diabetes* **2013**, *62*, 2997–3004. [CrossRef]
30. Cotillard, A.; Poitou, C.; Torcivia, A.; Bouillot, J.-L.; Dietrich, A.; Klöting, N.; Grégoire, C.; Lolmede, K.; Blüher, M.; Clément, K. Adipocyte Size Threshold Matters: Link with Risk of Type 2 Diabetes and Improved Insulin Resistance After Gastric Bypass. *J. Clin. Endocrinol. Metab.* **2014**, *99*, E1466–E1470. [CrossRef]
31. Divoux, A.; Tordjman, J.; Lacasa, D.; Veyrie, N.; Hugol, D.; Aissat, A.; Basdevant, A.; Guerre-Millo, M.; Poitou, C.; Zucker, J.D.; et al. Fibrosis in human adipose tissue: Composition, distribution, and link with lipid metabolism and fat mass loss. *Diabetes* **2010**, *59*, 2817–2825. [CrossRef]
32. Keophiphath, M.; Achard, V.; Henegar, C.; Rouault, C.; Clément, K.; Lacasa, D. Le Macrophage-secreted factors promote a profibrotic phenotype in human preadipocytes. *Mol. Endocrinol.* **2009**, *23*, 11–24. [CrossRef]
33. Crewe, C.; An, Y.A.; Scherer, P.E. The ominous triad of adipose tissue dysfunction: Inflammation, fibrosis, and impaired angiogenesis. *J. Clin. Investig.* **2017**, *127*, 74–82. [CrossRef] [PubMed]
34. Chabot, K.; Gauthier, M.-S.; Garneau, P.Y.; Rabasa-Lhoret, R. Evolution of subcutaneous adipose tissue fibrosis after bariatric surgery. *Diabetes Metab.* **2017**, *43*, 125–133. [CrossRef] [PubMed]
35. Henegar, C.; Tordjman, J.; Achard, V.; Lacasa, D.; Cremer, I.; Guerre-Millo, M.; Poitou, C.; Basdevant, A.; Stich, V.; Viguerie, N.; et al. Adipose tissue transcriptomic signature highlights the pathological relevance of extracellular matrix in human obesity. *Genome Biol.* **2008**, *9*, R14. [CrossRef]
36. Marcelin, G.; Ferreira, A.; Liu, Y.; Atlan, M.; Aron-Wisnewsky, J.; Pelloux, V.; Botbol, Y.; Ambrosini, M.; Fradet, M.; Rouault, C.; et al. A PDGFRα-Mediated Switch toward CD9high Adipocyte Progenitors Controls Obesity-Induced Adipose Tissue Fibrosis. *Cell Metab.* **2017**, *25*, 673–685. [CrossRef]
37. Muir, L.A.; Neeley, C.K.; Meyer, K.A.; Baker, N.A.; Brosius, A.M.; Washabaugh, A.R.; Varban, O.A.; Finks, J.F.; Zamarron, B.F.; Flesher, C.G.; et al. Adipose tissue fibrosis, hypertrophy, and hyperplasia: Correlations with diabetes in human obesity. *Obesity* **2016**, *24*, 597–605. [CrossRef]
38. Lehmann, S.; Linder, N.; Retschlag, U.; Schaudinn, A.; Stange, R.; Garnov, N.; Dietrich, A.; Oberbach, A.; Kahn, T.; Busse, H. MRI assessment of changes in adipose tissue parameters after bariatric surgery. *PLoS ONE* **2018**, *13*, e0206735. [CrossRef]
39. Scholz, T.D.; Fleagle, S.R.; Parrish, F.C.; Breon, T.; Skorton, D.J. Effect of tissue fat and water content on nuclear magnetic resonance relaxation times of cardiac and skeletal muscle. *Magn. Reson. Imaging* **1990**, *8*, 605–611. [CrossRef]
40. Katsogiannos, P.; Kamble, P.G.; Boersma, G.J.; Karlsson, F.A.; Lundkvist, P.; Sundbom, M.; Pereira, M.J.; Eriksson, J.W. Early Changes in Adipose Tissue Morphology, Gene Expression, and Metabolism After RYGB in Patients With Obesity and T2D. *J. Clin. Endocrinol. Metab.* **2019**, *104*, 2601–2613. [CrossRef]
41. García-Rubio, J.; León, J.; Redruello-Romero, A.; Pavón, E.; Cozar, A.; Tamayo, F.; Caba-Molina, M.; Salmerón, J.; Carazo, Á. Cytometric analysis of adipose tissue reveals increments of adipocyte progenitor cells after weight loss induced by bariatric surgery. *Sci. Rep.* **2018**, *8*, 1–12. [CrossRef] [PubMed]
42. Andersson, D.P.; Hogling, D.E.; Thorell, A.; Toft, E.; Qvisth, V.; Näslund, E.; Thörne, A.; Wirén, M.; Löfgren, P.; Hoffstedt, J.; et al. Changes in subcutaneous fat cell volume and insulin sensitivity after weight loss. *Diabetes Care* **2014**, *37*, 1831–1836. [CrossRef] [PubMed]
43. Hotamisligil, G.S. Inflammation and metabolic disorders. *Nature* **2006**, *444*, 860–867. [CrossRef] [PubMed]

44. Hosogai, N.; Fukuhara, A.; Oshima, K.; Miyata, Y.; Tanaka, S.; Segawa, K.; Furukawa, S.; Tochino, Y.; Komuro, R.; Matsuda, M.; et al. Adipose Tissue Hypoxia in Obesity and Its Impact on Adipocytokine Dysregulation. *Diabetes* **2007**, *56*, 901–911. [CrossRef] [PubMed]
45. Kusminski, C.M.; Bickel, P.E.; Scherer, P.E. Targeting adipose tissue in the treatment of obesity-associated diabetes. *Nat. Rev. Drug Discov.* **2016**, *15*, 639. [CrossRef]
46. Lumeng, C.N.; Bodzin, J.L.; Saltiel, A.R. Obesity induces a phenotypic switch in adipose tissue macrophage polarization. *J. Clin. Investig.* **2007**, *117*, 175–184. [CrossRef] [PubMed]
47. Shumer, D.E.; Nokoff, N.J. Metabolically activated adipose tissue macrophages perform detrimental and beneficial functions during diet-induced obesity. *Physiol. Behav.* **2017**, *176*, 139–148.
48. Ni, Y.; Ni, L.; Zhuge, F.; Xu, L.; Fu, Z.; Ota, T. Adipose Tissue Macrophage Phenotypes and Characteristics: The Key to Insulin Resistance in Obesity and Metabolic Disorders. *Obesity* **2020**, *28*, 225–234. [CrossRef]
49. Fried, S.K.; Bunkin, D.A.; Greenberg, A.S. Omental and Subcutaneous Adipose Tissues of Obese Subjects Release Interleukin-6: Depot Difference and Regulation by Glucocorticoid. *J. Clin. Endocrinol. Metab.* **1998**, *83*, 847–850. [CrossRef]
50. Ouchi, N.; Parker, J.L.; Lugus, J.J.; Walsh, K. Adipokines in inflammation and metabolic disease. *Nat. Rev. Immunol.* **2011**, *11*, 85–97. [CrossRef]
51. Kanmani, S.; Kwon, M.; Shin, M.K.; Kim, M.K. Association of C-Reactive Protein with Risk of Developing Type 2 Diabetes Mellitus, and Role of Obesity and Hypertension: A Large Population-Based Korean Cohort Study. *Sci. Rep.* **2019**, *9*, 1–8. [CrossRef]
52. Stanley, T.L.; Zanni, M.V.; Johnsen, S.; Rasheed, S.; Makimura, H.; Lee, H.; Khor, V.K.; Ahima, R.S.; Grinspoon, S.K. TNF-α antagonism with etanercept decreases glucose and increases the proportion of high molecular weight adiponectin in obese subjects with features of the metabolic syndrome. *J. Clin. Endocrinol. Metab.* **2011**, *96*, E146–E150. [CrossRef] [PubMed]
53. Lumeng, C.N.; Deyoung, S.M.; Saltiel, A.R. Macrophages block insulin action in adipocytes by altering expression of signaling and glucose transport proteins. *Am. J. Physiol. Endocrinol. Metab.* **2007**, *292*, E166. [CrossRef] [PubMed]
54. Murdolo, G.; Hammarstedt, A.; Sandqvist, M.; Schmelz, M.; Herder, C.; Smith, U.; Jansson, P.A. Monocyte chemoattractant protein-1 in subcutaneous abdominal adipose tissue: Characterization of interstitial concentration and regulation of gene expression by insulin. *J. Clin. Endocrinol. Metab.* **2007**, *92*, 2688–2695. [CrossRef] [PubMed]
55. Mine, S.; Okada, Y.; Tanikawa, T.; Kawahara, C.; Tabata, T.; Tanaka, Y. Increased expression levels of monocyte CCR2 and monocyte chemoattractant protein-1 in patients with diabetes mellitus. *Biochem. Biophys. Res. Commun.* **2006**, *344*, 780–785. [CrossRef] [PubMed]
56. Kanda, H.; Tateya, S.; Tamori, Y.; Kotani, K.; Hiasa, K.; Kitazawa, R.; Kitazawa, S.; Miyachi, H.; Maeda, S.; Egashira, K.; et al. MCP-1 contributes to macrophage infiltration into adipose tissue, insulin resistance, and hepatic steatosis in obesity1. Kanda H, Tateya S, Tamori Y, Kotani K, Hiasa K, Kitazawa R, Kitazawa S, Miyachi H, Maeda S, Egashira K, others. MCP-1 contributes to m. *J. Clin. Investig.* **2006**, *116*, 1494. [CrossRef]
57. Cancello, R.; Henegar, C.; Viguerie, N.; Taleb, S.; Poitou, C.; Rouault, C.; Coupaye, M.; Pelloux, V.; Hugol, D.; Bouillot, J.L.; et al. Reduction of macrophage infiltration and chemoattractant gene expression changes in white adipose tissue of morbidly obese subjects after surgery-induced weight loss. *Diabetes* **2005**, *54*, 2277–2286. [CrossRef]
58. Labrecque, J.; Laforest, S.; Michaud, A.; Biertho, L.; Tchernof, A. Impact of Bariatric Surgery on White Adipose Tissue Inflammation. *Can. J. Diabetes* **2017**, *41*, 407–417. [CrossRef]
59. Liu, Y.; Aron-Wisnewsky, J.; Marcelin, G.; Genser, L.; Le Naour, G.; Torcivia, A.; Bauvois, B.; Bouchet, S.; Pelloux, V.; Sasso, M.; et al. Accumulation and Changes in Composition of Collagens in Subcutaneous Adipose Tissue After Bariatric Surgery. *J. Clin. Endocrinol. Metab.* **2016**, *101*, 293–304. [CrossRef] [PubMed]
60. Cancello, R.; Tordjman, J.; Poitou, C.; Guilhem, G.; Bouillot, J.L.; Hugol, D.; Coussieu, C.; Basdevant, A.; Hen, A.B.; Bedossa, P.; et al. Increased infiltration of macrophages in omental adipose tissue is associated with marked hepatic lesions in morbid human obesity. *Diabetes* **2006**, *55*, 1554–1561. [CrossRef]
61. Askarpour, M.; Khani, D.; Sheikhi, A.; Ghaedi, E.; Alizadeh, S. Effect of Bariatric Surgery on Serum Inflammatory Factors of Obese Patients: A Systematic Review and Meta-Analysis. *Obes. Surg.* **2019**, *29*, 2631–2647. [CrossRef]
62. Cancello, R.; Clément, K. Review article: Is obesity an inflammatory illness? Role of low-grade inflammation and macrophage infiltration in human white adipose tissue. *BJOG Int. J. Obstet. Gynaecol.* **2006**, *113*, 1141–1147. [CrossRef]
63. O'Rourke, R.W.; Johnson, G.S.; Purnell, J.Q.; Courcoulas, A.P.; Dakin, G.F.; Garcia, L.; Hinojosa, M.; Mitchell, J.E.; Pomp, A.; Pories, W.J.; et al. Serum biomarkers of inflammation and adiposity in the LABS cohort: Associations with metabolic disease and surgical outcomes. *Int. J. Obes.* **2019**, *43*, 285–296. [CrossRef]
64. Carbone, F.; Nulli Migliola, E.; Bonaventura, A.; Vecchié, A.; De Vuono, S.; Ricci, M.A.; Vaudo, G.; Boni, M.; Dallegri, F.; Montecucco, F.; et al. High serum levels of C-reactive protein (CRP) predict beneficial decrease of visceral fat in obese females after sleeve gastrectomy. *Nutr. Metab. Cardiovasc. Dis.* **2018**, *28*, 494–500. [CrossRef]
65. Lasselin, J.; Magne, E.; Beau, C.; Ledaguenel, P.; Dexpert, S.; Aubert, A.; Layé, S.; Capuron, L. Adipose Inflammation in Obesity: Relationship With Circulating Levels of Inflammatory Markers and Association With Surgery-Induced Weight Loss. *J. Clin. Endocrinol. Metab.* **2014**, *99*, E53–E61. [CrossRef]
66. Wewer Albrechtsen, N.J.; Geyer, P.E.; Doll, S.; Treit, P.V.; Bojsen-Møller, K.N.; Martinussen, C.; Jørgensen, N.B.; Torekov, S.S.; Meier, F.; Niu, L.; et al. Plasma Proteome Profiling Reveals Dynamics of Inflammatory and Lipid Homeostasis Markers after Roux-En-Y Gastric Bypass Surgery. *Cell Syst.* **2018**, *7*, 601–612.e3. [CrossRef]

67. Considine, R.V.; Sinha, M.K.; Heiman, M.L.; Kriauciunas, A.; Stephens, T.W.; Nyce, M.R.; Ohannesian, J.P.; Marco, C.C.; Mckee, L.J.; Bauer, T.L.; et al. Serum immunoreactive-leptin concentrations in normal-weight and obese humans. *N. Engl. J. Med.* **1996**, *334*, 292–295. [CrossRef] [PubMed]
68. Münzberg, H.; Morrison, C.D. Structure, production and signaling of leptin. *Metabolism* **2015**, *64*, 13–23. [CrossRef]
69. Martin, T.L.; Alquier, T.; Asakura, K.; Furukawa, N.; Preitner, F.; Kahn, B.B. Diet-induced obesity alters AMP kinase activity in hypothalamus and skeletal muscle. *J. Biol. Chem.* **2006**, *281*, 18933–18941. [CrossRef] [PubMed]
70. Jung, C.H.; Kim, M.S. Molecular mechanisms of central leptin resistance in obesity. *Arch. Pharm. Res.* **2013**, *36*, 201–207. [CrossRef] [PubMed]
71. Ozcan, L.; Ergin, A.S.; Lu, A.; Chung, J.; Sarkar, S.; Nie, D.; Myers, M.G.; Ozcan, U. Endoplasmic Reticulum Stress Plays a Central Role in Development of Leptin Resistance. *Cell Metab.* **2009**, *9*, 35–51. [CrossRef] [PubMed]
72. Czupryniak, L.; Pawlowski, M.; Kumor, A.; Szymanski, D.; Loba, J.; Strzelczyk, J. Predicting maximum Roux-en-Y gastric bypass-induced weight reduction—Preoperative plasma leptin or body weight? *Obes. Surg.* **2007**, *17*, 162–167. [CrossRef] [PubMed]
73. Askarpour, M.; Alizadeh, S.; Hadi, A.; Symonds, M.E.; Miraghajani, M.; Sheikhi, A.; Ghaedi, E. Effect of Bariatric Surgery on the Circulating Level of Adiponectin, Chemerin, Plasminogen Activator Inhibitor-1, Leptin, Resistin, and Visfatin: A Systematic Review and Meta-Analysis. *Horm. Metab. Res.* **2020**, *52*, 207–215. [CrossRef] [PubMed]
74. Turer, A.T.; Scherer, P.E. Adiponectin: Mechanistic insights and clinical implications. *Diabetologia* **2012**, *55*, 2319–2326. [CrossRef]
75. Matsubara, M.; Maruoka, S.; Katayose, S. Inverse relationship between plasma adiponectin and leptin concentrations in normal-weight and obese women. *Eur. J. Endocrinol.* **2002**, *147*, 173–180. [CrossRef] [PubMed]
76. Meyer, L.K.; Ciaraldi, T.P.; Henry, R.R.; Wittgrove, A.C.; Phillips, S.A. Adipose tissue depot and cell size dependency of adiponectin synthesis and secretion in human obesity. *Adipocyte* **2013**, *2*, 217–226. [CrossRef] [PubMed]
77. Ryo, M.; Nakamura, T.; Kihara, S.; Kumada, M.; Shibazaki, S.; Takahashi, M.; Nagai, M.; Matsuzawa, Y.; Funahashi, T. Adiponectin as a biomarker of the metabolic syndrome. *Circ. J.* **2004**, *68*, 975–981. [CrossRef]
78. Mather, K.J.; Goldberg, R.B. Clinical Use of Adiponectin as a Marker of Metabolic Dysregulation. *Best Pract. Res. Clin. Endocrinol. Metab.* **2014**, *28*, 107–117. [CrossRef]
79. Herder, C.; Peltonen, M.; Svensson, P.A.; Carstensen, M.; Jacobson, P.; Roden, M.; Sjöström, L.; Carlsson, L. Adiponectin and bariatric surgery: Associations with diabetes and cardiovascular disease in the Swedish obese subjects study. *Diabetes Care* **2014**, *37*, 1401–1409. [CrossRef]
80. Wolf, R.M.; Jaffe, A.E.; Steele, K.E.; Schweitzer, M.A.; Magnuson, T.H.; Wolfe, A.; Wong, G.W. Cytokine, Chemokine, and Cytokine Receptor Changes Are Associated with Metabolic Improvements after Bariatric Surgery. *J. Clin. Endocrinol. Metab.* **2018**, *104*, 947–956. [CrossRef]
81. Haluzíková, D.; Lacinová, Z.; Kaválková, P.; Drápalová, J.; Křížová, J.; Bártlová, M.; Mráz, M.; Petr, T.; Vítek, L.; Kasalický, M.; et al. Laparoscopic sleeve gastrectomy differentially affects serum concentrations of FGF-19 and FGF-21 in morbidly obese subjects. *Obesity* **2013**, *21*, 1335–1342. [CrossRef]
82. Steppan, C.M.; Wang, J.; Whiteman, E.L.; Birnbaum, M.J.; Lazar, M.A. Activation of SOCS-3 by Resistin. *Mol. Cell. Biol.* **2005**, *25*, 1569–1575. [CrossRef]
83. Chen, B.H.; Song, Y.; Ding, E.L.; Roberts, C.K.; Manson, J.E.; Rifai, N.; Buring, J.E.; Gaziano, J.M.; Liu, S. Circulating levels of resistin and risk of type 2 diabetes in men and women: Results from two prospective cohorts. *Diabetes Care* **2009**, *32*, 329–334. [CrossRef]
84. Heidemann, C.; Sun, Q.; Van Dam, R.M.; Meigs, J.B.; Zhang, C.; Tworoger, S.S.; Mantzoros, C.S.; Hu, F.B. Total and high-molecular-weight adiponectin and resistin in relation to the risk for type 2 diabetes in women. *Ann. Intern. Med.* **2008**, *149*, 307–316. [CrossRef]
85. Panidis, D.; Koliakos, G.; Kourtis, A.; Farmakiotis, D.; Mouslech, T.; Rousso, D. Serum resistin levels in women with polycystic ovary syndrome. *Fertil. Steril.* **2004**, *81*, 361–366. [CrossRef] [PubMed]
86. Laudes, M.; Oberhauser, F.; Schulte, D.M.; Freude, S.; Bilkovski, R.; Mauer, J.; Rappl, G.; Abken, H.; Hahn, M.; Schulz, O.; et al. Visfatin/PBEF/Nampt and resistin expressions in circulating blood monocytes are differentially related to obesity and type 2 diabetes in humans. *Horm. Metab. Res.* **2010**, *42*, 268–273. [CrossRef] [PubMed]
87. Park, H.K.; Kwak, M.K.; Kim, H.J.; Ahima, R.S. Linking resistin, inflammation, and cardiometabolic diseases. *Korean J. Intern. Med.* **2017**, *32*, 239–247. [CrossRef] [PubMed]
88. Yang, Q.; Graham, T.E.; Mody, N.; Preitner, F.; Peroni, O.D.; Zabolotny, J.M.; Kotani, K.; Quadro, L.; Kahn, B.B. Serum retinol binding protein 4 contributes to insulin resistance in obesity and type 2 diabetes. *Nature* **2005**, *436*, 356–362. [CrossRef] [PubMed]
89. Graham, T.E.; Yang, Q.; Blüher, M.; Hammarstedt, A.; Ciaraldi, T.P.; Henry, R.R.; Wason, C.J.; Oberbach, A.; Jansson, P.A.; Smith, U.; et al. Retinol-binding protein 4 and insulin resistance in lean, obese, and diabetic subjects. *N. Engl. J. Med.* **2006**, *354*, 2552–2563. [CrossRef]
90. Lu, H.-Y.; Li, X.-F.; Mu, P.-W.; Jiang, W.; Zheng, L.-Y. Depot-specific Expression of Retinol-Binding Protein 4 in Human Adipose Tissue and Their Relationship With Obesity and Insulin Resistance. *Zhonghua Yi Xue Za Zhi* **2010**, *90*, 3395–3398.
91. Fan, J.; Yin, S.; Lin, D.; Liu, Y.; Chen, N.; Bai, X.; Ke, Q.; Shen, J.; You, L.; Lin, X.; et al. Association of serum retinol-binding protein 4 levels and the risk of incident type 2 diabetes in subjects with prediabetes. *Diabetes Care* **2019**, *42*, 1574–1581. [CrossRef]

92. Broch, M.; Gómez, J.M.; Auguet, M.T.; Vilarrasa, N.; Pastor, R.; Elio, I.; Olona, M.; García-España, A.; Richart, C. Association of retinol-binding protein-4 (RBP4) with lipid parameters in obese women. *Obes. Surg.* **2010**, *20*, 1258–1264. [CrossRef] [PubMed]
93. Terra, X.; Auguet, T.; Quesada, I.; Aguilar, C.; Luna, A.M.; Hernández, M.; Sabench, F.; Porras, J.A.; Martínez, S.; Lucas, A.; et al. Increased levels and adipose tissue expression of visfatin in morbidly obese women: The relationship with pro-inflammatory cytokines. *Clin. Endocrinol.* **2012**, *77*, 691–698. [CrossRef] [PubMed]
94. Unamuno, X.; Gómez-Ambrosi, J.; Rodríguez, A.; Becerril, S.; Frühbeck, G.; Catalán, V. Adipokine dysregulation and adipose tissue inflammation in human obesity. *Eur. J. Clin. Investig.* **2018**, *48*, e12997. [CrossRef]
95. Vargas-Castillo, A.; Fuentes-Romero, R.; Rodriguez-Lopez, L.A.; Torres, N.; Tovar, A.R. Understanding the Biology of Thermogenic Fat: Is Browning A New Approach to the Treatment of Obesity? *Arch. Med. Res.* **2017**, *48*, 401–413. [CrossRef] [PubMed]
96. Ouellet, V.; Labbé, S.M.; Blondin, D.P.; Phoenix, S.; Guérin, B.; Haman, F.; Turcotte, E.E.; Richard, D.; Carpentier, A.C. Brown adipose tissue oxidative metabolism contributes to energy expenditure during acute cold exposure in humans. *J. Clin. Investig.* **2012**, *122*, 545–552. [CrossRef] [PubMed]
97. Kajimura, S.; Spiegelman, B.M.; Seale, P. Brown and beige fat: Physiological roles beyond heat generation. *Cell Metab.* **2015**, *22*, 546–559. [CrossRef]
98. Ballestri, S.; Nascimbeni, F.; Baldelli, E.; Marrazzo, A.; Romagnoli, D.; Lonardo, A. NAFLD as a Sexual Dimorphic Disease: Role of Gender and Reproductive Status in the Development and Progression of Nonalcoholic Fatty Liver Disease and Inherent Cardiovascular Risk. *Adv. Ther.* **2017**, *34*, 1291–1326. [CrossRef]
99. Wu, J.; Boström, P.; Sparks, L.M.; Ye, L.; Choi, J.H.; Giang, A.H.; Khandekar, M.; Virtanen, K.A.; Nuutila, P.; Schaart, G.; et al. Beige adipocytes are a distinct type of thermogenic fat cell in mouse and human. *Cell* **2012**, *150*, 366–376. [CrossRef]
100. Lidell, M.E.; Betz, M.J.; Enerbäck, S. Two types of brown adipose tissue in humans. *Adipocyte* **2014**, *3*, 63–66. [CrossRef]
101. Tai, T.A.C.; Jennermann, C.; Brown, K.K.; Oliver, B.B.; MacGinnitie, M.A.; Wilkison, W.O.; Roger Brown, H.; Lehmann, J.M.; Kliewer, S.A.; Morris, D.C.; et al. Activation of the nuclear receptor peroxisome proliferator-activated receptor γ promotes brown adipocyte differentiation. *J. Biol. Chem.* **1996**, *271*, 29909–29914. [CrossRef] [PubMed]
102. Puigserver, P.; Wu, Z.; Park, C.W.; Graves, R.; Wright, M.; Spiegelman, B.M. A cold-inducible coactivator of nuclear receptors linked to adaptive thermogenesis. *Cell* **1998**, *92*, 829–839. [CrossRef]
103. Ghosh, P.M.; Shu, Z.J.; Zhu, B.; Lu, Z.; Ikeno, Y.; Barnes, J.L.; Yeh, C.K.; Zhang, B.X.; Katz, M.S.; Kamat, A. Role of β-adrenergic receptors in regulation of hepatic fat accumulation during aging. *J. Endocrinol.* **2012**, *213*, 251–261. [CrossRef] [PubMed]
104. Xu, H.; Barnes, G.T.; Yang, Q.; Tan, G.; Yang, D.; Chou, C.J.; Sole, J.; Nichols, A.; Ross, J.S.; Tartaglia, L.A.; et al. Chronic inflammation in fat plays a crucial role in the development of obesity-related insulin resistance. *J. Clin. Investig.* **2003**, *112*, 1821–1830. [CrossRef] [PubMed]
105. Wong, V.W.-S.; Wong, G.L.-H.; Yeung, D.K.-W.; Abrigo, J.M.; Kong, A.P.-S.; Chan, R.S.-M.; Chim, A.M.-L.; Shen, J.; Ho, C.-S.; Woo, J.; et al. Fatty Pancreas, Insulin Resistance, and β-Cell Function: A Population Study Using Fat-Water Magnetic Resonance Imaging. *Am. J. Gastroenterol.* **2014**, *109*, 589–597. [CrossRef]
106. Mingrone, G.; Panunzi, S.; De Gaetano, A.; Guidone, C.; Iaconelli, A.; Leccesi, L.; Nanni, G.; Pomp, A.; Castagneto, M.; Ghirlanda, G.; et al. Bariatric surgery versus conventional medical therapy for type 2 diabetes. *N. Engl. J. Med.* **2012**, *366*, 1577–1585. [CrossRef]
107. Jans, A.; Nä Slund Id, I.; Ottosson Id, J.; Szabo, E.; Nä Slund Id, E.; Stenbergid, E. Duration of type 2 diabetes and remission rates after bariatric surgery in Sweden 2007–2015: A registry-based cohort study. *PLoS Med.* **2019**, *16*, e1002985. [CrossRef]
108. Shashaj, B.; Luciano, R.; Contoli, B.; Morino, G.S.; Spreghini, M.R.; Rustico, C.; Sforza, R.W.; Dallapiccola, B.; Manco, M. Reference ranges of HOMA-IR in normal-weight and obese young Caucasians. *Acta Diabetol.* **2016**, *53*, 251–260. [CrossRef] [PubMed]
109. Aller, R.; De Luis, D.; Pacheco, D.; Velasco, M.C.; Izaola, O.; Sagrado, M.G. Insulin resistance predicts steatosis and fibrosis in morbidly obese patients undergoing bariatric surgery. *J. Investig. Med.* **2012**, *60*, 1005–1008. [CrossRef]
110. Still, C.D.; Wood, G.C.; Benotti, P.; Petrick, A.T.; Gabrielsen, J.; Strodel, W.E.; Ibele, A.; Seiler, J.; Irving, B.A.; Celaya, M.P.; et al. Preoperative prediction of type 2 diabetes remission after Roux-en-Y gastric bypass surgery: A retrospective cohort study. *Lancet Diabetes Endocrinol.* **2014**, *2*, 38–45. [CrossRef]
111. Mehaffey, J.H.; Mullen, M.G.; Mehaffey, R.L.; Turrentine, F.E.; Malin, S.K.; Kirby, J.L.; Schirmer, B.; Hallowell, P.T. Type 2 diabetes remission following gastric bypass: Does diarem stand the test of time? *Surg. Endosc.* **2017**, *31*, 538–542. [CrossRef]
112. Bojsen-Møller, K.N.; Dirksen, C.; Jørgensen, N.B.; Jacobsen, S.H.; Serup, A.K.; Albers, P.H.; Hansen, D.L.; Worm, D.; Naver, L.; Kristiansen, V.B.; et al. Early enhancements of hepatic and later of peripheral insulin sensitivity combined with increased postprandial insulin secretion contribute to improved glycemic control after Roux-en-Y gastric bypass. *Diabetes* **2014**, *63*, 1725–1737. [CrossRef]
113. Lim, E.L.; Hollingsworth, K.G.; Aribisala, B.S.; Chen, M.J.; Mathers, J.C.; Taylor, R. Reversal of type 2 diabetes: Normalisation of beta cell function in association with decreased pancreas and liver triacylglycerol. *Diabetologia* **2011**, *54*, 2506–2514. [CrossRef] [PubMed]
114. Jørgensen, N.B.; Dirksen, C.; Bojsen-Møller, K.N.; Jacobsen, S.H.; Worm, D.; Hansen, D.L.; Kristiansen, V.B.; Naver, L.; Madsbad, S.; Holst, J.J. Exaggerated glucagon-like peptide 1 response is important for improved β-cell function and glucose tolerance after roux-en-Y gastric bypass in patients with type 2 diabetes. *Diabetes* **2013**, *62*, 3044–3052. [CrossRef] [PubMed]

115. Habegger, K.M.; Heppner, K.M.; Amburgy, S.E.; Ottaway, N.; Holland, J.; Raver, C.; Bartley, E.; Müller, T.D.; Pfluger, P.T.; Berger, J.; et al. GLP-1R responsiveness predicts individual gastric bypass efficacy on glucose tolerance in rats. *Diabetes* **2014**, *63*, 505–513. [CrossRef]
116. Izaguirre, M.; Gómez-Ambrosi, J.; Rodríguez, A.; Ramírez, B.; Becerril, S.; Valentí, V.; Moncada, R.; Unamuno, X.; Silva, C.; de la Higuera, M.; et al. GLP-1 Limits Adipocyte Inflammation and Its Low Circulating Pre-Operative Concentrations Predict Worse Type 2 Diabetes Remission after Bariatric Surgery in Obese Patients. *J. Clin. Med.* **2019**, *8*, 479. [CrossRef]
117. Hutch, C.R.; Sandoval, D. The role of GLP-1 in the metabolic success of bariatric surgery. *Endocrinology* **2017**, *158*, 4139–4151. [CrossRef]
118. Sridharan, K.; Kalayarasan, R.; Kamalanathan, S.; Sahoo, J.; Kar, S.S.; Nandhini, L.P.; Palui, R.; Durgia, H. Change in insulin resistance, beta cell function, glucagon-like peptide-1 and calcitonin levels two weeks after bariatric surgery. *Diabetes Metab. Syndr. Clin. Res. Rev.* **2019**, *13*, 2142–2147. [CrossRef]
119. Martinussen, C.; Bojsen-Møller, K.N.; Dirksen, C.; Jacobsen, S.H.; Jørgensen, N.B.; Kristiansen, V.B.; Holst, J.J.; Madsbad, S. Immediate enhancement of first-phase insulin secretion and unchanged glucose effectiveness in patients with type 2 diabetes after Roux-en-Y gastric bypass. *Am. J. Physiol. Metab.* **2015**, *308*, E535–E544. [CrossRef]
120. Toro-Ramos, T.; Goodpaster, B.H.; Janumala, I.; Lin, S.; Strain, G.W.; Thornton, J.C.; Kang, P.; Courcoulas, A.P.; Pomp, A.; Gallagher, D. Continued loss in visceral and intermuscular adipose tissue in weight-stable women following bariatric surgery. *Obesity* **2015**, *23*, 62–69. [CrossRef] [PubMed]
121. Greco, A.V.; Mingrone, G.; Giancaterini, A.; Manco, M.; Morroni, M.; Cinti, S.; Granzotto, M.; Vettor, R.; Camastra, S.; Ferrannini, E. Insulin resistance in morbid obesity: Reversal with intramyocellular fat depletion. *Diabetes* **2002**, *51*, 144–151. [CrossRef] [PubMed]
122. Hui, S.C.N.; Wong, S.K.H.; Ai, Q.; Yeung, D.K.W.; Ng, E.K.W.; Chu, W.C.W. Observed changes in brown, white, hepatic and pancreatic fat after bariatric surgery: Evaluation with MRI. *Eur. Radiol.* **2019**, *29*, 849–856. [CrossRef] [PubMed]
123. Mummadi, R.R.; Kasturi, K.S.; Chennareddygari, S.; Sood, G.K. Effect of Bariatric Surgery on Nonalcoholic Fatty Liver Disease: Systematic Review and Meta-Analysis. *Clin. Gastroenterol. Hepatol.* **2008**, *6*, 1396–1402. [CrossRef] [PubMed]
124. Kashyap, S.R.; Daud, S.; Kelly, K.R.; Gastaldelli, A.; Win, H.; Brethauer, S.; Kirwan, J.P.; Schauer, P.R. Acute effects of gastric bypass versus gastric restrictive surgery on B-cell function and insulinotropic hormones in severely obese patients with type 2 diabetes. *Int. J. Obes.* **2010**, *34*, 462–471. [CrossRef] [PubMed]
125. Pournaras, D.J.; Osborne, A.; Hawkins, S.C.; Vincent, R.P.; Mahon, D.; Ewings, P.; Ghatei, M.A.; Bloom, S.R.; Welbourn, R.; Le Roux, C.W. Remission of type 2 diabetes after gastric bypass and banding: Mechanisms and 2 year outcomes. *Ann. Surg.* **2010**, *252*, 966–971. [CrossRef] [PubMed]
126. Lima, M.M.O.; Pareja, J.C.; Alegre, S.M.; Geloneze, S.R.; Kahn, S.E.; Astiarraga, B.D.; Chaim, É.A.; Geloneze, B. Acute effect of Roux-en-Y gastric bypass on whole-body insulin sensitivity: A study with the euglycemic-hyperinsulinemic clamp. *J. Clin. Endocrinol. Metab.* **2010**, *95*, 3871–3875. [CrossRef] [PubMed]
127. McTigue, K.M.; Wellman, R.; Nauman, E.; Anau, J.; Coley, R.Y.; Odor, A.; Tice, J.; Coleman, K.J.; Courcoulas, A.; Pardee, R.E.; et al. Comparing the 5-year diabetes outcomes of sleeve gastrectomy and gastric bypass the national patient-centered clinical research network (PCORNet) bariatric study. *JAMA Surg.* **2020**, *155*, 1–12. [CrossRef]
128. Benoit, S.C.; Hunter, T.D.; Francis, D.M.; De La Cruz-Munoz, N. Use of Bariatric outcomes longitudinal database (BOLD) to study variability in patient success after Bariatric surgery. *Obes. Surg.* **2014**, *24*, 936–943. [CrossRef]
129. Livhits, M.; Mercado, C.; Yermilov, I.; Parikh, J.A.; Dutson, E.; Mehran, A.; Ko, C.Y.; Gibbons, M.M. Preoperative predictors of weight loss following bariatric surgery: Systematic review. *Obes. Surg.* **2012**, *22*, 70–89. [CrossRef]
130. Nickel, F.; De La Garza, J.R.; Werthmann, F.S.; Benner, L.; Tapking, C.; Karadza, E.; Wekerle, A.L.; Billeter, A.T.; Kenngott, H.G.; Fischer, L.; et al. Predictors of Risk and Success of Obesity Surgery. *Obes. Facts* **2019**, *12*, 427–439. [CrossRef]
131. Gerber, P.; Anderin, C.; Gustafsson, U.O.; Thorell, A. Weight loss before gastric bypass and postoperative weight change: Data from the Scandinavian Obesity Registry (SOReg). *Surg. Obes. Relat. Dis.* **2016**, *12*, 556–562. [CrossRef]
132. Still, C.D.; Benotti, P.; Wood, G.C.; Gerhard, G.S.; Petrick, A.; Reed, M.; Strodel, W. Outcomes of preoperative weight loss in high-risk patients undergoing gastric bypass surgery. *Arch. Surg.* **2007**, *142*, 994–998. [CrossRef]
133. Hutcheon, D.A.; Hale, A.L.; Ewing, J.A.; Miller, M.; Couto, F.; Bour, E.S.; Cobb, W.S.; Scott, J.D. Short-Term Preoperative Weight Loss and Postoperative Outcomes in Bariatric Surgery. *J. Am. Coll. Surg.* **2018**, *226*, 514–524. [CrossRef] [PubMed]
134. Benaiges, D.; Goday, A.; Pedro-Botet, J.; Mas, A.; Chillaron, J.; Flores-Le-Roux, J. Bariatric surgery: To whom and when? *Minerva Endocrinol.* **2012**, *147*, 135–140.
135. Kaplan, U.; Penner, S.; Farrokhyar, F.; Andruszkiewicz, N.; Breau, R.; Gmora, S.; Hong, D.; Anvari, M. Bariatric Surgery in the Elderly Is Associated with Similar Surgical Risks and Significant Long-Term Health Benefits. *Obes. Surg.* **2018**, *28*, 2165–2170. [CrossRef] [PubMed]
136. Contreras, J.E.; Santander, C.; Court, I.; Bravo, J. Correlation between age and weight loss after bariatric surgery. *Obes. Surg.* **2013**, *23*, 1286–1289. [CrossRef] [PubMed]
137. Kinzl, J.F.; Schrattenecker, M.; Traweger, C.; Mattesich, M.; Fiala, M.; Biebl, W. Psychosocial predictors of weight loss after bariatric surgery. *Obes. Surg.* **2006**, *16*, 1609–1614. [CrossRef] [PubMed]
138. Kalarchian, M.A.; Marcus, M.D.; Levine, M.D.; Soulakova, J.N.; Courcoulas, A.P.; Wisinski, M.S.C. Relationship of psychiatric disorders to 6-month outcomes after gastric bypass. *Surg. Obes. Relat. Dis.* **2008**, *4*, 544–549. [CrossRef] [PubMed]

139. Goodarzi, M.O. Genetics of obesity: What genetic association studies have taught us about the biology of obesity and its complications. *Lancet Diabetes Endocrinol.* **2018**, *6*, 223–236. [CrossRef]
140. Yaghootkar, H.; Lotta, L.A.; Tyrrell, J.; Smit, R.A.J.; Jones, S.E.; Donnelly, L.; Beaumont, R.; Campbell, A.; Tuke, M.A.; Hayward, C.; et al. Genetic evidence for a link between favorable adiposity and lower risk of type 2 diabetes, hypertension, and heart disease. *Diabetes* **2016**, *65*, 2448–2460. [CrossRef]
141. Rinella, E.S.; Still, C.; Shao, Y.; Wood, G.C.; Chu, X.; Salerno, B.; Gerhard, G.S.; Ostrer, H. Genome-wide association of single-nucleotide polymorphisms with weight loss outcomes after Roux-en-Y gastric bypass surgery. *J. Clin. Endocrinol. Metab.* **2013**, *98*, 1131–1136. [CrossRef]
142. Aasbrenn, M.; Schnurr, T.M.; Have, C.T.; Svendstrup, M.; Hansen, D.L.; Worm, D.; Balslev-Harder, M.; Hollensted, M.; Grarup, N.; Burgdorf, K.S.; et al. Genetic Determinants of Weight Loss After Bariatric Surgery. *Obes. Surg.* **2019**, *29*, 2554–2561. [CrossRef] [PubMed]

Journal of
Clinical Medicine

MDPI

Article

Caspase-Cleaved Keratin 18 Measurements Identified Ongoing Liver Injury after Bariatric Surgery

Felix Hempel [1,†], Martin Roderfeld [1,†], Lucas John Müntnich [1], Jens Albrecht [2,3], Ziya Oruc [2], Borros Arneth [4,5], Thomas Karrasch [6], Jörn Pons-Kühnemann [7], Winfried Padberg [2], Harald Renz [4,5], Andreas Schäffler [6] and Elke Roeb [1,*]

1 Department of Gastroenterology, Justus Liebig University, D-35392 Giessen, Germany; felix.hempel@med.jlug.de (F.H.); martin.roderfeld@innere.med.uni-giessen.de (M.R.); lucas.j.muentnich@med.uni-giessen.de (L.J.M.)
2 Department of General, Visceral, Thoracic, Transplantation, and Pediatric Surgery, Justus Liebig University, D-35392 Giessen, Germany; j.albrecht@azhm.de (J.A.); z.oruc@web.de (Z.O.); winfried.padberg@chiru.med.uni-giessen.de (W.P.)
3 Department for Bariatric Surgery, Asklepios Hospital, D-35423 Lich, Germany
4 Institute of Laboratory Medicine, Pathobiochemistry and Molecular Diagnostics, Justus Liebig University, D-35392 Giessen, Germany; borros.arneth@klinchemie.med.uni-giessen.de (B.A.); renzh@med.uni-marburg.de (H.R.)
5 The German Lung Center (DZL) and the Universities of Giessen and Marburg Lung Center (UGMLC), D-35392 Giessen, Germany
6 Department of Internal Medicine III, Justus Liebig University, D-35392 Giessen, Germany; thomas.karrasch@innere.med.uni-giessen.de (T.K.); andreas.schaeffler@innere.med.uni-giessen.de (A.S.)
7 Institute of Medical Informatics, Justus Liebig University, D-35392 Giessen, Germany; Joern.Pons@informatik.med.uni-giessen.de
* Correspondence: elke.roeb@innere.med.uni-giessen.de; Tel.: +49-(0)-641-98542338
† These authors contributed equally.

Citation: Hempel, F.; Roderfeld, M.; Müntnich, L.J.; Albrecht, J.; Oruc, Z.; Arneth, B.; Karrasch, T.; Pons-Kühnemann, J.; Padberg, W.; Renz, H.; et al. Caspase-Cleaved Keratin 18 Measurements Identified Ongoing Liver Injury after Bariatric Surgery. *J. Clin. Med.* **2021**, *10*, 1233. https://doi.org/10.3390/jcm10061233

Academic Editor: David Benaiges Boix

Received: 18 February 2021
Accepted: 11 March 2021
Published: 16 March 2021

Abstract: Bariatric surgery has emerged as an effective treatment option in morbidly obese patients with non-alcoholic fatty liver disease (NAFLD). However, worsening or new onset of non-alcoholic steatohepatitis (NASH) and fibrosis have been observed. Caspase-cleaved keratin 18 (ccK18) has been established as a marker of hepatocyte apoptosis, a key event in NASH development. Thus, ccK18 measurements might be feasible to monitor bariatric surgery patients. Clinical data and laboratory parameters were collected from 39 patients undergoing laparoscopic Roux-en-Y gastric bypass at six timepoints, prior to surgery until one year after the procedure. ccK18 levels were measured and a high-throughput analysis of serum adipokines and cytokines was carried out. Half of the cohort's patients (20/39) presented with ccK18 levels indicative of progressed liver disease. 21% had a NAFLD-fibrosis score greater than 0.676, suggesting significant fibrosis. One year after surgery, a mean weight loss of 36.87% was achieved. Six and twelve months after surgery, ccK18 fragments were significantly reduced compared to preoperative levels ($p < 0.001$). Yet nine patients did not show a decline in ccK18 levels $\geq 10\%$ within one year postoperatively, which was considered a response to treatment. While no significant differences in laboratory parameters or ccK18 could be observed, they presented with a greater expression of leptin and fibrinogen before surgery. Consecutive ccK18 measurements monitored the resolution of NAFLD and identified non-responders to bariatric surgery with ongoing liver injury. Further studies are needed to elicit the pathological mechanisms in non-responders and study the potential of adipokines as prognostic markers.

Keywords: non-alcoholic fatty liver disease; NAFLD; NASH; keratin 18; cytokeratin 18; M30; gastric bypass; non-invasive biomarkers

1. Introduction

Non-alcoholic fatty liver disease (NAFLD) is considered the hepatic manifestation of metabolic syndrome. It comprises a spectrum of diseases from simple steatosis to nonalcoholic steatohepatitis (NASH), cirrhosis of the liver and complications such as hepatocellular carcinoma (HCC) [1,2]. NAFLD is extremely prevalent and its importance in the etiology of liver failure, HCC, and liver transplantation is increasing rapidly [3,4]. Although numerous studies have delineated the complex pathophysiological mechanisms of NAFLD in past decades, no approved drug treatment is available yet [5]. Established therapeutic concepts remain limited to the treatment of underlying metabolic dysregulations. Herein, bariatric surgery has emerged as an effective intervention in morbidly obese patients [6–8]. International guidelines and guidance statements recommend considering bariatric surgery, if lifestyle interventions fail [9–12].

Conversely, NAFLD is particularly common among patients undergoing bariatric surgery [13–15]. Thus, hepatologic counseling is needed for timely diagnosis, patient monitoring, and treatment optimization. This seems especially important in the context of the worsening or new onset of NAFLD, which has been observed in bariatric surgery trials. A recent meta-analysis found such a response in 5%–20% of patients [8]. Yet the concepts of these clinical trials rely on repeated liver biopsies. Although currently considered the gold standard in the diagnosis of NAFLD, risks and cost of the procedure and shortcomings of the technique itself (e.g., sampling error and interrater variability) forbid a widespread application in everyday clinical practice. Therefore, non-invasive biomarkers are needed to enable hepatologic surveillance, especially in bariatric surgery patients.

Among many potential candidates, caspase-cleaved keratin 18 (ccK18) is deemed a promising novel biomarker. During hepatocyte apoptosis, ccK18 fragments enter the bloodstream, allowing their detection by the M30 enzyme-linked immunosorbent assay (ELISA) [16,17]. Thus, elevated ccK18 levels were linked to chronic liver disease [18,19] and–as it became evident that apoptotic hepatocytes are a major pathophysiological feature of NAFLD–ccK18 was studied extensively as a non-invasive biomarker for NAFLD [20–27]. Thus far, a fair diagnostic accuracy has been demonstrated and ccK18, alone or in combined biomarker panels, is expected to enter clinical practice soon [28,29]. The marker's responsiveness following an intervention has been shown both after pharmacologic interventions and diet-induced weight loss [30–32]. In conclusion, ccK18 measurements might be a feasible way to monitor the disease progression in bariatric surgery patients.

We aimed to evaluate the use of ccK18 as a biomarker for NAFLD in the follow-up of a cohort undergoing bariatric surgery. We aimed to elucidate (1) the prevalence of NAFLD, based on ccK18 levels and established fibrosis scores, before and after surgery, (2) the natural history of ccK18 levels after bariatric surgery, and (3) whether inconsistencies in the response to bariatric surgery occur and if the addition of ccK18 to a standard follow-up laboratory panel might enable the prediction thereof.

2. Materials and Methods

2.1. Patients

Clinical data and serum samples were collected from consecutive patients undergoing laparoscopic Roux-en-Y gastric bypass (RYGB) at the Obesity Center at the University of Giessen, Germany. The decision for bariatric surgery was made in accordance with current guidelines, requiring a body mass index (BMI) > 40 kg/m^2 (or 35 kg/m^2 and type 2 diabetes mellitus), the failure of conservative weight loss efforts, and the absence of contraindications. Prior bariatric surgery led to the exclusion of patients from the current study. A medical history was obtained and patients were examined. Informed consent was obtained from all patients. The study was approved by the local ethics committee at the Justus Liebig University (AZ 60/16) and conducted in accordance with the declaration of Helsinki.

2.2. Surgery

The RYGB procedure was carried out by a single experienced surgeon at a single tertiary care center, embedded in a multidisciplinary treatment regimen. Gastric bypass and simultaneous fundectomy followed by a circular gastrojejunostomy were performed. An 8–10 cm pouch was created, and lengths of the biliopancreatic and alimentary limb were set to 70–90 cm and 140–160 cm, respectively.

2.3. Data Acquisition

Data were collected at six time points: several days prior to the surgery, 1–3 days after the surgery, 1, 3, 6 and 12 months postoperatively. Each time, anthropometric measurements and a routine laboratory panel were performed. Additional serum samples for the quantification of ccK18 levels were either drawn in clinic visits or provided by the Institute of Laboratory Medicine. At two timepoints, prior to the surgical procedure and six months after, blood samples were collected after a standard meal in addition to fasting samples.

2.4. Quantification of Serum ccK18 Levels

ccK18 levels were measured utilizing the Peviva® M30 Apoptosense® ELISA Kit (TECOmedical, Sissach, Switzerland). All measurements were performed in duplicate, according to the manufacturer's instructions. Concentrations were determined using an Infinite® 200 Pro microplate reader with Magellan™ data analysis software (TECAN, Männedorf, Switzerland), applying a four-parameter logistic regression.

2.5. Definition of Responders and Non-Responders to Bariatric Surgery

A reduction of ccK18 levels ≥10% one year after the RYGB procedure when compared to preoperative levels was defined as response to bariatric surgery. Responders and non-responders were compared during data analysis after the allocation was performed based on serum ccK18 levels.

2.6. Proteome Profiling

Human Adipokine and Cytokine Array Kits (ARY024 and ARY005B, R&D Systems, Minneapolis, MN, USA) were used to test pooled serum samples of responders and non-responders to bariatric surgery (n = 9 per group) before and one year after surgery. Experiments were performed and mean grey values retrieved as described earlier [33]. For each analyte, the expression relative to positive control dots as well as the difference of relative expressions preoperatively and one year postoperatively were calculated.

2.7. Statistical Analysis

Data collection, calculation of scores, and descriptive statistics were performed using SPSS Statistics, version 25 (IBM Corp., Armonk, NY, USA). Further statistical analysis was performed using Prism 8 for macOS, version 8.4.3 (GraphPad software, La Jolla, CA, USA). A fitted mixed effect model, accounting for the repeated measures design, using the Geisser-Greenhouse correction, was applied to evaluate the changes in readout parameters in all patients over time. For the comparison of responders and non-responders to bariatric surgery, two-way ANOVA was used for each individual timepoint. Sidak's multiple comparisons test was applied in all cases. The significance level α was set to 0.05.

3. Results

3.1. Preoperative Assessment of the Study Population

39 patients were included in the present study. Table 1 summarizes the baseline patient characteristics. The majority of participants was female, ranging from age 23 to 60. All of them were morbidly obese (BMI > 40 kg/m^2) with a mean BMI of 51.94 kg/m^2 before surgery. None of the patients had an established diagnosis of chronic liver disease. However, considering the additional moderate to high prevalence of diabetes mellitus or preconditions of impaired glucose tolerance, hyperlipidemia, and elevated liver transami-

nases (Table 1), our study population comprises major risk factors, especially for NAFLD. In fact, about half of the patients (20/39) presented with ccK18 levels that have been proposed indicative of progressed liver disease (>200 U/l) [18,24,25]. In order to further characterize our study population and evaluate the likelihood of advanced fibrosis, we applied established non-invasive biomarkers of liver fibrosis. While few or no patients exceeded the cutoff for the APRI or FIB-4 index [34,35], about 21% of the participants had a NAFLD-fibrosis score (NFS) greater than 0.676, suggesting significant (stage 3–4) fibrosis [36].

Table 1. Baseline parameters of the full cohort before and one year after surgery.

	Preoperative (n = 39)	**1 Year (n = 39)**	**p (Adjusted)**
Demographic			
Age (year)	39.44 (23 to 60)		
Female sex	35 (90%)		
Anthropometric			
BMI (kg/m^2)	51.94 (41.56 to 61.85)	32.64 (17.88 to 54.37)	<0.001
Body weight (kg)	146.54 (111.7 to 190.5)	91.84 (61.3 to 125)	<0.001
Total Body Weight Loss (%)		36.87 (17.88 to 54.37)	
Excess Weight Loss † (%)		71.89 (38.64 to 105.29)	
Metabolism			
HbA1c (%)	6.19 (4.7 to 9.6)	5.29 (4.5 to 6.7)	<0.001
Diabetes mellitus	10 (31%)	2 (5%)	
LDL cholesterol (mg/dl)	129.65 (53 to 233)	91.92 (20 to 153)	<0.001
HDL cholesterol (mg/dl)	46.32 (27 to 87)	50.79 (17 to 95)	0.021
Serum triglycerides (mg/dl)	173.12 (58 to 751)	88.1 (44 to 253)	<0.001
CRP (mg/l)	17.72 (2.09 to 146.61)	1.87 (0.5 to 14.6)	0.004
Liver-related			
Log ccK18 (U/l)	2.37 (2.01 to 3.17)	2.09 (1.64 to 2.62)	<0.001
ccK18 > 200 U/l	20 (51%)	5 (13%)	
ALT (U/l)	41.03 (11 to 126)	36.15 (10 to 186)	0.914
AST (U/l)	31.15 (10 to 136)	23.44 (8 to 137)	0.285
Alkaline Phosphatase (U/l)	77.44 (48 to 114)	82.74 (43 to 270)	0.836
GGT (U/l)	41 (9 to 162)	23.26 (6 to 279)	0.280
Bilirubin (mg/dl)	0.49 (0.3 to 1)	0.58 (0.2 to 1.5)	0.024
Albumine (g/dl)	4.29 (3.61 to 5.1)	4.41 (3.92 to 5)	0.213
Significant fibrosis?			
NFS	−0.24 (−3.01 to 2.78)	−2.36 (−5.44 to 0.4)	<0.001
NFS > 0.676	8 (21%)	0	
APRI	0.29 (0.06 to 0.99)	0.24 (0.05 to 1.25)	0.576
APRI > 0.7	2 (5%)	1 (3%)	
FIB-4	0.71 (0.23 to 1.67)	0.63 (0.21 to 1.51)	0.311
FIB-4 > 3.25	0	0	

Data are presented as Mean (range) or n (%) † Excess weight was calculated relative to BMI = 25. BMI, Body Mass Index; LDL, Low Density Lipoprotein; HDL, High Density Lipoprotein; CRP, C-reactive protein; ccK18, caspase-cleaved keratin 18 (M30); ALT, alanine-aminotransferase; AST, aspartate-aminotransferase; GGT, gamma-glutamyl-transferase; NFS, NAFLD fibrosis score; APRI, aspartate-aminotransferase to platelet ratio index.

3.2. *Roux-en-Y Gastric Bypass Induced Severe Weight Loss and Improved the Patient's Metabolic State*

Following bariatric surgery, all patients showed a steady loss of body weight (Figure 1A,B). One year after surgery, a mean total body weight loss (TBWL) of 36.87% (95% CI: 34.16%–39.57%) and an excessive weight loss (EWL) of 71.89% (66.87%–76.91%) were achieved (Table 1). The mean BMI was 32.64 (95% CI 31.38–34.1). The success of bariatric surgery was consistent throughout the entire patient collective, and the minimum

TBWL was 17.88%. Metabolic parameters, such as HbA1c, LDL-cholesterol, and serum triglycerides significantly improved as consequence of the intervention (Table 1).

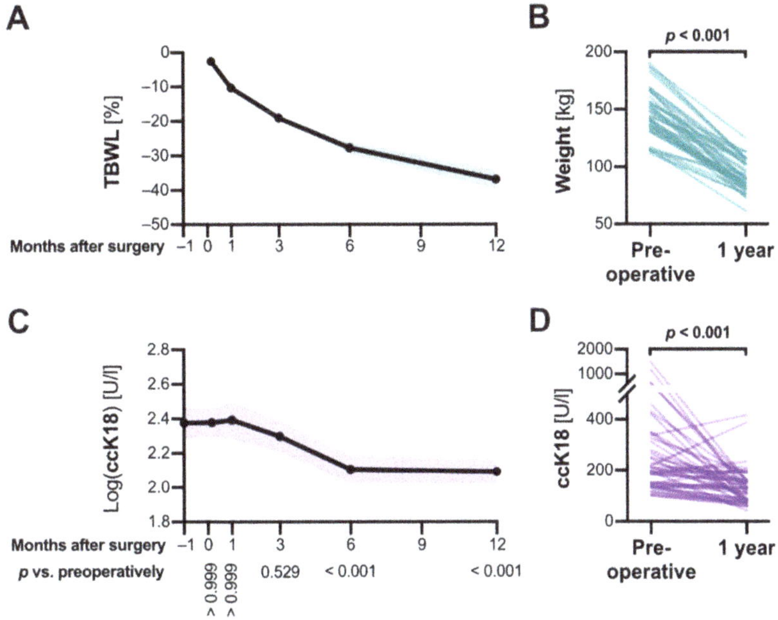

Figure 1. Roux-en-Y gastric bypass led to decreased body weight and caspase-cleaved keratin 18 levels. (**A**) Following the bariatric surgery, patients consistently lost weight with a mean total body weight loss (TBWL) of 37% after one year. Mean (line) and 95% confidence interval (colored area) are shown. (**B**) The reduction in body weight, affecting all included patients, was highly significant 12 months postoperatively when compared to preoperative levels ($p < 0.001$). (**C**) Caspase-cleaved keratin 18 (ccK18) fragments were measured utilizing a M30 enzyme-linked immunosorbent assay. Serum levels decreased significantly within 6 months after the procedure. Mean (line) and 95% confidence interval (colored area) are shown. (**D**) The individual course of ccK18 levels was, however, heterogenous among our cohort. A fitted mixed effect model was applied.

3.3. ccK18 Levels Decreased within Six Months after Surgery

To monitor the development of ccK18 levels after RYGB, we collected additional blood samples at six time points–several days before until one year after the surgery. Fasting blood samples were not required to obtain reliable ccK18 results. The coefficient of variation, comparing fasting and non-fasting blood samples at two time points (8.15% and 8.68%), undercut the inter-assay variability given by the manufacturer (<10%, see Supplementary Figure S1). Interestingly, the ccK18 levels we obtained followed a lognormal distribution, thus their respective logarithms were used for further analysis. During the first month after bariatric surgery, no alterations in mean ccK18 levels could be observed (Figure 1C). At both six and twelve months, ccK18 fragments were significantly reduced compared to preoperative levels ($p < 0.001$). Thereby, the natural history of ccK18 after bariatric surgery was distinct from other parameters of liver cell damage, such as alanine-aminotransferase, aspartate-aminotransferase, or gamma-glutamyl-transferase (GGT), which showed an initial increase subsequent to surgery, followed by a quick decline (Figure S2). One year after RYGB, only five out of the 39 patients had ccK18 levels greater than 200 U/l (Table 1).

3.4. The Response to Bariatric Surgery Was Inconsistent among Patients

Evaluating the individual courses of serum ccK18 levels, not all patients responded to the procedure with a reduction of ccK18 levels (Figure 1D). This observation falls in line with previous biopsy-controlled studies, which reported a worsening or new onset of NAFLD in 5%–20% of patients following bariatric surgery [8]. In our cohort, the reduction of ccK18 was not associated with total body- ($r = 0.32$, $p = 0.05$, Figure 2A) or excessive weight loss ($r = 0.12$, $p = 0.462$, Figure 2B). On the contrary, a rather modest weight loss of 20% was sufficient to induce the regression of ccK18 levels in some patients. To further investigate this issue, we categorized patients into two groups: A decrease in ccK18 levels by 10% or more one year after surgery when compared to preoperative values was considered a response to treatment. Out of the 39 patients analyzed, 30 met this criterium (Figure 2C). We compared those to the remaining nine patients, which were considered non-responders, to investigate whether the addition of ccK18 levels to a clinical follow-up including routine laboratory parameters could predict the eventual outcome. The results are summarized in Table 2. Preoperative serum triglyceride levels were greater in patients showing a response to bariatric surgery (+42.33 mg/dl, 95% CI 1.4–83.25 mg/dl, $p = 0.036$). In the one-year follow-up, non-responders presented with significantly higher mean GGT (+44.3 U/l, 95% CI 21.21–67.39 U/l, $p < 0.001$).

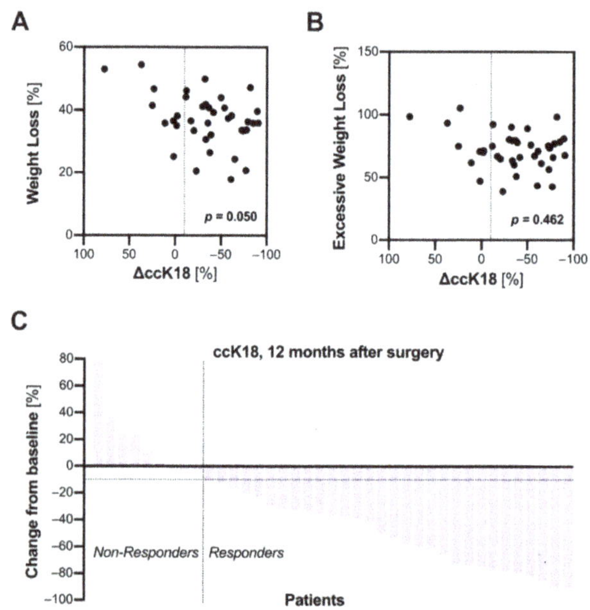

Figure 2. Consecutive ccK18 measurements identified non-responders to bariatric surgery. The individual changes in ccK18 levels during the one-year follow up (ΔccK18) were neither associated with (**A**) total body weight loss (r = 0.32), nor with (**B**) excessive weight loss (r = 0.12). Excessive weight loss was calculated relative to a body mass index of 25. Spearman's correlation coefficient was applied. Panel (**C**) shows a waterfall plot, depicting the individual change in ccK18 levels 12 months after surgery, compared to preoperative values, for each patient. While most patients experienced a decline, some presented unaltered or even increased ccK18 levels. For further analysis, we categorized patients into "Responders" and "Non-Responders", defining response as a decline in ccK18 levels $\geq$ 10% one year postoperatively.

Table 2. Comparison of responders and non-responders before and one year after surgery.

	Preoperative			1 Year		
	Responders (n = 30)	**Non-Responders** (n = 9)	p **(Adjusted)**	**Responders** (n = 30)	**Non-Responders** (n = 9)	p **(Adjusted)**
Demographic						
Age (year)	39.1 (23 to 60)	40.56 (27 to 51)	>0.999			
Female sex	27 (90%)	8 (89%)				
Anthropometric						
BMI (kg/m^2)	51.4 (41.56 to 61.85)	53.72 (44.92 to 59.88)	>0.999	32.89 (25.4 to 42.52)	31.81 (23.95 to 40.15)	>0.999
Body weight (kg)	145.51 (111.7 to 190.5)	149.98 (115 to 183)	>0.999	92.79 (73.4 to 125)	88.68 (61.3 to 108)	>0.999
Metabolism						
Diabetes mellitus	8 (33%)	2 (25%)		1 (3%)	1 (11%)	
LDL cholesterol (mg/dl)	128.15 (53 to 233)	134.5 (90 to 165)	>0.999	90.63 (20 to 145)	96.22 (65 to 153)	>0.999
HDL cholesterol (mg/dl)	44.5 (27 to 71)	52.25 (31 to 87)	>0.999	49.3 (17 to 83)	55.78 (38 to 95)	>0.999
Serum triglycerides (mg/dl)	183.08 (58 to 751)	140.75 (98 to 189)	0.036	90.53 (44 to 253)	80 (44 to 120)	0.962
CRP (mg/l)	15.25 (2.09 to 146.61)	25.94 (8.12 to 110.89)	>0.999	1.26 (0.5 to 7.91)	3.9 (0.5 to 14.6)	>0.999
Liver-related						
Log ccK18 (U/l)	2.4 (2.01 to 3.17)	2.27 (2.13 to 2.53)	>0.999	2.02 (1.64 to 2.28)	2.34 (2.21 to 2.62)	>0.999
ccK18 > 200 U/l	17 (57%)	3 (33%)		0	5 (56%)	
ALT (U/l)	45.5 (11 to 126)	26.11 (13 to 43)	0.921	34.47 (10 to 186)	41.78 (10 to 102)	>0.999
AST (U/l)	34.13 (10 to 136)	21.22 (12 to 30)	>0.999	22.87 (8 to 137)	25.33 (12 to 42)	>0.999
Alkaline Phosphatase (U/l)	76.87 (48 to 114)	79.33 (50 to 114)	>0.999	78.27 (43 to 122)	97.67 (60 to 270)	0.194
GGT (U/l)	45.33 (9 to 162)	26.56 (11 to 56)	0.939	13.03 (6 to 40)	57.33 (10 to 279)	< 0.001
Bilirubin (mg/dl)	0.49 (0.3 to 1)	0.5 (0.3 to 0.7)	>0.999	0.59 (0.2 to 1.5)	0.54 (0.3 to 0.9)	>0.999
Albumine (g/dl)	4.35 (3.8 to 5.1)	4.09 (3.6 to 4.6)	>0.999	4.47 (4.03 to 5)	4.24 (3.92 to 4.5)	>0.999
Significant fibrosis?						
NFS	−0.27	−0.164	>0.999	−2.21 (−4.68 to 0.4)	−2.87 (−5.44 to −0.44)	>0.999
NFS > 0.676	6 (20%)	2 (22%)		0	0	
APRI	0.318	0.187	>0.999	0.24 (0.05 to 1.25)	0.23 (0.09 to 0.48)	>0.999
APRI > 0.7	2 (7%)	0		1 (3%)	0	
FIB-4	0.74	0.594	>0.999	0.64 (0.21 to 1.51)	0.59 (0.36 to 1.33)	>0.999
FIB-4 > 3.25	0	0		0	0	

Data are given as Mean or Median (range) or n (%) LDL, Low Density Lipoprotein; HDL, High Density Lipoprotein; CRP, C-reactive protein; ccK18, caspase-cleaved Keratin 18 (M30); ALT, alanine-aminotransferase; AST, aspartate-aminotransferase; GGT, gamma-glutamyl-transferase; NFS, NAFLD fibrosis score; APRI, aspartate-aminotransferase to platelet ratio index.

3.5. The Expression of Adipokines and Cytokines Distinguished Responders and Non-Responders

Next, we aimed to evaluate possible differences in the molecular signatures of adipokines and cytokines between responders and non-responders. Before surgery, non-responders showed a strong expression of fibrinogen, while it was hardly detectable in the response group (Figure 3A,B). Non-responders, furthermore, presented with a 14% higher leptin expression and a reduced level of nidogen-1 (−25.6%). Repeated adipokine arrays demonstrated a distinct course of fibrinogen and insulin-like growth factor binding protein 6 (IGFBP-6) expression in responders and non-responders (Figure 3C): both increased in the response group one year after surgery but decreased in non-responders.

Leptin showed a greater decrease in non-responders, leading to a comparable expression one year after surgery. Adiponectin was unchanged in its expression in the response group. In non-responders, however, the expression decreased by 23.9% in the one-year follow up. Finally, cytokine arrays indicated a decreased preoperative expression of CXCL12, plasminogen activator inhibitor 1 (PAI-1), and macrophage migration inhibitory factor (MIF) in non-responders (Figure S3).

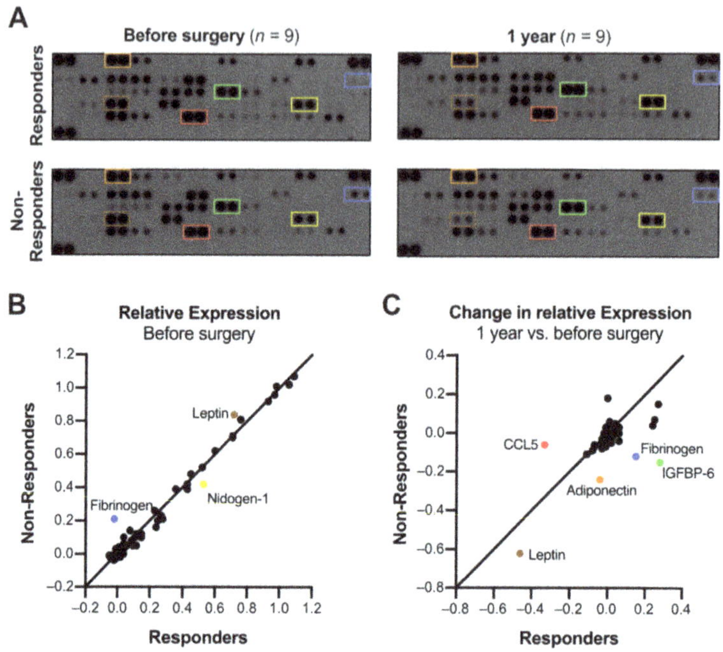

Figure 3. Distinct adipokine expression in responders and non-responders. (**A**) High resolution scans of the original arrays. Pooled serum samples of nine patients per group were subjected to adipokine arrays before and one year after surgery. (**B**) The analysis of the expression relative to positive control dots revealed a greater expression of fibrinogen and leptin in non-responders; nidogen-1 was less abundant in this group. (**C**) One year after surgery, fibrinogen and insulin-like growth factor binding protein 6 (IGFBP-6) expression increased in the response group but decreased in non-responders. Leptin also showed a greater decrease in non-responders. Adiponectin–unchanged in its expression in the response group–decreased by 23.9% in non-responders during the one-year follow up. Contrarily, CCL5 remained stable in non-responders but decreased in patients responding to the bariatric surgery. Correspondingly colored boxes in (**A**) label the protein's positions on the arrays.

4. Discussion

The present study elucidates the natural history of ccK18 levels and demonstrates its feasibility in the hepatic follow-up of a cohort undergoing Roux-en-Y gastric bypass. To our knowledge, this is the largest single-center study published to date in which all bariatric procedures were performed by the same surgeon. A significant decline in ccK18 levels was observed six months after surgery, falling in line with a previous report [23].

The high baseline levels of ccK18 and their marked decrease, following the surgery emphasize the extent of liver disease in our bariatric surgery cohort. Although no patient had been diagnosed with a chronic liver disease, the presence of NAFLD was likely in most subjects. According to the NALFD fibrosis score, advanced fibrosis was present in approximately 21% of patients preoperatively. The extent of ccK18 fragments and the high levels of established scores, such as the NFS, indicated progressed disease in some patients. The vigorous examination and thoughtful application of non-invasive biomarkers will be crucial to improve diagnosis, surveillance, and timely therapy of NAFLD in these patients.

Several authors stressed the imperfections of ccK18 as a biomarker for NAFLD. While combinations of liver stiffness measurements and other biomarkers seem promising [25,37], the inherent diagnostic accuracy of ccK18 has often been considered modest at best [38,39]. Furthermore, ideal ccK18 cut-offs are yet to be identified, as Kwok et al. accurately pointed out [28]. On the one hand, the approach presented herein addressed this issue by assessing the individual changes in ccK18 levels over time. Since the release of ccK18 reflects hepatocellular apoptosis as one of the underlying disease mechanisms, it seems especially well-suited to represent the spectrum of metabolism-associated liver disease, rather than imitating histological classifications [23–25]. In view of the multiple, short term, and close-knit checks before and after surgery, histological confirmation of the steatosis and fibrosis was not considered. Vuppalanchi et al., moreover, demonstrated that the decrease in ccK18 was correlated with histologic improvement of NAFLD [31]. On the other hand, in an unfiltered cohort without prior evaluation of NAFLD, this approach bears the risk of misinterpreting the lack of response in patients without serious liver disease in the first place. To this end, six out of our nine patients considered non-responders in this study presented with baseline ccK18 levels <200 U/l. In contrast, 13/30 patients, who responded to the intervention, also exhibited such ccK18 levels, and there was no significant difference in the preoperative ccK18 levels between the groups.

Consecutive ccK18 measurements revealed non-responders to bariatric surgery, which showed a decline <10% in ccK18 one year postoperatively when compared to baseline levels, in a similar magnitude as reported previously [8]. Great efforts have been made to reduce heterogeneity in our cohort: all patients were included in a structured, single center treatment regimen including a Roux-en-Y gastric bypass procedure performed by a single experienced surgeon. Yet responses were highly inconsistent. Lacking reduction in waist circumference, higher glucose levels, and insulin resistance have been postulated as possible modes of action [40–42]. However, neither the extent of weight loss nor HbA1c values significantly differed between responders and non-responders in our cohort. Further studies are needed to gain a comprehensive understanding of the underlying mechanisms. While the addition of ccK18 to a standard laboratory panel enabled the monitoring of the response to bariatric surgery, it did not increase its performance in predicting the eventual outcome.

However, the differences seen in the expression of adipokines imply promising perspectives. Fibrinogen, for instance, showed a greater expression in non-responders. In these, C-reactive protein was also increased in tendency, indicating a possible role of systemic inflammation. On the contrary, fibrinogen expression increased in responders, while it decreased in non-responders. The use of fibrinogen as a marker of systemic inflammation might also be confounded by the various changes in hemostasis, occurring post bariatric surgery [43]. Leptin was also overexpressed in non-responders. Although there have been conflicting results, a recent meta-analysis found higher circulating leptin levels to be associated with the severity of NAFLD, providing a possible explanation for the distinct course of disease in non-responders [44]. While the expression of adiponectin is comparable among the groups preoperatively, it decreased in non-responders. Adiponectin has been reported to negatively correlate with insulin resistance, visceral fat, advanced fibrosis, and the development of NASH [45–48]. Shorter intervals of adiponectin measurements might elucidate its potential to predict the response to bariatric surgery in future studies.

In summary, we demonstrated the successful clinical application of a ccK18-based follow-up to monitor the progression of liver disease in a bariatric surgery cohort. The use of non-invasive measures will be inevitable to establish a widespread application of NAFLD surveillance. We renounced histology in favor of close-knit non-invasive controls, as ccK18 has often been correlated with histological findings. The present study facilitates this development by clarifying the natural course of ccK18 in the first year post-bariatric surgery. To fully implement ccK18 in clinical practice, future studies investigating the influence of comorbidities and medication use will be necessary. Furthermore, a focus on the capability of biomarkers to predict outcomes in a subset of patients, rather than predicting the results of the imperfect gold standard liver biopsy, could provide new insights in this rapidly evolving field.

Supplementary Materials: The following are available online at https://www.mdpi.com/2077-0383/10/6/1233/s1, Figure S1: Fasting is not required to obtain reliable ccK18 serum levels, Figure S2: Natural history of parameters of liver injury following bariatric surgery, Figure S3: Cytokine expression in responders and non-responders.

Author Contributions: Conceptualization, E.R.; Data curation, T.K. and A.S.; Formal analysis, F.H. and J.P.-K.; Funding acquisition, E.R.; Investigation, F.H., M.R., L.J.M., and Z.O.; Resources, M.R., J.A., B.A., T.K., W.P., H.R., A.S., and E.R.; Supervision, M.R. and E.R.; Visualization, F.H. and J.P.-K.; Writing—original draft, F.H.; Writing—review & editing, F.H., M.R., and E.R. All authors have read and agreed to the published version of the manuscript.

Funding: This research was funded by the von-Behring-Röntgen Foundation, grant number 66-0008; German Research Foundation, grant number RO957/10-1 and The University Hospital Giessen and Marburg (UKGM), grant number 10/2013 GI.

Institutional Review Board Statement: The study was conducted according to the guidelines of the Declaration of Helsinki and approved by the Ethics Committee of the Justus Liebig University Giessen (AZ 60/16).

Informed Consent Statement: Informed consent was obtained from all subjects involved in the study.

Data Availability Statement: The data presented in this study are available on request from the corresponding author.

Acknowledgments: The authors thank Annette Tschuschner for excellent technical assistance.

Conflicts of Interest: The authors declare no conflict of interest. The funders had no role in the design of the study; in the collection, analyses, or interpretation of data; in the writing of the manuscript, or in the decision to publish the results.

References

1. Matteoni, C.A.; Younossi, Z.M.; Gramlich, T.; Boparai, N.; Liu, Y.C.; McCullough, A.J. Nonalcoholic fatty liver disease: A spectrum of clinical and pathological severity. *Gastroenterology* **1999**, *116*, 1413–1419. [CrossRef]
2. Vernon, G.; Baranova, A.; Younossi, Z.M. Systematic review: The epidemiology and natural history of non-alcoholic fatty liver disease and non-alcoholic steatohepatitis in adults. *Aliment. Pharmacol. Ther.* **2011**, *34*, 274–285. [CrossRef] [PubMed]
3. Younossi, Z.; Tacke, F.; Arrese, M.; Chander Sharma, B.; Mostafa, I.; Bugianesi, E.; Wai-Sun Wong, V.; Yilmaz, Y.; George, J.; Fan, J.; et al. Global Perspectives on Nonalcoholic Fatty Liver Disease and Nonalcoholic Steatohepatitis. *Hepatology* **2019**, *69*, 2672–2682. [CrossRef] [PubMed]
4. Younossi, Z.M.; Marchesini, G.; Pinto-Cortez, H.; Petta, S. Epidemiology of Nonalcoholic Fatty Liver Disease and Nonalcoholic Steatohepatitis: Implications for Liver Transplantation. *Transplantation* **2019**, *103*, 22–27. [CrossRef]
5. Friedman, S.L.; Neuschwander-Tetri, B.A.; Rinella, M.; Sanyal, A.J. Mechanisms of NAFLD development and therapeutic strategies. *Nat. Med.* **2018**, *24*, 908–922. [CrossRef]
6. De Ridder, R.J.; Schoon, E.J.; Smulders, J.F.; van Hout, G.C.; Stockbrugger, R.W.; Koek, G.H. Review article: Non-alcoholic fatty liver disease in morbidly obese patients and the effect of bariatric surgery. *Aliment. Pharmacol. Ther.* **2007**, *26*, 195–201. [CrossRef] [PubMed]
7. Mummadi, R.R.; Kasturi, K.S.; Chennareddygari, S.; Sood, G.K. Effect of bariatric surgery on nonalcoholic fatty liver disease: Systematic review and meta-analysis. *Clin. Gastroenterol. Hepatol.* **2008**, *6*, 1396–1402. [CrossRef] [PubMed]
8. Lee, Y.; Doumouras, A.G.; Yu, J.; Brar, K.; Banfield, L.; Gmora, S.; Anvari, M.; Hong, D. Complete Resolution of Nonalcoholic Fatty Liver Disease After Bariatric Surgery: A Systematic Review and Meta-analysis. *Clin. Gastroenterol. Hepatol.* **2019**, *17*, 1040–1060. [CrossRef]
9. Roeb, E.; Steffen, H.M.; Bantel, H.; Baumann, U.; Canbay, A.; Demir, M.; Drebber, U.; Geier, A.; Hampe, J.; Hellerbrand, C.; et al. S2k Guideline non-alcoholic fatty liver disease. *Z. Gastroenterol.* **2015**, *53*, 668–723. [CrossRef]
10. European Association for the Study of the Liver; European Association for the Study of Diabetes. Clinical Practice Guidelines for the management of non-alcoholic fatty liver disease. *J. Hepatol.* **2016**, *64*, 1388–1402. [CrossRef]
11. Chalasani, N.; Younossi, Z.; Lavine, J.E.; Charlton, M.; Cusi, K.; Rinella, M.; Harrison, S.A.; Brunt, E.M.; Sanyal, A.J. The diagnosis and management of nonalcoholic fatty liver disease: Practice guidance from the American Association for the Study of Liver Diseases. *Hepatology* **2018**, *67*, 328–357. [CrossRef] [PubMed]
12. Chitturi, S.; Wong, V.W.; Chan, W.K.; Wong, G.L.; Wong, S.K.; Sollano, J.; Ni, Y.H.; Liu, C.J.; Lin, Y.C.; Lesmana, L.A.; et al. The Asia-Pacific Working Party on Non-alcoholic Fatty Liver Disease guidelines 2017-Part 2: Management and special groups. *J. Gastroenterol. Hepatol.* **2018**, *33*, 86–98. [CrossRef]
13. Kroh, M.; Liu, R.; Chand, B. Laparoscopic bariatric surgery: What else are we uncovering? Liver pathology and preoperative indicators of advanced liver disease in morbidly obese patients. *Surg. Endosc.* **2007**, *21*, 1957–1960. [CrossRef]

14. Machado, M.; Marques-Vidal, P.; Cortez-Pinto, H. Hepatic histology in obese patients undergoing bariatric surgery. *J. Hepatol.* **2006**, *45*, 600–606. [CrossRef]
15. Harnois, F.; Msika, S.; Sabate, J.M.; Mechler, C.; Jouet, P.; Barge, J.; Coffin, B. Prevalence and predictive factors of non-alcoholic steatohepatitis (NASH) in morbidly obese patients undergoing bariatric surgery. *Obes. Surg.* **2006**, *16*, 183–188. [CrossRef]
16. Caulin, C.; Salvesen, G.S.; Oshima, R.G. Caspase cleavage of keratin 18 and reorganization of intermediate filaments during epithelial cell apoptosis. *J. Cell Biol.* **1997**, *138*, 1379–1394. [CrossRef]
17. Bantel, H.; Ruck, P.; Gregor, M.; Schulze-Osthoff, K. Detection of elevated caspase activation and early apoptosis in liver diseases. *Eur. J. Cell Biol.* **2001**, *80*, 230–239. [CrossRef] [PubMed]
18. Bantel, H.; Lugering, A.; Heidemann, J.; Volkmann, X.; Poremba, C.; Strassburg, C.P.; Manns, M.P.; Schulze-Osthoff, K. Detection of apoptotic caspase activation in sera from patients with chronic HCV infection is associated with fibrotic liver injury. *Hepatology* **2004**, *40*, 1078–1087. [CrossRef]
19. Kronenberger, B.; Wagner, M.; Herrmann, E.; Mihm, U.; Piiper, A.; Sarrazin, C.; Zeuzem, S. Apoptotic cytokeratin 18 neoepitopes in serum of patients with chronic hepatitis C. *J. Viral. Hepat.* **2005**, *12*, 307–314. [CrossRef] [PubMed]
20. Feldstein, A.E.; Canbay, A.; Angulo, P.; Taniai, M.; Burgart, L.J.; Lindor, K.D.; Gores, G.J. Hepatocyte apoptosis and fas expression are prominent features of human nonalcoholic steatohepatitis. *Gastroenterology* **2003**, *125*, 437–443. [CrossRef]
21. Wieckowska, A.; Zein, N.N.; Yerian, L.M.; Lopez, A.R.; McCullough, A.J.; Feldstein, A.E. In vivo assessment of liver cell apoptosis as a novel biomarker of disease severity in nonalcoholic fatty liver disease. *Hepatology* **2006**, *44*, 27–33. [CrossRef] [PubMed]
22. Younossi, Z.M.; Jarrar, M.; Nugent, C.; Randhawa, M.; Afendy, M.; Stepanova, M.; Rafiq, N.; Goodman, Z.; Chandhoke, V.; Baranova, A. A novel diagnostic biomarker panel for obesity-related nonalcoholic steatohepatitis (NASH). *Obes. Surg.* **2008**, *18*, 1430–1437. [CrossRef]
23. Diab, D.L.; Yerian, L.; Schauer, P.; Kashyap, S.R.; Lopez, R.; Hazen, S.L.; Feldstein, A.E. Cytokeratin 18 fragment levels as a noninvasive biomarker for nonalcoholic steatohepatitis in bariatric surgery patients. *Clin. Gastroenterol. Hepatol.* **2008**, *6*, 1249–1254. [CrossRef] [PubMed]
24. Feldstein, A.E.; Wieckowska, A.; Lopez, A.R.; Liu, Y.C.; Zein, N.N.; McCullough, A.J. Cytokeratin-18 fragment levels as noninvasive biomarkers for nonalcoholic steatohepatitis: A multicenter validation study. *Hepatology* **2009**, *50*, 1072–1078. [CrossRef] [PubMed]
25. Liebig, S.; Stoeckmann, N.; Geier, A.; Rau, M.; Schattenberg, J.M.; Bahr, M.J.; Manns, M.P.; Jaeckel, E.; Schulze-Osthoff, K.; Bantel, H. Multicenter Validation Study of a Diagnostic Algorithm to Detect NASH and Fibrosis in NAFLD Patients With Low NAFLD Fibrosis Score or Liver Stiffness. *Clin. Transl. Gastroenterol.* **2019**, *10*, e00066. [CrossRef]
26. Bantel, H.; John, K.; Schulze-Osthoff, K. Robust detection of liver steatosis and staging of NAFLD by an improved ELISA for serum cytokeratin-18 fragments. *Am. J. Gastroenterol.* **2014**, *109*, 140–141. [CrossRef]
27. Joka, D.; Wahl, K.; Moeller, S.; Schlue, J.; Vaske, B.; Bahr, M.J.; Manns, M.P.; Schulze-Osthoff, K.; Bantel, H. Prospective biopsy-controlled evaluation of cell death biomarkers for prediction of liver fibrosis and nonalcoholic steatohepatitis. *Hepatology* **2012**, *55*, 455–464. [CrossRef]
28. Kwok, R.; Tse, Y.K.; Wong, G.L.; Ha, Y.; Lee, A.U.; Ngu, M.C.; Chan, H.L.; Wong, V.W. Systematic review with meta-analysis: Non-invasive assessment of non-alcoholic fatty liver disease–the role of transient elastography and plasma cytokeratin-18 fragments. *Aliment. Pharmacol. Ther.* **2014**, *39*, 254–269. [CrossRef]
29. Musso, G.; Gambino, R.; Cassader, M.; Pagano, G. Meta-analysis: Natural history of non-alcoholic fatty liver disease (NAFLD) and diagnostic accuracy of non-invasive tests for liver disease severity. *Ann. Med.* **2011**, *43*, 617–649. [CrossRef]
30. Safarian, M.; Mohammadpour, S.; Shafiee, M.; Ganji, A.; Soleimani, A.; Nematy, M.; Bahari, A. Effect of diet-induced weight loss on cytokeratin-18 levels in overweight and obese patients with liver fibrosis. *Diabetes Metab. Syndr.* **2019**, *13*, 989–994. [CrossRef]
31. Vuppalanchi, R.; Jain, A.K.; Deppe, R.; Yates, K.; Comerford, M.; Masuoka, H.C.; Neuschwander-Tetri, B.A.; Loomba, R.; Brunt, E.M.; Kleiner, D.E.; et al. Relationship between changes in serum levels of keratin 18 and changes in liver histology in children and adults with nonalcoholic fatty liver disease. *Clin. Gastroenterol. Hepatol.* **2014**, *12*, 2121–2130. [CrossRef]
32. Tsutsui, M.; Tanaka, N.; Kawakubo, M.; Sheena, Y.; Horiuchi, A.; Komatsu, M.; Nagaya, T.; Joshita, S.; Umemura, T.; Ichijo, T.; et al. Serum fragmented cytokeratin 18 levels reflect the histologic activity score of nonalcoholic fatty liver disease more accurately than serum alanine aminotransferase levels. *J. Clin. Gastroenterol.* **2010**, *44*, 440–447. [CrossRef]
33. Hempel, F.; Roderfeld, M.; Savai, R.; Sydykov, A.; Irungbam, K.; Schermuly, R.; Voswinckel, R.; Kohler, K.; Churin, Y.; Kiss, L.; et al. Depletion of Bone Marrow-Derived Fibrocytes Attenuates TAA-Induced Liver Fibrosis in Mice. *Cells* **2019**, *8*, 1210. [CrossRef]
34. Lin, Z.H.; Xin, Y.N.; Dong, Q.J.; Wang, Q.; Jiang, X.J.; Zhan, S.H.; Sun, Y.; Xuan, S.Y. Performance of the aspartate aminotransferase-to-platelet ratio index for the staging of hepatitis C-related fibrosis: An updated meta-analysis. *Hepatology* **2011**, *53*, 726–736. [CrossRef] [PubMed]
35. Sterling, R.K.; Lissen, E.; Clumeck, N.; Sola, R.; Correa, M.C.; Montaner, J.; Sulkowski, M.S.; Torriani, F.J.; Dieterich, D.T.; Thomas, D.L.; et al. Development of a simple noninvasive index to predict significant fibrosis in patients with HIV/HCV coinfection. *Hepatology* **2006**, *43*, 1317–1325. [CrossRef] [PubMed]
36. Angulo, P.; Hui, J.M.; Marchesini, G.; Bugianesi, E.; George, J.; Farrell, G.C.; Enders, F.; Saksena, S.; Burt, A.D.; Bida, J.P. The NAFLD fibrosis score: A noninvasive system that identifies liver fibrosis in patients with NAFLD. *Hepatology* **2007**, *45*, 846–854. [CrossRef] [PubMed]

37. He, L.; Deng, L.; Zhang, Q.; Guo, J.; Zhou, J.; Song, W.; Yuan, F. Diagnostic Value of CK-18, FGF-21, and Related Biomarker Panel in Nonalcoholic Fatty Liver Disease: A Systematic Review and Meta-Analysis. *BioMed Res. Int.* **2017**, *2017*, e9729107. [CrossRef]
38. Cusi, K.; Chang, Z.; Harrison, S.; Lomonaco, R.; Bril, F.; Orsak, B.; Ortiz-Lopez, C.; Hecht, J.; Feldstein, A.E.; Webb, A.; et al. Limited value of plasma cytokeratin-18 as a biomarker for NASH and fibrosis in patients with non-alcoholic fatty liver disease. *J. Hepatol.* **2014**, *60*, 167–174. [CrossRef]
39. Wong, V.W.; Adams, L.A.; de Ledinghen, V.; Wong, G.L.; Sookoian, S. Noninvasive biomarkers in NAFLD and NASH—Current progress and future promise. *Nat. Rev. Gastroenterol. Hepatol.* **2018**, *15*, 461–478. [CrossRef]
40. Schwenger, K.J.P.; Fischer, S.E.; Jackson, T.; Okrainec, A.; Allard, J.P. In nonalcoholic fatty liver disease, Roux-en-Y gastric bypass improves liver histology while persistent disease is associated with lower improvements in waist circumference and glycemic control. *Surg. Obes. Relat. Dis.* **2018**, *14*, 1233–1239. [CrossRef] [PubMed]
41. Mathurin, P.; Gonzalez, F.; Kerdraon, O.; Leteurtre, E.; Arnalsteen, L.; Hollebecque, A.; Louvet, A.; Dharancy, S.; Cocq, P.; Jany, T.; et al. The evolution of severe steatosis after bariatric surgery is related to insulin resistance. *Gastroenterology* **2006**, *130*, 1617–1624. [CrossRef] [PubMed]
42. Mathurin, P.; Hollebecque, A.; Arnalsteen, L.; Buob, D.; Leteurtre, E.; Caiazzo, R.; Pigeyre, M.; Verkindt, H.; Dharancy, S.; Louvet, A.; et al. Prospective study of the long-term effects of bariatric surgery on liver injury in patients without advanced disease. *Gastroenterology* **2009**, *137*, 532–540. [CrossRef] [PubMed]
43. Tuovila, M.; Erkinaro, T.; Koivukangas, V.; Savolainen, E.R.; Laurila, P.; Ohtonen, P.; Ala-Kokko, T. Thromboelastography Values Remain Hypercoagulative 6 Months After Obesity Surgery: A Pilot Study. *Obes. Surg.* **2018**, *28*, 3943–3949. [CrossRef] [PubMed]
44. Polyzos, S.A.; Aronis, K.N.; Kountouras, J.; Raptis, D.D.; Vasiloglou, M.F.; Mantzoros, C.S. Circulating leptin in non-alcoholic fatty liver disease: A systematic review and meta-analysis. *Diabetologia* **2016**, *59*, 30–43. [CrossRef] [PubMed]
45. Jarrar, M.H.; Baranova, A.; Collantes, R.; Ranard, B.; Stepanova, M.; Bennett, C.; Fang, Y.; Elariny, H.; Goodman, Z.; Chandhoke, V.; et al. Adipokines and cytokines in non-alcoholic fatty liver disease. *Aliment. Pharmacol. Ther.* **2008**, *27*, 412–421. [CrossRef]
46. Polyzos, S.A.; Toulis, K.A.; Goulis, D.G.; Zavos, C.; Kountouras, J. Serum total adiponectin in nonalcoholic fatty liver disease: A systematic review and meta-analysis. *Metabolism* **2011**, *60*, 313–326. [CrossRef]
47. Balmer, M.L.; Joneli, J.; Schoepfer, A.; Stickel, F.; Thormann, W.; Dufour, J.F. Significance of serum adiponectin levels in patients with chronic liver disease. *Clin. Sci.* **2010**, *119*, 431–436. [CrossRef]
48. Boutari, C.; Mantzoros, C.S. Adiponectin and leptin in the diagnosis and therapy of NAFLD. *Metabolism* **2020**, *103*, e154028. [CrossRef] [PubMed]

Journal of
Clinical Medicine

MDPI

Review

Factors Related to Weight Loss Maintenance in the Medium–Long Term after Bariatric Surgery: A Review

Isabel Cornejo-Pareja [1,2,3], María Molina-Vega [1,2,*], Ana María Gómez-Pérez [1,2,*], Miguel Damas-Fuentes [1,2] and Francisco J. Tinahones [1,2,3]

1 Department of Endocrinology and Nutrition, Virgen de la Victoria University Hospital, 29010 Málaga, Spain; isabelmaria_cornejo@hotmail.com (I.C.-P.); migueldamasf@hotmail.com (M.D.-F.); fjtinahones@hotmail.com (F.J.T.)
2 Instituto de Investigación Biomédica de Málaga (IBIMA), Virgen de la Victoria University Hospital, 29010 Málaga, Spain
3 Centro de Investigación Biomédica en Red de la Fisiopatología de la Obesidad y Nutrición, Instituto de Salud Carlos III, 28029 Madrid, Spain
* Correspondence: molinavegamaria@gmail.com (M.M.-V.); anamgp86@gmail.com (A.M.G.-P.); Tel.: +34-95-1034-044 (M.M.-V. & A.M.G.-P.)

Abstract: Despite bariatric surgery being the most effective treatment for obesity, some individuals do not respond adequately, especially in the long term. Identifying the predictors of correct weight maintenance in the medium (from 1 to 3 years after surgery) and long term (from 3 years and above) is of vital importance to reduce failure after bariatric surgery; therefore, we summarize the evidence about certain factors, among which we highlight surgical technique, psychological factors, physical activity, adherence to diet, gastrointestinal hormones or neurological factors related to appetite control. We conducted a search in PubMed focused on the last five years (2015–2021). Main findings are as follows: despite Roux-en-Y gastric bypass being more effective in the long term, sleeve gastrectomy shows a more beneficial effectiveness–complications balance; pre-surgical psychological and behavioral evaluation along with post-surgical treatment improve long-term surgical outcomes; physical activity programs after bariatric surgery, in addition to continuous and comprehensive care interventions regarding diet habits, improve weight loss maintenance, but it is necessary to improve adherence; the impact of bariatric surgery on the gut–brain axis seems to influence weight maintenance. In conclusion, although interesting findings exist, the evidence is contradictory in some places, and long-term clinical trials are necessary to draw more robust conclusions.

Keywords: bariatric surgery; weight regain; surgical technique; psychological disorders; physical activity; diet; gut hormones; gut–brain axis

Citation: Cornejo-Pareja, I.; Molina-Vega, M.; Gómez-Pérez, A.M.; Damas-Fuentes, M.; Tinahones, F.J. Factors Related to Weight Loss Maintenance in the Medium–Long Term after Bariatric Surgery: A Review. *J. Clin. Med.* **2021**, *10*, 1739. https://doi.org/10.3390/jcm10081739

Academic Editors: David Benaiges Boix and Giuseppe Nisi

Received: 25 February 2021
Accepted: 9 April 2021
Published: 16 April 2021

1. Introduction

Obesity is defined as the pathological increase in adipose tissue associated with chronic low-grade inflammation and an increased risk of many pathological conditions such as type 2 diabetes mellitus (T2DM), cardiovascular disease, or cancer [1,2]. It is considered an epidemic disease and is expected to affect 44% of the adult population of the USA in 2031 and 31% of the adult population of Europe in 2037 [3].

The first-line treatment for obesity is lifestyle intervention, including a healthy diet and physical activity to produce a negative energy balance [2]. In those patients with moderate-risk or high-risk obesity, pharmacological therapy is indicated [2]. A weight loss of 5–10% can be easily attained and maintained for a time by lifestyle modification programs and anti-obesity medications. However, the weight usually recovers progressively from the first year after the intervention onwards [4].

Bariatric surgery is the most effective treatment for weight loss and weight-loss maintenance. Weight loss with bariatric surgery can reach 50–75% of excess body weight

(EBW) and can be maintained 10 years later [4]. Nevertheless, the efficacy of bariatric surgery is not uniform between patients, with some of them not obtaining satisfactory weight loss from the beginning (primary non-responders) or regaining weight in the long term (secondary non-responders) [5].

In this review, we will focus on the factors that influence weight loss in the medium–long term after bariatric surgery.

2. Surgical Technique

Since Edward Mason reported effective weight loss after the first gastric bypass in the mid-1960s, many bariatric procedures such as jejunoileal bypass, vertical banded gastroplasty, and laparoscopic adjustable gastric band (LAGB) have been used and later abandoned because of adverse events or inadequate long-term efficacy [6,7]. In 1994, the first report of the use of the laparoscopic technique was a landmark in bariatric surgical care as laparoscopic surgery reduces postoperative pain, time recovery, wound infection, and late ventral hernia formation in comparison to conventional techniques [6]. Nowadays, the most frequently performed bariatric procedures are laparoscopic Roux-en-Y gastric bypass (RYGB) and, especially, laparoscopic sleeve gastrectomy (SG), which accounts for 61% of primary bariatric procedures in the USA [7]. Therefore, we are going to analyze the evidence (clinical trials and meta-analysis) in the last 5 years comparing RYGB and SG regarding weight loss in the medium–long term.

In a recent meta-analysis, including 7443 patients from 23 studies, Hu et al. [8] found that there was no difference in excess weight loss (EWL)% between RYGB and SG in the short term (3 months–2 years), but RYGB was superior to SG in the mid-term (3 years) and long term (5 years) after surgery. However, RYBG showed more late complications than SG. Previously, Yang et al. [9] found similar results in a meta-analysis of 15 randomized controlled trials (1381 patients), concluding that SG and RYBG were similar regarding weight loss at <3 years but that EWL% was greater with RYBG 5 years after surgery, although with a higher incidence of complications. Other smaller meta-analyses found comparable results [10,11]. Likewise, King et al. [12] reported that weight regain seems to be higher after SG in comparison to RYGB. Conversely, other authors have concluded that there is no difference in weight loss between SG and RYBG at 1 year [13,14] and at 3 years [14,15] after surgery. Data from 10 or more years show that RYGB is able to maintain substantial weight loss, but data on SG are insufficient for a meta-analysis [16].

Results from clinical trials comparing weight loss between SG and RYGB published in the last 5 years are compiled in Table 1.

The Sleeve vs. Bypass (SLEEVEPASS) trial was a multicenter, multisurgeon, open-label randomized trial whose main aim was to determine if SG and RYGB were equivalent for weight loss in 240 patients. At five years since surgery, it was observed that EWL% after SG was 49% and after RYGB 57%, and this difference was not statistically significant despite that higher weight loss was achieved with RYGB [17]. Similar results were maintained at 7 years after surgery [18]. Regarding obesity co-morbidities, SG and RYGB were similar in T2DM remission and dyslipidemia resolution, where RYGB was better than SG in hypertension resolution at 5 years [17]. At 1 year after surgery, both Hofsø et al. [19] and Murphy et al. [20] reported RYGB to be superior to SG for weight loss (total weight loss 29% vs. 23%; $p < 0.001$ and EWL% 84.2% vs. 70.2%, $p = 0.002$, respectively). However, the primary outcome of these trials was T2DM remission, not weight loss, and although Hofsø et al. [19] found a higher remission of T2DM in RYGB in comparison to SG, Murphy et al. [20] observed both surgical procedures to be similar. In a small clinical trial, Schneider et al. [21] reported a higher EBMIL% (excess body mass index loss) with RYGB in comparison to SG (76.4% vs. 64.4%, $p = 0.046$) after 17 ± 5.6 months of follow-up. However, they also compared both surgical techniques regarding body composition and resting energy expenditure, not finding significant differences. In the Swiss Multicenter Bypass or Sleeve Study (SM-BOSS) trial, Peterli et al. [22,23] reported similar EBMIL% when comparing SG and RYGB at 1, 2, 3, and 5 years after surgery. Similarly, no statistically significant differences were observed between one anastomosis gastric bypass and SG at 1 year [24] and 3 years [25] after surgery. On the contrary, as that reported in the meta-analysis performed by Hu et al. [8], Ignat et al. [26] showed that, although EWL% was similar between SG and RYGB in the short term, a higher EWL% was achieved with RYBG vs. SG in the medium-term (at 3 years: 83% vs. 66.3%, $p = 0.024$) and long-term (at 5 years: 74.8% vs. 65.1%, $p = 0.045$) follow-up.

Table 1. Comparative clinical trials: SG vs. RY/OAGB.

	Sample Size (*n*)	Clinical Characteristics	Follow Up	Weight Loss (SG vs. RY/OAGB)	Conclusion
Grönroos [18] 2020	SG = 121 RYGB = 119	Female sex (%): SG: 71.9, RYGB: 67.2 Mean age (years): SG: 48.5, RYGB: 48.4 T2DM (%): SG: 52, RYGB: 49	7 years	EWL%: 47 vs. 55	GB = SG
Salminen [17] 2018			5 years	EWL%: 49 vs. 57	GB = SG
Hofsø [19] 2019	SG = 55 RYGB = 54	Female sex (%): SG: 58, RYGB: 74 Mean age (years): SG: 47.1, RYGB: 48.2 T2DM (%): 100	1 year	TWL%: 23 vs. 29	GB > SG
Murphy [20] 2018	SG = 58 RYGB = 56	Female sex (%): SG: 45, RYGB: 59 Mean age (years): SG: 45.5, RYGB: 46.6 T2DM (%): 100	1 year	EWL%: 70.2 vs. 84.2	GB > SG
Shivakumar [25] 2018	SG = 100 OAGB = 101	Female sex (%): SG: 65, RYGB: 61.4 Mean age (years): SG: 39.9, RYGB: 42.9 T2DM (%): SG: 47, RYGB: 49	3 years	EWL%: 61.1 vs. 66.5	GB = SG
Seetharamaiah [24] 2016			1 year	EWL%: 63.9 vs. 66.8	GB = SG
Ignat [26] 2017	SG = 55 RYGB = 45	Female sex (%): SG: 78.2, RYGB: 86.7 Mean age (years): SG: 35.1, RYGB: 32.2 T2DM (%): NR	1 year	EWL%: 83 vs. 80.4	GB = SG
			2 years	EWL%: 77.8 vs. 79.8	GB = SG
			3 years	EWL%: 66.3 vs. 83	GB > SG
			5 years	EWL%: 65.1 vs. 74.8	GB > SG
Peterli [22] 2017	SG = 107 RYGB = 110	Female sex (%): SG: 72, RYGB: 72 Mean age (years): SG: 43, RYGB: 42.1 T2DM (%): SG: 24, RYGB: 26	1 year 2 years 3 years	EBMIL%: 72 vs. 75 EBMIL%: 75 vs. 78 EBMIL%: 71 vs. 73	GB = SG GB = SG GB = SG
Peterli [23] 2018			5 years	EBMIL%: 61.1 vs. 68.3	GB = SG
Schneider [21] 2016	SG = 23 RYGB = 19	Female sex (%): SG: 87, RYGB: 84.2 Mean age (years): SG: 41.2, RYGB: 40.3 T2DM (%): SG: 57, RYGB: 42	17 months	EBMIL%: 64.4 vs. 76.4	GB > SG

SG: sleeve gastrectomy; RYGB: Roux-en-Y gastric bypass; OAGB: one anastomosis gastric bypass; T2DM: type 2 diabetes mellitus; EWL: excess weight loss; TWL: total weight loss; EBMIL: excess body mass index loss. GB > SG: gastric bypass better than sleeve gastrectomy; GB = SG: gastric bypass similar to sleeve gastrectomy.

In summary, despite many studies concluding that SG and RYGB are comparable at weight loss in the medium and long term, other studies have found RYGB to be better than

SG regarding this outcome and also in obesity-related co-morbidities (such as T2DM or hypertension, between others) resolution. However, SG seems to produce fewer complications than RYGB. Maybe new clinical trials [27] will be able to tip the balance in favor of RYBG or confirm the equivalence of both surgical procedures in weight loss at medium and long term.

3. Psychological Factors

Psychological difficulties and poorly treated mental health can negatively affect the results of bariatric surgery [28]. Mood, emotional dysregulation, depression, poor health literacy, and deficits in executive functioning, attention, and memory skills, among others, are likely to be important barriers to effective maintenance of weight loss [29], consistently finding deficiencies of these skills in the obese population compared to lean people [30].

A growing body of evidence suggests that deficits in executive function are common in obesity [31,32], finding a constant inverse association between obesity and executive function in children, adolescents, and the adult population [33].

Obese subjects show a pronounced impairment in decision-making and real-life learning in terms of reward and punishment (by the Iowa gambling task (IGT)) [34], and impaired central coherence (processing style centered on the details) that makes it impossible for them to see the "big picture" in a similar way to patients with anorexia nervosa [35,36]. In addition, the obese subject is impulsive and has poor performance on tests of global cognitive function and memory [37]. These deficits in executive function are considered the cause of inappropriate attitudes towards food and represent a trigger for both eating disorders and changes in BMI [38]. Likewise, obese individuals show an unregulated physiological response to intense emotion by tending to increase their food intake during periods of emotional arousal and/or stress, a response known as emotional eating [39]. However, the nature of this obesity-associated cognitive decline is unclear. Different explanations have been proposed including factors driven by inflammation, dopamine dysregulation implicated in hyperphagia, vascular diseases or neuroendocrine changes in ghrelin and leptin [40–42].

3.1. Cognitive Impairment

The presence of cognitive impairment in the obese subject can be particularly problematic in the population undergoing bariatric surgery, given the many lifestyle changes required after it. Up to 23% of subjects undergoing bariatric surgery have clinically significant cognitive impairment, and approximately 40% have more subtle cognitive deficits [43]. Such deficiencies in executive function have been associated with maladaptive eating behaviors, including uncontrolled or uninhibited eating along with sedentary behaviors, and may contribute to suboptimal weight loss after bariatric surgery [44] Spitznagel et al. found that preoperative baseline cognitive impairment predicted the outcome of weight at one year after bariatric surgery (RYGB) in 84 obese individuals. Poorer initial cognitive function in the domains of executive ability, attention, and memory predicted a lower percentage of weight loss and higher BMI at 12 months after bariatric surgery. Impairments in memory or executive function could interfere with the patient's ability to plan and follow postoperative guidelines for successful maintenance of weight loss [45]. Furthermore, cognition has been shown to improve shortly after bariatric surgery [46], and this initial improvement appears to be of substantial importance in its predictive ability for sustained weight loss. Supporting this notion, Spitznagel and colleagues [47,48] found that early postoperative cognitive dysfunction (at 12 postoperative weeks) predicted progression at 24 and 36 months. Poorer performance on cognitive tests at 12 weeks (lower performance in executive ability, attention, and memory) was indicative of a reduction in weight loss at 2- and 3-year follow-up after bariatric surgery. In this sense, Alosco et al. [49] evaluated 50 obese subjects who underwent RYGB, finding early cognitive benefits (12 weeks) that were generally maintained up to 36 months after surgery. Interestingly, it was observed in this work that the reduction in the domain of attention 24-36 months after the intervention was associated with weight recovery in this time. Kulendran et al. [50] in a study with 45 patients found that impulsivity measured as an inhibitory control of executive function together with the type of surgery (most effective RYGB vs. SG) were able to predict weight loss 6 months after bariatric surgery. The results found regarding the relationship between weight loss and executive performance in bariatric surgery may suggest that a reduction in body fat favors an improvement in executive function as a consequence of the resolution of metabolic alterations related to obesity. Likewise, a lower cognitive deficit at the beginning would lead to improvements in eating habits linked to a greater reduction in BMI, as we have seen. Similarly, cognitive function seems to be related to the durability of weight loss after bariatric surgery [47,48]. The cognitive skills that seem to best predict the results of weight loss included memory (particularly recognition memory) and executive functions (specifically working memory and generativity), and adherence behaviors could be the likely mechanism by which cognitive dysfunction leads to poorer performance in reducing long-term weight loss in bariatric surgery [33]. However, Bergh et al. [51], after evaluating 230 who underwent RYGB, found that while certain psychological factors such as self-esteem, planning, disposition to change behavior, or depressive symptoms, among others, were related to postoperative adherence to dietary recommendations and physical exercise. However, no associations were found in relation to weight loss one year after surgery.

3.2. Eating Disorders

Another important point in the failure of weight loss after bariatric surgery is related to the presence of eating disorders (EDs). Recent studies [52,53] have reported a higher prevalence of EDs among patients undergoing bariatric surgery with weight regain, with binge eating disorder especially prevalent in this population [54]. Conceição et al., [53] in a longitudinal study, found that up to 65% of patients who experienced weight regain between 17 and 20 months after surgery (both LAGB or RYGB) suffered from ED post-operatively. Furthermore, other studies have emphasized the role of other ED such as emotional eating, night eating syndrome (NES), or picking and nibling (P&N) in the results of bariatric surgery and how they contribute to suboptimal weight loss [55].

3.3. Depression

The reciprocal, longitudinal link between depression and obesity has been demonstrated in different studies [56]. Nevertheless, the exact nature of the relationship between depression and maintenance of obesity remains unclear, perhaps because clinical depression is a common exclusion criterion in weight loss intervention trials [57].

A recent meta-analysis [58] provides evidence for bariatric surgery, finding a reduction in depression symptoms at 6, 12, and 24 months after surgery. However, these symptoms increased after 36 months in a similar way to the baseline situation. Similar studies showed that improvements in depressive symptoms after bariatric surgery may not be maintained after 1–3 years after surgery, worsening again as in the starting point [59]. Weight regain and depression after surgery can act as a mutual risk factor. A depressed mood is associated with unhealthy lifestyle habits, emotional eating and loss of eating control [60], and weight regain after bariatric surgery [58,60,61]. Novelli et al. [62] found a higher score on emotional eating in obese women who underwent RYGB with insufficient weight loss 2 years after surgery. Feig et al. [63], in a cross-sectional study of 95 subjects undergoing RYGB and SG mainly, suggested that positive psychological states (positive affect or optimism) could be relevant in the state of well-being after bariatric surgery, finding greater adherence to healthy behaviors, physical activity, and weight loss. However, these associations lost statistical significance when factors such as depression were included.

3.4. Impulsive Behavior

Loss-of-control (LOC) eating is a common characteristic among subjects undergoing bariatric surgery [64], especially widespread in the adolescent population [65], and is associated with poorer weight outcomes. Goldschmidt et al. [64,66] and White et al. [67]

determined that postoperative LOC eating constitutes a phenotype that negatively affects the weight result, being prospectively related to greater long-term weight recovery after RYGB, while pre-surgical eating LOC was not related to changes in post-surgery BMI. The rates of LOC eating decreased in the period immediately after surgery (6 months) compared to baseline; however, these rates increased gradually over time (2–4 years) after surgery.

3.5. Other Psychological Factors

It has been investigated whether different personality types predict the results of weight after bariatric surgery, without being able to draw clear conclusions. While some showed no influence in this regard [68], Gordon et al. found that they could influence the amount of weight loss at 2 years of RYGB [69].

In conclusion, multiple physicological factors are related to weight loss after bariatric surgery. An integrative and multiple approach that includes pre-surgical psychological and behavioral evaluation along with post-surgical treatment can be corrective for weight regain and persistence of obesity. In addition, addressing depression and executive deficits before and after bariatric surgery is needed to improve long-term surgical outcomes. Future research should further explore the best way to consider cognitive deficits in preoperative detection and follow-up of candidates for bariatric surgery.

4. Physical Activity

National Institute for Health and Care Excellence (NICE) [70] recommends that the postoperative follow-up of the obese patient should incorporate counseling and support for physical activity.

4.1. Lack of Adherence to Exercise Training in Bariatric Surgery Patients

People with severe obesity can, generally, safely exercise vigorously [71]; however, candidates for bariatric surgery are generally less active than normal-weight subjects [72]. Additionally, candidates for bariatric surgery are more sedentary than the general obese population. Likewise, of all postoperative recommendations, those related to physical activity are commonly the most non-compliant [73]. King et al. [74] examined the physical activity of 310 patients who underwent bariatric surgery through the use of accelerometers, finding that most of the subjects increased their level of physical activity 1 year after bariatric surgery (RYGB mainly and other techniques included such as LAGB, SG, banded gastric bypass, or biliopancreatic diversion with duodenal switch) compared to baseline. However, most remained with poor physical activity according to the American Diabetes Association and the American College of Sports Medicine (<150 min per week), and some even decreased their activity compared to baseline. Bond et al. [75] compared self-reported estimates of physical activity vs. those based on objective measurements by an accelerometer in 20 patients who underwent bariatric surgery (65% LAGB and 35% RYGB) 6 months after surgery. Although in the postoperative period 55% of the participants self-reported adherence to the physical activity recommendations, only 5% were objectified by accelerometer measurement, with the changes in physical activity of moderate to vigorous intensity being much smaller than the self-reported. Ouellette et al. [76] also found no changes in early postoperative physical activity compared to baseline in subjects undergoing bariatric surgery (29% RYGB and 71% SG), with no correlation between the levels of physical activity self-reported by the patient and those observed by accelerometry. In addition, participants failed to adhere to the minimum recommended physical activity (150 min per week of moderate to vigorous intensity physical activity). Taken together, these data suggest that a high proportion of patients after bariatric surgery do not increase their physical activity, and some even decrease it, identifying a relevant area of intervention.

4.2. Aerobic and Resistance Training

Increased physical activity has been associated with greater weight loss after bariatric surgery [77–84]. Furthermore, close supervision and monitoring of exercise programs support greater weight loss compared to minimally supervised programs [85]. Egberts et al. [78] in a systematic review of observational studies (on 3852 patients) found a relationship between increased physical exercise (measured by physical activity questionnaires) and weight loss after bariatric surgery (LAGB and RYBG). In addition, the meta-analysis showed an average of 3.62 kg of greater weight loss with the practice of physical activity.

4.2.1. Aerobic Training

Carnero et al. [77] in a study carried out on 96 patients who underwent bariatric surgery (RYGB), monitored physical activity and effects on weight and body composition according to a 6 month structured exercise program, observing greater weight loss and more favorable body composition (less fat mass and greater muscle mass) in patients who performed moderate physical activity and decreased sedentary time. Furthermore, patients in the highest quartiles of physical activity achieved greater reductions in adiposity, reporting a dose–response association between exercise time and adiposity, already revealed by previous studies. In this sense, Woodlief et al. [86] demonstrated that patients who performed a greater amount of exercise (286 ± 40 min per week) after RYGB were those who obtained the greatest loss of weight and body fat compared to those who performed less physical activity. However, other studies have not supported this finding [87–90]. Coen et al. [88] examined the efficacy of a physical exercise program (120 min/week of treadmill walking for 6 months) in severely obese subjects, not observing any additional impact on RYGB-induced weight loss or fat mass. These findings are similar to those of Shah et al. [89] who showed how the prescription of a high-volume exercise program (energy expenditure in exercise > 2000 Kcal/week) with bariatric surgery (70% GB and 30% RYGB) at least 3 months earlier had no impact on the body weight or circumference of waist compared to the control group. The lack of effect of exercise on weight in these studies is probably due to the strong initial influence of surgery; thus, these data do not rule out the possibility that an exercise program may cause additional weight loss and improve body composition or adiposity favorably after surgery. Furthermore, after the initial large loss, weight tends to stabilize, and the long-term sustainability of this weight loss is probably more related to lifestyle changes such as avoiding sedentary behavior and regular physical activity [90].

4.2.2. Combination of Aerobic and Resistance Training

A randomized clinical trial introducing a 12-week structured and supervised physical exercise program in 24 post-bariatric surgery (surgical technique not specified) patients (at 12-24 months later) and 12 controls with the same characteristics demonstrated improvements in capacity/physical function and weight, among other parameters [91]. In this sense, Rothwell and colleagues [79] reported that weight loss after a semi-structured exercise program at 12 months of bariatric surgery (LAGB) improved, without observing this effect at 36 months. Hanvold and colleagues [81] found that patients undergoing RYGB who reported physical activity ≥150 min/week had a lower percentage of weight regain compared to less active participants. However, they found no differences when comparing the diet and physical activity-focused lifestyle intervention group vs. the usual care group at long-term (2 years). Coleman et al. [90] found that a structured post-bariatric exercise program improves the physical capacity of patients (strength, balance, flexibility, mobility, coordination) at 6–24 months post-surgery (GS, RYGB, LAGB), without finding additional effects on weight loss.

A recent meta-analysis [80] of 15 exercise training studies (aerobic training in 5 studies, resistance training in 2 studies, and a combination of aerobic and resistance training in 8 studies) also concluded that physical training programs carried out after bariatric surgery (RYGB and SB mainly) were effective in optimizing the loss of weight and fat mass and improving the physical condition of the patients, although no additional effect on lean mass loss was described.

4.3. Maintenance of Muscle Mass

The maintenance of muscle mass is vital to optimize physical functioning and preserve energy expenditure at rest. The latter represents 60–70% of total energy expenditure [70], finding greater reductions and less recovery of visceral abdominal fat when it is included physical exercise in weight loss programs [92]. Loss of fat free mass (FFM) can predispose to long-term weight regain. Metcalf et al. [93] found that duodenal switch surgery in patients adhering to an exercise program (30 min per session, with > 3 sessions a week) achieved 28% more loss of fat mass and 8% more gain of lean mass compared to sedentary patients at 18 months postoperatively. A systematic review by Chaston et al. [94] suggests that loss of FFM (skeletal muscle, bone, and organs) represents a weight percentage of 31.3% of weight loss after RYGB. Although the significance of the loss of this FFM is not well known, excessive loss may be undesirable. Specifically, in older patients, the loss of muscle mass and bone mineral density may have a negative impact on their physical function, sarcopenia, and quality of life [95]. Physical exercise, and specifically endurance exercise, is effective in maintaining muscle mass [96].

In summary, despite that physical activity programs after bariatric surgery have been shown to be associated with a higher weight loss and a more beneficial body composition, most patients do not increase, and may even decrease, physical activity. However, most of the papers refer to the early postoperative stages, and the evidence is very limited in the long term. More interventional clinical trials with long-term structured exercise programs are needed to determine whether exercise is important in preventing weight regain in bariatric surgery patients.

5. Dietary Factors

In the bariatric population in particular, the diet is often poor, and caloric intake often increases progressively after bariatric surgery [97]. Sawer et al. [98] found an increase in caloric intake 2 years after bariatric surgery compared to the first 5 months (1172.9 ± 46.5 Kcal/day vs. 1358.1 ± 60.5 Kcal/day), finding greater weight loss and maintenance in those with greater dietary adherence.

In the National Weight Control Registry (NWCR), a large-scale prospective study to investigate the maintenance of long-term weight loss, among the dietary strategies adopted for the stable maintenance of weight loss, the following stand out: Adherence to a low-calorie and low-fat diet, eating breakfast regularly, and maintaining a consistent eating pattern throughout the week [99]. However, the literature on dietary advice to improve weight after bariatric surgery is limited. In addition, the studies in this regard present a small sample size, as well as heterogeneity of dietary support, settings, times, duration, type of surgery, etc.

The main macronutrients in food (carbohydrates, proteins, and fats) stimulate oxygen consumption in different ways, which can influence changes in body weight and possibly subsequent weight regain. Bray et al. [100] in the POUNDS LOST Study and Grave et al. [101] found no effect of diet composition on body weight or energy expenditure [100]. However, Reid et al. [102] found higher carbohydrate and alcohol consumption in those subjects who had regained weight after an average of 12 years since bariatric surgery, compared to those who had maintained weight loss. Frequent consumption of high-fat and high-sugar snacks can lead to excessive energy intake from carbohydrates, and this behavior may reduce the maintenance of weight loss [103]. Restricting the consumption of soft drinks or carbonated beverages is another important aspect that has been related to the stability of postsurgical weight [104]. Likewise, different studies [105,106] have found that a diet high in protein and with a low glycemic index was the best option to maintain weight loss, and this macronutrient composition could be related to a lower decrease in energy expenditure in the subjects who followed it [105].

Regarding dietary behavior, and more specifically behaviors related to reduced rations and frequency of intake, they have been related to more favorable weight 3 years after bariatric surgery [107]. Similar findings have been described in a cohort of 50 adolescents undergoing bariatric surgery [87].

It is likely that numerous mechanisms contribute to changes in lifestyle after bariatric surgery. Continuous and comprehensive care interventions appear to be the most successful approaches to maintaining weight loss. However, more long-term randomized clinical trials are needed to clarify these issues.

6. Gut Hormones and Neuronal Factors

6.1. Gut Hormones

Bariatric surgery produces changes in gastrointestinal anatomy and functionality that may be implicated in different ways in weight loss after the procedure and weight maintenance in the long-term. Regulation of appetite and eating is a complex process that depends on the integration of signals from the digestive tract to the central nervous system (CNS). Specifically, there are regions in the hypothalamus and brainstem that integrate peripheral signals to coordinate orexigenic and anorexigenic responses. Those signals provide information about energy availability depending on nutritional state and energy storage in adipose tissue. There is a very intricate system of signals between the gut, vagal afferents, hypothalamus, brainstem, and reward centers in response to nutrient ingestion to regulate energy homeostasis [108].

The main gut hormones implicated in energy homeostasis are ghrelin, which is orexigenic, peptide tyrosin-tyrosin (PYY), glucagon-like peptide 1 (GLP-1), oxyntomodulin (OXM), glicentin, pancreatic polypeptide (PP), amylin and cholecystokinin (CCK), which are anorexigenic [109]. Ghrelin increases appetite and food intake, accelerates gastric emptying, increases gastric acid secretion, decreases insulin secretion, and stimulates hepatic glucose production. Its levels are higher just before nutrient intake, and there is a ghrelin suppression after a meal; this suppression is greater following a high-carbohydrate meal compared to a high-fat meal [108]. On the contrary, PYY reduces food intake and appetite, increases insulin secretion, and delays gastric emptying. The peak in PYY secretion takes place typically 15–30 min after food intake, and protein and fat-rich foods stimulate greater peaks of this hormone compared to carbohydrates [110]. GLP-1 has a biphasic secretion after nutrients intake with an early phase 15 min after ingestion and a second peak at 30–60 min [111]. Its effects are similar to PYY—suppressing appetite, reducing food intake, and delaying gastric emptying—but it also promotes glucose-dependent insulin secretion [112]. OXM is co-secreted with GLP-1 in response to food ingestion, and it reduces energy intake, increases energy expenditure related to physical activity, delays gastric emptying, and also stimulates glucose-dependent insulin secretion. Glicentin seems to have a role in stimulating insulin secretion, and decreasing gut motility and acid secretion in animals, but its biological role is not fully elucidated yet. PP is secreted after nutrients ingestion depending on caloric load, and its main functions are the inhibition of gastric emptying, pancreatic exocrine secretion, and gallbladder motility. Amylin levels reach a peak one hour after nutrient ingestion and remain high for four hours, slowing gastric emptying, suppressing glucagon postprandial secretion, inhibiting energy intake, and increasing energy expenditure [108]. Finally, CCK promotes gallbladder contraction and pancreatic exocrine secretion favoring food digestion, but it also slows gastric emptying, inhibits acid gastric secretion, decreases energy intake, and stimulates insulin secretion [113].

Some alterations in the normal function of these hormones have been reported in obese patients compared to lean subjects, also in syndromic obesity. Some changes in these hormones have been identified following different weight loss strategies, including bariatric surgery (Table 2). For example, an increase in postprandial levels of GLP-1 in patients after SG and RYGB has been reported in several studies, and this change may persist in the long-term (at least 1–2 years). In the case of GIP (Gastric inhibitory polypeptide), data are more controversial, as some studies have reported an increase in postprandial levels after bariatric surgery, but some others did not find any change, especially after RYGB. Similar effects have been observed in a lot of studies for OXM and PYY, with increases in postprandial levels after RYGB and for PYY also after SG. Regarding ghrelin, the only orexigenic gut hormone of those previously mentioned, its suppression is usually improved after bariatric surgery. However, the mechanism seems to be different depending on the technique, as in RYGB the effect observed is in postprandial ghrelin, and in SG the effect observed is in fasting ghrelin. Although this is controversy, lower ghrelin levels may have beneficial effects on appetite regulation and in body weight [114].

Table 2. Summary of main changes in gut hormones after RYGB and SG.

Hormones	SG	RYGB
GLP-1	Increase	Increase
GIP	Increase/no changes	Increase/no changes
OXM	Increase	Increase
PYY	Increase	Increase
Glicentin	Increase	Increase
Ghrelin *	Suppression	Suppression

* All hormone levels refer to postprandial levels, except for ghrelin, whose changes occurred mainly in fasting levels. RYGB: Roux-en-Y gastric bypass. SG: sleeve gastrectomy. GLP-1: glucagon polypeptide like 1. GIP: glucose-dependent insulinotropic peptide OXM: oxyntomodulin. PYY: polypeptide tyrosine-tyrosine.

Differential behaviors of gut hormones depending on surgical technique could be related with anatomical changes (duodenum exclusion in RYGB and restriction of the gastric fundus in SG) produced in the surgery and with different exposure to carbohydrates and fat. Based on this idea, there are three hypothesis that try to explain weight control. The hindgut hypothesis poses that the accelerated delivery of nutrients to the distal gut increases insulinotropic signals that are mediated, among others, by GLP-1, and that improves postprandial glucose and free fatty acids metabolism, favoring body weight control [115]. Besides, nutrient delivery to the distal intestine also may produce an increase in intestinal gluconeogenesis and may activate a hepato-portal sensor that leads to neural signals for reduced food intake and decreased glucose output from the liver, as the midgut hypothesis proposes [116]. Finally, foregut hypothesis suggests that bypassing the duodenum may reduce some factors that induce insulin resistance and β-cell dysfunction, decreasing diabetogenic signals [117].

Among the studies published in last five years regarding gut hormones and weight maintenance after bariatric surgery, there are some interesting results, though the majority of them are observational studies. Perakakis et al. performed two independent trials to assess circulating levels of gut hormones in response to different types of bariatric surgery and its influence on weight loss after a year of follow up. They compared the fasting and postprandial levels of nine gut hormones after a mixed meal test, before and after bariatric surgery (laparoscopic gastric banding, SG and RYGB), and they related them with weight loss, looking for predictors of long-term weight loss. Their most robust results referred to OXM and glicentin, which showed a significant increase 3 months after the surgery (SG and RYGB) that was maintained at one year. The percentage of weight change was related to this increase at 6 months (OXM: $p = 0.004$; glicentin: $p = 0.001$) and at 12 months (OXM: $p = 0.053$; glicentin: $p = 0.049$). For GLP-1, changes were more profound and significant for SG than for RYGB, in contrast with other studies. For GIP they only found a decrease after RYGB and no changes for SG, and finally for ghrelin there was a significant decrease after SG but no changes after RYGB. They concluded that glicentin increase may predict weight loss at 12 months better than GLP-1, and these effects seemed to be related with better satiety control [118]. In another comparative study, Santo et al. compared postprandial secretion of ghrelin, GIP, GLP-1, and leptin in patients with maintenance of more than 50% of the EWL (group A) versus patients with regain of more than 50% of the EWL (group B), with a follow up of 26 months. Although the sample size was very small and all patients had undergone RYGB, they found some interesting results. There was a decrease in postprandial ghrelin levels in both groups, suggesting better appetite control. GIP showed a relatively larger increase (with respect to baseline) in postprandial levels at 30 min in group A compared to group B ($p = 0.01$), and GLP-1 also showed a greater increase at 30 min in group A compared to group B ($p = 0.05$) as well as a greater relative increase with respect to baseline ($p = 0.01$). Finally, leptin showed greater basal levels in group B compared to group A ($p = 0.02$), suggesting that energetic reserves could have been larger in group B. Thus, they concluded that the increase in GLP-1 and GIP after nutrient intake may show the influence of these hormones in weight maintenance after RYGB [119]. Another similar prospective observational study led by Alamuddin analyzed postprandial GLP-1, PYY, ghrelin, and leptin levels at 6 and 18 months after bariatric surgery (SG and RYGB), and they compared with a control group. Despite the low number of patients who completed the 18 months of follow up, the results are interesting to understand gut hormone changes in the long term. They reported a decrease in fasting ghrelin levels, especially in the SG group at 6 months ($p = 0.0199$) and 18 months ($p = 0.0003$), and an exaggerated postprandial increase in GLP-1 and PYY at 6 months (RYGB: $p < 0.0001$; SG: $p = 0.006$) that lasted until 18 months only for GLP-1 [120]. With some differences, the results of these studies suggest that the increase in anorexigenic hormones levels and the decrease in orexigenic hormones may be related to weight loss and weight maintenance after bariatric surgery in the short and long-term.

Other Hormonal Factors

On the other hand, bile acids also may have a role in weight loss and weight maintenance after bariatric surgery. A lower increase in circulating levels of postprandial bile acids has been reported in obese individuals, and this fact may play a role in energetic metabolism and weight control because they have some hormonal effects, and they stimulate brown adipose tissue activity for thermogenic effects. Some studies have shown an increase in postprandial bile acids levels after RYGB, and this increase seems to be grater in the long-term. The exact mechanism is not known, but it could be related to the nutrient delivery to the distal small intestine [121]. In addition, the alterations in gut microbiota after RYGB could have a role because microbiota are a key regulator of bile acids conjugation and secondary bile acids formation [122]. Bile acid fasting levels correlate with GLP-1 peak levels and stimulate GLP-1 secretion, probably contributing to satiety and ß-cell insulin secretion [123]. Insulin secretion also may be facilitated via farnesoid X receptor (FXR), which directly responds to bile acid increase [124]. Moreover, there are bile acid receptors (TGR5 receptors) in skeletal muscle and brown adipose tissue. Thus, the binding of bile acids to these receptors may increase energy expenditure, facilitating thyroid hormone action. However, data are controversial, and it is not clear if energy expenditure contributes to weight maintenance after bariatric surgery [125].

6.2. Neuronal Factors

Several studies have suggested that changes in taste preferences after bariatric surgery, especially after RYGB and alterations in the reward system, may have an influence in weight maintenance after surgical treatment of obesity, though data are inconclusive [126].

The mesolimbic reward pathway is a dopaminergic pathway that is key in substance abuse disorders, and there is evidence that it is also important in obesity. Although food intake regulation is a very complex system with many actors implied, dopamine may mediate some aspects of eating behaviors. It is known that food reward and dopamine functions are altered in obesity [127]. Bariatric surgery (SG and RYGB) may increase striatal dopamine transmission, improving reward sensitivity. This improved sensitivity, along with other factors, may help to modify eating behaviors enhancing the preference for non-highly stimulating food. These changes in striatal dopamine transmission seem to be related to changes in gut hormone levels after bariatric surgery, such as the decrease in ghrelin levels and the increase in GLP-1 or PYY levels. Gut hormones are key in the connection of the gut and brain as well as microbiota, as some gut bacteria are also implicated in dopamine release, and the shift in gut microbiota after bariatric procedures may improve dopaminergic signaling. This microbiota–gut–brain axis is an important regulator of weight control, including after bariatric surgery [126].

Finally, another interesting point is the connection between appetite, taste preferences, and eating behavior since some changes in appetite and taste preferences have been reported after bariatric surgery [128]. A recent study by Zhang et al. [129] investigated the association between presurgical taste preferences and postsurgical weight regain. They included patients who underwent RYGB or SG and had at least 2 years of follow up, and they assessed preoperative taste preferences with a multichoice questionnaire. They found that patients with sweet food preferences had 5.5 kg of weight regain (p = 0.038), and patients with salty food preferences had 6.1 kg of weight regain (p = 0.048) compared to patients with no taste preferences. After adjustment, patients with salty food preferences showed the greater weight regain with 6.8 kg (p = 0.027) compared to patients with no preferences. Though these results from just one study do not allow to establish robust evidence, it is a very interesting approach to identify more factors related to weight maintenance in the long-term after bariatric surgery.

In summary, there are very complex and intricate systems connecting gut hormones, microbiota, and the CNS that play an important role in appetite control and energy homeostasis. Thus, the changes produced by SG and RYGB in this complex gut–brain axis seem to influence weight maintenance in the medium- and long-term after surgery.

7. Conclusions

Bariatric surgery is the most effective intervention for weight loss in obese patients, although it is not exempt from possible long-term failure and weight regain. Multiple factors that may be related to long-term weight maintenance have been described, ranging from the surgical technique itself to anatomical and functional modifications that lead to changes in the microbiota–gut–brain axis through gastrointestinal hormones, bile acids, and FXR-TGR5 influence on skeletal muscle and brown adipose tissue or dopaminergic pathways related to appetite control and energy homeostasis. Similarly, factors such as changes in lifestyle related to diet and physical activity, psychological factors such as executive function disorders, and the coexistence of depressive symptoms and eating disorders can play important roles in maintaining long-term weight loss. Therefore, numerous mechanisms may contribute to changes in lifestyle and weight maintenance after bariatric surgery; thus, continuous and comprehensive care interventions appear to be the most successful approaches to maintaining. However, some data are discordant, and more long-term studies are necessary in order to clearly identify predictive factors of weight regain that allow us to optimize the management and follow-up of the obese patient undergoing bariatric surgery.

Author Contributions: Conceptualization, F.J.T. and I.C.-P.; methodology, M.M.-V.; investigation, I.C.-P., A.M.G.-P. and M.M.-V.; resources, M.D.-F. and A.M.G.-P.; writing—original draft preparation, I.C.-P., M.M.-V. and A.M.G.-P.; writing—review and editing, I.C.-P., M.M.-V. and A.M.G.-P.; visualization, M.D.-F.; supervision, F.J.T. All authors have read and agreed to the published version of the manuscript.

Funding: ICP was supported by Rio Hortega, and Juan Rodes from the Spanish Ministry of Economy and Competitiveness (ISCIII), and cofounded by Fondo Europeo de Desarrollo Regional-FEDER (CM 17/00169, JR 19/00054). MMV was supported by Rio Hortega from the Spanish Ministry of Economy and Competitiveness (ISCIII) and cofounded by Fondo Europeo de Desarrollo Regional-FEDER (CM18/00120). AMGP was supported by a research contract from Servicio Andaluz de Salud (B-0033-2014). MDF was supported by Rio Hortega from the Spanish Ministry of Economy and Competitiveness (ISCIII) and cofounded by Fondo Europeo de Desarrollo Regional-FEDER (CM20/00183). This study was supported by the "Centros de Investigación Biomédica en Red" (CIBER) of the Institute of Health Carlos III (ISCIII) (CB06/03/0018), research grants from the ISCIII (PI18/01160), and co-financed by the European Regional Development Fund (ERDF). The funders had no role in the manuscript.

Institutional Review Board Statement: Not applicable.

Informed Consent Statement: Not applicable.

Data Availability Statement: Not applicable.

Conflicts of Interest: The authors declare no conflict of interest.

References

1. Bischoff, S.C.; Schweinlin, A. Obesity therapy. *Clin. Nutr. ESPEN* **2020**, *38*, 9–18. [CrossRef] [PubMed]
2. González-Muniesa, P.; Mártinez-González, M.A.; Hu, F.B.; Després, J.P.; Matsuzawa, Y.; Loos, R.J.F.; Moreno, L.A.; Bray, G.A.; Martinez, J.A. Obesity. *Nat. Rev. Dis. Primers* **2017**, *15*, 17034. [CrossRef]
3. Janssen, F.; Bardoutsos, A.; Vidra, N. Obesity prevalence in the long-term future in 18 european countries and in the USA. *Obes. Facts* **2020**, *13*, 514–527. [CrossRef]
4. Petroni, M.L.; Caletti, M.T.; Calugi, S.; Dalle Grave, R.; Marchesini, G. Long-term treatment of severe obesity: Are lifestyle interventions still an option? *Expert Rev. Endocrinol. Metab.* **2017**, *12*, 391–400. [CrossRef] [PubMed]
5. Belligoli, A.; Bettini, S.; Segato, G.; Busetto, L. Predicting responses to bariatric and metabolic surgery. *Curr. Obes. Rep.* **2020**, *9*, 373–379. [CrossRef]
6. Nguyen, N.T.; Varela, J.E. Bariatric surgery for obesity and metabolic disorders: State of the art. *Nat. Rev. Gastroenterol. Hepatol.* **2017**, *14*, 160–169. [CrossRef] [PubMed]
7. Arterburn, D.E.; Telem, D.A.; Kushner, R.F.; Courcoulas, A.P. Benefits and risks of bariatric surgery in adults: A review. *JAMA* **2020**, *324*, 879–887. [CrossRef]
8. Hu, Z.; Sun, J.; Li, R.; Wang, Z.; Ding, H.; Zhu, T.; Wang, G.A. Comprehensive comparison of LRYGB and LSG in obese patients including the effects on QoL, comorbidities, weight loss, and complications: A systematic review and meta-analysis. *Obes. Surg.* **2020**, *30*, 819–827. [CrossRef] [PubMed]
9. Yang, P.; Chen, B.; Xiang, S.; Lin, X.F.; Luo, F.; Li, W. Long-term outcomes of laparoscopic sleeve gastrectomy versus Roux-en-Y gastric bypass for morbid obesity: Results from a meta-analysis of randomized controlled trials. *Surg. Obes. Relat. Dis.* **2019**, *15*, 546–555. [CrossRef]
10. Hayoz, C.; Hermann, T.; Raptis, D.A.; Brönnimann, A.; Peterli, R.; Zuber, M. Comparison of metabolic outcomes in patients undergoing laparoscopic Roux-en-Y gastric bypass versus sleeve gastrectomy—A systematic review and meta-analysis of randomised controlled trials. *Swiss Med. Wkly.* **2018**, *148*, 14633.
11. Osland, E.; Yunus, R.M.; Khan, S.; Memon, B.; Memon, M.A. Weight loss outcomes in laparoscopic vertical sleeve gastrectomy (LVSG) versus laparoscopic Roux-en-Y gastric bypass (LRYGB) procedures: A meta-analysis and systematic review of randomized controlled trials. *Surg. Laparosc. Endosc. Percutan. Tech.* **2017**, *27*, 8–18. [CrossRef]
12. King, W.C.; Hinerman, A.S.; Courcoulas, A.P. Weight regain after bariatric surgery: A systematic literature review and comparison across studies using a large reference sample. *Surg. Obes. Relat. Dis.* **2020**, *16*, 1133–1144. [CrossRef]
13. Kang, J.H.; Le, Q.A. Effectiveness of bariatric surgical procedures: A systematic review and network meta-analysis of randomized controlled trials. *Medicine* **2017**, *96*, e8632. [CrossRef] [PubMed]
14. Zhao, H.; Jiao, L. Comparative analysis for the effect of Roux-en-Y gastric bypass vs. sleeve gastrectomy in patients with morbid obesity: Evidence from 11 randomized clinical trials (meta-analysis). *Int. J. Surg.* **2019**, *72*, 216–223. [CrossRef]
15. Park, C.H.; Nam, S.J.; Choi, H.S.; Kim, K.O.; Kim, D.H.; Kim, J.W.; Sohn, W.; Yoon, J.H.; Jung, S.H.; Hyun, Y.S.; et al. Korean research group for endoscopic management of metabolic disorder and obesity. comparative efficacy of bariatric surgery in the treatment of morbid obesity and diabetes mellitus: A systematic review and network meta-analysis. *Obes. Surg.* **2019**, *29*, 2180–2190. [CrossRef]
16. O'Brien, P.E.; Hindle, A.; Brennan, L.; Skinner, S.; Burton, P.; Smith, A.; Crosthwaite, G.; Brown, W. Long-term outcomes after bariatric surgery: A systematic review and meta-analysis of weight loss at 10 or more years for all bariatric procedures and a single-centre review of 20-year outcomes after adjustable gastric banding. *Obes. Surg.* **2019**, *29*, 3–14. [CrossRef]
17. Salminen, P.; Helmiö, M.; Ovaska, J.; Juuti, A.; Leivonen, M.; Peromaa-Haavisto, P.; Hurme, S.; Soinio, M.; Nuutila, P.; Victorzon, M. Effect of laparoscopic sleeve gastrectomy vs. laparoscopic Roux-en-Y gastric bypass on weight loss at 5 years among patients with morbid obesity: The SLEEVEPASS randomized clinical trial. *JAMA* **2018**, *16*, 241–254. [CrossRef] [PubMed]
18. Grönroos, S.; Helmiö, M.; Juuti, A.; Tiusanen, R.; Hurme, S.; Löyttyniemi, E.; Ovaska, J.; Leivonen, M.; Peromaa-Haavisto, P.; Mäklin, S.; et al. Effect of laparoscopic sleeve gastrectomy vs. Roux-en-Y gastric bypass on weight loss and quality of life at 7 years in patients with morbid obesity: The SLEEVEPASS randomized clinical trial. *JAMA Surg.* **2020**, *9*, e205666.
19. Hofsø, D.; Fatima, F.; Borgeraas, H.; Birkeland, K.I.; Gulseth, H.L.; Hertel, J.K.; Johnson, L.K.; Lindberg, M.; Nordstrand, N.; Småstuen, M.C.; et al. Gastric bypass versus sleeve gastrectomy in patients with type 2 diabetes (Oseberg): A single-centre, triple-blind, randomised controlled trial. *Lancet Diabetes Endocrinol.* **2019**, *7*, 912–924. [CrossRef]
20. Murphy, R.; Clarke, M.G.; Evennett, N.J.; John, R.S.; Lee, H.M.; Hammodat, H.; Jones, B.; Kim, D.D.; Cutfield, R.; Johnson, M.H.; et al. Laparoscopic sleeve gastrectomy versus banded Roux-en-Y gastric bypass for diabetes and obesity: A prospective randomised double-blind trial. *Obes. Surg.* **2018**, *28*, 293–302. [CrossRef] [PubMed]
21. Schneider, J.; Peterli, R.; Gass, M.; Slawik, M.; Peters, T.; Wölnerhanssen, B.K. Laparoscopic sleeve gastrectomy and Roux-en-Y gastric bypass lead to equal changes in body composition and energy metabolism 17 months postoperatively: A prospective randomized trial. *Surg. Obes. Relat. Dis.* **2016**, *12*, 563–570. [CrossRef] [PubMed]

22. Peterli, R.; Wölnerhanssen, B.K.; Vetter, D.; Nett, P.; Gass, M.; Borbély, Y.; Peters, T.; Schiesser, M.; Schultes, B.; Beglinger, C.; et al. Laparoscopic sleeve gastrectomy versus Roux-Y-gastric bypass for morbid obesity-3-year outcomes of the prospective randomized Swiss multicenter bypass or sleeve study (SM-BOSS). *Ann. Surg.* **2017**, *265*, 466–473. [CrossRef]
23. Peterli, R.; Wölnerhanssen, B.K.; Peters, T.; Vetter, D.; Kröll, D.; Borbély, Y.; Schultes, B.; Beglinger, C.; Drewe, J.; Schiesser, M.; et al. Effect of laparoscopic sleeve gastrectomy vs. laparoscopic Roux-en-Y gastric bypass on weight loss in patients with morbid obesity: The SM-BOSS randomized clinical trial. *JAMA* **2018**, *319*, 255–265. [CrossRef]
24. Seetharamaiah, S.; Tantia, O.; Goyal, G.; Chaudhuri, T.; Khanna, S.; Singh, J.P.; Ahuja, A. LSG vs. OAGB-1 year follow-up data—A randomized control trial. *Obes. Surg.* **2017**, *27*, 948–954. [CrossRef]
25. Shivakumar, S.; Tantia, O.; Goyal, G.; Chaudhuri, T.; Khanna, S.; Ahuja, A.; Poddar, A.; Majumdar, K. LSG vs. MGB-OAGB-3-year follow-up data: A randomised control trial. *Obes. Surg.* **2018**, *28*, 2820–2828. [CrossRef] [PubMed]
26. Ignat, M.; Vix, M.; Imad, I.; D'Urso, A.; Perretta, S.; Marescaux, J.; Mutter, D. Randomized trial of Roux-en-Y gastric bypass versus sleeve gastrectomy in achieving excess weight loss. *Br. J. Surg.* **2017**, *104*, 248–256. [CrossRef]
27. Hedberg, S.; Olbers, T.; Peltonen, M.; Österberg, J.; Wirén, M.; Ottosson, J.; Thorell, A.; BEST Study Group. BEST: Bypass equipoise sleeve trial; rationale and design of a randomized, registry-based, multicenter trial comparing Roux-en-Y gastric bypass with sleeve gastrectomy. *Contemp. Clin. Trials* **2019**, *84*, 105809. [CrossRef] [PubMed]
28. Rudolph, A.; Hilbert, A. Cognitive-behavioral therapy for postbariatric surgery patients with mental disorders: A pilot study. *Front. Psychiatry* **2020**, *11*, 14. [CrossRef]
29. Raman, J.; Smith, E.; Hay, P. The clinical obesity maintenance model: An integration of psychological constructs including mood, emotional regulation, disordered overeating, habitual cluster behaviours, health literacy and cognitive function. *J. Obes.* **2013**. [CrossRef]
30. Gunstad, J.; Paul, R.H.; Cohen, R.A.; Tate, D.F.; Spitznagel, M.B.; Gordon, E. Elevated body mass index is associated with executive dysfunction in otherwise healthy adults. *Compr. Psychiatry* **2007**, *48*, 57–61. [CrossRef]
31. Stuss, D.T.; Benson, D.F. *The Frontal Lobes*; Ravan Press: New York, NY, USA, 1996.
32. Smith, E.; Hay, P.; Campbell, L.; Trollor, J.N. A review of the association between obesity and cognitive function across the lifespan: Implications for novel approaches to prevention and treatment. *Obes. Rev.* **2011**, *12*, 740–755. [CrossRef]
33. Favieri, F.; Forte, G.; Casagrande, M. The executive functions in overweight and obesity: A systematic review of neuropsychological cross-sectional and longitudinal studies. *Front. Psychol.* **2019**, *10*, 2126. [CrossRef]
34. Yang, Y.; Shields, G.S.; Guo, C.; Liu, Y. Executive function performance in obesity and overweight individuals: A meta-analysis and review. *Neurosci. Biobehav. Rev.* **2018**, *84*, 225–244. [CrossRef]
35. Pignatti, R.; Bertella, L.; Albani, G.; Mauro, A.; Molinari, E.; Semenza, C. Decision-making in obesity: A study using the gambling task. *Eat. Weight Disord. Stud. Anorex. Bulim. Obes.* **2006**, *11*, 126–132. [CrossRef] [PubMed]
36. Tchanturia, K.; Liao, P.-C.; Uher, R.; Lawrence, N.; Treasure, J.; Campbell, I.C. An investigation of decision making in anorexia nervosa using the Iowa gambling task and skin conductance measurements. *J. Int. Neuropsychol. Soc. JINS* **2007**, *13*, 635–641. [CrossRef] [PubMed]
37. Tchanturia, K.; Davies, H.; Lopez, C.; Schmidt, U.; Treasure, J.; Wykes, T. Neuropsychological task performance before and after cognitive remediation in anorexia nervosa: A pilot case-series. *Psychol. Med.* **2008**, *38*, 1371–1373. [CrossRef]
38. Roberts, M.E.; Demetriou, L.; Treasure, J.L.; Tchanturia, K. Neuropsychological profile in the overweight population: An exploratory study of set-shifting and detail focused processing styles. *Therapy* **2007**, *4*, 821–824. [CrossRef]
39. Dohle, S.; Diel, K.; Hofmann, W. Executive functions and the self-regulation of eating behavior: A review. *Appetite* **2018**, *124*, 4–9. [CrossRef]
40. Small, D.M. Dopamine adaptations as a common pathway for neurocognitive impairment in diabetes and obesity: A neuropsychological perspective. *Front. Neurosci.* **2017**, *11*, 134. [CrossRef]
41. Rashidian, H.; Rosenblat, J.D.; McIntyre, R.S.; Mansur, R.B. Leptin, obesity, and response to ketamine. *Prog. Neuro Psychopharmacol. Biol. Psychiatry* **2020**, *98*, 109773. [CrossRef] [PubMed]
42. Alosco, M.L.; Spitznagel, M.B.; Strain, G.; Devlin, M.; Cohen, R.; Crosby, R.D.; Mitchell, J.E.; Gunstad, J. Improved serum leptin and ghrelin following bariatric surgery predict better postoperative cognitive function. *J. Clin. Neurol.* **2015**, *11*, 48–56. [CrossRef]
43. Luppino, F.S.; Leonore, M.; Wit, D.L.M.; Bouvy, P.F.; Stijnen, T.; Cuijpers, P.; Penninx, B.W.J.H.P.; Frans, G.Z. Overweight, obesity, and depression: A systematic review and meta-analysis of longitudinal studies. *Arch. Gen. Psychiatry* **2010**, *67*, 220–229. [CrossRef] [PubMed]
44. Linde, J.A.; Simon, G.E.; Ludman, E.J.; Ichikawa, L.E.; Operskalski, B.H.; Arterburn, D.; Rohde, P.; Finch, E.A.; Jeffery, R.W. A randomized controlled trial of behavioral weight loss treatment versus combined weight loss/depression treatment among women with comorbid obesity and depression. *Ann. Behav. Med.* **2011**, *41*, 119–130. [CrossRef]
45. Spitznagel, M.B.; Garcia, S.; Miller, L.A.; Strain, G.; Devlin, M.; Wing, R.; Cohen, R.; Paul, R.; Crosby, R.; Mitchell, J.E.; et al. Cognitive function predicts weight loss following bariatric surgery. *Surg. Obes. Relat. Dis.* **2013**, *9*, 453–459. [CrossRef] [PubMed]
46. Handley, J.D.; Williams, D.M.; Caplin, S.; Stephens, J.W.; Barry, J. Changes in cognitive function following bariatric surgery: A systematic review. *Obes. Surg.* **2016**, *26*, 2530–2537. [CrossRef] [PubMed]
47. Spitznagel, M.B.; Alosco, M.; Strain, G.; Devlin, M.; Cohen, R.; Paul, R.; Crosby, R.D.; Mitchell, J.E.; Gunstad, P.D.J. Cognitive function predicts 24-month weight loss success following bariatric surgery. *Surg. Obes. Relat. Dis.* **2013**, *9*, 765–770. [CrossRef]

48. Spitznagel, M.B.; Alosco, M.; Galioto, R.; Strain, G.; Devlin, M.; Sysko, R.; Crosby, R.D.; Mitchell, J.E.; Gunstad, J. The role of cognitive function in postoperative weight loss outcomes: 36-month follow-up. *Obes. Surg.* **2014**, *24*, 1078–1084. [CrossRef]
49. Alosco, M.L.; Galioto, R.; Spitznagel, M.B.; Strain, G.; Devlin, M.; Cohen, R.; Crosby, R.D.; Mitchell, J.E.; Gunstad, J. Cognitive function following bariatric surgery: Evidence for improvement 3 years post-surgery. *Am. J. Surg.* **2014**, *207*, 870–876. [CrossRef] [PubMed]
50. Kulendran, M.; Borovoi, L.; Purkayastha, S.; Darzi, A.; Vlaev, I. Impulsivity predicts weight loss after obesity surgery. *Surg. Obes. Relat. Dis.* **2017**, *13*, 1033–1040. [CrossRef]
51. Bergh, I.; Kvalem, L.I.; Risstad, H.; Sniehotta, F.F. Preoperative predictors of adherence to dietary and physical activity recommendations and weight loss one year after surgery. *Surg. Obes. Relat. Dis.* **2016**, *12*, 910–918. [CrossRef] [PubMed]
52. Mauro, M.F.F.P.; Papelbaum, M.; Brasil, M.A.A.; Carneiro, J.R.I.; Coutinho, E.S.F.; Coutinho, W.; Appolinario, J.C. Is weight regain after bariatric surgery associated with psychiatric comorbidity? A systematic review and meta-analysis. *Obes. Rev.* **2019**, *20*, 1413–1425. [CrossRef]
53. Conceição, E.M.; Mitchell, J.E.; Pinto-Bastos, A.; Arrojado, F.; Brandão, I.; Machado, P.P. Stability of problematic eating behaviors and weight loss trajectories after bariatric surgery: A longitudinal observational study. *Surg. Obes. Relat.* **2017**, *13*, 1063–1070. [CrossRef] [PubMed]
54. Smith, K.E.; Orcutt, M.; Steffen, K.J.; Crosby, R.D.; Cao, L.; Garcia, L.; Mitchell, J.E. Loss of control eating and binge eating in the 7 years following bariatric surgery. *Obes. Surg.* **2019**, *29*, 1773–1780. [CrossRef]
55. Brode, C.S.; Mitchell, J.E. Problematic eating behaviors and eating disorders associated with bariatric surgery. *Psychiatr. Clin.* **2019**, *42*, 287–297. [CrossRef]
56. Gunstad, J.; Strain, G.; Devlin, M.J.; Wing, R.; Cohen, R.A.; Paul, R.H.; Crosby, R.D.; Mitchell, J.E. Improved memory function 12 weeks after bariatric surgery. *Surg. Obes. Relat. Dis. Off. J. Am. Soc. Bariatr. Surg.* **2011**, *7*, 465–472. [CrossRef]
57. Calvo, D.; Galioto, R.; Gunstad, J.; Spitznagel, M.B. Uncontrolled eating is associated with reduced executive functioning. *Clin. Obes.* **2014**, *4*, 172–179. [CrossRef]
58. Müller, A.; Hase, C.; Pommnitz, M.; Zwaan, D.M. Depression and suicide after bariatric surgery. *Curr. Psychiatry Rep.* **2019**, *21*, 84. [CrossRef]
59. Ribeiro, G.A.N.A.; Giapietro, H.B.; Belarmino, L.B.; Salgado-Junior, W. Depression, anxiety, and binge eating before and after bariatric surgery: Problems that remain. *ABCD. Arq. Bras. Cir. Dig.* **2018**, *31*, e1356. [CrossRef] [PubMed]
60. Romain, A.; Marleau, J.; Baillot, A. Impact of obesity and mood disorders on physical comorbidities, psychological well-being, health behaviours and use of health services. *J Affect. Disord.* **2017**, *225*, 381–388. [CrossRef]
61. Freire, C.C.; Zanella, M.T.; Segal, A.; Arasaki, C.H.; Matos, M.I.R.; Carneiro, G. Associations between binge eating, depressive symptoms and anxiety and weight regain after Roux-en-Y gastric bypass surgery. *Eat. Weight Disord.* **2020**, 191–199. [CrossRef] [PubMed]
62. Novelli, I.R.; Fonseca, L.G.; Gomes, D.L.; Dutra, E.S.; Carvalho, D.B.K.M. Emotional eating behavior hinders body weight loss in women after Roux-en-Y gastric bypass surgery. *Nutrition* **2018**, *49*, 13–16. [CrossRef]
63. Feig, E.H.; Golden, J.; Huffman, J.C. Emotional impact on health behavior adherence after bariatric surgery: What about positive psychological constructs? *Obes. Surg.* **2019**, *29*, 2238–2246. [CrossRef] [PubMed]
64. Goldschmidt, A.B.; Conceição, E.M.; Thomas, J.G.; Mitchell, J.E.; Raynor, H.A.; Bond, D.S. Conceptualizing and studying binge and loss of control eating in bariatric surgery patients-time for a paradigm shift? *Surg. Obes. Relat.Dis.* **2016**, *12*, 1622–1625. [CrossRef] [PubMed]
65. He, J.; Cai, Z.; Fan, X. Prevalence of binge and loss of control eating among children and adolescents with overweight and obesity: An exploratory meta-analysis. *Int. J. Eat. Disord.* **2017**, *50*, 91–103. [CrossRef]
66. Goldschmidt, A.B.; Khoury, J.; Jenkins, T.M.; Bond, D.S.; Thomas, J.G.; Utzinger, L.M.; Zeller, M.H.; Inge, T.H.; Mitchell, J.E. Adolescent loss-of-control eating and weight loss maintenance after bariatric surgery. *Pediatrics* **2018**, *141*. [CrossRef]
67. White, M.A.; Kalarchian, M.A.; Masheb, R.M.; Marcus, M.D.; Grilo, C.M. Loss of control over eating predicts outcomes in bariatric surgery patients: A prospective, 24-month follow-up study. *J. Clin. Psychiatry* **2010**, *71*, 175–184. [CrossRef] [PubMed]
68. Peterhänsel, C.; Linde, K.; Wagner, B.; Dietrich, A.; Kersting, A. Subtypes of personality and "locus of control" in bariatric patients and their effect on weight loss, eating disorder and depressive symptoms, and quality of life. *Eur. Eat Disord. Rev.* **2017**, *25*, 397–405. [CrossRef]
69. Gordon, P.C.; Sallet, J.A.; Sallet, P.C. The impact of temperament and character inventory personality traits on long-term outcome of Roux-en-Y Gastric Bypass. *Obes. Surg.* **2014**, *24*, 1647–1655. [CrossRef] [PubMed]
70. National Institute for Health and Care Excelence (NICE). Obesity: Identification, Assessment and Management of Overweight and Obesity in Children, Young People and Adults. In *NICE Clinical Guideline*, 189th ed.; NICE: London, UK, 2014; p. 37.
71. Goodpaster, B.H.; Delany, J.P.; Otto, A.D.; Kuller, L.; Vockley, J.; South-Paul, J.E.; Thomas, S.B.; Brown, J.; McTigue, K.; Hames, K.C.; et al. Effects of diet and physical activity interventions on weight loss and cardiometabolic risk factors in severely obese adults: A randomized trial. *JAMA* **2010**, *304*, 1795–1802. [CrossRef]
72. Bond, D.S.; Jakicic, J.M.; Vithiananthan, S.; Thomas, J.G.; Leahey, T.M.; Sax, H.C.; Pohl, D.; Roye, G.D.; Ryder, B.A.; Wing, R.R. Objective quantification of physical activity in bariatric surgery candidates and normal-weight controls. *Surg. Obes. Relat. Dis.* **2010**, *6*, 72–78. [CrossRef]

73. Elkins, G.; Whitfield, P.; Marcus, J.; Symmonds, R.; Rodriguez, J.; Cook, T. Noncompliance with behavioral recommendations following bariatric surgery. *Obes. Surg.* **2005**, *15*, 546–551. [CrossRef] [PubMed]
74. King, W.C.; Hsu, J.Y.; Belle, S.H.; Courcoulas, A.P.; Eid, G.M.; Flum, D.R.; Mitchell, J.E.; Pender, J.R.; Smith, M.D.; Steffen, K.J.; et al. Pre- to postoperative changes in physical activity: Report from the longitudinal assessment of bariatric surgery-2 (LABS-2). *Surg. Obes. Relat.* **2012**, *8*, 522–532. [CrossRef]
75. Bond, D.S.; Jakicic, J.M.; Unick, J.L.; Vithiananthan, S.; Pohl, D.; Roye, G.D.; Ryder, B.A.; Sax, H.C.; Wing, R.R. Pre-to post-operative physical activity changes in bariatric surgery patients: Self-report vs. objective measures. *Obesity* **2010**, *18*, 2395–2397. [CrossRef]
76. Ouellette, K.A.; Mabey, J.G.; Eisenman, P.A.; Shaw, J.M.; Brusseau, T.A.; Hatfield, D.L.; Ford, C.N.; Davidson, L.E. Physical activity patterns among individuals before and soon after bariatric surgery. *Obes. Surg.* **2020**, *30*, 416–422. [CrossRef]
77. Carnero, E.A.; Dubis, G.S.; Hames, K.C.; Jakicic, J.M.; Houmard, J.A.; Coen, P.M.; Goodpaster, B.H. Randomized trial reveals that physical activity and energy expenditure are associated with weight and body composition after RYGB. *Obesity* **2017**, *25*, 1206–1216. [CrossRef]
78. Egberts, K.; Brown, W.A.; Brennan, L.; O'Brien, P.E. Does exercise improve weight loss after bariatric surgery? A systematic review. *Obes. Surg.* **2012**, *22*, 335–341. [CrossRef] [PubMed]
79. Rothwell, L.; Kow, L.; Toouli, J. Effect of a post-operative structured exercise programme on short-term weight loss after obesity surgery using adjustable gastric bands. *Obes. Surg.* **2015**, *25*, 126–128. [CrossRef]
80. Bellicha, A.; Ciangura, C.; Poitou, C.; Portero, P.; Oppert, J.-M. Effectiveness of exercise training after bariatric surgery-a systematic literature review and meta-analysis. *Obes. Rev.* **2018**, *19*, 1544–1556. [CrossRef] [PubMed]
81. Hanvold, S.E.; Vinknes, K.J.; Løken, E.B.; Hjartåker, A.; Klungsøyr, O.; Birkeland, E.; Risstad, H.; Gulseth, H.L.; Refsum, H.; Aas, A.M. Does lifestyle intervention after gastric bypass surgery prevent weight regain? A randomized clinical trial. *Obes. Surg.* **2019**, *29*, 3419–3431. [CrossRef]
82. Vatier, C.; Henegar, C.; Ciangura, C.; Poitou-Bernert, C.; Bouillot, J.-L.; Basdevant, A.; Oppert, J.M. Dynamic relations between sedentary behavior, physical activity, and body composition after bariatric surgery. *Obes. Surg.* **2012**, *22*, 1251–1256. [CrossRef]
83. Evans, R.K.; Bond, D.S.; Wolfe, L.G.; Meador, J.G.; Herrick, J.E.; Kellum, J.M.; Maher, J.W. Participation in 150 min/wk of moderate or higher intensity physical activity yields greater weight loss after gastric bypass surgery. *Surg. Obes. Relat. Dis.* **2007**, *3*, 526–530. [CrossRef]
84. Herman, K.M.; Carver, T.E.; Christou, N.V.; Andersen, R.E. Keeping the weight off: Physical activity, sitting time, and weight loss maintenance in bariatric surgery patients 2 to 16 years post-surgery. *Obes. Surg.* **2014**, *24*, 1064–1072. [CrossRef] [PubMed]
85. Kaviani, S.; Dadgostar, H.; Mazaherinezhad, A.; Adib, H.; Solaymani-Dodaran, M.; Soheilipour, F.; Hakiminezhad, M. Comparing minimally supervised home-based and closely supervised gym-based exercise programs in weight reduction and insulin resistance after bariatric surgery: A randomized clinical trial. *Med. J. Islam. Repub. Iran* **2017**, *31*, 34. [CrossRef] [PubMed]
86. Woodlief, T.L.; Carnero, E.A.; Standley, R.A.; Distefano, G.; Anthony, S.J.; Dubis, G.S.; Jakicic, J.M.; Houmard, J.A.; Coen, P.M.; Goodpaster, B.H. Dose response of exercise training following roux-en-Y gastric bypass surgery: A randomized trial. *Obesity* **2015**, *23*, 2454–2461. [CrossRef]
87. Ryder, J.R.; Gross, A.C.; Fox, C.K.; Kaizer, A.M.; Rudser, K.D.; Jenkins, T.M.; Ratcliff, M.B.; Kelly, A.S.; Kirk, S.; Siegel, R.M.; et al. Factors associated with long-term weight-loss maintenance following bariatric surgery in adolescents with severe obesity. *Int. J. Obes.* **2005**, *42*, 102–107. [CrossRef] [PubMed]
88. Coen, P.M.; Tanner, C.J.; Helbling, N.L.; Dubis, G.S.; Hames, K.C.; Xie, H.; Eid, G.M.; Stefanovic-Racic, M.; Toledo, F.G.; Jakicic, J.M.; et al. Clinical trial demonstrates exercise following bariatric surgery improves insulin sensitivity. *J. Clin. Invest.* **2015**, *125*, 248–257. [CrossRef] [PubMed]
89. Shah, M.; Snell, P.G.; Rao, S.; Adams-Huet, B.; Quittner, C.; Livingston, E.H.; Garg, A. High-volume exercise program in obese bariatric surgery patients: A randomized, controlled trial. *Obesity (Silver Spring)* **2011**, *19*, 1826–1834. [CrossRef]
90. Coleman, K.J.; Caparosa, S.L.; Nichols, J.F.; Fujioka, K.; Koebnick, C.; McCloskey, K.N.; Ngor, E.; Levy, S. Understanding the capacity for exercise in post-bariatric patients. *Obes. Surg.* **2017**, *27*, 51–58. [CrossRef]
91. Herring, L.Y.; Stevinson, C.; Carter, P.; Biddle, S.J.H.; Bowrey, D.; Sutton, C.; Davies, M.J. The effects of supervised exercise training 12-24 months after bariatric surgery on physical function and body composition: A randomised controlled trial. *Int. J. Obes.* **2017**, *41*, 909–916. [CrossRef]
92. Shaw, K.; O'Rourke, P.; Del Mar, C.; Kenardy, J. Psychological interventions for overweight or obesity. *Cochrane Database Syst. Rev.* **2005**. CD003818. [CrossRef]
93. Metcalf, B.; Rabkin, R.A.; Rabkin, J.M.; Metcalf, L.J.; Lehman-Becker, L.B. Weight loss composition: The effects of exercise following obesity surgery as measured by bioelectrical impedance analysis. *Obes. Surg.* **2005**, *15*, 183–186. [CrossRef]
94. Chaston, T.B.; Dixon, J.B.; O'Brien, P.E. Changes in fat-free mass during significant weight loss: A systematic review. *Int. J. Obes.* **2007**, *31*, 743–750. [CrossRef]
95. Miller, S.L.; Wolfe, R.R. The danger of weight loss in the elderly. *J. Nutr. Health Aging* **2008**, *12*, 487–491. [CrossRef]
96. Churchward-Venne, T.A.; Tieland, M.; Verdijk, L.B.; Leenders, M.; Dirks, M.L.; Groot, D.L.C.; Van Loon, L.J. There are no nonresponders to resistance-type exercise training in older men and women. *J. Am. Med. Dir. Assoc.* **2015**, *16*, 400–411. [CrossRef]
97. Forman, E.M.; Butryn, M.L.; Manasse, S.M.; Crosby, R.D.; Goldstein, S.P.; Wyckoff, E.P.; Thomas, J.G. Acceptance-based versus standard behavioral treatment for obesity: Results from the mind your health randomized controlled trial. *Obesity (Silver Spring)* **2016**, *24*, 2050–2056. [CrossRef]

98. Sarwer, D.B.; Wadden, T.A.; Moore, R.H.; Baker, A.W.; Gibbons, L.M.; Raper, S.E.; Williams, N.N. Preoperative eating behavior, postoperative dietary adherence, and weight loss after gastric bypass surgery. *Surg. Obes. Relat. Dis.* **2008**, *4*, 640–646. [CrossRef] [PubMed]
99. Thomas, J.G.; Bond, D.S.; Phelan, S.; Hill, J.O.; Wing, R.R. Weight-loss maintenance for 10 years in the national weight control registry. *Am. J. Prev. Med.* **2014**, *46*, 17–23. [CrossRef] [PubMed]
100. Bray, G.; Smith, S.; Jonge, D.L.; Souza, D.R.; Rood, J.; Champagne, C.; Laranjo, N.; Carey, V.; Obarzanek, E.; Loria, C.M.; et al. Effect of diet composition on energy expenditure during weight loss: The POUNDS LOST Study. *Int. J. Obes.* **2012**, *36*, 448–455. [CrossRef] [PubMed]
101. Grave, D.R.; Calugi, S.; Gavasso, I.; El Ghoch, M.; Marchesini, G. A randomized trial of energy-restricted high-protein versus high-carbohydrate, low-fat diet in morbid obesity. *Obesity (Silver Spring)* **2013**, *21*, 1774–1781. [CrossRef]
102. Reid, R.E.R.; Oparina, E.; Plourde, H.; Andersen, R.E. Energy intake and food habits between weight maintainers and regainers, five years after Roux-en-Y gastric bypass. *Can. J. Diet. Pract. Res.* **2016**, *77*, 195–198. [CrossRef]
103. Faria, S.L.; Oliveira, D.K.E.; Faria, O.P.; Ito, M.K. Snack-eating patients experience lesser weight loss after Roux-en-Y gastric bypass surgery. *Obes. Surg.* **2009**, *19*, 1293–1296. [CrossRef]
104. Spaggiari, G.; Santi, D.; Budriesi, G.; Dondi, P.; Cavedoni, S.; Leonardi, L.; Delvecchio, C.; Valentini, L.; Bondi, M.; Miloro, C.; et al. Eating behavior after bariatric surgery (EBBS) questionnaire: A new validated tool to quantify the patients' compliance to post-bariatric dietary and lifestyle suggestions. *Obes. Surg.* **2020**, *30*, 3831–3838. [CrossRef] [PubMed]
105. Ebbeling, C.B.; Swain, J.F.; Feldman, H.A.; Wong, W.W.; Hachey, D.L.; Garcia-Lago, E.; Ludwig, D.S. Effects of dietary composition on energy expenditure during weight-loss maintenance. *JAMA* **2012**, *307*, 2627–2634. [CrossRef]
106. Larsen, T.M.; Dalskov, S.-M.; Van Baak, M.; Jebb, S.A.; Papadaki, A.; Pfeiffer, A.F.H.; Martinez, J.A.; Handjieva-Darlenska, T.; Kunešová, M.; Pihlsgård, M.; et al. Diets with high or low protein content and glycemic index for weight-loss maintenance. *N. Engl. J. Med.* **2010**, *363*, 2102–2113. [CrossRef]
107. Mitchell, J.E.; Christian, N.J.; Flum, D.R.; Pomp, A.; Pories, W.J.; Wolfe, B.M.; Courcoulas, A.P.; Belle, S.H. Postoperative behavioral variables and weight change 3 years after bariatric surgery. *JAMA Surg.* **2016**, *151*, 752–757. [CrossRef]
108. Koliaki, C.; Liatis, S.; Dalamaga, M.; Kokkinos, A. The implication of gut hormones in the regulation of energy homeostasis and their role in the pathophysiology of obesity. *Curr. Obes. Rep.* **2020**, *9*, 255–271. [CrossRef] [PubMed]
109. Karra, E.; Batterham, R.L. The role of gut hormones in the regulation of body weight and energy homeostasis. *Mol. Cell Endocrinol.* **2010**, *316*, 120–128. [CrossRef] [PubMed]
110. Da Silva, A.; Salem, V.; Long, C.J.; Makwana, A.; Newbould, R.D.; Rabiner, E.A.; Ghatei, M.A.; Bloom, S.R.; Matthews, P.M.; Beaver, J.D.; et al. The gut hormones PYY 3-36 and GLP-17-36 amide reduce food intake and modulate brain activity in appetite centers in humans. *Cell Metab.* **2011**, *14*, 700–706. [CrossRef] [PubMed]
111. Madsbad, S. The role of glucagon-like peptide-1 impairment in obesity and potential therapeutic implications. *Diabetes Obes. Metab.* **2014**, *16*, 9–21. [CrossRef]
112. Steinert, R.E.; Feinle-Bisset, C.; Asarian, L.; Horowitz, M.; Beglinger, C.; Geary, N.; Ghrelin, C.C.K. GLP-1, and PYY (3–36): Secretory controls and physiological roles in eating and glycemia in health, obesity, and after RYGB. *Physiol Rev.* **2017**, *97*, 411–463. [CrossRef]
113. Dockray, G.J. Cholecystokinin. *Curr. Opin. Endocrinol. Diabetes Obes.* **2012**, *19*, 8–12. [CrossRef] [PubMed]
114. Malin, S.K.; Kashyap, S.R. Differences in weight loss and gut hormones: Rouen-Y gastric bypass and sleeve gastrectomy surgery. *Curr. Obes. Rep.* **2015**, *4*, 279–286. [CrossRef] [PubMed]
115. Cummings, D.E. Endocrine mechanisms mediating remission of diabetes after gastric bypass surgery. *Int. J. Obes.* **2009**, *33*, 33–40. [CrossRef]
116. Mithieux, G. A novel function of intestinal gluconeogenesis: Central signaling in glucose and energy homeostasis. *Nutrition* **2009**, *25*, 881–884. [CrossRef] [PubMed]
117. Salinari, S.; Debard, C.; Bertuzzi, A.; Durand, C.; Zimmet, P.; Vidal, H.; Mingrone, G. Jejunal proteins secreted by db/db mice or insulin-resistant humans impair the insulin signaling and determine insulin resistance. *PLoS ONE* **2013**, *8*, e56258. [CrossRef]
118. Perakakis, N.; Kokkinos, A.; Peradze, N.; Tentolouris, N.; Ghaly, W.; Pilitsi, E.; Upadhyay, J.; Alexandrou, A.; Mantzoros, C.S. Circulating levels of gastrointestinal hormones in response to the most common types of bariatric surgery and predictive value for weight loss over one year: Evidence from two independent trials. *Metabolism* **2019**, *101*, 153997. [CrossRef] [PubMed]
119. Santo, M.A.; Riccioppo, D.; Pajecki, D.; Kawamoto, F.; Cleva, D.R.; Antonangelo, L.; Marçal, L.; Cecconello, I. Weight regain after gastric bypass: Influence of gut hormones. *Obes. Surg.* **2016**, *26*, 919–925. [CrossRef] [PubMed]
120. Alamuddin, N.; Vetter, M.L.; Ahima, R.S.; Hesson, L.; Ritter, S.; Minnick, A.; Faulconbridge, L.F.; Allison, K.C.; Sarwer, D.B.; Chittams, J.; et al. Changes in fasting and prandial gut and adiposity hormones following vertical sleeve gastrectomy or Roux-en-Y-gastric bypass: An 18-month prospective study. *Obes. Surg.* **2017**, *27*, 1563–1572. [CrossRef]
121. Ahmad, N.N.; Pfalzer, A.; Kaplan, L.M. Roux-en-Y gastric bypass normalizes the blunted postprandial bile acid excursion associated with obesity. *Int. J. Obes.* **2013**, *37*, 1553–1559. [CrossRef]
122. Liou, A.P.; Pazik, M.; Luevano, J.M., Jr.; Machineni, S.; Turnbaugh, P.J.; Kaplan, L.M. Conserved shifts in the gut microbiota due to gastric bypass reduce host weight and adiposity. *Sci. Transl. Med.* **2013**, *5*, 178ra41. [CrossRef] [PubMed]

123. Thomas, C.; Gioiello, A.; Noriega, L.; Strehle, A.; Oury, J.; Rizzo, G.; Macchiarulo, A.; Yamamoto, H.; Mataki, C.; Pruzanski, M.; et al. TGR5-mediated bile acid sensing controls glucose homeostasis. *Cell Metab.* **2009**, *10*, 167–177. [CrossRef] [PubMed]
124. Duüfer, M.; Hörth, K.; Wagner, R.; Schittenhelm, B.; Prowald, S.; Wagner, T.F.; Oberwinkler, J.; Lukowski, R.; Gonzalez, F.J.; Krippeit-Drews, P.; et al. Bile acids acutely stimulate insulin secretion of mouse β-cells via farnesoid X receptor activation and K(ATP) channel inhibition. *Diabetes* **2012**, *61*, 1479–1489.
125. Carrasco, F.; Papapietro, K.; Csendes, A.; Salazar, G.; Echenique, C.; Lisboa, C.; Díaz, E.; Rojas, J. Changes in resting energy expenditure and body composition after weight loss following Roux-en-Y gastric bypass. *Obes. Surg.* **2007**, *17*, 608–616. [CrossRef] [PubMed]
126. Orellana, E.R.; Covasa, M.; Hajnal, A. Neuro-hormonal mechanisms underlying changes in reward related behaviors following weight loss surgery: Potential pharmacological targets. *Biochem. Pharmacol.* **2019**, *164*, 106–114. [CrossRef] [PubMed]
127. Kroemer, N.B.; Small, D.M. Fuel not fun: Reinterpreting attenuated brain responses to reward in obesity. *Physiol. Behav.* **2016**, *162*, 37–45. [CrossRef] [PubMed]
128. Pepino, M.Y.; Bradley, D.; Eagon, J.C.; Sullivan, S.; Abumrad, N.A.; Klein, S. Changes in taste perception and eating behavior after bariatric surgery-induced weight loss in women. *Obesity* **2014**, *22*, E13–E20. [CrossRef]
129. Zhang, Y.; Nagarajan, N.; Portwood, C.; Smith, K.R.; Kamath, V.; Carnell, S.; Moran, T.H.; Steele, K.E. Does taste preference predict weight regain after bariatric surgery? *Surg. Endosc.* **2020**, *34*, 2623–2629. [CrossRef] [PubMed]

Journal of
Clinical Medicine

MDPI

Review

Bariatric Surgery and Hypertension

Elisenda Climent [1,2,3], Anna Oliveras [2,4,5,6], Juan Pedro-Botet [1,2,3], Albert Goday [1,2,3,7] and David Benaiges [1,2,3,8,*]

1 Endocrinology Department, Hospital Universitari del Mar, 08003 Barcelona, Spain; ecliment@parcdesalutmar.cat (E.C.); 86620@parcdesalutmar.cat (J.P.-B.); agoday@parcdesalutmar.cat (A.G.)
2 IMIM (Hospital del Mar Medical Research Institute), 08003 Barcelona, Spain; 87052@parcdesalutmar.cat
3 Department of Medicine, Universitat Autònoma de Barcelona, 08139 Barcelona, Spain
4 Nephrology Department, Hospital Universitari del Mar, 08003 Barcelona, Spain
5 Department of Experimental and Health Sciences, Area of Medicine, Universitat Pompeu Fabra, 08002 Barcelona, Spain
6 Red de Investigación Renal (REDINREN), Instituto Carlos III-FEDER, 28029 Madrid, Spain
7 Centro de Investigaciones Biomédicas en Red de Obesidad y Nutrición, CIBERobn, 28029 Madrid, Spain
8 Consorci Sanitari de l'Alt Penedès i Garraf, 08720 Vilafranca del Penedès, Spain
* Correspondence: 96002@parcdesalutmar.cat; Tel.: +34-93-248-3902; Fax: +34-93-248-3254

Abstract: A clear pathogenetic association exists between obesity and arterial hypertension, becoming even more evident in subjects with severe obesity. Bariatric surgery has proved to be the most effective treatment for severe obesity, with its benefits going beyond weight loss. The present review aimed to determine the effects of bariatric surgery on arterial hypertension evident in short- and long-term follow-ups. Moreover, the differences between surgical techniques regarding hypertension remission are described as well as the possible pathophysiologic mechanisms involved. In addition, the effects of bariatric surgery beyond blood pressure normalization are also analyzed, including those on target organs and cardiovascular morbidity and mortality.

Keywords: bariatric surgery; obesity; severe obesity; hypertension; blood pressure; modifications of structural changes

Citation: Climent, E.; Oliveras, A.; Pedro-Botet, J.; Goday, A.; Benaiges, D. Bariatric Surgery and Hypertension. *J. Clin. Med.* **2021**, *10*, 4049. https://doi.org/10.3390/jcm10184049

Academic Editor: Emmanuel Andrès

Received: 23 July 2021
Accepted: 7 September 2021
Published: 7 September 2021

1. Introduction

Hypertension (HTN) is one of the best known and most widely studied cardiovascular risk factors, and a close correlation between obesity and HTN has been extensively demonstrated [1]. Thus, HTN prevalence in subjects with obesity varies between 60 and 77%, and it is clearly higher than the 34% observed in subjects with normal weight [2]. The mechanisms by which obesity raises the risk of developing HTN are multifactorial, involving structural, functional, and hemodynamic changes in the cardiovascular system [3].

Conventional medical treatment for morbid obesity has previously achieved mild outcomes, which are probably related to limited long-term adherence to lifestyle modifications in some patients [1]. By contrast, bariatric surgery (BS) has proved to be the most effective therapy for these patients when both weight loss and comorbidity remission after surgery, including HTN, were evaluated [2,3].

In this respect, owing to the widely known systematic review published by Buchwald et al. [3] in 2004, which included a total of 22,094 patients, it has been accepted that approximately three of every five subjects undergoing BS achieve HTN remission. However, it must be considered that this meta-analysis mainly included studies with a short-term follow-up, with the surgical procedures performed at that time (gastric bypass (GB), gastric band, and biliopancreatic diversion), and most studies were retrospective and with great heterogeneity regarding HTN remission definition. In recent years, several prospective studies have reported mid- and long-term results after surgery, with laparoscopic sleeve gastrectomy (LSG) emerging as the most used BS technique worldwide [4]. Moreover, the possible underlying mechanisms responsible for HTN improvement after BS have been further evaluated, together with the possible benefits beyond weight loss. The present narrative review aimed to delve into these newly acquired data.

2. Bariatric Surgery Effects on Blood Pressure

2.1. Short-Term Effects on Blood Pressure

HTN remission in the short term (<3 years) after BS has been widely analyzed in observational studies, some meta-analyses, and a few randomized controlled trials (RCT) [5–9]. Schiavon et al. [10] in 2018 published the first RCT specifically aimed at evaluating the effect of BS on HTN remission. The GATEWAY (Gastric Bypass to Treat Obese Patients with Steady Hypertension) trial [10] included patients with HTN (using $\geq$2 medications at maximum doses or >2 at moderate doses) and a body mass index between 30.0 and 39.9 kg/m^2. Subjects were randomized to GB plus medical therapy or medical therapy alone. The primary endpoint ($\geq$30% reduction in the total number of antihypertensive medications while maintaining systolic and diastolic blood pressure < 140 and 90 mmHg, respectively, at 12 months) occurred more frequently in the GB group (83.7%) compared to the control group (12.8%). Moreover, HTN remission 1 year after surgery, defined as systolic and diastolic blood pressure < 140 and 90 mmHg, respectively, with previous withdrawal of all medication, occurred in approximately one-half of the patients in the GB group and none in the conventional treatment group. It is noteworthy that the HTN remission rate after BS obtained in the GATEWAY trial [10] was lower than those described in other previous reports [5,6,9], including the Buchwald et al. meta-analysis [3]. This was probably due to the first including patients who required an "aggressive" antihypertensive treatment, in comparison to the other studies where the included patients needed one or no antihypertensive medication. Hence, taking these results into account, if BS were primarily indicated to control refractory HTN, the chance of achieving remission would probably be close to 50% in the short term. In accordance with these data, it has been reported that the number of antihypertensive drugs prior to surgery was associated with a lower remission rate during the first year [9]. Another relevant result obtained from the GATEWAY study was that no differences in systolic and diastolic blood pressure levels were observed between groups during follow-up. This seems to indicate that if good titration of the medication is made during follow-up considering blood pressure levels, the effects of BS on HTN are mainly reflected in the reduction in the number of antihypertensive medications.

2.2. Mid- and Long-Term Effects

Less evidence exists on the mid- (3–5 years) and long-term (>5 years) effects of BS on HTN remission compared to other obesity comorbidities such as type 2 diabetes, and this evidence is mainly available from observational studies [2,11,12].

The results obtained in the mid- and long-term after BS were more modest compared to those achieved with a shorter-term follow-up. Regarding this, our group had previously evaluated HTN remission after BS with a 36-month follow-up, observing that 68.1% of hypertensive patients showed HTN remission 1 year after the surgical procedure, 21.9% of whom had relapsed at 3 years [9]. A possible justification for these less favorable results seems to be explained, at least in part, by weight regain after surgery. It must be taken into account that maximum weight loss is achieved during the first 12 months post-surgery, and from this point onwards, weight regain and worsening of certain metabolic parameters usually emerge. This coincides with the results obtained in our cohort, where milder weight loss during the first year was also associated with increased HTN recurrence at 3 years [9].

However, BS still presents more beneficial outcomes in the mid- and long-term follow-up compared to conventional treatment. In this respect, various RCT [13–15] compared BS to conventional treatment with a 5-year follow-up. Mingrone et al. [13] found that the BS group and conventional treatment maintained similar blood pressure levels 60 months after surgery. Nevertheless, more subjects in the latter group required antihypertensive medication (73% with conventional treatment versus 58% after GB and 32% after biliopancreatic diversion). Similarly, Ikramuddin et al. [15] also found a favorable trend toward BS. In that study, primary systolic blood pressure < 130 mm Hg at 5 years was obtained in 73% in the GB group versus 49% in the lifestyle and intensive medical management group (odds ratio (OR), 2.71; 95% CI, 0.95–7.78; $p = 0.06$).

The superior results obtained with a surgical approach compared to lifestyle modifications have also been further confirmed with a longer-term follow-up. In this respect, the Swedish Obese Subjects cohort [2] observed a greater reduction in blood pressure levels after GB compared to a non-surgical approach, with a mean follow-up of 10 years. Moreover, the percentage of patients requiring antihypertensive treatment was also lower after BS compared to the control group (35% vs. 53%; $p < 0.001$), with these results being in line with other previous studies [11,16].

Systematic reviews and meta-analyses also confirmed the superiority of BS, which was previously observed with a short-term follow-up. In this respect, Vest et al. [17] in 2012 (including 70 observational studies and three RCT) reported a 63% resolution or improvement in HTN with a mean follow-up of approximately 5 years. Similarly, Wilhelm et al. [8] in 2014 (including 31 prospective and 26 retrospective studies) observed 50% and 63.7% HTN resolution or improvement, respectively, with a mean follow-up varying from 1 week to 7 years post-surgery. Of the 57 studies included, 32 reported HTN improvement (OR, 13.24; 95% CI, 7.73–22.68; $p < 0.00001$) and 46 reported HTN resolution (OR, 1.70; 95% CI, 1.13–2.58; $p = 0.01$).

However, although studies with a longer follow-up confirmed the beneficial outcomes after BS in comparison to conventional treatment regarding HTN evolution, an RCT specifically focused on evaluating HTN remission at mid- and long-term after BS is lacking. Moreover, the possible differences among the most used surgical procedures (including malabsortive, restrictive, or both surgical approaches) must not be ignored, as detailed below.

2.3. Differences among Surgical Procedures

Considering the different BS procedures, GB has been considered, until recently, the gold standard technique owing to its favorable results in both weight loss and comorbidity remission [18]. However, in recent years, LSG also proved to achieve comparable promising results to GB, hence becoming the most used BS procedure in 2014 [4]. Moreover, LSG is a technically easier procedure compared to GB [19,20], with a presumably lower risk of perioperative complications [18].

In order to shed light on the effects of both BS techniques, our group carried out a meta-analysis to evaluate 1 and 5-year HTN remission after both procedures [21]. Thirty-two articles were involved, with a higher HTN remission rate being observed with GB compared to LSG both at 1 year (RR, 1.14, 95% CI, 1.06–1.21) and at 5 years (RR, 1.26, 95% CI, 1.07–1.48) after surgery. Blood pressure improvement after surgery was also evaluated. No differences were found between GB and LSG in terms of systolic or diastolic blood pressure changes at both 1 and 5 years. Thus, we could speculate that although patients in the LSG group were less likely to present HTN remission after BS, and hence not all the antihypertensive medication could be withdrawn, overall blood pressure levels in both groups were equivalent after surgery. It is also important to highlight the fact that the superiority of GB over LSG was observed when all studies were included, as well as when only the highest evidence studies (RCT) were evaluated.

Thus, although some studies obtained more promising results regarding HTN remission after GB compared to LSG, the superiority of GB must be further confirmed with longer-term follow-up (>5 years).

2.4. Metabolic Surgery and HTN

Owing to the favorable results (which go beyond weight loss) of BS in obese subjects, the concept of metabolic surgery has gained importance in recent years [22], with the focus on the physiologic modifications that occur after surgery, which lead to comorbidity improvement [23]. Moreover, the metabolic effects of the surgical procedure become more evident when obesity comorbidities improve within days after BS and when significant weight loss has not yet been achieved [8].

This fact has opened debate on whether BS should be indicated in patients with body mass index < 35 kg/m^2 for comorbidity improvement, which was addressed in previous observational publications mainly aimed at glycemic improvement after surgery but also at achieving hopeful results regarding HTN remission [24,25].

Five RCT [5,26–29] also assessed the effects of BS in subjects with class I obesity, observing positive results in blood pressure evolution, nearly equivalent to those obtained in patients with body mass index > 35 kg/m^2 (Table 1). However, the main limitation when evaluating these data was the heterogeneity of the definitions used for remission or improvement in the different studies, as some considered total withdrawal of antihypertensive medication and others only blood pressure normalization. In order to standardize all studies evaluating comorbidity remission with grade I obesity, the International Federation for the Surgery of Obesity and Metabolic Disorders (IFSO) realized a position statement in 2014 [30] summarizing the scientific background concerning BS in class I obesity. They concluded that a clinical decision of whether to deny BS to these patients should be based on a more comprehensive evaluation of the patient's current global health and on a more reliable prediction of future morbidity and mortality. Hence, future observational studies and RCT with a longer-term follow-up are necessary.

Table 1. Randomized trials of bariatric surgery including patients with body mass index <35 kg/m^2.

Study	*N*	BMI (kg/m^2)	Follow-Up (Months)	Intervention Groups	Weight Loss	HTN-Related Outcomes
O'Brien et al.	80	30–35	24	LAGB Conventional therapy	87.2% EWL 21.8% EWL	−10.8% decrease in SBP/−10.9% decrease in DBP −7.2% decrease in SBP/−1.58% decrease in DBP
Dixon et al.	60	30–40 (21.7% BMI < 35)	24	LAGB Conventional therapy	20.7 TWL 1.7 TWL	−6.0 mmHg decrease in SBP/−0.7 mmHg decrease in DBP −1.7 mmHg decrease in SBP/−0.9 mmHg decrease in DBP
Lee et al.	60	25–35	12	Minigastric bypass LSG	94% EWL 76% EWL	12 months: SBP 119.6 mmHg/DBP 74.2 mmHg 12 months: SBP 123.5 mmHg/DBP 75.4 mmHg
Schauer et al.	150	27–43 (34% BMI < 35)	12	LRYGB LSG Intensive medical therapy	88% EWL 81% EWL 13% EWL	78% subjects antiHTN medication baseline/33% at 12 months 67% subjects antiHTN medication baseline/27% at 12 months 76% subjects antiHTN medication baseline/77% at 12 months
Ikramunddin et al.	120	30–40 (59.2% BMI < 35)	12	LRYGB Intensive medical therapy	26.1 TWL 7.9 TWL	Remission: 84% subjects SBP < 130 mmHg at 12 months 12 months: SBP 115 mmHg/DBP 68 mmHg Remission: 79% subjects SBP < 130 mmHg at 12 months 12 months: SBP 124 mmHg/DBP 74 mmHg

BMI: body mass index; DBP: diastolic blood pressure; EWL: excess weight loss; HTN: hypertension; LABG: laparoscopic adjustable gastric banding; LRYGB: laparoscopic Roux-en Y gastric bypass; LSG: laparoscopic sleeve gastrectomy; SBP: systolic blood pressure; TWL: total weight loss.

2.5. Possible Mechanisms Related to HTN Improvement

Although weight loss has proved to be a key factor in comorbidity improvement after BS, other underlying factors may also play an important role. With regard to blood pressure improvement after BS, the reasons are probably multifactorial and remain under debate (Figure 1) [31,32].

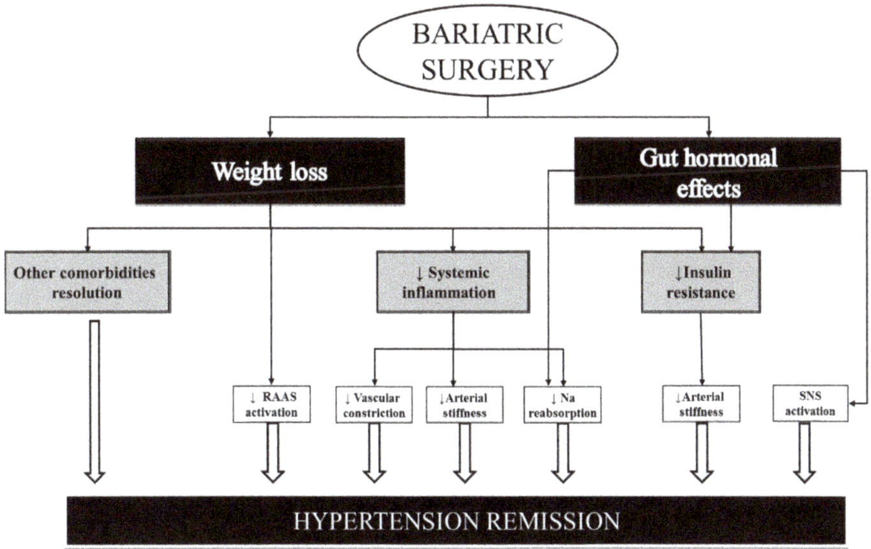

Figure 1. Mechanisms related to HTN remission. RAAS = Renin–angiotensin–aldosterone system; Na = Sodium; SNS ≠ sympathetic nervous system. ↑ ≠ increase; ↓ ≠ decrease.

It has been speculated that a decreased inflammatory response together with an improvement in insulin resistance could reduce arterial stiffness and sodium reabsorption and hence lead to normalization of blood pressure levels [33]. Patients with central obesity are known to have increased activation of the renin–angiotensin–aldosterone system, which may also normalize after surgery [34].

In addition, an increase in gastrointestinal gut hormones such as peptide YY (PYY) and glucagon-like peptide-1 (GLP-1) could also play an important part due to their effects on the gastrointestinal system together with a diuretic and natriuretic effect on the kidney [35]. Furthermore, a possible effect of GLP-1 on the sympathetic nervous system, which may play a part in the blood pressure-lowering effect after BS, has also been described [36]. Ghrelin may also aid in normalizing blood pressure levels, although its levels may raise, fall, or remain unchanged after BS, depending on the surgical procedure [37].

Furthermore, adipokines and other inflammatory cytokines also appear to be related to HTN recovery. In this respect, previous studies observed a decline in leptin levels from 1 week up to 1 year after BS together with increasing adiponectin concentrations [38]. Moreover, as insulin sensitivity increases, C-reactive protein and interleukin-6 levels decrease, thus ameliorating adipocyte inflammation and in turn preventing vascular constriction [39].

Finally, the resolution of other obesity comorbidities (which share pathophysiologic mechanisms with HTN) such as obstructive sleep apnea could also play a part in blood pressure improvement [40,41].

The underlying mechanisms related to the possible superiority of GB over LSG are also worth mentioning. The main accepted hypothesis is that these differences could be explained by the superior weight loss after GB in the mid- and long-term follow-up. As mentioned previously, the possible role of gastrointestinal hormones in HTN improvement after surgery gains value, as some studies observed a decrease in blood pressure levels within the first week post-BS and when weight loss was minimal [8]. In this respect, a previous study found significant reductions in both systolic (9 mm Hg) and diastolic (7 mm Hg) blood pressure 1 week after GB, and these were maintained 1 year after surgery [42]. Considering the different surgical procedures, GLP-1 and PYY are known to increase after both, but they increase more intensely after GB [42,43], which may account for the more favorable results after this procedure.

3. Bariatric Surgery Benefits beyond Blood Pressure Improvement

3.1. Organ Damage Changes

Patients with morbid obesity have a higher prevalence of target organ damage than patients of normal weight, and HTN is clearly related to its development. These target organ alterations mostly refer to changes in heart, vessels, and kidney structure and function [44].

3.1.1. Cardiac Changes

Regarding cardiac changes, several works reported echocardiographic alterations, both morphologic and functional, in obese patients [45,46]. The main alterations consisted of left ventricular (LV) hypertrophy and impaired LV diastolic function, while LV systolic dysfunction was less common and, on these lines, reports concerning the ejection fraction in obese patients were contradictory [47]. Morphologic LV alterations have been described in patients with morbid obesity, with 56% of LV hypertrophy being reported from a meta-analysis of 22 studies including 5486 obese subjects [45]. Many of these changes are precursors of more overt forms of cardiac dysfunction and heart failure [48]. Indeed, obesity clearly increases the risk of atrial fibrillation, myocardial infarction, heart failure, and sudden death [49]. Beyond findings from observational epidemiology, Larsson et al. [50] recently found evidence that a genetically instrumented 1 kg/m^2 higher body mass index is associated with an increased risk of aortic stenosis, heart failure, deep venous thrombosis, HTN, peripheral artery disease, coronary artery disease, atrial fibrillation, and pulmonary embolism (estimates in the range of 6–13% higher risk). The findings for fat mass were broadly consistent. Specifically, the link between obesity and heart failure is known to be stronger than those for other cardiovascular disease subtypes and is uniquely unexplained by traditional risk factors [51]. However, the findings apparently diverged from observational studies for ischemic stroke, and this field merits further investigation [50].

In relation to the mechanisms responsible for cardiac improvement after BS, several authors concur in that the effects of weight-loss surgery on cardiac function and morphology are either hormonally or centrally regulated, probably with an important role for leptin and other adipokines [52], as well as for the renin–angiotensin–aldosterone axis [53]; however, further insight needs to be gained into the mechanisms underlying changes in cardiovascular function after weight loss.

Importantly, these cardiovascular structure and function alterations have also proved to be reversible with weight loss strategies such as BS, resulting in lowered cardiovascular risk [54]. The effects of BS on cardiac structure and function were recorded in a systematic review of 23 studies and meta-analysis [55], showing that in obese patients with preserved LV systolic function, BS induced significant decrements of absolute LV mass and relative wall thickness (RWT), which are all reliable indexes of LV hypertrophy and LV geometry that have been shown to predict cardiovascular outcomes. Furthermore, that meta-analysis showed improvements in LV diastolic function, as reflected by a clear-cut increase in the mitral flow ratio of the early (E) to late (A) ventricular filling velocities (E/A ratio), as well as decreases in left atrium size, which is an indirect marker of chronically elevated LV filling pressure and diastolic dysfunction. As for LV hypertrophy and RWT, similar results were reported by Owan et al. [56] 2 years after BS. Those authors found that the decreases in LV mass index and RWT correlated with body mass index reduction but not with changes in blood pressure. Of note, one of the most salient observations of the BARIHTA study by our group was that even severely-obese patients with strictly normal blood pressure experience an improvement in morphologic and functional LV parameters after BS [53].

3.1.2. Vessel Changes

One of the main manifestations of vessel alteration is the development of arterial stiffness (AS). It is considered to be an independent cardiovascular risk factor [57] and is defined as the diminished ability of an artery to expand and contract in response to a given pressure change [58]. Pulse wave velocity (PWV) is the gold standard for AS measurement [59]. In the last two decades, excess body weight has been found to be associated with greater aortic stiffness in young and older adults [60]. Therefore, increased AS may be one of the mechanisms by which obesity raises cardiovascular risk independently of traditional risk factors. Indeed, high PWV predicts outcomes independent of the Framingham Risk Score, and it is associated with increased cardiovascular disease risk regardless of HTN status [61]. On the same lines, some authors suggested that AS may precede rises in systolic blood pressure and incident HTN in obese individuals [62].

Regarding the effect of BS on AS, several studies reported a significant decrease in both PWV and the augmentation index, another marker of AS, several months after BS [63–65]. The potential mechanisms responsible for the reduction in AS after weight loss are not clear. Some authors [66] found a correlation between weight loss and reduction in PWV independently of changes in established hemodynamic and cardiometabolic risk factors, and other groups [64], but not all [60], suggested that this correlation is mediated by the drop in blood pressure. On the other hand, elevated cardiac volume and output in obese individuals were also noted as possible mediators of AS, more importantly than elevated BP [67].

3.1.3. Renal Changes

Obesity is an independent risk factor for kidney disease, regardless of diabetes and HTN, both of which are driven largely by obesity [68]. Hyperfiltration is the hallmark of obesity-associated kidney dysfunction, and the main proposed mechanisms for this association are hemodynamic factors, inflammatory cytokines, and renal lipotoxicity [68,69]. As regards hemodynamic factors [70], excessive weight initially causes functional renal vasodilation and increases in renal blood flow and glomerular hyperfiltration prior to nephron injury. These changes are later followed by declines in renal blood flow and the glomerular filtration rate (GFR) as a result of kidney injury and gradual loss of nephrons. Increased extracellular fluid volume results from the obesity-associated increase in tubular sodium reabsorption. This may be related to the elevated levels of anti-natriuretic hormones such as angiotensin II and aldosterone, as a consequence of both kidney compression by visceral, perirenal, and renal sinus fat and of the increased renal sympathetic nerve activity. These and other contributors may be linked by the altered macula densa feedback (tubuloglomerular feedback) to the observed afferent arteriola vasodilation. Sodium balance may be re-established despite increased sodium chloride reabsorption in the loop of Henle through compensatory increases in the GFR and blood pressure elevation. Furthermore, mineralocorticoid receptor (MR) activation may also contribute to renal vasodilation. MR expressed on macula densa cells are activated by aldosterone, thereby increasing their production of nitric oxide and leading to renal vasodilation and glomerular hyperfiltration. Despite the adaptative value of glomerular hyperfiltration in offsetting renal sodium reabsorption, this increase in glomerular hydrostatic pressure probably contributes greatly to the renal injury observed in obesity.

Obesity also favors a deleterious adipocytokine pattern [68,69] characterized by the overproduction of angiotensinogen and angiotensin II as well as the upregulation of pro-inflammatory cytokines such as interleukin-6, C-reactive protein, and tumor necrosis factor-α. These factors induce renal fibrosis via the transforming growth factor-β (TGF-β) pathway and via oxidative stress, as shown by experimental models. Moreover, obese individuals are known to have high levels of serum leptin and high expression of leptin receptors in the kidney, which also stimulate cellular proliferation and expression of the prosclerotic TGF-β1 cytokine implicated in the early scarring formation of renal failure. Finally, reduced levels of another adipokine, adiponectin, have been implicated as a mechanism of obesity-related renal impairment through podocyte damage leading to albuminuria. Pathologic changes due to long-lasting hyperfiltration include the development of glomerulomegaly and renal lesions of focal segmental glomerulosclerosis, leading to obesity-related glomerulopathy [71]. Thus, hyperfiltration, i.e., GFR higher than 120 mL/min/1.73 m^2, and albuminuria, biomarkers of kidney function and damage, respectively, characterize renal alterations in obese patients.

The gold-standard method to assess the GFR is measurement of the renal clearance of an exogenous filtration tracer (inulin, 51 Cr-EDTA, 125 I-iothalamat, iohexol); however, most studies use GFR (eGFR) estimations derived from prediction equations. These equations were obtained by regression analyses in various populations with body mass index < 30 kg/m^2, where the GFR was measured by the gold standard method, but these are not accurate in obesity classes II and III [68]. Thus, it is unclear how reliably creatinine-based eGFR equations perform among those with obesity, especially when faced with results normalized to a body surface area of 1.73 m^2 since, after BS, patients lose not only fat but also muscle mass, which generates creatinine [72]. Furthermore, although body surface area, which is considered in the eGFR equations, is vastly reduced after BS, it is not reflected in the eGFR results routinely available [73]. Cystatin C has been suggested as a potential alternative since, unlike creatinine, it does not come strictly from muscle. However, it has not been validated as a reliable biomarker of GFR in obese patients, nor has its laboratory assay been standardized as for creatinine. On the other hand, measurement of albumin excretion rates via albumin-to-creatinine ratios (ACR) in fresh spot urines or absolute excretion rates in timed urine collection has become a more reliable measurement of renal damage [74].

Overall, patients with complicated obesity will likely benefit from the weight loss after BS [75]. Li et al. [76] reported a systematic review and meta-analysis from 32 studies showing significant reductions in hyperfiltration (measured GFR, eGFR, and creatinine clearance with and without adjustment for body surface area), albuminuria (defined as an ACR of more than 30 mg/g of creatinine), and proteinuria after BS. They reported a reduction in hyperfiltration (RR: 0.46, 95% CI 0.26–0.82, $p = 0.008$) after surgery when analyzed as a dichotomous variable as well as statistically significant decreases. Moreover, drops were observed in the incidences of albuminuria and proteinuria after BS of 58% and 69%, respectively ($p < 0.0001$ for both). Data on the 4047 patients included in the Swedish Obese Subjects study [77], comparing patients undergoing BS and controls followed up for a median time of 18 years, showed a lower incidence of chronic kidney disease (CKD) stages 4 and 5 in patients in the surgery group (adjusted HR = 0.33; 95% CI 0.18–0.62; $p < 0.001$). Similarly, O'Brien et al. [78] in a retrospective analysis reported a 59% lower incidence of nephropathy at 5 years in a cohort of 4000 diabetic patients undergoing BS compared to 11,000 matched non-surgically treated patients. Friedman et al. [75] analyzed 2144 obese patients who underwent BS and found an improvement in CKD risk categories in a large proportion of patients over a 7-year follow-up period. They reported that the reduction in risk was most pronounced in persons with high baseline risk.

As regards renal protective factors, Favre et al. [68] reported that low C-reactive protein levels, high fat mass, lack of HTN, and young age predicted kidney protection in severely obese patients undergoing BS.

The mechanisms behind the improvement in risk factors following BS are not well understood. Glomerular function may be related to restoration in homeostasis of the renin–angiotensin system through better renal perfusion and to the restitution of normal insulin signaling in glomerular podocytes and attenuation of hyperfiltration. Additionally, this improvement may also be secondary to reductions in the pro-inflammatory state related to obesity [74] as measured by urinary monocyte-chemoattractant protein-1/creatinine ratios [73]. It has recently been shown that the glucagon-like peptide 1 (GLP-1), an incretin hormone released by intestinal endocrine L cells, exerts renoprotective effects by inhibiting tubular reabsorption of sodium. These effects increase after BS, suggesting a role in the improvement in glomerular function. As for albuminuria remission, at least in obese diabetics, the restitution of podocyte health may be a key cellular event contributing to the benefits of BS.

Obese patients who undergo BS may also experience some renal complications. Lieske et al. [72] reported that up to 50% of these patients might be hyperoxaluric one year after surgery, and the risk of new kidney stone events doubled compared with unoperated obese controls. Nevertheless, the net effect on long-term kidney health is potentially positive for most patients.

3.2. Implications in Cardiovascular Morbidity and Mortality

Moving a step forward, the next question to answer is: what is the real impact of HTN improvement after BS in terms of cardiovascular morbidity and mortality reduction? It has previously been reported that BS reduces the number of cardiovascular events and mortality rates in patients with morbid obesity. For instance, the Swedish Obese Subjects Study Group [79] observed a reduced number of cardiovascular deaths in the surgical group compared to the control group (28 events among 2010 patients vs. 49 events among 2037 patients; adjusted hazard ratio (HR), 0.47; 95% CI, 0.29–0.76; $p = 0.002$) during a median follow-up of 14.7 years. In that same cohort, the number of total fatal or non-fatal cardiovascular events (myocardial infarction or stroke) was also lower in patients undergoing BS. Other studies yielded similar results, thereby confirming the beneficial effects of BS on cardiovascular morbidity and mortality [80,81].

Although the observed reduction in cardiovascular disease prevalence after BS is probably multifactorial, it can be assumed that HTN improvement probably plays a key role, although this remains to be confirmed. In fact, the Swedish Cohort [79] failed to find an association between weight loss and cardiovascular event reduction, thus highlighting the possible role of other factors that could explain the improvement in cardiovascular outcomes. In this respect, the decline in cardiovascular risk following the improvement in blood pressure levels after BS could be related to a reduction in target organ damage (including cardiac, vessel, and renal changes), as described previously in the present review [44,82].

However, the possible "obesity paradox" must also be acknowledged. This refers to a more favorable evolution regarding cardiovascular or renal outcomes in patients with a higher body mass index. This possible paradoxical effect observed in some studies could be explained by increased tumor necrosis factor (TNF-α) receptors in adipose tissue or an earlier diagnosis of cardiovascular events in the obese population, among others. Despite this, the underlying mechanisms of this possible paradox in obese population are still being investigated in order to achieve more solid conclusions [83].

4. Conclusions

BS has proved to be a highly effective treatment for obesity-associated HTN, achieving HTN remission in more than half of patients. However, a greater need for antihypertensive medication prior to BS and less weight loss during follow-up are both factors that may hinder the achievement of complete HTN remission.

Moreover, a decline in cardiovascular morbidity and mortality has also been observed after BS in morbidly obese subjects. These favorable results regarding cardiovascular outcomes may be mediated by multiple mechanisms that go beyond weight loss, one of which may be improved blood pressure levels together with a decline in target organ damage. However, future studies are required in this field for more solid conclusions to be drawn.

Author Contributions: All authors contributed equally to this review. All authors have read and agreed to the published version of the manuscript.

Funding: This research received no external funding.

Institutional Review Board Statement: Not applicable.

Informed Consent Statement: Not applicable.

Data Availability Statement: Not applicable.

Acknowledgments: We thank Christine O'Hara for review of the English version of the manuscript.

Conflicts of Interest: The authors declare no conflict of interest.

References

1. Dansinger, M.L.; Tatsioni, A.; Wong, J.B.; Chung, M.; Balk, E.M. Meta-analysis: The effect of dietary counseling for weight loss. *Ann. Intern. Med.* **2007**, *147*, 41–50. [CrossRef]
2. Sjöström, L.; Lindroos, A.-K.; Peltonen, M.; Torgerson, J.; Bouchard, C.; Carlsson, B.; Dahlgren, S.; Larsson, B.; Narbro, K.; Sjöström, C.D.; et al. Lifestyle, Diabetes, and Cardiovascular Risk Factors 10 Years after Bariatric Surgery. *N. Engl. J. Med.* **2004**, *351*, 2683–2693. [CrossRef]
3. Buchwald, H.; Avidor, Y.; Braunwald, E.; Jensen, M.D.; Pories, W.; Fahrbach, K.; Schoelles, K. Bariatric surgery: A systematic review and meta-analysis. *JAMA* **2004**, *292*, 1724–1737. [CrossRef] [PubMed]
4. Angrisani, L.; Santonicola, A.; Iovino, P.; Vitiello, A.; Zundel, N.; Buchwald, H.; Scopinaro, N. Bariatric Surgery and Endoluminal Procedures: IFSO Worldwide Survey 2014. *Obes. Surg.* **2017**, *27*, 2279–2289. [CrossRef] [PubMed]
5. Schauer, P.R.; Kashyap, S.R.; Wolski, K.; Brethauer, S.A.; Kirwan, J.P.; Pothier, C.E.; Thomas, S.; Abood, B.; Nissen, S.E.; Bhatt, D.L. Bariatric surgery versus intensive medical therapy in obese patients with diabetes. *N. Engl. J. Med.* **2012**, *366*, 1567–1576. [CrossRef] [PubMed]
6. Mingrone, G.; Panunzi, S.; De Gaetano, A.; Guidone, C.; Iaconelli, A.; Leccesi, L.; Nanni, G.; Pomp, A.; Castagneto, M.; Ghirlanda, G.; et al. Bariatric surgery versus conventional medical therapy for type 2 diabetes. *N. Engl. J. Med.* **2012**, *109*, 1155. [CrossRef] [PubMed]
7. Zhang, Y.; Zhao, H.; Cao, Z.; Sun, X.; Zhang, C.; Cai, W.; Liu, R.; Hu, S.; Qin, M. A randomized clinical trial of laparoscopic Roux-en-Y gastric bypass and sleeve gastrectomy for the treatment of morbid obesity in China: A 5-year outcome. *Obes. Surg.* **2014**, *24*, 1617–1624. [CrossRef]
8. Wilhelm, S.M.; Young, J.; Kale-Pradhan, P.B. Effect of Bariatric Surgery on Hypertension: A Meta-analysis. *Ann. Pharmacother.* **2014**, *48*, 674–682. [CrossRef]
9. Benaiges, D.; Saguéa, M.; Flores-Le Roux, J.A.; Pedro-Botet, J.; Ramón, J.M.; Villatoro, M.; Chillarón, J.J.; Pera, M.; Más, A.; Grande, L.; et al. Predictors of Hypertension Remission and Recurrence after Bariatric Surgery. *Am. J. Hypertens.* **2016**, *29*, 653–659. [CrossRef]
10. Schiavon, C.A.; Bersch-Ferreira, A.C.; Santucci, E.V.; Oliveira, J.D.; Torreglosa, C.R.; Bueno, P.T.; Frayha, J.C.; Santos, R.N.; Damiani, L.P.; Noujaim, P.M.; et al. Effects of bariatric surgery in obese patients with hypertension the GATEWAY randomized trial (gastric bypass to treat obese patients with steady hypertension). *Circulation* **2018**, *137*, 1132–1142. [CrossRef]
11. Adams, T.D.; Davidson, L.E.; Litwin, S.E.; Kim, J.; Kolotkin, R.L.; Nanjee, M.N.; Gutierrez, J.M.; Frogley, S.J.; Ibele, A.R.; Brinton, E.A.; et al. Weight and metabolic outcomes 12 years after gastric bypass. *N. Engl. J. Med.* **2017**, *377*, 1143–1155. [CrossRef] [PubMed]
12. Hallersund, P.; Sjöström, L.; Olbers, T.; Lönroth, H.; Jacobson, P.; Wallenius, V.; Näslund, I.; Carlsson, L.M.; Fändriks, L. Gastric Bypass Surgery Is Followed by Lowered Blood Pressure and Increased Diuresis—Long Term Results from the Swedish Obese Subjects (SOS) Study. *PLoS ONE* **2012**, *7*, e49696. [CrossRef] [PubMed]
13. Mingrone, G.; Panunzi, S.; De Gaetano, A.; Guidone, C.; Iaconelli, A.; Nanni, G.; Castagneto, M.; Bornstein, S.; Rubino, F. Bariatric-metabolic surgery versus conventional medical treatment in obese patients with type 2 diabetes: 5 Year follow-up of an open-label, single-centre, randomised controlled trial. *Lancet* **2015**, *386*, 964–973. [CrossRef]
14. Schauer, P.R.; Bhatt, D.L.; Kirwan, J.P.; Wolski, K.; Aminian, A.; Brethauer, S.A.; Navaneethan, S.D.; Singh, R.P.; Pothier, C.E.; Nissen, S.E.; et al. Bariatric surgery versus intensive medical therapy for diabetes—5-year outcomes. *N. Engl. J. Med.* **2017**, *376*, 641–651. [CrossRef]
15. Ikramuddin, S.; Korner, J.; Lee, W.J.; Thomas, A.J.; Connett, J.E.; Bantle, J.P.; Leslie, D.B.; Wang, Q.; Inabnet, W.B.; Jeffery, R.W.; et al. Lifestyle intervention and medical management with vs without roux-en-y gastric bypass and control of hemoglobin a1c, ldl cholesterol, and systolic blood pressure at 5 years in the diabetes surgery study. *JAMA-J. Am. Med. Assoc.* **2018**, *319*, 266–278. [CrossRef]
16. Jakobsen, G.S.; Småstuen, M.C.; Sandbu, R.; Nordstrand, N.; Hofsø, D.; Lindberg, M.; Hertel, J.K.; Hjelmesæth, J. Association of bariatric surgery vs medical obesity treatment with long-term medical complications and obesity-related comorbidities. *JAMA-J. Am. Med. Assoc.* **2018**, *319*, 291–301. [CrossRef]
17. Vest, A.R.; Heneghan, H.M.; Agarwal, S.; Schauer, P.R.; Young, J.B. Bariatric surgery and cardiovascular outcomes: A systematic review. *Heart* **2012**, *98*, 1763–1777. [CrossRef] [PubMed]
18. Vidal, P.; Ramón, J.M.; Goday, A.; Benaiges, D.; Trillo, L.; Parri, A.; González, S.; Pera, M.; Grande, L. Laparoscopic gastric bypass versus laparoscopic sleeve gastrectomy as a definitive surgical procedure for morbid obesity. Mid-term results. *Obes. Surg.* **2013**, *23*, 292–299. [CrossRef]

19. Osland, E.; Yunus, R.M.; Khan, S.; Memon, B.; Memon, M.A. Weight loss outcomes in Laparoscopic Vertical Sleeve Gastrectomy (LVSG) versus laparoscopic Roux-en-Y Gastric Bypass (LRYGB) procedures: A meta-analysis and systematic review of randomized controlled trials. *Surg. Laparosc. Endosc. Percutaneous Tech.* **2017**, *27*, 8–18. [CrossRef] [PubMed]
20. Zhang, Y.; Ju, W.; Sun, X.; Cao, Z.; Xinsheng, X.; Daquan, L.; Xiangyang, X.; Qin, M. Laparoscopic Sleeve Gastrectomy Versus Laparoscopic Roux-En-Y Gastric Bypass for Morbid Obesity and Related Comorbidities: A Meta-Analysis of 21 Studies. *Obes. Surg.* **2015**, *25*, 19–26. [CrossRef]
21. Climent, E.; Goday, A.; Pedro-Botet, J.; Solà, I.; Oliveras, A.; Ramón, J.M.; Flores-Le Roux, J.A.; Checa, M.Á.; Benaiges, D. Laparoscopic Roux-en-Y gastric bypass versus laparoscopic sleeve gastrectomy for 5-year hypertension remission in obese patients: A systematic review and meta-analysis. *J. Hypertens.* **2020**, *38*, 185–195. [CrossRef]
22. Rubino, F.; Nathan, D.M.; Eckel, R.H.; Schauer, P.R.; Alberti, K.G.M.; Zimmet, P.Z.; Del Prato, S.; Ji, L.; Sadikot, S.M.; Herman, W.H.; et al. Metabolic surgery in the treatment algorithm for type 2 diabetes: A joint statement by international diabetes organizations. *Diabetes Care* **2016**, *39*, 861–877. [CrossRef]
23. Vidal, J.; Corcelles, R.; Jiménez, A.; Flores, L.; Lacy, A.M. Metabolic and Bariatric Surgery for Obesity. *Gastroenterology* **2017**, *152*, 1780–1790. [CrossRef]
24. Cohen, R.V.; Pinheiro, J.C.; Schiavon, C.A.; Salles, J.E.; Wajchenberg, B.L.; Cummings, D.E. Effects of gastric bypass surgery in patients with type 2 diabetes and only mild obesity. *Diabetes Care* **2012**, *35*, 1420–1428. [CrossRef]
25. Lee, W.J.; Hur, K.Y.; Lakadawala, M.; Kasama, K.; Wong, S.K.H.; Lee, Y.C. Gastrointestinal Metabolic Surgery for the Treatment of Diabetic Patients: A Multi-Institutional International Study. *J. Gastrointest. Surg.* **2012**, *16*, 45–52. [CrossRef] [PubMed]
26. O'Brien, P.E.; Dixon, J.B.; Laurie, C.; Skinner, S.; Proietto, J.; McNeil, J.; Strauss, B.; Marks, S.; Schachter, L.; Chapman, L.; et al. Treatment of mild to moderate obesity with laparoscopic adjustable gastric banding or an intensive medical program: A randomized trial. *Ann. Intern. Med.* **2006**, *144*, 625–633. [CrossRef]
27. Dixon, J.B.; O'Brien, P.E.; Playfair, J.; Chapman, L.; Schachter, L.M.; Skinner, S.; Proietto, J.; Bailey, M.; Anderson, M. Adjustable gastric banding and conventional therapy for type 2 diabetes: A randomized controlled trial. *JAMA-J. Am. Med. Assoc.* **2008**, *299*, 316–323. [CrossRef]
28. Lee, W.J.; Chong, K.; Ser, K.H.; Lee, Y.C.; Chen, S.C.; Chen, J.C.; Tsai, M.H.; Chuang, L.M. Gastric bypass vs sleeve gastrectomy for type 2 diabetes mellitus: A randomized controlled trial. *Arch. Surg.* **2011**, *146*, 143–148. [CrossRef] [PubMed]
29. Ikramuddin, S.; Korner, J.; Lee, W.J.; Connett, J.E.; Inabnet, W.B.; Billington, C.J.; Thomas, A.J.; Leslie, D.B.; Chong, K.; Jeffery, R.W.; et al. Roux-en-Y gastric bypass vs intensive medical management for the control of type 2 diabetes, hypertension, and hyperlipidemia: The diabetes surgery study randomized clinical trial. *JAMA-J. Am. Med. Assoc.* **2013**, *309*, 2240–2249. [CrossRef]
30. Busetto, L.; Dixon, J.; De Luca, M.; Shikora, S.; Pories, W.; Angrisani, L. Bariatric surgery in class i obesity: A position statement from the international federation for the surgery of obesity and metabolic disorders (IFSO). *Obes. Surg.* **2014**, *24*, 487–519. [CrossRef] [PubMed]
31. Flores, L.; Vidal, J.; Núñez, I.; Rueda, S.; Viaplana, J.; Esmatjes, E. Longitudinal changes of blood pressure after weight loss: Factors involved. *Surg. Obes. Relat. Dis.* **2015**, *11*, 215–221. [CrossRef]
32. Schiavon, C.A.; Drager, L.F.; Bortolotto, L.A.; Amodeo, C.; Ikeoka, D.; Berwanger, O.; Cohen, R.V. The Role of Metabolic Surgery on Blood Pressure Control. *Curr. Atheroscler. Rep.* **2016**, *18*, 1–8. [CrossRef]
33. Bueter, M.; Ahmed, A.; Ashrafian, H.; le Roux, C.W. Bariatric surgery and hypertension. *Surg. Obes. Relat. Dis.* **2009**, *5*, 615–620. [CrossRef] [PubMed]
34. Landsberg, L.; Aronne, L.J.; Beilin, L.J.; Burke, V.; Igel, L.I.; Lloyd-Jones, D.; Sowers, J. Obesity-related hypertension: Pathogenesis, cardiovascular risk, and treatment-a position paper of the the obesity society and the American society of hypertension. *Obesity* **2013**, *21*, 8–24. [CrossRef] [PubMed]
35. Le Roux, C.W.; Welbourn, R.; Werling, M.; Osborne, A.; Kokkinos, A.; Laurenius, A.; Lönroth, H.; Fändriks, L.; Ghatei, M.A.; Bloom, S.R.; et al. Gut hormones as mediators of appetite and weight loss after Roux-en-Y gastric bypass. *Ann. Surg.* **2007**, *246*, 780–785. [CrossRef] [PubMed]
36. Yamamoto, H.; Kishi, T.; Lee, C.E.; Choi, B.J.; Fang, H.; Hollenberg, A.N.; Drucker, D.J.; Elmquist, J.K. Glucagon-like peptide-1-responsive catecholamine neurons in the area postrema link peripheral glucagon-like peptide-1 with central autonomic control sites. *J. Neurosci.* **2003**, *23*, 2939–2946. [CrossRef]
37. Virdis, A.; Lerman, L.O.; Regoli, F.; Ghiadoni, L.; Lerman, A.; Taddei, S. Human Ghrelin: A Gastric Hormone with Cardiovascular Properties. *Curr. Pharm. Des.* **2015**, *22*, 52–58. [CrossRef]
38. Woelnerhanssen, B.; Peterli, R.; Steinert, R.E.; Peters, T.; Borbély, Y.; Beglinger, C. Effects of postbariatric surgery weight loss on adipokines and metabolic parameters: Comparison of laparoscopic Roux-en-Y gastric bypass and laparoscopic sleeve gastrectomya prospective randomized trial. *Surg. Obes. Relat. Dis.* **2011**, *7*, 561–568. [CrossRef]
39. Kopp, H.P.; Kopp, C.W.; Festa, A.; Krzyzanowska, K.; Kriwanek, S.; Minar, E.; Roka, R.; Schernthaner, G. Impact of weight loss on inflammatory proteins and their association with the insulin resistance syndrome in morbidly obese patients. *Arterioscler. Thromb. Vasc. Biol.* **2003**, *23*, 1042–1047. [CrossRef]
40. Pedrosa, R.P.; Krieger, E.M.; Lorenzi-Filho, G.; Drager, L.F. Recent advances of the impact of obstructive sleep apnea on systemic hypertension. *Arq. Bras. Cardiol.* **2011**, *97*, e40–e47. [CrossRef]
41. Gottlieb, D.J.; Punjabi, N.M.; Mehra, R.; Patel, S.R.; Quan, S.F.; Babineau, D.C.; Tracy, R.P.; Rueschman, M.; Blumenthal, R.S.; Lewis, E.F.; et al. CPAP versus Oxygen in Obstructive Sleep Apnea. *N. Engl. J. Med.* **2014**, *370*, 2276–2285. [CrossRef]

42. Ahmed, A.R.; Rickards, G.; Coniglio, D.; Xia, Y.; Johnson, J.; Boss, T.; O'Malley, W. Laparoscopic Roux-en-Y Gastric Bypass and Its Early Effect on Blood Pressure. *Obes. Surg.* **2009**, *19*, 845–849. [CrossRef] [PubMed]
43. Ramón, J.M.; Salvans, S.; Crous, X.; Puig, S.; Goday, A.; Benaiges, D.; Trillo, L.; Pera, M.; Grande, L. Effect of Roux-en-Y Gastric Bypass vs Sleeve Gastrectomy on Glucose and Gut Hormones: A Prospective Randomised Trial. *J. Gastrointest. Surg.* **2012**, *16*, 1116–1122. [CrossRef] [PubMed]
44. Reisin, E.; Jack, A.V. Obesity and Hypertension: Mechanisms, Cardio-Renal Consequences, and Therapeutic Approaches. *Med. Clin. N. Am.* **2009**, *93*, 733–751. [CrossRef] [PubMed]
45. Cuspidi, C.; Rescaldani, M.; Sala, C.; Grassi, G. Left-ventricular hypertrophy and obesity: A systematic review and meta-analysis of echocardiographic studies. *J. Hypertens.* **2014**, *32*, 16–25. [CrossRef] [PubMed]
46. Aggarwal, R.; Harling, L.; Efthimiou, E.; Darzi, A.; Athanasiou, T.; Ashrafian, H. The Effects of Bariatric Surgery on Cardiac Structure and Function: A Systematic Review of Cardiac Imaging Outcomes. *Obes. Surg.* **2016**, *26*, 1030–1040. [CrossRef] [PubMed]
47. Alpert, M.A.; Omran, J.; Bostick, B.P. Effects of Obesity on Cardiovascular Hemodynamics, Cardiac Morphology, and Ventricular Function. *Curr. Obes. Rep.* **2016**, *5*, 424–434. [CrossRef] [PubMed]
48. Abel, E.D.; Litwin, S.E.; Sweeney, G. Cardiac remodeling in obesity. *Physiol. Rev.* **2008**, *88*, 389–419. [CrossRef]
49. Kotsis, V.; Jordan, J.; Micic, D.; Finer, N.; Leitner, D.R.; Toplak, H.; Tokgozoglu, L.; Athyros, V.; Elisaf, M.; Filippatos, T.D.; et al. Obesity and cardiovascular risk: A call for action from the European Society of Hypertension Working Group of Obesity, Diabetes and the High-risk Patient and European Association for the Study of Obesity: Part A: Mechanisms of obesity induced hypertension, diabetes and dyslipidemia and practice guidelines for treatment. *J. Hypertens.* **2018**, *36*, 1427–1440. [CrossRef]
50. Larsson, S.C.; Bäck, M.; Rees, J.M.B.; Mason, A.M.; Burgess, S. Body mass index and body composition in relation to 14 cardiovascular conditions in UK Biobank: A Mendelian randomization study. *Eur. Heart J.* **2020**, *41*, 221–226. [CrossRef]
51. Ndumele, C.E.; Matsushita, K.; Lazo, M.; Bello, N.; Blumenthal, R.S.; Gerstenblith, G.; Nambi, V.; Ballantyne, C.M.; Solomon, S.D.; Selvin, E.; et al. Obesity and Subtypes of Incident Cardiovascular Disease. *J. Am. Heart Assoc.* **2016**, *5*. [CrossRef]
52. Von Jeinsen, B.; Short, M.I.; Xanthakis, V.; Carneiro, H.; Cheng, S.; Mitchell, G.F.; Vasan, R.S. Association of circulating adipokines with echocardiographic measures of cardiac structure and function in a community-based cohort. *J. Am. Heart Assoc.* **2018**, *7*, e008997. [CrossRef]
53. Oliveras, A.; Molina, L.; Goday, A.; Sans, L.; Riera, M.; Vazquez, S.; Benaiges, D.; Granados, A.M.; Ramon, J.M.; Pascual, J. Effect of bariatric surgery on cardiac structure and function in obese patients: Role of the renin-angiotensin system. *J. Clin. Hypertens.* **2021**, *23*, 181–192. [CrossRef] [PubMed]
54. Karimian, S.; Stein, J.; Bauer, B.; Teupe, C. Improvement of impaired diastolic left ventricular function after diet-induced weight reduction in severe obesity. *Diabetes Metab. Syndr. Obes. Targets Ther.* **2017**, *10*, 19–25. [CrossRef] [PubMed]
55. Cuspidi, C.; Rescaldani, M.; Tadic, M.; Sala, C.; Grassi, G. Effects of bariatric surgery on cardiac structure and function: A systematic review and meta-analysis. *Am. J. Hypertens.* **2014**, *27*, 146–156. [CrossRef]
56. Owan, T.; Avelar, E.; Morley, K.; Jiji, R.; Hall, N.; Krezowski, J.; Gallagher, J.; Williams, Z.; Preece, K.; Gundersen, N.; et al. Favorable changes in cardiac geometry and function following gastric bypass surgery: 2-year follow-up in the Utah obesity study. *J. Am. Coll. Cardiol.* **2011**, *57*, 732–739. [CrossRef]
57. Safar, M.E. Arterial stiffness as a risk factor for clinical hypertension. *Nat. Rev. Cardiol.* **2018**, *15*, 97–105. [CrossRef] [PubMed]
58. Cecelja, M.; Chowienczyk, P. Role of arterial stiffness in cardiovascular disease. *JRSM Cardiovasc. Dis.* **2012**, *1*, 1–10. [CrossRef] [PubMed]
59. Laurent, S.; Cockcroft, J.; Van Bortel, L.; Boutouyrie, P.; Giannattasio, C.; Hayoz, D.; Pannier, B.; Vlachopoulos, C.; Wilkinson, I.; Struijker-Boudier, H. Expert consensus document on arterial stiffness: Methodological issues and clinical applications. *Eur. Heart J.* **2006**, *27*, 2588–2605. [CrossRef]
60. Wildman, R.P.; Mackey, R.H.; Bostom, A.; Thompson, T.; Sutton-Tyrrell, K. Measures of obesity are associated with vascular stiffness in young and older adults. *Hypertension* **2003**, *42*, 468–473. [CrossRef]
61. Niiranen, T.J.; Kalesan, B.; Hamburg, N.M.; Benjamin, E.J.; Mitchell, G.F.; Vasan, R.S. Relative contributions of arterial stiffness and hypertension to cardiovascular disease: The Framingham heart study. *J. Am. Heart Assoc.* **2016**, *5*, e004271. [CrossRef] [PubMed]
62. Weisbrod, R.M.; Shiang, T.; Al Sayah, L.; Fry, J.; Bajpai, S.; Reinhart-King, C.A.; Lob, H.E.; Santhanam, L.; Mitchell, G.; Cohen, R.A.; et al. Arterial stiffening precedes systolic hypertension in diet-induced obesity. *Hypertension* **2013**, *62*, 1105–1110. [CrossRef]
63. Cooper, J.N.; Buchanich, J.M.; Youk, A.; Brooks, M.M.; Barinas-Mitchell, E.; Conroy, M.B.; Sutton-Tyrrell, K. Reductions in arterial stiffness with weight loss in overweight and obese young adults: Potential mechanisms. *Atherosclerosis* **2012**, *223*, 485–490. [CrossRef]
64. Samaras, K.; Viardot, A.; Lee, P.N.; Jenkins, A.; Botelho, N.K.; Bakopanos, A.; Lord, R.V.; Hayward, C.S. Reduced arterial stiffness after weight loss in obese type 2 diabetes and impaired glucose tolerance: The role of immune cell activation and insulin resistance. *Diabetes Vasc. Dis. Res.* **2013**, *10*, 40–48. [CrossRef] [PubMed]
65. Petersen, K.S.; Blanch, N.; Keogh, J.B.; Clifton, P.M. Effect of weight loss on pulse wave velocity: Systematic review and meta-analysis. *Arterioscler. Thromb. Vasc. Biol.* **2015**, *35*, 243–252. [CrossRef]
66. Frey, S.; Jacobi, D.; Pichelin, M.; Cariou, B.; Mirallié, E.; Blanchard, C. Improvement in arterial stiffness (pOpmètre®) after bariatric surgery. Results from a prospective study. *Ann. Endocrinol.* **2020**, *81*, 44–50. [CrossRef] [PubMed]

67. Ikonomidis, I.; Mazarakis, A.; Papadopoulos, C.; Patsouras, N.; Kalfarentzos, F.; Lekakis, J.; Kremastinos, D.T.; Alexopoulos, D. Weight loss after bariatric surgery improves aortic elastic properties and left ventricular function in individuals with morbid obesity: A 3-year follow-up study. *J. Hypertens.* **2007**, *25*, 439–447. [CrossRef]
68. Favre, G.; Anty, R.; Canivet, C.; Clément, G.; Ben-Amor, I.; Tran, A.; Gugenheim, J.; Gual, P.; Esnault, V.L.M.; Iannelli, A. Determinants associated with the correction of glomerular hyper-filtration one year after bariatric surgery. *Surg. Obes. Relat. Dis.* **2017**, *13*, 1760–1766. [CrossRef]
69. Currie, A.; Chetwood, A.; Ahmed, A.R. Bariatric surgery and renal function. *Obes. Surg.* **2011**, *21*, 528–539. [CrossRef]
70. Hall, J.E.; do Carmo, J.M.; da Silva, A.A.; Wang, Z.; Hall, M.E. Obesity, kidney dysfunction and hypertension: Mechanistic links. *Nat. Rev. Nephrol.* **2019**, *15*, 367–385. [CrossRef]
71. Rosenstock, J.L.; Pommier, M.; Stoffels, G.; Patel, S.; Michelis, M.F. Prevalence of proteinuria and albuminuria in an obese population and associated risk factors. *Front. Med.* **2018**, *5*, 122. [CrossRef]
72. Lieske, J.C. Bariatric surgery and kidney health. *J. Am. Soc. Nephrol.* **2018**, *29*, 1085–1086. [CrossRef]
73. Naira, M.; Le Roux, C.W.; Docherty, N.G. Mechanisms underpinning remission of albuminuria following bariatric surgery. *Curr. Opin. Endocrinol. Diabetes Obes.* **2016**, *23*, 366–372. [CrossRef]
74. Tham, J.C.; le Roux, C.W.; Docherty, N.G. Cardiovascular, Renal and Overall Health Outcomes After Bariatric Surgery. *Curr. Cardiol. Rep.* **2015**, *17*, 1–8. [CrossRef]
75. Friedman, A.N.; Wahed, A.S.; Wang, J.; Courcoulas, A.P.; Dakin, G.; Hinojosa, M.W.; Kimmel, P.L.; Mitchell, J.E.; Pomp, A.; Pories, W.J.; et al. Effect of bariatric surgery on CKD risk. *J. Am. Soc. Nephrol.* **2018**, *29*, 1289–1300. [CrossRef] [PubMed]
76. Li, K.; Zou, J.; Ye, Z.; Di, J.; Han, X.; Zhang, H.; Liu, W.; Ren, Q.; Zhang, P. Effects of bariatric surgery on renal function in obese patients: A systematic review and meta analysis. *PLoS ONE* **2016**, *11*, e0163907. [CrossRef] [PubMed]
77. Shulman, A.; Peltonen, M.; Sjöström, C.D.; Andersson-Assarsson, J.C.; Taube, M.; Sjöholm, K.; Le Roux, C.W.; Carlsson, L.M.S.; Svensson, P.A. Incidence of end-stage renal disease following bariatric surgery in the Swedish Obese Subjects Study. *Int. J. Obes.* **2018**, *42*, 964–973. [CrossRef]
78. O'Brien, R.; Johnson, E.; Haneuse, S.; Coleman, K.J.; O'Connor, P.J.; Fisher, D.P.; Sidney, S.; Bogart, A.; Theis, M.K.; Anau, J.; et al. Microvascular outcomes in patients with diabetes after bariatric surgery versus usual care. *Ann. Intern. Med.* **2018**, *169*, 300–310. [CrossRef]
79. Sjöström, L.; Peltonen, M.; Jacobson, P.; Sjöström, C.D.; Karason, K.; Wedel, H.; Ahlin, S.; Anveden, Å.; Bengtsson, C.; Bergmark, G.; et al. Bariatric surgery and long-term cardiovascular events. *JAMA-J. Am. Med. Assoc.* **2012**, *307*, 56–65. [CrossRef]
80. Christou, N.V.; Sampalis, J.S.; Liberman, M.; Look, D.; Auger, S.; McLean, A.P.H.; MacLean, L.D.; Pories, W.J.; Wolfe, B.M.; Thirlby, R.C. Surgery decreases long-term mortality, morbidity, and health care use in morbidly obese patients. *Ann. Surg.* **2004**, *240*, 416–424. [CrossRef] [PubMed]
81. Adams, T.D.; Gress, R.E.; Smith, S.C.; Halverson, R.C.; Simper, S.C.; Rosamond, W.D.; LaMonte, M.J.; Stroup, A.M.; Hunt, S.C. Long-Term Mortality after Gastric Bypass Surgery. *N. Engl. J. Med.* **2007**, *357*, 753–761. [CrossRef] [PubMed]
82. Wong, C.Y.; O'Moore-Sullivan, T.; Leano, R.; Byrne, N.; Beller, E.; Marwick, T.H. Alterations of left ventricular myocardial characteristics associated with obesity. *Circulation* **2004**, *110*, 3081–3087. [CrossRef] [PubMed]
83. Morse, S.A.; Gulati, R.; Reisin, E. The obesity paradox and cardiovascular disease. *Curr. Hypertens. Rep.* **2010**, *12*, 120–126. [CrossRef] [PubMed]

Journal of
Clinical Medicine

MDPI

Review

Sleeve Gastrectomy and Roux-En-Y Gastric Bypass. Two Sculptors of the Pancreatic Islet

Gonzalo-Martín Pérez-Arana [1,2,3,*], José Fernández-Vivero [1], Alonso Camacho-Ramírez [1,3,4], Alfredo Díaz Gómez [5], José Bancalero de los Reyes [6], Antonio Ribelles-García [1], David Almorza-Gomar [2,7], Carmen Carrasco-Molinillo [1] and José-Arturo Prada-Oliveira [1,2,3,*]

1 Department of Human Anatomy and Embryology, Faculty of Medicine, University of Cadiz, 11003 Cadiz, Spain; jose.vivero@uca.es (J.F.-V.); alonso.camacho@uca.es (A.C.-R.); Antonio.ribelles@uca.es (A.R.-G.); carmen.carrasco@uca.es (C.C.-M.)
2 Institute for Biomedical Science Research and Innovation (INIBICA), University of Cadiz, 11003 Cadiz, Spain; david.almorza@uca.es
3 Asociación Gaditana de Apoyo al Investigador (AGAI), 11012 Cadiz, Spain
4 Surgery Unit, Puerta del Mar Universitary Hospital, University of Cadiz, 11003 Cadiz, Spain
5 San Carlos Hospital, Andalusian Health System, 28040 Madrid, Spain; diazgomez.a@gmail.com
6 Badajoz Hospital, Extremadura Health System, 06001 Badajoz, Spain; josebancalerodelosreyes@gmail.com
7 Operative Statistic and Research Department, University of Cadiz, 11003 Cadiz, Spain
* Correspondence: gonzalo.perez@uca.es (G.-M.P.-A.); arturo.prada@uca.es (J.-A.P.-O.)

Citation: Pérez-Arana, G.-M.; Fernández-Vivero, J.; Camacho-Ramírez, A.; Díaz Gómez, A.; Bancalero de los Reyes, J.; Ribelles-García, A.; Almorza-Gomar, D.; Carrasco-Molinillo, C.; Prada-Oliveira, J.-A. Sleeve Gastrectomy and Roux-En-Y Gastric Bypass. Two Sculptors of the Pancreatic Islet. *J. Clin. Med.* **2021**, *10*, 4217. https://doi.org/10.3390/jcm10184217

Academic Editor: David Benaiges Boix

Received: 22 July 2021
Accepted: 14 September 2021
Published: 17 September 2021

Publisher's Note: MDPI stays neutral with regard to jurisdictional claims in published maps and institutional affiliations.

Abstract: Several surgical procedures are performed for the treatment of obesity. A main outcome of these procedures is the improvement of type 2 diabetes mellitus. Trying to explain this, gastrointestinal hormone levels and their effect on organs involved in carbohydrate metabolism, such as liver, gut, muscle or fat, have been studied intensively after bariatric surgery. These effects on endocrine-cell populations in the pancreas have been less well studied. We gathered the existing data on these pancreatic-cell populations after the two most common types of bariatric surgery, the sleeve gastrectomy (SG) and the roux-en-Y gastric bypass (RYGB), with the aim to explain the pathophysiological mechanisms underlying these surgeries and to improve their outcome.

Keywords: sleeve gastrectomy; roux-en-Y gastric bypass; beta-cell; alpha-cell; epsilon-cell; islet; trans-differentiation

1. Introduction

Bariatric/metabolic surgery has been a powerful tool for the treatment of diabetes mellitus for a long time. Sleeve gastrectomy (SG) and roux-en-Y gastric bypass (RYGB) are two of the most performed ones [1,2] as Figure 1 shows.

Changes in energy homeostasis and body fat mass have been proposed as a primary mechanism to explain these phenomena [3,4], but other mechanisms such as changes in several gastrointestinal hormones also seem to be involved with a large number of publications written on the topic. Many of them have related the anatomical changes in the gastrointestinal tract after surgery with the modification of serum levels of glucagon like peptide-1 (GLP-1) [5], ghrelin [6], peptide tyrosine-tyrosine (PYY) [7], gastrointestinal inhibitory peptide (GIP) [8], or even leptin [9], among others, in humans and animal models. Their involvement is clear, but the exact mechanisms and their degree of participation remain partially unknown.

At the other end of the entero-pancreatic axis, the endocrine pancreas containing Langerhans islets determines changes in carbohydrate metabolism after bariatric/metabolic surgery. Their hormonal secretions before and after bariatric/metabolic surgery have been widely studied in plasma or serum from animals and humans [10,11] but the islet cell composition and its paracrine interactions have been studied less. We will attempt to summarize what we know about the subject by means of a bibliographical review of the most relevant works published on the subject.

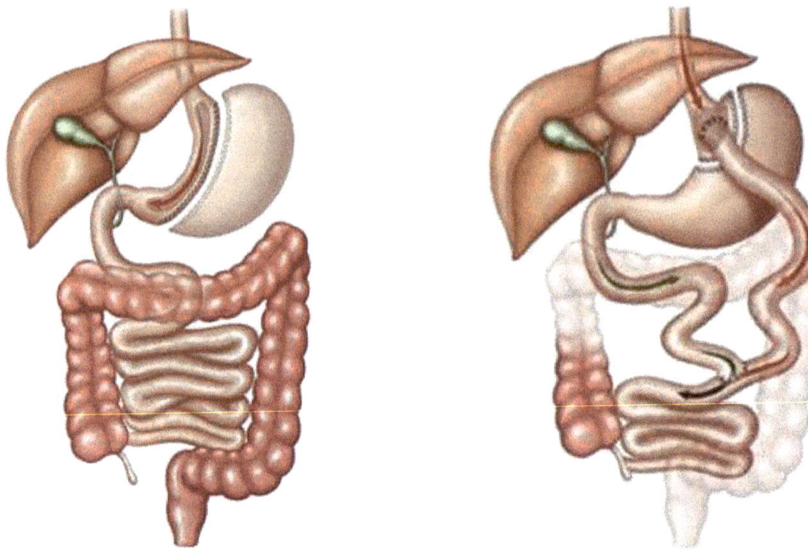

(A) (B)

Figure 1. Schematic drawing of Sleeve Gastrectomy and Roux-en-Y Gastric bypass. (**A**) Sleeve Gastrectomy (SG). Representation of a common human sleeve gastrectomy (SG) procedure. The SG is a surgical procedure including a reduction of final gastric volume, since most of the gastric major curvature is resected. The stomach is reduced to a cylindrical pouch removing most of the fundus, stomach-corpus and antrum. The pylorus and minor curvature is preserved. SG reduces the initial stomach volume by approximately 15–20%. In animal models this configuration is maintained since the final gastric pouch volume and valves are preserved. (**B**) Roux-en-Y Gastric Bypass (RYGB). Representation of a common human roux-en-Y gastric bypass (RYGB) surgery. This includes a transverse section of the stomach performed from the major to the minor curvature, configuring a gastric pouch. This pouch of the stomach continues to the food handle with an alimentary bulb, which continues with the medium portion of the jejunum. RYGB, a mixed malabsorptive and restrictive technique, excludes the antrum and the proximal intestine to aliments by bypassing the duodenum and the initial part of the jejunum. This includes biliopancreatic secretion, which determines the malabsorptive component. The biliopancreatic bulb connects with the mid jejunum. In rats, the model was reproduced similarly with minor modifications according to the animal anatomy. Exempli gratia, the jejunal alimentary bulb was 10 cm due to the usual intestinal medium extension of 80 cm. Original figure seen in https://sagebariatric.com/about-surgery-home/sleeve-gastrectomy (accessed on 22 July 2021).

2. Methods and Results

This paper is a narrative literature review text that aims to expose the framework surrounding the effects of RYGB and SG on endocrine-cell populations in the pancreas. We performed a selective search of numerous articles in different databases, as well as books.

The literature of the main scientific databases was reviewed. The search was limited to documents published between 2001 and 2021. These databases were Medline, PubMed, Chochrane and Scopus. In addition, a search was carried out on academic websites, such as Google Scholar, SciELO and Dialnet. The main Boolean operators used were: AND, OR and NOT, and the key words were sleeve gastrectomy; roux-en-Y gastric bypass; beta-cell, alpha-cell; epsilon-cell; islet; trans-differentiation. Due to the large number of studies found, the following criteria were applied to filter the results and work with the most relevant studies.

Inclusion criteria: Original articles, systematic reviews and meta-analyses concerning modifications of the endocrine pancreas after bariatric or metabolic surgery in humans or animal models. Papers published in English in the last 20 years (2001–2021). We prioritised information from systematic reviews and meta-analyses with high scientific evidence.

Exclusion criteria: Papers not related to the topic or not meeting the inclusion criteria.

In the end, a total of 435 articles were found that met the search criteria. Of these, 47 were selected for the preparation of this manuscript. As Table 1 shows, a large number of disciplines are involved in the study of the topic.

Table 1. Search Results. Break down of the total number of articles used to prepare the work. The left column represents the different fields of research of each journal citation (Journal Citation Report categories). The central column contains the number of citations found in each category and the right column contains the number and percentage of citations selected for the manuscript.

Research Field (JCR)	Number of Articles Obtained	Number and % of Articles Selected
Endocrinology & Metabolism	223	22 (46.80%)
Surgery	91	6 (12.76%)
Cell Biology	29	4 (8.50%)
Medicine General & Internal	27	4 (8.50%)
Biochemistry & Molecular Biology	21	2 (4.25%)
Multidisciplinary Sciences	14	2 (4.25%)
Medical Research & Experimental	11	2 (4.25%)
Gastroenterology & Hepatology	11	2 (4.25%)
Genetics & Heredity	4	1 (2.12%)
Pediatrics	3	1 (2.12%)
Peripheral Vascular disease	1	1 (2.12%)
Total of Research fields	435	47 (100%)

3. Discussion

3.1. The Sleeve Gastrectomy and the Islet Architecture

Bariatric/metabolic surgery involves different techniques leading to different effects on pancreatic cell populations. Currently, sleeve gastrectomy (SG) is one of the most performed techniques. A consequence of this procedure is the drastic removal of the gastric fundus and corpus ghrelin-producing cell population. This situation leads to 35–45% reduction of blood ghrelin levels after gastrectomy in humans [12–14]. However, a recent study described the expansion of the pancreatic residual postnatal epsilon-cell population with recovery of plasma ghrelin levels in rats twelve weeks after SG. This expansion takes place at the expense of pancreatic cell progenitors that differentiate into epsilon-cells showing a high expression of lineage markers such as neurogenin-3 (Ngn-3) but not homeodomain protein Nkx2.2 (Figure 2) [15].

This leads us to believe in an adaptive response of the endocrine pancreas to low circulating ghrelin levels and in a possible explanation of the improvement of beta cell function after SG if we take into account the protective role of ghrelin on it [16].

Furthermore, this surgery does not only affect the epsilon-cells in the islets. It is clear that SG preserves the beta-cell function, at least for a while [17,18]. This could be explained by the increase of GLP-1 receptor expression in beta cells after SG, implying an increase in paracrine sensitivity to GLP-1 [19,20]. However, there are doubts about this due to a recent study with a modified mouse model involving an inducible knockdown of GLP-1r in beta-cells (GLP1rβ-cell-ko), which showed improved glycemic profiles, to the wild-nature level, after SG [21]. Other researchers have linked the maintenance of beta-cell mass and beta-cell identity markers such as PDX-1 or MafA [22] (Picture 2) to high levels of gastrin after SG, as well as to correction of long-term blood glucose levels in rodents [23].

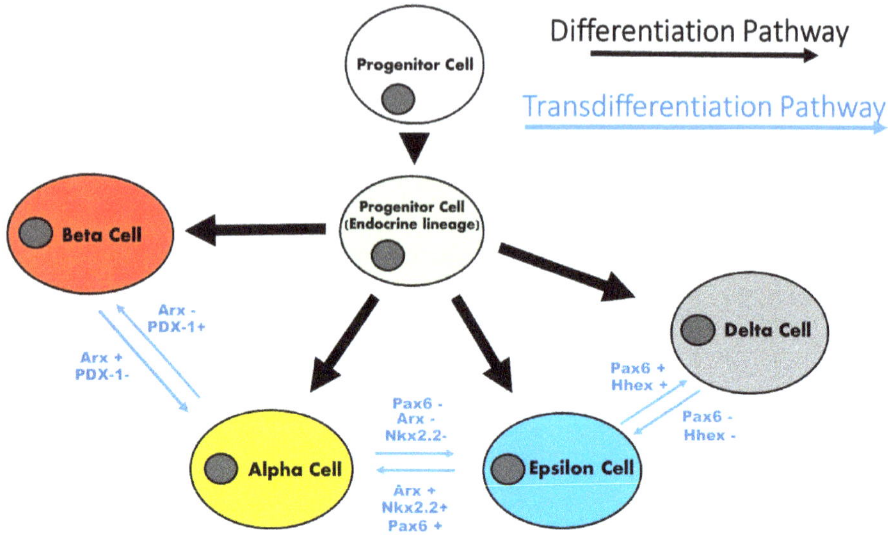

Figure 2. Pancreatic endocrine cell identity markers and possible cell trans/differentiation pathways after SG/RYGB. Pancreatic endocrine-cell identity markers and possible cell differentiation pathways from progenitor-cells (Black arrows) or trans-differentiation from other pancreatic endocrine-cells (Blue arrows) after sleeve gastrectomy or roux-en-Y gastric bypass.

This brings us to the problem of diabetes relapse after SG, which is as high as 41.6% of cases five years after surgery [2]. Liu et al. proposed long-term recovery of insulin sensitivity without beta-cell dysfunction as an answer to the question [24], but a recent work showed loss of beta-cell mass and a strong increase in alpha-cell mass in Wistar rats twelve weeks after SG. Trans-differentiation of the beta-cell population under stressful situations with loss of beta-cell markers such as PDX-1 and gain of alpha-cell markers such as Pax-6 and Arx has been shown [25] (Figure 2). Moreover, this is supported by studies performed on mice outside the scope of bariatric surgery where alpha-cell populations labeled with Gcg-Cre lineage tracers showed a dilution of the marker at the expense of the beta-cell population throughout life [26]. Therefore, the appearance of alpha-cells at the expense of the beta-cell population may explain the long-term relapses in diabetes after SG.

Finally, the protective effect of the somatostatin-14 isoform on Min6 pancreatic beta cells of mice has recently been verified, limiting the stress markers HSPa1 and Ddit3 and apoptosis [27]. This together with the occurrence of delta-cell hyperplasia in Goto-Kakizaki diabetic mice [28] makes us think about a possible role of this delta population in the mechanisms underlying SG. This seems to be reinforced by the ability of ghrelin to activate the paracrine secretion of somatostatin [29] as mentioned above. However, due to the difficulty in carrying out these studies in humans and the ethical aspects, further investigation on animal models is needed to clarify this issue and the possible involvement of other pancreatic endocrine populations.

3.2. The Roux-en-Y Gastric Bypass and the Islet Architecture

Roux-en-Y gastric bypass appears to be the most powerful tool for the management of obesity and hyperglycemia in patients [30]. This procedure has demonstrated its efficiency in increasing beta-cell function in animal models and patients [31,32]. It also appears to increase beta-cell mass after surgery in both animal models and patients [33,34]. GLP-1 activity has been proposed as responsible for these effects on beta-cell mass after RYGB [35]. On the other hand, glucose improvement after RYGB has long been reported in mice models of functional GLP-1 and GLP-1 receptor deficiency, suggesting a GLP-1 independent mechanism for glycemic control after surgery [36]. Another very interesting candidate is intra-islet PYY. Guida et al. reported a large increase in islet PYY content after RYGB, mediated by locally produced PYY but not GLP-1 glucose-stimulated insulin secretion. Furthermore, interleukin-22 (IL-22) seems to play a key role in the increase of intra-islet expression of PYY after RYGB. This situation would imply that non-surgical treatment for diabetes is possible [37].

An interesting study would be to determine the participation of pancreatic delta-cells in the maintenance of beta-cell mass after RYGB surgery since a recent study demonstrated that delta-cells become insulin-expressing cells after the ablation of insulin-secreting beta-cells in human islets [38] (Figure 2). This should be investigated in the future.

Other cell types, such as pancreatic epsilon-cells, do not seem to be affected after RYGB [15]. However, high plasma ghrelin levels were detected in obese mice six weeks after RYGB, probably due to an expansion of ghrelin-producing cells in the duodenum and stomach of these mice [39].

On the contrary, the plasticity of the pancreatic alpha-cell population under stressful circumstances is well known. Pregnancy or intermittent fasting are capable of enhancing the alpha-cell mass in mice [40,41]. Some factors related to the functionality of hepatic glucagon receptors (GCgr) have been proposed as brakes and regulators of alpha-cell population expansion in animal models [42]. In this sense, RYGB is also able to cause an increase in the alpha-cell population in mice six months after the operation, including a loss of beta identity markers such as PDX-1 and a gain of alpha-cell markers such as ARX in the islets (Figure 2). All of this suggests long-term trans-differentiation of beta-cells into alpha-cells after surgery [25].

This brings us to long-term relapse of diabetes again. Like SG, the outcomes of RYGB published in relevant trials have shown a progressive worsening of diabetes-related parameters such as glycated hemoglobin, reaching a 50% relapse in diabetes at five years [2]. Patel et al. proposed weak beta-cell function and peripheral insulin resistance as possible causes of relapse after RYGB [43]. An decrease in beta-cell mass and an increase in alpha-cell mass could explain this, but what is the mechanism that triggers trans-differentiation? Hyperinsulinism and subsequent hypoglycemia have been a problem after RYGB but also may be the answer [44]. In this sense, RYGB seems to cause an extreme requirement and stressful situation to the beta-cell population, triggering conversion to alpha-cells [45]. According to this, a study in patients reported hyperinsulinism but elevated postprandial glucagon secretion after RYGB. However, the same study did not report extremely increased beta cell function [46]. The landscape is complex and exciting and could be a good line of research to improve the efficiency of these surgeries in the remission of diabetes.

4. Conclusions

SG and RYGB are a therapeutic option not only for overweight but also for diabetes. The effects of these surgeries on enterohormonal levels have been extensively studied but on another level, further research on endocrine pancreatic cell populations is also needed. Nevertheless, it seems that different pathophysiological mechanisms underlie each of these surgeries, at least in reference to their pancreatic involvement. This is a complicated issue in humans. However, a better understanding of the mechanisms and cellular dynamics governing these populations after these two surgeries would allow us to limit hypoglycemic episodes, the relapse of diabetes over time or even the development of pharmacological alternatives to the use of bariatric/metabolic surgery.

Author Contributions: Writing—original draft preparation, J.F.-V., A.C.-R., A.D.G., J.B.d.l.R., A.R.-G., D.A.-G. and C.C.-M.; writing—review and editing, G.-M.P.-A. and J.-A.P.-O. All authors have read and agreed to the published version of the manuscript.

Funding: This research received no external funding.

Institutional Review Board Statement: Not applicable.

Informed Consent Statement: Not applicable.

Data Availability Statement: The scientific articles consulted for the preparation of this review were obtained from the following databases: Pubmed, Science Direct, Google Academic and Rodin: (UCA Institutional Repository): It is a database of teaching and research objects of the University of Cadiz.

Conflicts of Interest: The authors declare no conflict of interest.

References

1. Mingrone, G.; Panunzi, S.; De Gaetano, A.; Guidone, C.; Iaconelli, A.; Leccesi, L.; Nanni, G.; Pomp, A.; Castagneto, M.; Ghirlanda, G.; et al. Bariatric surgery versus conventional medical therapy for type 2 diabetes. *N. Engl. J. Med.* **2012**, *366*, 1577–1585. [CrossRef] [PubMed]
2. Schauer, P.R.; Bhatt, D.L.; Kirwan, J.P.; Wolski, K.; Aminian, A.; Brethauer, S.A.; Navaneethan, S.D.; Singh, R.P.; Pothier, C.E.; Nissen, S.E.; et al. Bariatric surgery versus intensive medical therapy for diabetes 5-year outcomes. *N. Engl. J. Med.* **2017**, *376*, 641–651. [CrossRef] [PubMed]
3. Heneghan, H.M.; Nissen, S.; Schauer, P.R. Gastrointestinal Surgery for Obesity and Diabetes: Weight Loss and Control of Hyperglycemia. *Curr. Atheroscler. Rep.* **2012**, *14*, 579–587. [CrossRef] [PubMed]
4. Miras, A.D.; le Roux, C.W. Mechanisms underlying weight loss after bariatric surgery. *Nat. Rev. Gastroenterol. Hepatol.* **2013**, *10*, 575–584. [CrossRef]
5. Larraufie, P.; Roberts, G.P.; McGavigan, A.K.; Kay, R.G.; Li, J.; Leiter, A.; Melvin, A.; Biggs, E.K.; Ravn, P.; Davy, K.; et al. Important Role of the GLP-1 Axis for glucose homeostasis after bariatric surgery. *Cell. Rep.* **2019**, *26*, 1399–1408. [CrossRef]
6. Frezza, E.E.; Chiriva-Internati, M.; Wachtel, M.S. Analysis of the results of sleeve gastrectomy for morbid obesity and the role of ghrelin. *Surg. Today* **2008**, *38*, 481–483. [CrossRef]
7. Camacho-Ramírez, A.; Prada-Oliveira, J.A.; Ribelles-García, A.; Almorza-Gomar, D.; Pérez-Arana, G.M. The leading role of peptide tyrosine tyrosine in glycemic control after roux-en-y gastric bypass in rats. *Obes. Surg.* **2020**, *30*, 697–706. [CrossRef]
8. Honka, H.; Koffert, J.; Kauhanen, S.; Kudomi, N.; Hurme, S.; Mari, A.; Lindqvist, A.; Wierup, N.; Parkkola, R.; Groop, L.; et al. Liver blood dynamics after bariatric surgery: The effects of mixed-meal test and incretin infusions. *Endocr. Connect.* **2018**, *7*, 888–896. [CrossRef]
9. Münzberg, H.; Laque, A.; Yu, S.; Rezai-Zadeh, K.; Berthou, H.R. Appetite and body weight regulation after bariatric surgery. *Obes. Rev.* **2015**, *16*, 77–90. [CrossRef] [PubMed]
10. Dimitriadis, G.K.; Randeva, M.S.; Miras, A.D. Potential Hormone Mechanisms of Bariatric Surgery. *Curr. Obes. Rep.* **2017**, *6*, 253–265. [CrossRef]
11. Meek, C.L.; Lewis, H.B.; Reimann, F.; Gribble, F.M.; Park, A.J. The effect of bariatric surgery on gastrointestinal and pancreatic peptide hormones. *Peptides* **2016**, *77*, 28–37. [CrossRef] [PubMed]
12. Ariyasu, H.; Takaya, K.; Tagami, T.; Ogawa, Y.; Hosoda, K.; Akamizu, T.; Suda, M.; Koh, T.; Natsui, K.; Toyooka, S. Stomach is a major source of circulating ghrelin, and feeding state determines plasma ghrelin-like immunoreactivity levels in humans. *J. Clin. Endocrinol. Metab.* **2001**, *86*, 4753–4758. [CrossRef]
13. Kalinowski, P.; Paluszkiewicz, R.; Wróblewski, T.; Remiszewski, P.; Grodzicki, M.; Bartoszewicz, Z.; Krawczyk, M. Ghrelin, leptin, and glycemic control after sleeve gastrectomy versus Roux-en-Y gastric bypass-results of a randomized clinical trial. *Surg. Obes. Relat. Dis.* **2017**, *13*, 181–188. [CrossRef]
14. Popovic, V.; Miljic, D.; Pekic, S.; Pesko, P.; Djurovic, M.; Doknic, M.; Damjanovic, S.; Micic, D.; Cvijovic, G.; Glodic, J.; et al. Low plasma ghrelin level in gastrectomized patients is accompanied by enhanced sensitivity to the ghrelin-induced growth hormone release. *J. Clin. Endocrinol. Metab.* **2005**, *90*, 2187–2191. [CrossRef] [PubMed]
15. Camacho-Ramírez, A.; Mayo-Ossorio, M.A.; Pacheco-García, J.M.; Almorza-Gomar, D.; Ribelles-García, A.; Belmonte-Núñez, A.; Prada-Oliveira, J.A.; Pérez-Arana, M. Pancreas is a preeminent source of ghrelin after sleeve gastrectomy in Wistar rats. *Histol. Histopathol.* **2020**, *35*, 801–809. [CrossRef]
16. Baena-Nieto, G.; Lomas-Romero, I.M.; Mateos, R.M.; Leal-Cosme, N.; Perez-Arana, G.; Aguilar-Diosdado, M. Ghrelin mitigates β-cell mass loss during insulitis in an animal model of autoimmune diabetes mellitus, the BioBreeding/Worcester rat. *Diabetes Metab. Res. Rev.* **2017**, *33*, e2813. [CrossRef] [PubMed]
17. Mullally, J.A.; Febres, G.J.; Bessler, M.; Korner, J. Sleeve Gastrectomy and Roux-en-Y gastric bypass achieve similar early improvements in beta-cell function in obese patients with Type 2 Diabetes. *Sci. Rep.* **2019**, *9*, 1880. [CrossRef]
18. Ugi, S.; Morino, K.; Yamaguchi, T.; Yamamoto, H.; Kaida, S.; Miyazawa, I.; Sato, D.; Sekine, O.; Fujita, Y.; Kashiwagi, A.; et al. Preserving beta-cell function is the major determinant of diabetes remission following laparoscopic sleeve gastrectomy in Japanese obese diabetic patients. *Endocr. J.* **2019**, *66*, 817–826. [CrossRef] [PubMed]
19. Garibay, D.; McGavigan, A.K.; Lee, S.A.; Ficorilli, J.V.; Cox, A.L.; Michael, M.D.; Sloop, K.W.; Cummings, B.P. Beta-cell glucagon-like peptide-1 receptor contributes to improved glucose tolerance after vertical sleeve gastrectomy. *Endocrinology* **2016**, *157*, 3405–3409. [CrossRef]
20. Garibay, D.; Lou, J.; Lee, S.A.; Zaborska, K.E.; Weissman, M.H.; Sloma, E.; Donahue, L.; Miller, A.D.; White, A.C.; Michael, A.D.; et al. β Cell GLP-1R signaling alters α cell proglucagon processing after vertical sleeve gastrectomy in mice. *Cell Rep.* **2018**, *23*, 967–973. [CrossRef] [PubMed]

21. Douros, J.D.; Lewis, A.G.; Smith, E.P.; Niu, J.; Capozzi, M.; Wittmann, A.; Campbell, J.; Tong, J.; Wagner, C.; Mahbod, P.; et al. Share enhanced glucose control following vertical sleeve gastrectomy does not require a beta-Cell Glucagon-Like Peptide 1 Receptor. *Diabetes* **2018**, *67*, 1504–1511. [CrossRef]
22. Li, F.; Cao, H.; Sheng, C.; Sun, H.; Song, K.; Qu, S. Upregulated Pdx1 and MafA contribute to β-cell function improvement by sleeve gastrectomy. *Obes. Surg.* **2016**, *26*, 904–909. [CrossRef] [PubMed]
23. Grong, E.; Kulseng, B.; Arbo, I.B.; Nord, C.; Eriksson, M.; Ahlgren, U.; Mårvik, R. Sleeve gastrectomy, but not duodenojejunostomy, preserves total beta-cell mass in Goto-Kakizaki rats evaluated by three-dimensional optical projection tomography. *Surg. Endosc.* **2016**, *30*, 532–542. [CrossRef] [PubMed]
24. Liu, T.; Zhong, M.W.; Liu, Y.; Sun, D.; Wei, M.; Huang, X.; Cheng, Y.G.; Wu, Q.Z.; Wu, D.; Zhang, X.Q.; et al. Diabetes recurrence after metabolic surgeries correlates with re-impaired insulin sensitivity rather than beta-cell function. *World J. Gastroenterol.* **2017**, *23*, 3468–3479. [CrossRef]
25. Bancalero-de los Reyes, J.; Camacho-Ramírez, A.; Fernández-Vivero, J.; Ribelles-García, A.; Macías-Rodríguez, M.; Almorza-Gomar, D.; Carrasco-Molinillo, C.; Mayo-Ossorio, M.A.; Prada-Oliveira, J.A.; Perez-Arana, G. Glucagon-producing cell expansion in Wistar rats. Changes to islet architecture after sleeve gastrectomy. *Obes. Surg.* **2021**, *31*, 2241–2249. [CrossRef]
26. Huising, M.O.; Lee, S.; Van der Meulen, T. Evidence for a neogenic niche at the periphery of pancreatic islets. *Bioessays* **2018**, *40*, e1800119. [CrossRef] [PubMed]
27. Damsteegt, E.L.; Hassan, Z.; Hewawasam, N.V.; Sarnsamak, K.; Jones, P.M.; Hauge-Evans, A. Novel Role for Somatostatin in the Survival of Mouse Pancreatic Beta Cells AC. *Cell Physiol. Biochem.* **2019**, *52*, 486–502. [CrossRef]
28. Alán, L.; Olejár, T.; Cahová, M.; Zelenka, J.; Berková, Z.; Smětáková, M.; Saudek, F.; Matěj, R.; Ježek, P. Delta Cell Hyperplasia in Adult Goto-Kakizaki (GK/MolTac) Diabetic Rats. *J. Diabetes Res.* **2015**, *2015*, 385395. [CrossRef]
29. DiGruccio, M.R.; Mawla, A.M.; Donaldson, C.J.; Noguchi, G.M.; Vaughan, J.; Cowing-Zitron, C.; van der Meulen, T.; Huising, M.O. Comprehensive alpha, beta and delta cell transcriptomes reveal that ghrelin selectively activates delta cells and promotes somatostatin release from pancreatic islets. *Mol. Metab.* **2016**, *5*, 449–458. [CrossRef]
30. Hayoz, C.; Hermann, T.; Raptis, D.A.; Brönnimann, A.; Peterli, R.; Zuber, M. Comparison of metabolic outcomes in patients undergoing laparoscopic roux-en-Y gastric bypass versus sleeve gastrectomy -a systematic review and meta-analysis of randomised controlled trials. *Swiss Med. Wkly.* **2018**, *148*, w14633. [CrossRef]
31. Inge, T.H.; Prigeon, R.L.; Elder, D.A.; Jenkins, T.M.; Cohen, R.M.; Xanthakos, S.A.; Benoit, S.C.; Dolan, L.M.; Daniels, S.R.; D'Alessio, D.A. Share insulin sensitivity and beta-cell function improve after gastric bypass in severely obese adolescents. *J. Pediatr.* **2015**, *167*, 1042–1048.e1. [CrossRef] [PubMed]
32. Lindqvist, A.; Spégel, P.; Ekelund, M.; Garcia Vaz, E.; Pierzynowski, S.; Gomez, M.F.; Mulder, H.; Hedenbro, J.; Groop, L.; Wierup, N. Gastric bypass improves β-cell function and increases β-cell mass in a porcine model. *Diabetes* **2014**, *63*, 1665–1671. [CrossRef]
33. Patti, M.E.; Goldfine, A.B.; Hu, J.; Hoem, D.; Molven, A.; Goldsmith, J.; Schwesinger, W.H.; La Rosa, S.; Folli, F.; Kulkarni, R.N. Heterogeneity of proliferative markers in pancreatic beta-cells of patients with severe hypoglycemia following Roux-en-Y gastric bypass. *Acta Diabetol.* **2017**, *54*, 737–747. [CrossRef] [PubMed]
34. Zhang, S.; Guo, W.; Wu, J.; Gong, L.; Li, Q.; Xiao, X.; Zhang, J.; Wang, Z. Increased β-cell mass in obese rats after gastric bypass: A potential mechanism for improving glycemic control. *Med. Sci. Monit.* **2017**, *23*, 2151–2158. [CrossRef] [PubMed]
35. Shah, M.; Laurenti, M.C.; Man, C.D.; Ma, J.; Cobelli, C.; Rizza, R.A.; Vella, A. Contribution of endogenous glucagon-like peptide-1 to changes in glucose metabolism and islet function in people with type 2 diabetes four weeks after Roux-en-Y gastric bypass (RYGB). *Metabolism* **2019**, *93*, 10–17. [CrossRef] [PubMed]
36. Mokadem, M.; Zechner, J.F.; Margolskee, R.F.; Drucker, D.J.; Aguirre, V. Effects of Roux-en-Y gastric bypass on energy and glucose homeostasis are preserved in two mouse models of functional glucagon-like peptide-1 deficiency. *Mol. Metab.* **2013**, *3*, 191–201. [CrossRef]
37. Guida, C.; Stephen, S.D.; Watson, M.; Dempster, N.; Larraufie, P.; Marjot, T.; Cargill, T.; Rickers, L.; Pavlides, M.; Tomlinson, J.; et al. PYY plays a key role in the resolution of diabetes following bariatric surgery in humans. *EBioMedicine* **2019**, *40*, 67–76. [CrossRef]
38. Furuyama, K.; Chera, S.; van Gurp, L.; Oropeza, D.; Ghila, L.; Damond, N.; Vethe, H.; Paulo, J.A.; Joosten, A.M.; Berney, T.; et al. Diabetes relief in mice by glucose-sensing insulin-secreting human alpha-cells. *Nature* **2019**, *567*, 43–48. [CrossRef]
39. Uchida, A.; Zechner, J.F.; Mani, B.K.; Park, W.M.; Aguirre, V.; Zigman, J.M. Altered ghrelin secretion in mice in response to diet-induced obesity and Roux-en-Y gastric bypass. *Mol. Metab.* **2014**, *3*, 717–730. [CrossRef]
40. Quesada-Candela, C.; Tudurí, E.; Marroquí, L.; Alonso-Magdalena, P.; Quesada, I.; Nadal, A. Morphological and functional adaptations of pancreatic alpha-cells during late pregnancy in the mouse. *Metabolism* **2020**, *102*, 153963. [CrossRef] [PubMed]
41. Marinho, T.S.; Borges, C.C.; Aguila, M.B.; Mandarim-de-Lacerda, C.A. Intermittent fasting benefits on alpha- and beta-cell arrangement in diet-induced obese mice pancreatic islet. *J. Diabetes Complicat.* **2019**, *26*, 107497. [CrossRef] [PubMed]
42. Longuet, C.; Robledo, A.M.; Dean, E.D.; Dai, C.; Ali, S.; McGuinness, I.; de Chavez, V.; Vuguin, P.M.; Charron, M.J.; Powers, A.C.; et al. Liver-specific disruption of the murine glucagon receptor produces alpha-cell hyperplasia: Evidence for a circulating alpha-cell growth factor. *Diabetes* **2013**, *62*, 1196–1205. [CrossRef]
43. Patel, K.; Levesque, K.; Mark, V.; Pierini, E.; Rojas, B.; Ahlers, M.; Shah, A.; Laferrère, B. Proinsulin associates with poor β-cell function, glucose-dependent insulinotropic peptide, and insulin resistance in persistent type 2 diabetes after Roux-en-Y gastric bypass in humans. *J. Diabetes* **2020**, *12*, 77–86. [CrossRef] [PubMed]

44. Malik, S.; Mitchell, J.E.; Steffen, K.; Engel, S.; Wiisanen, R.; Garcia, L.; Malik, S.A. Recognition and management of hyperinsulinemic hypoglycemia after bariatric surgery. *Obes. Res. Clin. Pract.* **2016**, *10*, 1–14. [CrossRef]
45. Swisa, A.; Glaser, B.; Dor, Y. Metabolic stress and compromised identity of pancreatic beta cells. *Front. Genet.* **2017**, *8*, 21. [CrossRef] [PubMed]
46. Georgia, A.; Asnis, M.C.C.; Febres, G.; Tsang, A.; Bessler, M.; Korner, J. Roux-en-Y Gastric Bypass is associated with hyperinsulinemia but not increased maximal β-cell. *Funct. J. Endocr. Soc.* **2019**, *3*, 632–642. [CrossRef] [PubMed]

Journal of
Clinical Medicine

MDPI

Article

Dental Erosion in Obese Patients before and after Bariatric Surgery: A Cross-Sectional Study

Cui Yang [1,*], Frederik Johannes Hammer [1,2], Christoph Reissfelder [1], Mirko Otto [1] and Georgi Vassilev [1]

[1] Department of Surgery, Medical Faculty Mannheim, University of Heidelberg, Theodor-Kutzer-Ufer 1-3, 68167 Mannheim, Germany; christoph.reissfelder@umm.de (F.J.H.); mirko.otto@umm.de (C.R.); georgi.vassilev@umm.de (M.O.); frederik.hammer@web.de (G.V.)

[2] Faculty of Dentistry, University of Heidelberg, 68167 Mannheim, Germany

* Correspondence: cui.yang@umm.de; Tel.: +49-621-383-2226

Abstract: Obese patients are at risk of dental erosion due to micronutrient deficiency, consumption of soft drinks, gastric reflux disease and vomiting. The present study evaluates the presence of dental erosion in obese patients before and after bariatric surgery using the BEWE (basic erosive wear examination) scoring system. A total of 62 patients with severe obesity were included in the analysis, 31 in the control group (without bariatric surgery) and 31 in the surgery group (after bariatric surgery). BEWE scores did not vary between groups. Vitamin D deficiency was detected in 19 patients in the control group and three in the surgery group ($p < 0.001$). The serum calcium and vitamin D values were significantly higher in the surgery group ($p = 0.003$, $p < 0.001$ consecutively). All patients after bariatric surgery showed compliance with supplements, including vitamin D and calcium daily. Patients after bariatric surgery were less likely to drink soft drinks regularly ($p = 0.026$). Obese patients, before or after bariatric surgery, are at risk for erosive dental wear. However, with sufficient education prior to surgery and consistent intake of vitamin and mineral supplements, significant erosive dental wear after bariatric surgery could be avoided. Regular dental examination should be included in the check-up and follow-up program.

Keywords: obesity; follow-up; substitution; micronutrient deficiency; dental health; RYGB; VSG; sleeve gastrectomy

Citation: Yang, C.; Hammer, F.J.; Reissfelder, C.; Otto, M.; Vassilev, G. Dental Erosion in Obese Patients before and after Bariatric Surgery: A Cross-Sectional Study. *J. Clin. Med.* **2021**, *10*, 4902. https://doi.org/10.3390/jcm10214902

Academic Editor: David Benaiges Boix

Received: 24 September 2021
Accepted: 21 October 2021
Published: 24 October 2021

1. Introduction

Among patients with poorly managed obesity, metabolic/bariatric surgery has been proven to be the most effective and durable therapy for obesity [1]. Obesity and bariatric surgery have been shown to be associated with a higher risk for dental wear [2,3], which is multifactorial: frequent consumption of soft drinks is associated with obesity and dental problems [4–6]; unhealthy food choices might have led to micronutrient deficiency before surgery, e.g., iron, vitamin D and calcium [7–10]; aversion to special foods and taste changes were often reported after surgery [11–14]; and the reduced intestinal absorptive surface area affected hormonal mediators, which can lead to micronutrient deficiency postoperatively, including lower vitamin D and calcium in serum [15–17].

Erosive tooth wear is defined as a chemical–mechanical condition with an increasing prevalence worldwide, which results in a loss of hard dental tissue [18,19]. The erosion of enamel, the outer surface layer of the teeth, leads to an exposure of the dentin [20]. Unprotected dentin creates hypersensitivity to physical stimuli, such as heat and cold [21]. With progressive degradation processes, exposure of the pulp and thus avitalization of the teeth can occur [20]. As an important biological factor, saliva buffers the pH in the oral cavity and decelerates the process of dental erosion [22]. Low pH is a risk factor for hypersensitivity and erosion: dietary acids (e.g., soft drinks) have been associated with erosive tooth wear [23,24], and a clear impact on erosion prevalence was found in patients with gastro-esophageal reflux (GERD) and eating disorders associated with vomiting [25].

In contrast, normal calcium concentration is considered as a major protective factor in determining the erosive potential [19].

GERD and vomiting are potential obesity-related problems and complications after bariatric surgery [26]. Considering the fact that patients are at further risk for calcium and vitamin D deficiency after bariatric surgery, it is suggested that the oral impactions of bariatric surgery might have consequences such as dental erosion. A recent review based on five Brazilian studies concluded that patients undergoing bariatric surgery had a higher incidence of dental complications [27]. The changes of saliva after bariatric surgery are also contradictory in the literature. Robust evidence, especially for dental erosion, is still lacking.

This study aimed to compare the dental erosion in obese patients before and after bariatric surgery. Potential dietary and health factors associating with erosive tooth wear were also evaluated.

2. Materials and Methods

2.1. Study Design

The study was designed as a single-center, cross-sectional analysis observing the effects of bariatric procedures on the severity of tooth erosion. The study was approved by the university faculty ethics committee and institutional review board (#2020-598N) and was conducted at a university hospital. The trial is registered in the German Clinical Trials Register (DRKS00025580).

2.2. Sample Size Calculation and Inclusion

Based on the described changes of dental wear and salivary flow after bariatric surgery in a previous study [28], we used G * Power sample size calculator [29] and set alpha to 0.05 and power to 0.9, resulting in a sample size of 30 participants per group.

The control group was composed of patients who possessed poorly managed obesity (body mass index (BMI) $\geq$ 35 kg/m^2 and one or more comorbidities (e.g., diabetes, arterial hypertension, or sleep apnea), or BMI $\geq$ 40 kg/m^2) who presented for bariatric surgery in the outpatient clinic; the surgery group consisted of patients who had already underwent bariatric surgery at least 3 months previously. Participation for all patients was predicated on their written informed consent.

2.3. Dental Examination

2.3.1. BEWE Score

The BEWE (basic erosive wear examination) is a simple tool designed to assess the level of dental erosion [30]. The teeth are divided into sextants. Only the value of the tooth surface with the highest BEWE value per sextant is documented. A value from 0 to 3 is determined in each sextant. Table 1 shows the criteria for sextant scores from 0 to 3, which are summed to obtain a cumulative score (0–18), which is the basis for determining interventions. The BEWE categories define the severity of erosion in 4 groups: group 0: 0–2 points; group 1: 3–8 points; group 2: 9–13 points; and group 3: 14–18 points. The BEWE categories can be further divided into the low-risk group (group 0 and 1) and the high-risk group (group 2 and 3). Patients in the high-risk group require dental health interventions.

Table 1. BEWE (basic erosive wear examination) scores and criteria.

Score	Criteria
0	No erosion
1	Initial loss of surface texture
2	Distinct defect; hard tissue loss involving <50% of the surface area
3	Hard tissue loss $\geq$50% of the surface area

2.3.2. Sialometry

To determine the saliva flow rate, a measurement of the unstimulated saliva production within 5 min as the "spitting method" was used [31]. Using the unstimulated method, the naturally produced saliva is gathered in the floor of the mouth and spat into a collecting tube at certain time intervals. A hyposalivation is defined as salivary flow below 0.25 mL/min.

Blood samples were collected on the same day of dental examination. Vitamins and minerals, including vitamin D and calcium in serum, were measured in a routine diagnostic setting.

2.4. Questionnaire

Using an investigative questionnaire, the following data were collected: sociodemographic data (age, gender, education level, income, and migrant status), preexisting comorbidities (e.g., diabetes, arterial hypertension, and thyroid disease), dietary habits (soft drinks, eating frequencies, smoking, alcohol consumption and eating disorders), gastrointestinal discomforting (regurgitation, gastroesophageal reflux and vomiting) and dental health (hypersensitivity, history of dental or periodontal disease) as well as dental health awareness (dentist visit frequency and oral hygiene).

2.5. Statistical Analysis

All statistical calculations were performed with the RStudio Version 1.2.5042, "Double Marigold" (Boston, MA, USA) and Python 3.9.5. (Wilmington, DE, USA) For quantitative variables, the mean and standard deviations were assessed. For qualitative factors, absolute and relative frequencies were given. For non-normally distributed data, the Wilcoxon rank-sum test was used. Pearson correlation coefficient measured correlations between two metric variables, Spearman correlation between an ordinal and a metric variable, and Chi^2-test between a nominal and an ordinal variable. In general, the result of a statistical test was considered statistically significant for a p-value < 0.05.

3. Results

The study was conducted at our university hospital between January and March 2021. All operations were performed laparoscopically by two of the co-authors (M.O. and G.V.) and the dental examinations were carried out by a dentist (co-author F.J.H.).

3.1. Demographics

Obese patients who presented for bariatric surgery or a follow-up after bariatric surgery were included. Sixty-two patients were enrolled (thirty-one in each group), with an average age of 40 years old. The majority of the participants are females. Participants in the control group are younger and more obese. Other sociodemographic characteristics did not differ between groups (Table 2).

Table 2. Sociodemographic characteristics of 62 patients.

Variables	Control	Surgery	p-Value
Number of patients	31	31	n.s.
Female (%)	22 (71)	28 (90)	n.s.
Age (years), Mean ± SD	37.5 ± 9.6	42.7 ± 10.1	$p = 0.038$
BMI (kg/m^2), Mean ± SD	46.1 ± 7.5	32.5 ± 5.9	$p < 0.0001$
Education classification (%)			n.s.
low	11 (35.5)	7 (22.4)	
middle	16 (51.6)	16 (51.6)	
high	4 (12.9)	8 (25.8)	
Income (%)			n.s.
low	6 (19.4)	3(9.7)	
middle	22(71.0)	20 (64.5)	
high	3(9.6)	8 (25.8)	
Migration (%)	8 (25.8)	3 (9.7)	n.s.

BMI, body mass index; n.a., not available; n.s., not significant; SD, Standard Deviation. Significant p-values are highlighted in bold (Wilcoxon, Chi^2 and Fisher's exact tests, $p < 0.05$). The education was classified based on ISCED 2011 (International Standard Classification of Education [32]). The income was classified by statistic data in Germany [33,34].

3.2. Oral Health Related Parameters

Patients after bariatric surgery were less likely to drink soft drinks regularly ($p = 0.026$) and reported less GERD ($p = 0.012$). Other parameters, including hypersensitivity of the teeth, eating disorders and vomiting, were similar among the groups (Table 3).

Table 3. Oral health related parameters.

Variables	Control	Surgery	*p*-Value
Smoking (%)	10 (32.2)	8 (25.8)	n.s.
Alcohol consumption (%)	2 (6.4)	1 (3.2)	n.s.
Soft drinks (%)	14 (45.2)	5 (16.1)	$p = 0.026$
Eating frequency			n.s.
1–3 meals/d (%)	22 (71.0)	15 (48.4)	
≥4 meals/d (%)	9 (29.0)	16 (51.6)	
Eating disorder (%)	6 (19.4)	4 (12.9)	n.s.
GERD (%)			$p = 0.012$
never	15 (48.4)	26 (83.9)	
maximal once/week	11 (35.5)	3 (9.7)	
>once/week	5 (16.1)	2 (6.4)	
Vomiting (%)			n.s.
never	28 (90.3)	27 (87.1)	
maximal once/week	3 (9.7)	3 (9.7)	
>once/week	0 (0)	1 (3.2)	
Hypersensitivity of teeth (%)	12 (38.7)	11 (35.5)	n.s.

GERD, gastroesophageal reflux disease; n.s., not significant. Significant *p*-values are highlighted in bold (Chi^2 and Fisher's exact tests).

3.3. Dental Examination and Level of Serum Vitamin D/Calcium

All patients after bariatric surgery have taken the recommended supplements, including vitamin D and calcium citrate, daily. Among all patients, three patients had a hypocalcaemia (<2.18 mmol/L), who were all in the control group. No hypocalcaemia was found in the surgery group. Vitamin D deficiency (<20 µg/L) was detected in 19 patients in the control group and three in the surgery group ($p < 0.001$). The serum calcium and vitamin D values were significantly higher in the surgery group ($p = 0.003$, $p < 0.001$ consecutively).

BEWE scores, BEWE category and BEWE risk groups did not vary between groups. Of the preoperative obese patients, 22.6% were classified in BEWE category 2 and 3, therefore they had a high risk for further exposure of the pulp and consequential avitalization of the teeth (Figure 1). In the surgery group, the percentage was even higher (32.2%), but the difference was not significant. Neither was there a significant difference in the salivary flow (Table 4).

3.4. Correlation

Sociodemographic parameters, such as age, education level, migration status and comorbidities, did not show significant correlations with BEWE scores, risk and salivary flow.

3.5. VSG versus RYGB

In the surgery group, seven patients underwent a vertical sleeve gastrectomy (VSG), 21 underwent a Roux-en-Y gastric bypass (RYGB) and three others underwent a single-anastomosis duodeno-ileal bypass (S.A.D.I-S) or bilio-pancreatic diversion with duodenal switch (BPD-DS). The frequency of GERD, vomiting, BEWE scores, BEWE categories, risk, salivary flow, salivary flow categories, calcium and vitamin D did not differ between patients who underwent VSG and RYGB.

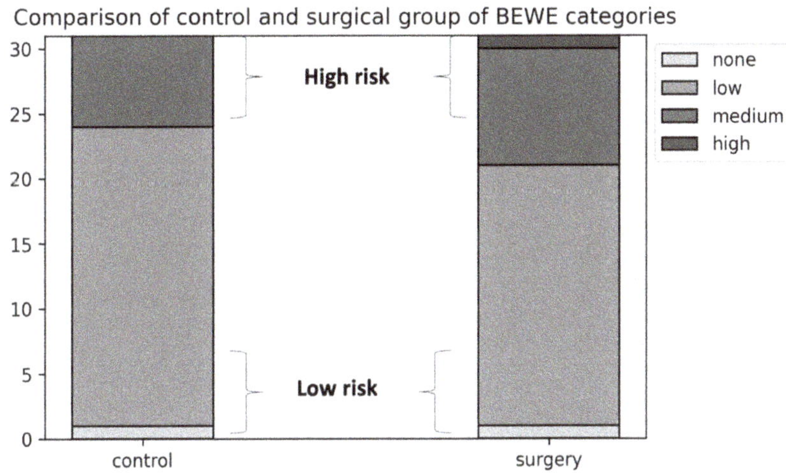

Figure 1. Portion of BEWE categories in control and surgery group.

Table 4. Results of dental examinations.

Variables	Control	Surgery	p-Value
Calcium, mmol/L	2.34 ± 0.11	2.42 ± 0.10	$p = 0.003$
Vitamin D, μg/L	18.0 ± 9.2	31.0 ± 12.1	$p < 0.001$
BEWE score	7.0 ± 2.2	7.4 ± 2.8	n.s.
BEWE category (%)			n.s.
0	1 (3.2)	1 (3.2)	
1	23 (74.2)	20 (64.5)	
2	7 (22.6)	9 (29.0)	
3	0 (0)	1 (3.2)	
BEWE risk categories (%)			n.s.
low risk	24 (77.4)	21 (67.7)	
high risk	7 (22.6)	10 (32.2)	
Salivary flow, mL/min	0.32 ± 0.1	0.32 ± 0.1	n.s.
Classification of salivary flow			n.s.
hyposalivation (%)	10 (32.2)	10 (32.2)	
normal salivary flow (%)	21 (67.8)	21 (67.8)	

BEWE (basic erosive wear examination); n.s., not significant. All values are shown as means and standard deviation or frequency and percentage. Significant p-values ($p < 0.05$) are highlighted in bold.

3.6. Short-Term Follow-Up versus Long-Term Follow-Up

In the surgery group, the period between bariatric surgery and dental examination was 11 (3–142) months. Patients with a shorter follow-up (<11 months) had significantly higher calcium levels in the serum ($p = 0.014$). Vitamin D, BEWE scores and salivary flow did not differ between patients with a short-term (<11 months) and long-term (>11 months) follow-up.

4. Discussion

The prevalence of obesity is increasing, along with the number of bariatric surgeries. Accordingly, the side effects of obesity and bariatric surgery are gaining growing attention. Several factors associated with bariatric surgery might lead to dental health problems: micronutrient deficiency, as vitamin D and calcium deficiency accompanies the great severity of oral disease [35,36]; increased prevalence of gastroesophageal reflux and vomiting, which lowers the pH in oral cavity, and is consequently a major risk factor for erosive dental wear [23,24]; and the postoperative, recommended, small yet frequent meals (4–6 meals/day), which shorten the regeneration period for the saliva [28,37], which is of great importance for the hard tissue protection.

The current study confirmed that a significant number of obese patients are at a high risk for erosive dental wear and can experience further exposure of the pulp and thus avitalization of the teeth. However, the condition of dental wear did not worsen significantly after bariatric surgery. This is not in line with the limited data in the literature which have evaluated the effect of bariatric surgery on dental erosion. Quintella et al. reviewed five Brazilian studies and concluded that patients undergoing bariatric surgery had a higher incidence of dental wear [27]. Of these studies, one focused on erosive damage, and showed more severe dental erosion in patients after bariatric surgery [38]. The divergence of conclusions might be multifactorial. Firstly, the entire population in our surgery group have taken recommended supplements, including calcium citrate and vitamin D3, which was confirmed by the significantly higher serum levels of calcium and vitamin D after surgery. Calcium and vitamin D are known to have a protective effect on hard tooth tissues [39]. The recommended supplement of vitamins and minerals was not mentioned in the Brazilian studies. Secondly, GERD and vomiting were not increased after bariatric surgery in our observation. On the contrary, GERD was significantly less reported in the surgery group, which can be explained by two facts: postoperative patients were less obese (significant lower BMI) and therefore possessed a decreased risk for GERD [40], and, in the majority of the postoperative patients, RYGB was performed. After RYGB, gastric reflux remission is more frequently observed than after VSG [41]. Thus, RGYB could be a protective factor for dental health. Thirdly, the daily consumption of soft drinks, another potential factor to lower pH in oral cavity, was significantly reduced in our surgery group. Previous investigations showed that soft drink consumption can contribute to detrimental oral health, especially due to the erosive potential [6]. Postoperative taste changes might explain the altered dietary habits [11,13]. Moreover, patients were required to take part in a minimally 6-month long, multimodal concept, including intensive consultation by nutritional therapist before the surgery. Nutritional therapists assess and correct their nutritional status and, more importantly, educate the patients on how to establish healthy dietary habits (fewer soft drinks, less carbohydrates, and more proteins, etc.). The presurgical education seemed to have a lasting effect in the patients, which was not mentioned in the Brazilian studies. Fourthly, the spans between the bariatric surgery and the survey differ. Interestingly, studies confirming a worsening of dental wear in patients after bariatric surgery were performed with a relatively short flow-up (3–6 months) [28,42]. Even with a longer follow-up span (with a median of 11 months), no significant difference was detected in our study population. Moreover, patients with a longer follow-up did not present with a higher risk for erosive dental wear than patients with a short-term follow-up in our study. It can be assumed that the risk of erosive dental wear would not increase if patients were compliant with supplements and follow-up.

Saliva is an important biological factor, which buffers the pH in the oral cavity and decelerates the process of dental erosion [22]. The impact of bariatric surgery on saliva production remains unclear. Some studies showed an improvement in the salivary flow rate, while others found no change or even a worsening in saliva production after the surgery [43]. In our study, the salivary rate did not differ between the groups. The inconsistency might be partially due to different measuring methods. We preferred the unstimulated spitting method to the stimulated measurement, since the unstimulated saliva flow, which occurs around 14 to 16 h per day, is primarily responsible for the maintenance of oral health and the protection of our teeth. The stimulated saliva flow rate, on the other hand, embodies the functional capacity of the salivary glands and is only present for around two hours a day [31]. Furthermore, our measurement was performed in two different groups, and interindividual differences might preexist for salivary production.

To the best of our knowledge, this is the first study evaluating erosive dental ware in obese patients before and after bariatric surgery in Europe. Bariatric surgery might be associated with risks of erosive dental wear due to multiple factors. However, with sufficient education prior to surgery, consistent intake of vitamin and mineral supplements, and regular follow-ups, significant erosive dental wear after bariatric surgery could be avoided. Regular dental examination should be included in the follow-up program after bariatric surgery. A remineralization solution might help to prevent dental erosions from occurring [44].

5. Limitations

The majority of patients in the surgery group received a Roux-en-Y gastric bypass. The results might be different in patients after sleeve gastrectomy. Overall, there are more female than male participants in our study. Patients were not perfectly paired in both groups due to different BMIs and ages. To minimize the bias, dental examination should be performed in patients indicated for bariatric surgery before and after surgery in further trials.

6. Conclusions

Obesity and bariatric surgery might be associated with risks for erosive dental wear due to multiple factors. However, with sufficient education prior to surgery and consistent intake of vitamin and mineral supplements, significant erosive dental wear after bariatric surgery could be avoided. Regular dental examination should be included in the check-up and follow-up program in obese patients before and after bariatric surgery.

Author Contributions: Conceptualization, C.Y., F.J.H., M.O. and G.V.; methodology, C.Y., F.J.H. and G.V.; formal analysis, C.Y.; investigation, F.J.H.; data curation, C.Y.; writing—original draft preparation, C.Y. and F.J.H.; writing—review and editing, C.R., M.O. and G.V.; supervision, C.R., M.O. and G.V.; project administration, C.Y. All authors have read and agreed to the published version of the manuscript.

Funding: This research received no external funding.

Institutional Review Board Statement: The study was conducted according to the guidelines of the Declaration of Helsinki and approved by the university faculty ethics committee and institutional review board (#2020-598N).

Informed Consent Statement: Informed consent was obtained from all subjects involved in the study.

Data Availability Statement: The data presented in this study are available on request from the corresponding author.

Conflicts of Interest: The authors declare no conflict of interest.

References

1. Wadden, T.A.; Bantle, J.P.; Blackburn, G.L.; Bolin, P.; Brancati, F.L.; Bray, G.A.; Clark, J.M.; Coday, M.; Dutton, G.R.; Egan, C.; et al. Eight-Year Weight Losses with an Intensive Lifestyle Intervention: The Look AHEAD Study. *Obesity* **2014**, *22*, 5–13. [CrossRef]
2. Castilho, A.V.S.S.; Foratori-Junior, G.A.; Sales-Peres, S.H.D.C. Bariatric surgery impact on gastroesophageal reflux and dental wear: A systematic review. *Arquivos Brasileiros de Cirurgia Digestiva* **2019**, *32*, e1466. [CrossRef]
3. Tschammler, C.; Simon, A.; Brockmann, K.; Röbl, M.; Wiegand, A. Erosive Tooth Wear and Caries Experience in Children and Adolescents with Obesity. *J. Dent.* **2019**, *83*, 77–86. [CrossRef] [PubMed]
4. Khadri, F.A.; Gopinath, V.K.; Hector, M.P.; Davenport, E.S. Evaluating the Risk Factors That Link Obesity and Dental Caries in 11-17-Year-Old School Going Children in the United Arab Emirates. *Eur. J. Dent.* **2018**, *12*, 217–224. [CrossRef] [PubMed]
5. Marro, F.; De Smedt, S.; Rajasekharan, S.; Martens, L.; Bottenberg, P.; Jacquet, W. Associations between Obesity, Dental Caries, Erosive Tooth Wear and Periodontal Disease in Adolescents: A Case-Control Study. *Eur. Arch. Paediatr. Dent.* **2021**, *22*, 99–108. [CrossRef] [PubMed]
6. Basha, S.; Enan, E.T.; Mohamed, R.N.; Ashour, A.A.; Alzahrani, F.S.; Almutairi, N.E. Association between Soft Drink Consumption, Gastric Reflux, Dental Erosion, and Obesity among Special Care Children. *Spec. Care Dent.* **2020**, *40*, 97–105. [CrossRef]
7. Costa, T.L.; Paganotto, M.; Radominski, R.B.; Kulak, C.M.; Borba, V.C. Calcium Metabolism, Vitamin D and Bone Mineral Density after Bariatric Surgery. *Osteoporos. Int.* **2015**, *26*, 757–764. [CrossRef] [PubMed]

8. Schweiger, C.; Weiss, R.; Berry, E.; Keidar, A. Nutritional Deficiencies in Bariatric Surgery Candidates. *Obes. Surg.* **2010**, *20*, 193–197. [CrossRef] [PubMed]
9. Arshad, M.; Jaberian, S.; Pazouki, A.; Riazi, S.; Rangraz, M.A.; Mokhber, S. Iron Deficiency Anemia and Megaloblastic Anemia in Obese Patients. *Rom. J. Intern. Med.* **2017**, *55*, 3–7. [CrossRef] [PubMed]
10. Tan, B.C.; Park, Y.S.; Won, Y.; Lee, S.; Kang, S.H.; Ahn, S.-H.; Park, D.J.; Kim, H.-H. Preoperative Nutritional Deficiencies in Bariatric Surgery Candidates in Korea. *Obes. Surg.* **2021**, *31*, 2660–2668. [CrossRef] [PubMed]
11. Ahmed, K.; Penney, N.; Darzi, A.; Purkayastha, S. Taste Changes after Bariatric Surgery: A Systematic Review. *Obes. Surg.* **2018**, *28*, 3321–3332. [CrossRef]
12. Zerrweck, C.; Zurita, L.; Álvarez, G.; Maydón, H.G.; Sepúlveda, E.M.; Campos, F.; Caviedes, A.; Guilbert, L. Taste and Olfactory Changes Following Laparoscopic Gastric Bypass and Sleeve Gastrectomy. *Obes. Surg.* **2016**, *26*, 1296–1302. [CrossRef] [PubMed]
13. Nance, K.; Acevedo, M.B.; Pepino, M.Y. Changes in Taste Function and Ingestive Behavior Following Bariatric Surgery. *Appetite* **2020**, *146*, 104423. [CrossRef] [PubMed]
14. Graham, L.; Murty, G.; Bowrey, D.J. Taste, Smell and Appetite Change after Roux-En-Y Gastric Bypass Surgery. *Obes. Surg.* **2014**, *24*, 1463–1468. [CrossRef]
15. Gehrer, S.; Kern, B.; Peters, T.; Christoffel-Courtin, C.; Peterli, R. Fewer Nutrient Deficiencies after Laparoscopic Sleeve Gastrectomy (LSG) than after Laparoscopic Roux-Y-Gastric Bypass (LRYGB)-a Prospective Study. *Obes. Surg.* **2010**, *20*, 447–453. [CrossRef]
16. Coupaye, M.; Puchaux, K.; Bogard, C.; Msika, S.; Jouet, P.; Clerici, C.; Larger, E.; Ledoux, S. Nutritional Consequences of Adjustable Gastric Banding and Gastric Bypass: A 1-Year Prospective Study. *Obes. Surg.* **2009**, *19*, 56–65. [CrossRef] [PubMed]
17. Ledoux, S.; Calabrese, D.; Bogard, C.; Dupré, T.; Castel, B.; Msika, S.; Larger, E.; Coupaye, M. Long-Term Evolution of Nutritional Deficiencies after Gastric Bypass: An Assessment According to Compliance to Medical Care. *Ann. Surg.* **2014**, *259*, 1104–1110. [CrossRef] [PubMed]
18. Lussi, A.; Carvalho, T.S. Erosive Tooth Wear: A Multifactorial Condition of Growing Concern and Increasing Knowledge. *Monogr. Oral Sci.* **2014**, *25*, 1–15. [CrossRef] [PubMed]
19. Carvalho, T.S.; Colon, P.; Ganss, C.; Huysmans, M.-C.; Lussi, A.; Schlueter, N.; Schmalz, G.; Shellis, P.R.; Björg Tveit, A.; Wiegand, A. Consensus Report of the European Federation of Conservative Dentistry: Erosive Tooth Wear—Diagnosis and Management. *Swiss Dent. J.* **2016**, *126*, 342–346. [CrossRef] [PubMed]
20. Sivasithamparam, K.; Harbrow, D.; Vinczer, E.; Young, W.G. Endodontic Sequelae of Dental Erosion. *Aust. Dent. J.* **2003**, *48*, 97–101. [CrossRef]
21. Bartlett, D.W. The Role of Erosion in Tooth Wear: Aetiology, Prevention and Management. *Int. Dent. J.* **2005**, *55*, 277–284. [CrossRef]
22. Buzalaf, M.A.R.; Hannas, A.R.; Kato, M.T. Saliva and Dental Erosion. *J. Appl. Oral Sci. Rev.* **2012**, *20*, 493–502. [CrossRef]
23. O'Toole, S.; Bernabé, E.; Moazzez, R.; Bartlett, D. Timing of Dietary Acid Intake and Erosive Tooth Wear: A Case-Control Study. *J. Dent.* **2017**, *56*, 99–104. [CrossRef] [PubMed]
24. Bartlett, D.W.; Lussi, A.; West, N.X.; Bouchard, P.; Sanz, M.; Bourgeois, D. Prevalence of Tooth Wear on Buccal and Lingual Surfaces and Possible Risk Factors in Young European Adults. *J. Dent.* **2013**, *41*, 1007–1013. [CrossRef] [PubMed]
25. Schlueter, N.; Luka, B. Erosive Tooth Wear—A Review on Global Prevalence and on Its Prevalence in Risk Groups. *Br. Dent. J.* **2018**, *224*, 364–370. [CrossRef] [PubMed]
26. Gu, L.; Chen, B.; Du, N.; Fu, R.; Huang, X.; Mao, F.; Khadaroo, P.A.; Zhao, S. Relationship Between Bariatric Surgery and Gastroesophageal Reflux Disease: A Systematic Review and Meta-Analysis. *Obes. Surg.* **2019**, *29*, 4105–4113. [CrossRef] [PubMed]
27. Quintella, M.C.M.; Farias, T.M.C.P.; Soutomaior, J.R.; Casado, B.G.D.S.; Leão, R.D.S.; De Moraes, S.L.D. Relationship between Bariatric Surgery and Dental Erosion: A Systematic Review. *Surg. Obes. Relat. Dis.* **2020**, *16*, 1283–1290. [CrossRef]
28. Marsicano, J.A.; Grec, P.G.D.M.; Belarmino, L.B.; Ceneviva, R.; Peres, S.H.D.C.S. Interfaces between Bariatric Surgery and Oral Health: A Longitudinal Survey. *Acta Cirurgica Brasileira* **2011**, *26* (Suppl. 2), 79–83. [CrossRef] [PubMed]
29. Faul, F.; Erdfelder, E.; Buchner, A.; Lang, A.-G. Statistical power analyses using G*Power 3.1: Tests for correlation and regression analyses. *Behav. Res. Methods* **2009**, *41*, 1149–1160. [CrossRef]
30. Bartlett, D.; Ganss, C.; Lussi, A. Basic Erosive Wear Examination (BEWE): A New Scoring System for Scientific and Clinical Needs. *Clin. Oral Investig.* **2008**, *12* (Suppl. 1), S65–S68. [CrossRef] [PubMed]
31. Sreebny, L.M.; Vissink, A. *Dry Mouth, the Malevolent Symptom: A Clinical Guide*; John Wiley & Sons: Hoboken, NJ, USA, 2010; ISBN 978-0-8138-1623-4.
32. UNESCO Institute for Statistics. *International Standard Classification of Education: ISCED 2011*; UNESCO Institute for Statistics: Montreal, QC, Canada, 2012; ISBN 978-92-9189-123-8.
33. Armutsgrenze in Deutschland. Available online: https://de.statista.com/statistik/daten/studie/510/umfrage/einstufung-in-arm-und-reich-fuer-singles-und-paare/ (accessed on 16 May 2021).
34. Armutsgrenzen laut Armutsbericht und Reich für Familien. Available online: https://de.statista.com/statistik/daten/studie/515/umfrage/einstufung-in-arm-und-reich-fuer-familien/ (accessed on 16 May 2021).
35. Antonenko, O.; Bryk, G.; Brito, G.; Pellegrini, G.; Zeni, S.N. Oral Health in Young Women Having a Low Calcium and Vitamin D Nutritional Status. *Clin. Oral Investig.* **2015**, *19*, 1199–1206. [CrossRef] [PubMed]

36. Uwitonze, A.M.; Murererehe, J.; Ineza, M.C.; Harelimana, E.I.; Nsabimana, U.; Uwambaye, P.; Gatarayiha, A.; Haq, A.; Razzaque, M.S. Effects of Vitamin D Status on Oral Health. *J. Steroid Biochem. Mol. Biol.* **2018**, *175*, 190–194. [CrossRef]
37. Marsh, P.D.; Lewis, M.A.O.; Rogers, H.; Williams, D.W.; Wilson, M. *Marsh and Martin's Oral Microbiology—E-Book*; Elsevier: Amsterdam, The Netherlands, 2016; ISBN 978-0-7020-6174-5.
38. Alves, M.D.S.C.; Da Silva, F.A.C.C.; Araújo, S.G.; De Carvalho, A.C.A.; Santos, A.M.; De Carvalho, A.L.A. Tooth Wear in Patients Submitted to Bariatric Surgery. *Braz. Dent. J.* **2012**, *23*, 160–166. [CrossRef]
39. Cagetti, M.G.; Wolf, T.G.; Tennert, C.; Camoni, N.; Lingström, P.; Campus, G. The Role of Vitamins in Oral Health. A Systematic Review and Meta-Analysis. *Int. J. Environ. Res. Public. Health* **2020**, *17*, 938. [CrossRef] [PubMed]
40. Maret-Ouda, J.; Markar, S.R.; Lagergren, J. Gastroesophageal Reflux Disease: A Review. *JAMA* **2020**, *324*, 2536–2547. [CrossRef]
41. Peterli, R.; Wölnerhanssen, B.K.; Peters, T.; Vetter, D.; Kröll, D.; Borbély, Y.; Schultes, B.; Beglinger, C.; Drewe, J.; Schiesser, M.; et al. Effect of Laparoscopic Sleeve Gastrectomy vs Laparoscopic Roux-En-Y Gastric Bypass on Weight Loss in Patients With Morbid Obesity: The SM-BOSS Randomized Clinical Trial. *JAMA* **2018**, *319*, 255–265. [CrossRef]
42. De Moura-Grec, P.G.; Yamashita, J.M.; Marsicano, J.A.; Ceneviva, R.; de Souza Leite, C.V.; de Brito, G.B.; Brienze, S.L.A.; de Carvalho Sales-Peres, S.H. Impact of Bariatric Surgery on Oral Health Conditions: 6-Months Cohort Study. *Int. Dent. J.* **2014**, *64*, 144–149. [CrossRef] [PubMed]
43. Schwenger, K.J.P.; Alghamdi, M.M.; Ghorbani, Y.; Jackson, T.D.; Okrainec, A.; Allard, J.P. Hyposalivation Is Prevalent in Bariatric Patients but Improves after Surgery. *Surg. Obes. Relat. Dis.* **2020**, *16*, 1407–1413. [CrossRef]
44. Scribante, A.; Farahani, M.R.D.; Marino, G.; Matera, C.; Baena, R.R.Y.; Lanteri, V.; Butera, A. Biomimetic Effect of Nano-Hydroxyapatite in Demineralized Enamel before Orthodontic Bonding of Brackets and Attachments: Visual, Adhesion Strength, and Hardness in In Vitro Tests. *BioMed Res. Int.* **2020**, *2020*, e6747498. [CrossRef]

Journal of
Clinical Medicine

MDPI

Article

Long-Term Weight Outcomes after Bariatric Surgery: A Single Center Saudi Arabian Cohort Experience

Assim A. Alfadda [1,2,*], Mohammed Y. Al-Naami [3], Afshan Masood [1], Ruba Elawad [1], Arthur Isnani [1], Shaik Shaffi Ahamed [4] and Nora A. Alfadda [5]

1 Obesity Research Center, College of Medicine, King Saud University, P.O. Box 2925 (98), Riyadh 11461, Saudi Arabia; afsmasood@ksu.edu.sa (A.M.); r.elawad@gmail.com (R.E.); aisnani@ksu.edu.sa (A.I.)
2 Department of Medicine, College of Medicine, King Saud University, P.O. Box 2925 (38), Riyadh 11461, Saudi Arabia
3 Department of Surgery, College of Medicine, King Saud University, Riyadh 11461, Saudi Arabia; alnaami@ksu.edu.sa
4 Department of Family and Community Medicine, College of Medicine, King Saud University, P.O. Box 7065, Riyadh 12372, Saudi Arabia; sshaik@ksu.edu.sa
5 Clinical Nutrition Program, Department of Community Health Sciences, College of Applied Medical Sciences, King Saud University, P.O. Box 10219, Riyadh 11433, Saudi Arabia; noraalfadda@gmail.com
* Correspondence: aalfadda@ksu.edu.sa; Tel./Fax: +966-11-467-1315

Citation: Alfadda, A.A.; Al-Naami, M.Y.; Masood, A.; Elawad, R.; Isnani, A.; Ahamed, S.S.; Alfadda, N.A. Long-Term Weight Outcomes after Bariatric Surgery: A Single Center Saudi Arabian Cohort Experience. *J. Clin. Med.* **2021**, *10*, 4922. https://doi.org/10.3390/jcm10214922

Academic Editor: David Benaiges Boix

Received: 12 October 2021
Accepted: 22 October 2021
Published: 25 October 2021

Abstract: Background: Obesity is considered a global chronic disease requiring weight management through lifestyle modification, pharmacotherapy, or weight loss surgery. The dramatic increase in patients with severe obesity in Saudi Arabia is paralleled with those undergoing bariatric surgery. Although known to be beneficial in the short term, the long-term impacts of surgery within this group and the sustainability of weight loss after surgery remains unclear. Objectives: We aimed to assess the long-term weight outcomes after bariatric surgery. Setting: The study was conducted at King Khalid University Hospital (KKUH), King Saud University Medical City (KSUMC) in Riyadh, Saudi Arabia. Methods: An observational prospective cohort study on adult patients with severe obesity undergoing bariatric surgery (sleeve gastrectomy (SG) or Roux-en Y gastric bypass (RYGB)) during the period between 2009 and 2015 was conducted. Weight loss patterns were evaluated pre- and post-surgery through clinical and anthropometric assessments. Absolute weight loss was determined, and outcome variables: percent excess weight loss (%EWL), percent total weight loss (%TWL), and percent weight regain (%WR), were calculated. Statistical analysis using univariate and multivariate general linear modelling was carried out. Results: A total of 91 (46 males and 45 females) patients were included in the study, with the majority belonging to the SG group. Significant weight reductions were observed at 1 and 3 years of follow-up ($p < 0.001$) from baseline. The %EWL and %TWL were at their maximum at 3 years (72.4% and 75.8%) and were comparable between the SG and RYGB. Decrements in %EWL and %TWL and increases in %WR were seen from 3 years onwards from bariatric surgery until the study period ended. The yearly follow-up attrition rate was 20.8% at 1 year post-surgery, 26.4% at year 2, 31.8% at year 3, 47.3% at year 4, 62.6% at year 5, and 79.1% at end of study period (at year 6). Conclusion: The major challenge to the successful outcome of bariatric surgery is in maintaining weight loss in the long-term and minimizing weight regain. Factors such as the type of surgery and gender need to be considered before and after surgery, with an emphasis on the need for long-term follow-up to enssure the optimal benefits from this intervention.

Keywords: weight regain; bariatric surgery; obesity; long-term follow-up; weight loss

1. Introduction

Obesity has become a worldwide epidemic: according to the 2016 World Health Organization statistics, 1.9 billion adults were overweight, and more than 650 million were obese [1]. This increase in the number of individuals with overweight and obesity is also reflected in the Saudi population [2,3], where the estimated rate of overweight and obesity is 24.1% in men and 33.5% in women [3]. Obesity management aims at achieving weight loss, utilizing a multifactorial stepwise approach consisting of behavioral therapy, lifestyle and dietary interventions, and medical pharmacotherapy. Weight loss through bariatric surgery is an adjunct to the former strategies in patients who did not benefit from them or who have additional comorbidities associated with obesity.

Presently, bariatric surgery is globally considered among the most effective management modalities for patients with obesity. The Saudi clinical practice guidelines, similar to the American Society for Metabolic and Bariatric Surgery, recommends that bariatric surgery should be conducted for patients with obesity who have a body mass index (BMI) $\geq$40 or $\geq$35 kg/m^2 and the presence of comorbidities [4] to diminish the risk of the associated comorbidities and to improve quality of life [5,6]. In Saudi Arabia, the number of patients with obesity who undergo bariatric surgery has noticeably grown [7], and $\geq$15,000 procedures are estimated to be performed annually [8]. These procedures are known to be effective and lead to major weight loss, with the maximum weight loss occurring at 12–18 months post-surgery [9]. The Swedish Obese Subjects (SOS) study, the largest non-randomized intervention trial that compared weight loss outcome over 10 years, reported a maximal total body weight change in patients after 1 year after receiving Roux-en-Y gastric bypass (RYGB) and vertical banded gastroplasty surgeries, with reductions of 38 $\pm$ 7% and 26 $\pm$ 10%, respectively [5]. A successful outcome of bariatric surgery is one that achieves a loss of 50–70% of excess weight (EWL) or the 20–30% loss of the patient's initial weight, or a BMI < 35 kg/m^2 [9,10]. Although many studies have documented the competence and effectiveness of bariatric surgery in reducing excess weight in the short term, mid- and long-term studies have reported weight regain as an index for failure of the surgery, regardless of the surgical procedure [5,11]. According to the SOS study, patients were noted to have regained around 20–25% of their lost weight at 10 years post-surgery. A weight regain of 12% total body weight was observed in patients who underwent RYGB, while those reported for sleeve gastrectomy (SG) were variable, ranging from 6% at as early as two years post-surgery to 76% at six years post-surgery [12]. Previous studies have addressed different factors that contribute to weight regain and the failure of bariatric surgery, including dilation of the gastric pouch or gastro-jejunal anastomosis, pre-surgery BMI, eating behaviors, increases in energy intake, level of physical activity, the patient's lack of commitment to follow-up visits, and psychological factors [13–18].

Obesity, similar to other chronic diseases, persists for prolonged durations and requires a continuous close follow-up to re-assess the efficacy of treatments, including bariatric surgeries. Compared to the number of surgeries being performed, there are few mid-long-term studies assessing the effectiveness and changes in weight loss. This is even more true in case of the Saudi population, where only a few studies have addressed bariatric surgery outcomes [4,7,8,19,20] and fewer have evaluated the long-term weight loss outcomes. In this study, we aim to observe and evaluate the weight evolution pattern in Saudi patients during a six-year follow-up period following bariatric surgery.

2. Materials and Methods

2.1. Study Design, Setting and Subjects

An observational prospective cohort study of adult patients with obesity (age $\geq$ 18 years) who underwent SG and RYGB was conducted at King Khalid University Hospital (KKUH), King Saud University Medical City (KSUMC) in Riyadh, Saudi Arabia, between 2009 and 2015. All procedures and protocols were reviewed and approved by the Research Ethics Committee of the College of Medicine, King Saud University. Written informed consent was obtained from all participants. The bariatric procedures were conducted under the supervision of a single bariatric surgeon. Patients who underwent bariatric surgery and who had follow-up visits at the Obesity Clinic at KKUH and the Obesity Research Center for a period of 6 years were included in the study. Their pre and postoperative clinical data and anthropometric measurements were collected and recorded during follow-up.

Weight (in kilograms) was measured in light clothing and without shoes to the nearest 0.1 kg. Height was measured using a stadiometer, and BMI was calculated. The variables analyzed were age, sex, BMI, absolute weight loss, %EWL, percent total weight loss (%TWL), and percent weight regain (%WR).

2.2. Calculated Variables

We calculated the absolute weight loss as ((follow-up weight − pre-surgery weight/pre-surgery weight) × 100) for all of the different time points. The outcome variables in the study included %EWL, %TWL, and %WR. The %EWL was calculated as ((pre-surgery weight − follow-up weight)/(operative excess weight)) × 100, where the operative excess weight equaled (pre-surgery weight − ideal weight) and where the ideal weight was based on the metropolitan tables [21]. A %EWL of ≥50% represented successful weight loss; a %EWL of ≤50% was considered as a failure [22]. In other studies, the rates indicating failure were reported to be ≤25% at ≥5 years [23,24]. Given the variability of %EWL depending on the definition of the ideal body weight, we used %TWL, as it is reported to be less influenced by BMI and other anthropometric measures. The %TWL was calculated as follows: ((preceding year weight − current weight)/preceding year weight) × 100 [25]. The %WR, which is the percentage of weight regained from the nadir weight (lowest measured post-surgery weight), was calculated using the following formula: ((current weight − nadir weight))/(pre-surgery weight − nadir weight) × 100), where ≥25% weight gain from nadir was considered to be excessive weight regain [22]. After surgery, the patients were prospectively followed up with in the clinic for 6 years. A comprehensive anthropometric measurement (weight, height, and BMI) was performed before surgery and post-surgery at each time point annually until the end of the study period. The yearly attrition rate (in %) was derived by dividing the number of withdrawn participants (calculated as the number of participants retained in the study subtracted from the total number of participants originally included in the study at pre-surgery) by the number of participants originally included in the study × 100 [26].

2.3. Statistical Analysis

Data were analyzed using the SPSS 24.0 Advanced statistics module (IBM Inc., Chicago, IL, USA). Categorical variables (gender and type of surgery) were reported as numbers and percentages, whereas continuous variables (age, anthropometric measurements, %EWL, %TWL and %WR) were reported as mean, standard deviation, and range. The mean weights for all patients from pre-surgery and across the six follow-up time points were graphically presented according to gender and type of surgery.

Changes in the mean values of three outcome variables: %EWL, %TWL, and %WR, over the six time points were compared using the repeated measures analysis of variance (ANOVA), and F values were reported to represent the systematic variance of %EWL, %TWL, and %WR across the six time points. Repeated measures of analysis for the outcome variables (%EWL, %TWL, and %WR) with each of the independent variables (gender and type of surgery) were also conducted.

A generalized linear mixed model for repeated measures for univariate and multivariate analysis were used to evaluate the changes in the quantitative outcome variables, which were observed at the six observation time points (1 to 6 years post-surgery). The fixed effects used in the model were time points, gender, and type of surgery. Akaike-corrected information criteria were used to identify the model of best fit. The least significant difference criterion was used to calculate the adjusted p-values in a pairwise comparison of the mean values. A p-value of <0.05 was used to report the statistically significant results.

3. Results

A total of 91 (50.5% male) patients with the mean age of 33.3 ± 9.7 years who underwent bariatric surgery were included in the study at baseline. The mean pre-surgery weight and BMI were 134.4 ± 33.8 kg and 49.7 ± 9.9 kg/m^2, respectively. Table 1 shows a detailed demographic profile of the total study population.

Table 1. Overall demographic data and baseline characteristics of patients with obesity who underwent bariatric surgery. The values are represented as mean ± SD (standard deviation).

Demographic Variables	
Gender	
Male	46 (50.5%)
Female	45 (49.5%)
Type of Surgery	
Sleeve Gastrectomy	62 (68.1%)
Roux-en-Y Gastric Bypass	29 (31.9%)
Age at baseline, in years	
Mean ± SD	33.3 ± 9.7
Range	17–60
Height, in meters	
Mean ± SD	1.64 ± 0.1
Range	1.45–1.90
Pre-surgery weight, in kilograms	
Mean ± SD	134.4 ± 33.8
Range	78.1–300.7
Pre-surgery BMI, in kg/m^2	
Mean ± SD	49.7 ± 9.9
Range	29.4–83.3

The overall annual follow-up rate of the patients was 79.1% (33 males/39 females) at 1 year, 81.3% (35 males/39 females) at 2 years, 68.1% (30 males/33 females) at 3 years, 54.9% (27 males and 23 females), 42.9% (17 males and 17 females), and 20.9% (7 males, 12 females) at 6 years. The yearly follow-up attrition rate was 20.8% at year 1 post-surgery, 26.4% at year 2, 31.8% at year 3, 47.3% at year 4, 62.6% at year 5, and 79.1% at end of the study period, i.e., year 6 post-surgery.

To characterize the weight change patterns in our cohort, a subgrouping of the patients according to the type of surgery and gender was conducted. Based on the type of surgery, the patients in the RYGB group accounted for 31.9% of patients (n = 29, 11 males and 18 females) while the SG group comprised 68.1% of patients (n = 62, 35 males and 27 females). The maximum mean weight-loss percentage in the RYGB and SG groups was seen at 3 years post-surgery and was similar (54.3% and 54.4%, respectively). Increments in weight were observed in both the bariatric surgery groups beyond the 3-year follow-up period. Both the groups also showed an increasing weight gain trend from year 4 post-surgery and onwards (Figure 1).

Based on gender, we noticed that the maximum mean percentage weight loss occurred at 3 years post-surgery by as much as −65.07% in males, while it was −43.48% at 4 years post-surgery for females (Figure 2). The rate of weight regain was seen to increase gradually from 3 years post-surgery onwards until the end of the study period. Significant weight regain (defined as ≥25% weight gain from nadir weight) was seen in 53.3% of the patients after 6 years.

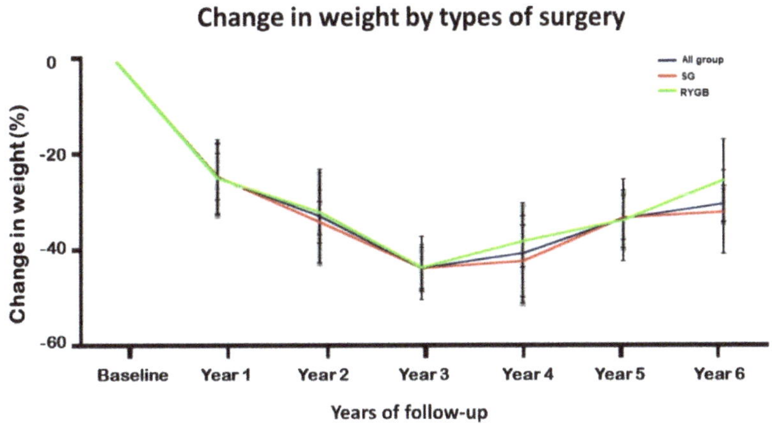

Figure 1. Graphical representations of changes in weight (%), with the error bars representing the ±2 SD during the 6-year follow-up period for all patients who underwent bariatric surgery (blue line), for those who underwent SG (red line), and those who underwent RYGB (green line).

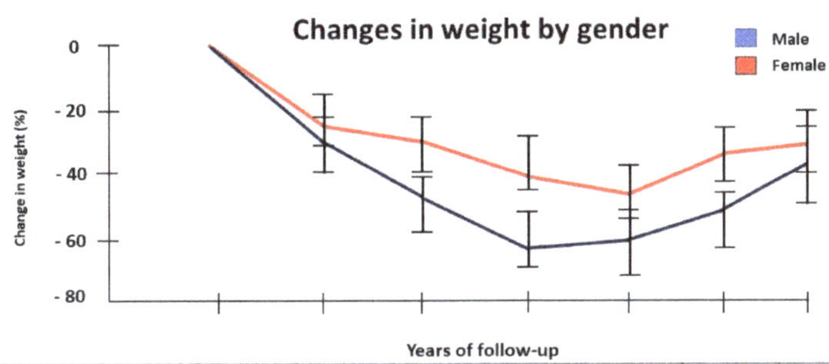

	Baseline	Year 1	Year 2	Year 3	Year 4	Year 5	Year 6
N Males	46	33	35	30	24	17	7
N Females	45	39	32	32	24	17	12
Weight change (%), Males	0	-31.4	-50.75	-65.07	-59.47	-51.40	-38.94
Weight change (%), Females	0	-28.63	-36.49	-40.13	-43.48	-30.16	-33.07

Figure 2. Graphical representation of weight change (%), with the error bars representing the ±2 SD, according to gender of the patients post bariatric surgery during the 6-year follow-up period. The number of patients at each time point and the mean percentage weight loss in male and female participants is shown. SD-standard deviation.

Three outcome variables (%EWL, %TWL, and %WR) were considered for the analysis. A total of 314, 308, and 98 repeated measures were used in the analysis for these outcome variables. Table 2 shows the comparison of the mean values of %EWL, %TWL, and %WR across the six observation time points, and Table 3 shows the comparison of mean values of %EWL, %TWL, and % WR across the observation time points in male and female patients and in those who had undergone RYGB and SG surgeries. A similar comparison is shown for %EWL (Figure 3A–C), %TWL (Figure 3D–F), and %WR (Figure 3G–I).

Table 2. Comparison of repeated measure (%EWL, %TWL, and %WR) mean (SD) values of study subjects across the six time points and the difference between each time point and at the end observation time point.

Outcome Variables	Time Points (in Years)						F-Value	p-Value
	1st	2nd	3rd	4th	5th	6th		
%EWL	45.46 (21.9)	65.71 (32.0)	73.14 (28.8)	75.12 (43.4)	58.04 (22.5)	54.11 (20.3)	10.82	<0.0001
%TWL	22.87 (10.0)	16.07 (15.6)	3.47 (13.2)	−0.73 (14.1)	−7.08 (16.4)	−0.49 (12.1)	43.99	<0.0001
%WR	–	10.20 (12.9)	13.32 (12.1)	17.58 (29.1)	20.81 (18.7)	30.38 (20.9)	2.72	0.034

%EWL—percentage excess weight loss, %TWL—percentage total weight loss, %WR—percentage weight regain.

Table 3. Comparison of repeated measure (%EWL, %TWL, and %WR) mean values across the six time points in male and female subjects and in relation to type of surgery.

Outcome Variables, Type of Surgery and Gender		Time Points (in Years)						F-Value	p-Value
		1st	2nd	3rd	4th	5th	6th		
%EWL	RYGB	51.21 (21.0)	71.18 (40.2)	79.0 (41.1)	80.04 (52.8)	60.7 (23.1)	54.20 (20.3)	2.89	0.018
	SG	42.64 (21.9)	62.80 (26.7)	69.91 (18.8)	72.20 (37.3)	56.78 (22.6)	54.02 (21.5)	9.27	<0.0001
%TWL	RYGB	24.41 (9.1)	17.23 (14.4)	8.04 (14.1)	−1.43 (15.6)	−9.96 (13.1)	−0.23 (14.9)	20.53	<0.0001
	SG	22.12 (10.5)	15.4 (16.4)	1.01 (12.1)	−0.24 (13.2)	−5.58 (18.0)	−0.755 (9.3)	27.63	<0.0001
WR	RYGB	–	5.42 (6.1)	9.41 (7.5)	11.31 (12.5)	17.91 (16.2)	26.25 (19.9)	2.28	0.080
	SG	–	14.97 (17.6)	15.55 (13.8)	21.76 (36)	22.44 (20.2)	35.1 (22.9)	1.27	0.294
%EWL	Male	42.96 (24.1)	74.34 (38.2)	80.54 (36.1)	76.26 (48.1)	63.15 (26.3)	49.64 (20.5)	7.22	<0.0001
	Female	47.52 (19.9)	58.15 (23.3)	66.21 (17.3)	73.84 (38.4)	52.93 (17.1)	56.71 (20.7)	4.74	<0.0001
%TWL	Male	21.32 (10.8)	22.72 (17.0)	4.20 (15.5)	−0.23 (17.9)	−0.51 (14.2)	0.62 (8.6)	16.67	<0.0001
	Female	24.13 (9.2)	10.29 (11.7)	2.84 (10.9)	−1.34 (7.5)	−13.3 (16.3)	−1.24 (14.3)	39.15	<0.0001
%WR	Male	–	7.42 (7.1)	13.28 (13.4)	20.0 (37.4)	16.61 (13.4)	28.33 (18.0)	1.54	0.209
	Female	–	11.59 (15.9)	13.36 (11.3)	14.42 (12.8)	23.62 (21.4)	31.75 (23.6)	1.74	0.156

3.1. Univariate Analysis: Generalized Linear Mixed Effects Model Analysis for the Outcome Variables %EWL, %TWL and %WR for Each of the Independent Variables (Time Points, Type of Surgery and Gender)

The univariate repeated measures and generalized linear mixed effects model for the outcome variables %EWL, %TWL, and % WR across the six time points showed statistically significant differences (F = 10.82, $p < 0.0001$; F = 43.99, $p < 0.0001$; F = 2.72; $p = 0.034$) (Table 2).

The mean %EWL values were significantly increased at 3 and 4 years post-surgery when compared to the mean values at 6 years post-surgery ($p < 0.0001$), where the coefficients at 3 (19.04, $t = 3.21$, $p = 0.001$) and 4 (21.02, $t = 2.74$, $p = 0.006$) years indicate that %EWL increased by 19.04 and 21.02 units when compared to the mean value of %EWL at 6 years post-surgery.

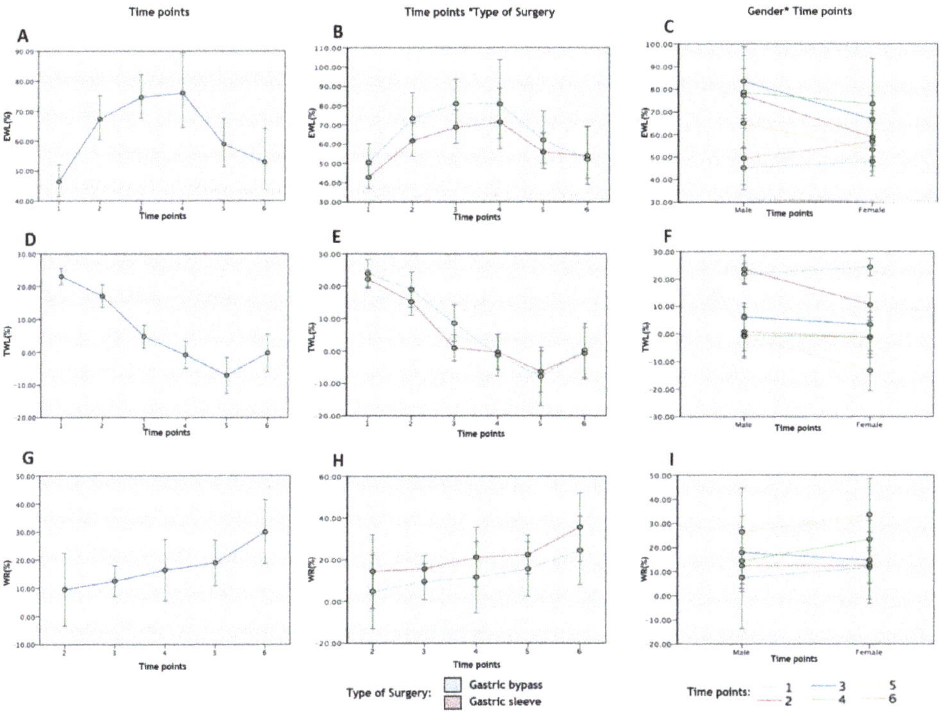

Figure 3. The figure shows a line graph with 95% confidence intervals and depicts the changes in the estimated mean of outcome variables with the predictors over the study duration at the different time points. The changes in %EWL with (**A**) different time points, (**B**) time points and type of surgery, and (**C**) time points and gender; the changes in %TWL with (**D**) different time points, (**E**) time points and type of surgery, and (**F**) time points and gender; and the changes in %WR with (**G**) different time points, (**H**) time points and type of surgery, and (**I**) time points and gender are shown.

The mean %TWL values were significantly higher at 1 and 2 years post-surgery when compared to the mean values at 6 years post-surgery ($p < 0.0001$), where the coefficients at 1 (23.35, $t = 7.90$, $p < 0.0001$) and 2 years (16.57, $t = 5.08$, $p < 0.001$) showed that the %TWL mean values increased by 23.35 and 16.57 units when compared to the mean value of %TWL at 6 years post-surgery.

The mean %WR values were significantly decreased at 2 (−20.18, $t = -2.67$, $p = 0.009$) and 3 (−17.06, $t = -2.85$, $p = 0.005$) years post-surgery when compared to the mean values at 6 years post-surgery, indicating that the %WR mean values decreased by 20.18 and 17.06 units when compared to the mean value of %WR at 6 years post-surgery.

The comparison of the mean values of %EWL in each of the surgery groups (RYGB and SG) across the six time points showed highly statistically significant differences (F = 2.89, $p = 0.018$ and F = 9.27, $p < 0.0001$), respectively (Table 3). The mean values of %EWL in patients who underwent RYGB surgery at 3 years was increased by 24.82 units ($t = 2.24$, $p = 0.027$), while it increased by 15.89 units ($t = 2.14$, $p = 0.033$) in those who underwent SG when compared to the mean value of %EWL at 6 years post-surgery.

Similarly, high statistically significant difference was observed for the mean values of % TWL in each of the surgery groups (RYGB and SG) across the six time points (F = 20.53; $p < 0.0001$ and F = 27.63; $p < 0.0001$) (Table 3). The mean values of %TWL in patients who underwent RYGB surgery was higher at 1 and 2 years by 24.64 units ($t = 4.85$, $p < 0.001$) and 17.47 units ($t = 3.19$, $p = 0.002$), while it was higher by 22.87 units ($t = 6.90$, $p < 0.001$) and by 16.15 units ($t = 4.24$, $p < 0.001$) in those who underwent SG when compared to the mean value of %TWL at 6 years post-surgery. Hence, it can be inferred that the mean %TWL values were significantly lower after 6 years in patients who had undergone either surgery when compared to the mean values at 1 and 2 years post-surgery.

However, for the mean values of % WR, a non-significance was observed in each of the surgery groups (RYGB and SG) across the six time points (F = 2.28; $p = 0.080$ and F = 1.27, $p = 0.294$) (Table 3). However, the pairwise compassion of the time points shows that patients who underwent RYGB surgery had significantly decreased mean values of %WR at 2 and 3 years by −20.82 units ($t = -2.64$, $p = 0.012$) and 16.83 units ($t = -2.24$, $p = 0.031$), while those who underwent SG showed a significant decrease in the mean value of %WR at 3 years by 19.55 units ($t = -2.10$, $p = 0.041$) when compared to the mean value of %WR at 6 years post-surgery.

The comparison of the mean values of %EWL in each of the gender groups (male and female) across the six time points showed highly statistically significant differences (F = 7.22; $p < 0.0001$ and F = 4.74; $p < 0.0001$) (Table 3). The mean %EWL values in males were significantly increased at 2 (24.70, $t = 2.45$, $p = 0.015$), 3 (38.90, $t = 10.18$, $p = 0.003$), and 4 (26.61, $t = 2.21$, $p = 0.029$) years when compared to the mean value at 6 years post-surgery. In female subjects, the mean values of %EWL across the six time points were statistically significantly different, whereas the comparison of each time point with the mean values at 6 years post-surgery did not show any statistically significant differences.

Additionally, highly statistically significant differences were observed for the mean values of % TWL in both male and female subjects across the six time points (F = 16.67; $p < 0.0001$ and F = 39.15; $p < 0.0001$) (Table 3). The pairwise comparison showed that the mean %TWL values in males was significantly higher at 1 (20.69, $t = 5.75$, $p < 0.001$) and at 2 (22.10, $t = 5.23$, $p < 0.001$) years when compared to the mean value at 6 years post-surgery. This was also noted in the female subjects, and the mean values of %TWL were found to be significantly higher at 1 (25.37, $t = 4.38$, $p < 0.001$) and 2 (11.53, $t = 4.53$, $p = 0.012$) years when compared to the mean values of %TWL at 6 years post-surgery.

In each of the gender groups (male and female) the comparison of the mean values of %WR across the five time points of observations showed no statistically significant differences (F = 1.54, $p = 0.209$ and F = 1.74, $p = 0.156$) (Table 3). However, the pairwise comparison of the time points indicated that the mean %WR values in males were significantly decreased at 2 years (−20.91, $t = -2.34$, $p = 0.024$) while in females, they were significantly decreased at 3 years (−18.39, $t = 4–2.14$, $p = 0.037$) when compared to the mean values of %WR at 6 years post-surgery (Figure S1I).

3.2. Multivariate Analysis: General Linear Mixed Effects Modelling for Each of the Outcome Variables, %EWL, %TWL and %WR with Independent Variables (Time Points, Type of Surgery and Gender)

The multivariate repeated-measures generalized linear mixed effects model for the outcome variables %EWL and %TWL was significant for the overall model (F = 4.49, dff = 17, $p < 0.0001$ and F = 14.78, dff = 17, $p < 0.0001$). Significance was also noted with time points (F = 10.70, $p < 0.001$ and F = 40.05, $p < 0.0001$), gender (F = 3.53, $p = 0.068$ and F = 7.35, $p = 0.007$) and type of surgery (F = 4.14, $p = 0.043$ and F = 1.160, $p = 0.282$), time points × gender (F = 2.05, $p = 0.071$ and F = 3.36, $p = 0.006$), and time points × type of surgery (F = 0.310, $p = 0.91$ and F = 0.695, $p = 0.628$) were used as predictors of the model.

Taking the time point predictors into consideration, significant differences ($p < 0.001$) in %EWL were observed at 2 (15.06), 3 (22.12), and 4 (23.09) years and for %TWL at 1 (23.34) and 2 (17.30) years in comparison to the mean value at 6 years post-surgery. The %EWL mean values in males were observed to be statistically significant at 2 (27.97), 3 (34.15), and 4 years (29.20) when compared to the mean value at 6 years post-surgery. Males showed significantly higher %EWL at 2 years post-surgery by 25.81 units ($p = 0.045$) compared to the females, while no significant differences were noted for the coefficients for the other terms in the model. The %TWL mean values in males were observed to be significant at 1 (21.07) and 2 years (22.70) and for females at 1 (25.60) and 2 (11.85) years when compared to the mean value at 6 years post-surgery. Similar to %EWL, %TWL in males was significantly higher at 2 years post-surgery compared to females.

Considering surgery as a predictor, %EWL was significantly higher in male subjects who had undergone RYGB at 2 (21.91), 3 (29.18) and 4 (28.59) years post-surgery, while no statistically significant differences were observed in female subjects and in subjects who had undergone SG. Mean values of %TWL were statistically significant at 1 and 2 years post-surgery in patients who had undergone RYGB (23.75 and 18.73 units) and in SG the group (22.93 and 15.87) when compared to the mean values of %TWL at 6 years post-surgery.

The multivariate analysis for the outcome variable %WR with time points, gender, and type of surgery as predictors showed no statistical significance for the overall model (F = 1.10, dff = 14, $p = 0.370$). Among all of the coefficients, at 3 years post-surgery, the %WR mean value decreased by 23.59 units ($p = 0.044$) when compared to the mean value of %WR at 6 years post-surgery, whereas the coefficients for other terms in the model were not statistically significant. For the time points predictor, significant differences were observed at 2 (−20.53) and 3 years (−17.56) post-surgery when compared to the mean value at 6 years post-surgery.

No statistically significant differences in the %WR pattern were observed in male subjects in the comparison of the mean values of %WR between the pair of time points (2 to 6 years post-surgery), whereas in female subjects, the mean values of %WR at 2 (−22.02) and at 3 years (−21.08) were significantly decreased when compared to the mean value at 6 years. Statistically significant differences were observed at 3 years in patients who had undergone SG surgery, where the mean values of %WR decreased by −20.06 units when compared to the mean values at 6 years post-surgery, while no significant differences were observed in patients who had undergone RYGB surgery (Figure S1).

4. Discussion

Being a chronic disease, managing or treating severe obesity is challenging and requires constant close clinical and nutritional monitoring to reduce the recurrence of weight gain after weight loss. A large body of literature has shown that weight loss, even at a modest level of 5–10%, is beneficial and helps in the resolution of obesity associated comorbidities including, T2DM, hypertension, and fatty liver disease, among others, and in improving the overall quality of life [27–29]. Attaining a weight loss change of ≥5 and/or ≥10% of initial body weight has also been shown to be strongly correlated with a reduction in the risk of cardiovascular disease [30]. Surgical intervention techniques such as bariatric surgery were instated to provide a more permanent weight loss solution. Regardless of the type of surgery or the mechanisms by which weight loss is achieved, bariatric surgery has proven to lead to a significant amount of weight loss immediately post-surgery [31], but its long-term efficacy needs to be evaluated. The general metrics to assess the success of the surgeries includes calculating %EWL (>50%), %TWL, and %WR post-surgery [32–36]. Different studies have shown a large amount of variability within these values, which have been attributed to either the type of surgery, the preoperative BMI, and to the race and ethnicity that the patients belong to [29,30]. To date, only a limited number of studies have looked at differences in weight loss patterns across different populations and specifically in the Saudi population, where bariatric procedures are presently being performed routinely. In our present study, we conducted a longitudinal follow-up of patients undergoing bariatric surgery and observed the weight evolution patterns through annual follow ups for a period of 6 years post-surgery.

4.1. Weight Evolution in the Overall Bariatric Group

All of the patients demonstrated a uniform annual incremental increase in the weight loss outcome measures (i.e., absolute weight change, %EWL, and %TWL) as early as 1 year post-surgery, and significant changes in these parameters were seen from baseline to up to 3 years post-surgery. Our findings are different from those of the previous studies that have reported maximum weight loss to occur at 1–2 years post-surgery. The %EWL and %TWL showed a similar pattern across the cohort, where incremental increases in weight loss were seen from the baseline, peaking at the 3-year post surgery. The calculated %EWL values observed in our study population were higher than those reported by Bohdjalian et al. at the 3-year annual follow up, and while long-term weight outcomes were similar to theirs [37], they were higher than those observed in other cohorts [37,38]. Weight change patterns beyond 3 years showed a decrease in the propensity for further weight loss followed by a plateauing phase and then a slow and gradual increase in the patients' weight. Our findings are in line with the findings of the SM-BOSS study that also showed an increased BMI at 5 years [39].

Weight regain remains a major challenge in relation to the long-term success of bariatric surgery [40]. Numerous studies have previously shown a higher tendency for patients to regain their weight after an initial impressive weight loss until the midterm (>3 years), which was not substantiated in the long term (>5 years). Although weight regain is a consistent finding among studies, there are considerable inter-individual variations in the magnitude and rate of weight regain depending on factors ranging from behavioral, dietary, lifestyle, psychological, ethnic, and racial differences [22,40–43]. One of the reasons for the weight regain has been attributed to the influences of gastrointestinal hormones, including glucagon-like peptide 1 (GLP-1) ghrelin, glucose-dependent insulinotropic polypeptide (GIP), and the adipokine leptin. These hormones have been shown to regulate feelings of satiety, influence hunger and energy balance by regulating the intake and storage, and energy expenditure through the actions of the entero–hypothalamic axis [44,45]. In our study, we observed a gradual and consistent increase in the number of patients who experienced weight regain across the follow-up period. Significant weight regain (defined as $\geq$25% weight gain from nadir weight) was seen in 53.3% of the patients at 6 years post-surgery. The %WR was significantly higher in the 6th year in comparison to the 2nd and 3rd years of follow-up post-surgery. Our findings indicate that, similar to lifestyle and medical management of obesity, bariatric surgery is also successful in yielding short term weight loss. The notion that bariatric surgery provides a permanent solution for resolution in the long term has to be made with caution.

4.2. Weight Loss Patterns between SG and RYGB

The two most common weight loss surgical procedures that are performed are SG and RYGB, which differ in terms of the irreversible anatomical alterations created surgically at specific sites in the gastrointestinal tract (GIT). These anatomical changes in the GIT lead to many physiological and biochemical variations that produce differences in the regulation of the food and appetite, gut hormones, bile acids, and gut microbiota and consequently lead to weight loss by reducing appetite [46–49]. Few studies have claimed better weight loss outcomes with RYGB, while another study that conducted a head to head comparison between these two techniques suggests that in the long-term, only a subtle weight loss difference exists in favor of RYGB [49]. In our study, we found that the trajectories of weight loss in both the RYGB and SG demonstrated a similar trend when measured in terms of changes in weight % and %EWL from baseline up to 3 years post-surgery, at which point, the weight loss started decreasing. On the other hand, %TWL showed a steeper decline in weight loss in the RYGB group up until 4 years post-surgery compared to the SG group. Beyond the 4-year mark, both surgeries showed a similar weight pattern. Compared to SG, RYGB is considered to be the intervention that results in far greater weight loss. Our findings indicate that this assumption holds true with regard to weight loos in the short term, but the effects of both surgical procedures are similar in the long term. Our results are in line with the SLEEVEPASS and the SM-BOSS studies, which also reported no significant differences between the two bariatric methods with regard to weight loss in both the short or long term [48].

Previous studies have shown that on average, patients regain 7% of their total body weight from their lowest post-operative weight over the course of 10 years [50]. This weight regain pattern in our study was similar between the SG and RYGB groups. The RYGB group demonstrated an increase in the %WR in the 3-year post-surgery follow up, while weight regain in the SG group was seen from the 4-year follow-up onwards. Previously, the weight regain in patients who had undergone RYGB, was shown to be about 15% within two years of the surgery, which subsequently increased to 70% of patients between two and five years and to 85% at after five years post-surgery [51]. However, in our study, significant weight regain was noted at 3-year post-surgery follow up. The causes for weight regain have been shown to be due to homeostatic changes in the body post-surgery that lead to biochemical, physiological, hormonal, and metabolic adaptations to weight loss that support weight regain. These changes include perturbations in the levels of circulating appetite-related hormones and energy homoeostasis. In addition, the alterations in nutrient metabolism and subjective appetite are rather dependent on factors that depend on the physiology of the body and the metabolism. RYGB and SG induce similar changes in leptin, PYY, and GLP-1 levels, but not in the levels of ghrelin, whose levels are reduced after SG, while they are known to change over time after RYGB and may be the reason for the differences in weight regain between these methods [52]. The high prevalence of weight regain after bariatric surgery has also been a reason for an increase in the number of revisional bariatric surgeries that pose an increased surgical risk to the patient [53].

4.3. Weight Loss Changes According to Gender

In our study we also looked at the pattern of change in the weight loss patterns among the male and female participants at the different post-surgery time points. We found that males lost significantly more weight in terms of the mean values of %EWL in the 2, 3, and 4-year post-surgery follow ups, while the weight loss in the female subjects at each time point did not show any statistically significant differences with mean value of %EWL 6 years post-surgery. On the other hand, the mean %TWL values in both males and females were significantly higher at 1 and at 2 years post-surgery when compared to the mean values of %TWL at 6 years post-surgery. The differences in weight loss patterns among the genders were also seen in previous report by Tymitz et al., who showed that men had a higher absolute weight loss [54] while females showed a greater BMI loss post bariatric surgery [55]. This difference between the genders has been suggested to be the result of higher loss percentage of fat mass and an increase in fat free mass in men [56]. With regard to weight regain, we observed that males started to show an increase in weight earlier than their female counterparts, i.e., at the 3 years post-surgery. On the other hand, the weight regain seen in the females started at 4 years post-surgery, but both groups showed the same pattern at 6 years post-surgery. In their study, Meguid et al. attributed higher weight regain in females to differences in eating habits, diet, and probably a failure in developing and sustaining a large amount of plasma peptide YY levels, a hormone that regulates satiety and suppresses hunger [57]. The differences in the weight regain pattern of the males compared to the females within the two groups highlights the fact that gender is an important factor that affects the outcome of these surgeries. Additional studies to study the changes in the levels of these hormones in relation to differences in gender as well as with the type of surgery will be conducted in the future. Emphasis should be placed on regular follow ups post-surgery along with the implementation of a multidisciplinary approach to track weight regain to provide the best outcomes.

To our knowledge, the present study is the first to have looked at the long-term weight changes that occur post bariatric surgery in patients with obesity from Saudi Arabia. As previously mentioned, a lack of standardization in the reporting measures used for weight loss outcomes has been noted in the literature, which has hindered direct comparisons of weight loss among various studies. Therefore, we used two weight loss measures or outcome variables, EWL% and TWL%, in the present study to provide a broader representation of the measures of weight loss that will allow our results to be more easily compared to those of other studies [32,33,58]. Our study has a number of limitations, specifically with regard to the attrition rate and number of patients that followed up, even after being given clinical appointments. One of the reasons for this could be the increased weight regain due to unhealthy dietary habits and behavioral lifestyle practices [17], which could have deterred the patients from attending their follow-up appointments. Although our follow-up rate is low, it is similar to that found by other groups attempting long-term follow-up studies [33,59,60]. All of the patients undergoing bariatric surgery were included without any prior stratification of their preoperative weight that could have affected the results.

5. Conclusions

The weight loss results that occur after bariatric surgery can be considered profound, as seen at 3 years post-surgery, but they are not consistent in the long run. Weight regain remains a major challenge post bariatric surgery, and long-term follow-up is required to ensure gaining the optimal benefits from this intervention.

Supplementary Materials: The following are available online at https://www.mdpi.com/article/10.3390/jcm10214922/s1, Figure S1: The figure shows a bar graph with 95% confidence intervals depicting changes in the outcome variables with the predictors over the study duration at the different time points. The changes in %EWL with (A) different time points, (B) time points and type of surgery, and (C) time points and gender are shown. The changes in %TWL with (D) different time points, (E) time points and type of surgery, and (F) time points and gender are shown. The changes in %WR with (G) different time points, (H) time points and type of surgery, and (I) time points and gender are shown. The horizontal line represents the estimated mean of the outcome variables at time point = 6. The vertical bars are the simple contrasts of the outcome variables at each level of time points minus the outcome variable at time point = 6. Significant contrasts are shaded in gold. The least significant difference adjusted significance level is 0.05.

Author Contributions: Conceptualization and clinical and surgical follow up, A.A.A. and M.Y.A.-N.; methodology and software, A.M. and A.I.; statistical analysis, S.S.A.; formal analysis, A.M., A.I., A.A.A. and M.Y.A.-N.; data curation, R.E., A.I. and N.A.A.; writing—original draft preparation, A.M., A.A.A. and A.I.; review and editing, A.A.A., N.A.A. and S.S.A.; funding acquisition, A.A.A. All authors have read and agreed to the published version of the manuscript.

Funding: This work was funded by the National Plan for Science, Technology and Innovation MAARIFAH), King Abdulaziz City for Science and Technology, Kingdom of Saudi Arabia. (Project No. 08-MED513-02).

Institutional Review Board Statement: Ethical clearance was obtained from the Research Ethics Committee of College of Medicine, King Saud University.

Informed Consent Statement: Written informed consent was obtained from all participants. This study was conducted at the Obesity Research Center, College of Medicine and King Khalid University Hospital, King Saud University, Riyadh, Saudi Arabia.

Data Availability Statement: All data generated or analyzed in the current study are included in this article.

Acknowledgments: We would like to thank Hadeel M. Awwad for assisting in reviewing the weight loss data and the manuscript. This work was funded by the National Plan for Science, Technology and Innovation (MAARIFAH), King Abdulaziz City for Science and Technology, Kingdom of Saudi Arabia (Project No. 08-MED513-02).

Conflicts of Interest: The authors have no commercial associations that might be conflicts of interest in relation to this article.

References

1. World Health Organization. Facts about Overweight and Obesity. Available online: https://www.who.int/news-room/fact-sheets/detail/obesity-and-overweight (accessed on 1 March 2021).
2. Memish, Z.A.; El Bcheraoui, C.; Tuffaha, M.; Robinson, M.; Daoud, F.; Jaber, S.; Mikhitarian, S.; Al Saeedi, M.; AlMazroa, M.A.; Mokdad, A.H.; et al. Obesity and associated factors—Kingdom of Saudi Arabia, 2013. *Prev. Chronic Dis.* **2014**, *11*, E174. [CrossRef]
3. Alqarni, S.S.M. A Review of Prevalence of Obesity in Saudi Arabia. *J. Obes. Eat. Disord.* **2016**, 1–6. [CrossRef]
4. Alfadda, A.A.; Al-Dhwayan, M.M.; Alharbi, A.A.; Al Khudhair, B.K.; Al Nozha, O.M.; Al-Qahtani, N.M.; Alzahrani, S.H.; Bardisi, W.M.; Sallam, R.M.; Riva, J.J.; et al. The Saudi clinical practice guideline for the management of overweight and obesity in adults. *Saudi Med. J.* **2016**, *37*, 1151–1162. [CrossRef] [PubMed]

5. Sjostrom, L.; Narbro, K.; Sjostrom, C.D.; Karason, K.; Larsson, B.; Wedel, H.; Lystig, T.; Sullivan, M.; Bouchard, C.; Carlsson, B.; et al. Effects of bariatric surgery on mortality in Swedish obese subjects. *N. Engl. J. Med.* **2007**, *357*, 741–752. [CrossRef]
6. Geraci, A.A.; Brunt, A.; Marihart, C. The Work behind Weight-Loss Surgery: A Qualitative Analysis of Food Intake after the First Two Years Post-Op. *ISRN Obes.* **2014**, *2014*, 427062. [CrossRef] [PubMed]
7. Mofti, A.B.; Al-Saleh, M.S. Bariatric surgery in Saudi Arabia. *Ann. Saudi Med.* **1992**, *12*, 440–445. [CrossRef] [PubMed]
8. Al-Khaldi, Y.M. Bariatric surgery in Saudi Arabia: The urgent need for standards. *Saudi J. Obes.* **2016**, *4*, 1. [CrossRef]
9. Chou, J.J.; Lee, W.J.; Almalki, O.; Chen, J.C.; Tsai, P.L.; Yang, S.H. Dietary Intake and Weight Changes 5 Years After Laparoscopic Sleeve Gastrectomy. *Obes. Surg.* **2017**, *27*, 3240–3246. [CrossRef] [PubMed]
10. Al-Bader, I.; Khoursheed, M.; Al Sharaf, K.; Mouzannar, D.A.; Ashraf, A.; Fingerhut, A. Revisional Laparoscopic Gastric Pouch Resizing for Inadequate Weight Loss After Roux-en-Y Gastric Bypass. *Obes. Surg.* **2015**, *25*, 1103–1108. [CrossRef] [PubMed]
11. Adams, T.D.; Davidson, L.E.; Litwin, S.E.; Kolotkin, R.L.; LaMonte, M.J.; Pendleton, R.C.; Strong, M.B.; Vinik, R.; Wanner, N.A.; Hopkins, P.N.; et al. Health benefits of gastric bypass surgery after 6 years. *JAMA* **2012**, *308*, 1122–1131. [CrossRef]
12. Lauti, M.; Kularatna, M.; Hill, A.G.; MacCormick, A.D. Weight Regain Following Sleeve Gastrectomy—A Systematic Review. *Obes. Surg.* **2016**, *26*, 1326–1334. [CrossRef]
13. Kanerva, N.; Larsson, I.; Peltonen, M.; Lindroos, A.K.; Carlsson, L.M. Changes in total energy intake and macronutrient composition after bariatric surgery predict long-term weight outcome: Findings from the Swedish Obese Subjects (SOS) study. *Am. J. Clin. Nutr.* **2017**, *106*, 136–145. [CrossRef] [PubMed]
14. Thompson, C.C.; Slattery, J.; Bundga, M.E.; Lautz, D.B. Peroral endoscopic reduction of dilated gastrojejunal anastomosis after Roux-en-Y gastric bypass: A possible new option for patients with weight regain. *Surg. Endosc.* **2006**, *20*, 1744–1748. [CrossRef] [PubMed]
15. McGrice, M.; Don Paul, K. Interventions to improve long-term weight loss in patients following bariatric surgery: Challenges and solutions. *Diabetes Metab. Syndr. Obes. Targets Ther.* **2015**, *8*, 263–274. [CrossRef] [PubMed]
16. Shah, M.; Simha, V.; Garg, A. Review: Long-term impact of bariatric surgery on body weight, comorbidities, and nutritional status. *J. Clin. Endocrinol. Metab.* **2006**, *91*, 4223–4231. [CrossRef]
17. Masood, A.; Alsheddi, L.; Alfayadh, L.; Bukhari, B.; Elawad, R.; Alfadda, A.A. Dietary and Lifestyle Factors Serve as Predictors of Successful Weight Loss Maintenance Postbariatric Surgery. *J. Obes.* **2019**, *2019*, 7295978. [CrossRef] [PubMed]
18. Hsu, L.K.; Benotti, P.N.; Dwyer, J.; Roberts, S.B.; Saltzman, E.; Shikora, S.; Rolls, B.J.; Rand, W. Nonsurgical factors that influence the outcome of bariatric surgery: A review. *Psychosom. Med.* **1998**, *60*, 338–346. [CrossRef]
19. Alqahtani, A.R. Reply to Letter to Editor RE: Laparoscopic Sleeve Gastrectomy After Endoscopic Sleeve Gastroplasty: Technical Aspects and Short-Term Outcomes. *Obes. Surg.* **2020**, *30*, 338. [CrossRef]
20. Alqahtani, A.R.; Elahmedi, M.; Alqahtani, Y.A.; Al-Darwish, A. Laparoscopic Sleeve Gastrectomy After Endoscopic Sleeve Gastroplasty: Technical Aspects and Short-Term Outcomes. *Obes. Surg.* **2019**, *29*, 3547–3552. [CrossRef]
21. Carrasco, F.; Papapietro, K.; Csendes, A.; Salazar, G.; Echenique, C.; Lisboa, C.; Diaz, E.; Rojas, J. Changes in resting energy expenditure and body composition after weight loss following Roux-en-Y gastric bypass. *Obes. Surg.* **2007**, *17*, 608–616. [CrossRef]
22. Cooper, T.C.; Simmons, E.B.; Webb, K.; Burns, J.L.; Kushner, R.F. Trends in Weight Regain Following Roux-en-Y Gastric Bypass (RYGB) Bariatric Surgery. *Obes. Surg.* **2015**, *25*, 1474–1481. [CrossRef] [PubMed]
23. Aminian, A.; Jamal, M.; Augustin, T.; Corcelles, R.; Kirwan, J.P.; Schauer, P.R.; Brethauer, S.A. Failed Surgical Weight Loss Does Not Necessarily Mean Failed Metabolic Effects. *Diabetes Technol. Ther.* **2015**, *17*, 682–684. [CrossRef] [PubMed]
24. Mann, J.P.; Jakes, A.D.; Hayden, J.D.; Barth, J.H. Systematic review of definitions of failure in revisional bariatric surgery. *Obes. Surg.* **2015**, *25*, 571–574. [CrossRef]
25. Sabench Pereferrer, F.; Molina Lopez, A.; Vives Espelta, M.; Raga Carceller, E.; Blanco Blasco, S.; Buils Vilalta, F.; Paris Sans, M.; Pinana Campon, M.L.; Hernandez Gonzalez, M.; Sanchez Marin, A.; et al. Weight Loss Analysis According to Different Formulas after Sleeve Gastrectomy With or Without Antral Preservation: A Randomised Study. *Obes. Surg.* **2017**, *27*, 1254–1260. [CrossRef]
26. Cooper, C.L.; Whitehead, A.; Pottrill, E.; Julious, S.A.; Walters, S.J. Are pilot trials useful for predicting randomisation and attrition rates in definitive studies: A review of publicly funded trials. *Clin. Trials* **2018**, *15*, 189–196. [CrossRef] [PubMed]
27. Schauer, P.R.; Bhatt, D.L.; Kirwan, J.P.; Wolski, K.; Aminian, A.; Brethauer, S.A.; Navaneethan, S.D.; Singh, R.P.; Pothier, C.E.; Nissen, S.E.; et al. Bariatric Surgery versus Intensive Medical Therapy for Diabete—5-Year Outcomes. *N. Engl. J. Med.* **2017**, *376*, 641–651. [CrossRef]
28. Carlsson, L.M.S.; Sjoholm, K.; Karlsson, C.; Jacobson, P.; Andersson-Assarsson, J.C.; Svensson, P.A.; Larsson, I.; Hjorth, S.; Neovius, M.; Taube, M.; et al. Long-term incidence of microvascular disease after bariatric surgery or usual care in patients with obesity, stratified by baseline glycaemic status: A post-hoc analysis of participants from the Swedish Obese Subjects study. *Lancet. Diabetes Endocrinol.* **2017**, *5*, 271–279. [CrossRef]
29. Sjoholm, K.; Pajunen, P.; Jacobson, P.; Karason, K.; Sjostrom, C.D.; Torgerson, J.; Carlsson, L.M.; Sjostrom, L.; Peltonen, M. Incidence and remission of type 2 diabetes in relation to degree of obesity at baseline and 2 year weight change: The Swedish Obese Subjects (SOS) study. *Diabetologia* **2015**, *58*, 1448–1453. [CrossRef]
30. Kroes, M.; Osei-Assibey, G.; Baker-Searle, R.; Huang, J. Impact of weight change on quality of life in adults with overweight/obesity in the United States: A systematic review. *Curr. Med. Res. Opin.* **2016**, *32*, 485–508. [CrossRef]
31. Ionut, V.; Bergman, R.N. Mechanisms responsible for excess weight loss after bariatric surgery. *J. Diabetes Sci. Technol.* **2011**, *5*, 1263–1282. [CrossRef]

32. Buchwald, H.; Buchwald, J.N.; McGlennon, T.W. Systematic review and meta-analysis of medium-term outcomes after banded Roux-en-Y gastric bypass. *Obes. Surg.* **2014**, *24*, 1536–1551. [CrossRef] [PubMed]
33. Puzziferri, N.; Roshek, T.B., 3rd; Mayo, H.G.; Gallagher, R.; Belle, S.H.; Livingston, E.H. Long-term follow-up after bariatric surgery: A systematic review. *JAMA* **2014**, *312*, 934–942. [CrossRef]
34. Christou, N.V.; Look, D.; Maclean, L.D. Weight gain after short- and long-limb gastric bypass in patients followed for longer than 10 years. *Ann. Surg.* **2006**, *244*, 734–740. [CrossRef]
35. Diniz Mde, F.; Passos, V.M.; Barreto, S.M.; Linares, D.B.; de Almeida, S.R.; Rocha, A.L.; Diniz, M.T. Different criteria for assessment of Roux-en-Y gastric bypass success: Does only weight matter? *Obes. Surg.* **2009**, *19*, 1384–1392. [CrossRef] [PubMed]
36. Admiraal, W.M.; Celik, F.; Gerdes, V.E.; Dallal, R.M.; Hoekstra, J.B.; Holleman, F. Ethnic differences in weight loss and diabetes remission after bariatric surgery: A meta-analysis. *Diabetes Care* **2012**, *35*, 1951–1958. [CrossRef]
37. Bohdjalian, A.; Langer, F.B.; Shakeri-Leidenmuhler, S.; Gfrerer, L.; Ludvik, B.; Zacherl, J.; Prager, G. Sleeve gastrectomy as sole and definitive bariatric procedure: 5-year results for weight loss and ghrelin. *Obes. Surg.* **2010**, *20*, 535–540. [CrossRef]
38. Ochner, C.N.; Jochner, M.C.; Caruso, E.A.; Teixeira, J.; Xavier Pi-Sunyer, F. Effect of preoperative body mass index on weight loss after obesity surgery. *Surg. Obes. Relat. Dis. Off. J. Am. Soc. Bariatr. Surg.* **2013**, *9*, 423–427. [CrossRef] [PubMed]
39. Bastos, E.C.; Barbosa, E.M.; Soriano, G.M.; dos Santos, E.A.; Vasconcelos, S.M. Determinants of weight regain after bariatric surgery. *Arq. Bras. Cir. Dig. ABCD Braz. Arch. Dig. Surg.* **2013**, *26* (Suppl. 1), 26–32. [CrossRef]
40. Thomas, D.D.; Anderson, W.A.; Apovian, C.M.; Hess, D.T.; Yu, L.; Velazquez, A.; Carmine, B.; Istfan, N.W. Weight Recidivism After Roux-en-Y Gastric Bypass Surgery: An 11-Year Experience in a Multiethnic Medical Center. *Obesity* **2019**, *27*, 217–225. [CrossRef]
41. Nicoletti, C.F.; de Oliveira, B.A.; de Pinhel, M.A.; Donati, B.; Marchini, J.S.; Salgado Junior, W.; Nonino, C.B. Influence of excess weight loss and weight regain on biochemical indicators during a 4-year follow-up after Roux-en-Y gastric bypass. *Obes. Surg.* **2015**, *25*, 279–284. [CrossRef]
42. Still, C.D.; Wood, G.C.; Chu, X.; Manney, C.; Strodel, W.; Petrick, A.; Gabrielsen, J.; Mirshahi, T.; Argyropoulos, G.; Seiler, J.; et al. Clinical factors associated with weight loss outcomes after Roux-en-Y gastric bypass surgery. *Obesity* **2014**, *22*, 888–894. [CrossRef]
43. Wood, M.H.; Carlin, A.M.; Ghaferi, A.A.; Varban, O.A.; Hawasli, A.; Bonham, A.J.; Birkmeyer, N.J.; Finks, J.F. Association of Race With Bariatric Surgery Outcomes. *JAMA Surg.* **2019**, *154*, e190029. [CrossRef]
44. Santo, M.A.; Riccioppo, D.; Pajecki, D.; Kawamoto, F.; de Cleva, R.; Antonangelo, L.; Marcal, L.; Cecconello, I. Weight Regain After Gastric Bypass: Influence of Gut Hormones. *Obes. Surg.* **2016**, *26*, 919–925. [CrossRef]
45. Ionut, V.; Burch, M.; Youdim, A.; Bergman, R.N. Gastrointestinal hormones and bariatric surgery-induced weight loss. *Obesity* **2013**, *21*, 1093–1103. [CrossRef] [PubMed]
46. Jirapinyo, P.; Jin, D.X.; Qazi, T.; Mishra, N.; Thompson, C.C. A Meta-Analysis of GLP-1 After Roux-En-Y Gastric Bypass: Impact of Surgical Technique and Measurement Strategy. *Obes. Surg.* **2018**, *28*, 615–626. [CrossRef] [PubMed]
47. Tsouristakis, A.I.; Febres, G.; McMahon, D.J.; Tchang, B.; Conwell, I.M.; Tsang, A.J.; Ahmed, L.; Bessler, M.; Korner, J. Long-Term Modulation of Appetitive Hormones and Sweet Cravings After Adjustable Gastric Banding and Roux-en-Y Gastric Bypass. *Obes. Surg.* **2019**, *29*, 3698–3705. [CrossRef]
48. Benaiges, D.; Climent, E.; Goday, A.; Julia, H.; Flores-Le Roux, J.A.; Pedro-Botet, J. Mid-term results of laparoscopic Roux-en-Y gastric bypass and laparoscopic sleeve gastrectomy compared-results of the SLEEVEPASS and SM-BOSS trials. *Ann. Transl. Med.* **2018**, *6*, S83. [CrossRef] [PubMed]
49. Pucci, A.; Batterham, R.L. Mechanisms underlying the weight loss effects of RYGB and SG: Similar, yet different. *J. Endocrinol. Investig.* **2019**, *42*, 117–128. [CrossRef] [PubMed]
50. Kaouk, L.; Hsu, A.; Tanuseputro, P.; Jessri, M. Modifiable factors associated with weight regain after bariatric surgery: A scoping review. *F1000Research* **2019**, *8*, 615. [CrossRef] [PubMed]
51. Freire, R.H.; Borges, M.C.; Alvarez-Leite, J.I.; Toulson Davisson Correia, M.I. Food quality, physical activity, and nutritional follow-up as determinant of weight regain after Roux-en-Y gastric bypass. *Nutrition* **2012**, *28*, 53–58. [CrossRef]
52. Xu, H.C.; Pang, Y.C.; Chen, J.W.; Cao, J.Y.; Sheng, Z.; Yuan, J.H.; Wang, R.; Zhang, C.S.; Wang, L.X.; Dong, J. Systematic Review and Meta-analysis of the Change in Ghrelin Levels After Roux-en-Y Gastric Bypass. *Obes. Surg.* **2019**, *29*, 1343–1351. [CrossRef] [PubMed]
53. Roth, A.E.; Thornley, C.J.; Blackstone, R.P. Outcomes in Bariatric and Metabolic Surgery: An Updated 5-Year Review. *Curr. Obes. Rep.* **2020**, *9*, 380–389. [CrossRef] [PubMed]
54. Tymitz, K.; Kerlakian, G.; Engel, A.; Bollmer, C. Gender differences in early outcomes following hand-assisted laparoscopic Roux-en-Y gastric bypass surgery: Gender differences in bariatric surgery. *Obes. Surg.* **2007**, *17*, 1588–1591. [CrossRef]
55. Ranasinghe, W.K.; Wright, T.; Attia, J.; McElduff, P.; Doyle, T.; Bartholomew, M.; Hurley, K.; Persad, R.A. Effects of bariatric surgery on urinary and sexual function. *BJU Int.* **2011**, *107*, 88–94. [CrossRef]
56. Infanger, D.; Baldinger, R.; Branson, R.; Barbier, T.; Steffen, R.; Horber, F.F. Effect of significant intermediate-term weight loss on serum leptin levels and body composition in severely obese subjects. *Obes. Surg.* **2003**, *13*, 879–888. [CrossRef]
57. Meguid, M.M.; Glade, M.J.; Middleton, F.A. Weight regain after Roux-en-Y: A significant 20% complication related to PYY. *Nutrition* **2008**, *24*, 832–842. [CrossRef] [PubMed]

58. Vennapusa, A.; Panchangam, R.B.; Kesara, C.; Chivukula, T. Response: Factors Predicting Weight Loss after "Sleeve Gastrectomy with Loop Duodenojejunal Bypass" Surgery for Obesity. *J. Obes. Metab. Syndr.* **2020**, *29*, 327–329. [CrossRef]
59. Barhouch, A.S.; Padoin, A.V.; Casagrande, D.S.; Chatkin, R.; Sussenbach, S.P.; Pufal, M.A.; Rossoni, C.; Mottin, C.C. Predictors of Excess Weight Loss in Obese Patients After Gastric Bypass: A 60-Month Follow-up. *Obes. Surg.* **2016**, *26*, 1178–1185. [CrossRef] [PubMed]
60. Higa, K.; Ho, T.; Tercero, F.; Yunus, T.; Boone, K.B. Laparoscopic Roux-en-Y gastric bypass: 10-year follow-up. *Surg. Obes. Relat. Dis. Off. J. Am. Soc. Bariatr. Surg.* **2011**, *7*, 516–525. [CrossRef] [PubMed]

Journal of
Clinical Medicine

MDPI

Article

Changes in Trimethylamine-N-oxide Levels in Obese Patients following Laparoscopic Roux-en-Y Gastric Bypass or Sleeve Gastrectomy in a Korean Obesity Surgical Treatment Study (KOBESS)

Soo Jin Lee [1], Young Suk Park [2], Yong-Jin Kim [3], Sang-Uk Han [4], Geum-Sook Hwang [5], Yeyoung Han [5,6], Yoonseok Heo [7], Eunyoung Ha [8,*] and Tae Kyung Ha [9,*]

1 Department of Nuclear Medicine, Hanyang University Medical Center, Seoul 04763, Korea; suji76@hanmail.net
2 Department of Surgery, Seoul National University Bundang Hospital, Seongnam 13620, Korea; youngsukmd@gmail.com
3 Department of Surgery, H Plus Yangji Hospital, Seoul 08779, Korea; yjgs1997@gmail.com
4 Department of Surgery, Ajou University Hospital, Suwon 16499, Korea; hansu@ajou.ac.kr
5 Integrated Metabolomics Research Group, Western Seoul Center, Korea Basic Science Institute, Seoul 24341, Korea; gshwang@kbsi.re.kr (G.-S.H.); tblove519@gmail.com (Y.H.)
6 Department of Chemistry, Sungkyunkwan University, 2066 Seobu-ro, Jangan-gu, Suwon-si 16419, Korea
7 Department of Surgery, College of Medicine, Inha University, Incheon 22212, Korea; gshur@inha.ac.kr
8 Department of Biochemistry, School of Medicine, Keimyung University, Daegu 42601, Korea
9 Department of Surgery, Hanyang University College of Medicine, 222 Wangsimni-ro, Seongdong-gu, Seoul 04764, Korea
* Correspondence: eyha@dsmc.or.kr (E.H.); missurgeon@hanyang.ac.kr (T.K.H.); Tel.: +82-2-2290-8444 (T.K.H.); Fax: +82-2-2281-0224 (T.K.H.)

Citation: Lee, S.J.; Park, Y.S.; Kim, Y.-J.; Han, S.-U.; Hwang, G.-S.; Han, Y.; Heo, Y.; Ha, E.; Ha, T.K. Changes in Trimethylamine-N-oxide Levels in Obese Patients following Laparoscopic Roux-en-Y Gastric Bypass or Sleeve Gastrectomy in a Korean Obesity Surgical Treatment Study (KOBESS). *J. Clin. Med.* **2021**, *10*, 5091. https://doi.org/10.3390/jcm10215091

Academic Editor: David Benaiges Boix

Received: 13 September 2021
Accepted: 28 October 2021
Published: 29 October 2021

Abstract: Trimethylamine N-oxide (TMAO), a gut microbe-dependent metabolite, has been implicated as a novel risk factor for cardiovascular events related to obesity and type 2 diabetes mellitus (T2DM). The aim of the study was to test the hypothesis if TMAO is associated with the reduction of cardiovascular disease in the Korean obese patients who underwent bariatric surgery. From a subgroup of a multicenter, nonrandomized, controlled trial, titled KOBESS, 38 obese patients, 18 with and 20 without T2DM, who underwent Roux-en-Y gastric bypass (RYGB) or sleeve gastrectomy (SG) were investigated. Bariatric surgery is indicated for Korean patients with a body mass index (BMI) ≥ 35 kg/m^2 or for Korean patients with a BMI ≥ 30 kg/m^2 who have comorbidities. Serum levels of TMAO and its precursors, betaine, carnitine, and choline were measured before and six months after bariatric surgery. The levels of TMAO and its precursors did not differ between obese patients with T2DM and non-T2DM at baseline. However, TMAO increased more than twofold in patients with T2DM after RYGB surgery, but not in patients without T2DM. Choline levels were decreased by half in all patients after RYGB. In patients with T2DM who underwent SG, TMAO, betaine, and carnitine levels did not change after the surgery. Furthermore, in obese patients who underwent bariatric surgery, increased TMAO levels were associated with both T2DM and RYGB, while reduced choline levels were associated with RYGB. These associations need to be further elucidated in follow-up studies to gain further insights into the relationship between TMAO levels and bariatric surgery outcomes.

Keywords: trimethylamine N-oxide; cardiovascular disease; obesity; bariatric surgery; diabetes mellitus

1. Introduction

Obesity is an ever-growing disease that is strongly associated with metabolic syndrome, characterized by insulin resistance, hyperglycemia, hyperlipidemia, and hypertension. Patients with obesity and diabetes mellitus (DM) are at an increased risk of cardiovascular morbidity and mortality. Several clinical trials have shown the significant effects of bariatric surgery, including weight loss, improvements in serum glucose control, and reduced risk of cardiovascular diseases [1,2].

Trimethylamine N-oxide (TMAO), a gut microbe-dependent metabolite, is a small organic compound derived from dietary choline, betaine, and L-carnitine through metabolic processes of gut microbiota and subsequently by hepatic flavin monooxygenases [3–5]. Evidence suggests that TMAO induces platelet hyperactivity and thrombosis, thereby increasing the atherosclerotic burden [6]. These findings are replicated in other clinical studies that showed an association between elevated TMAO levels and an increased risk of atherosclerosis and cardiovascular disease (CVD) [7,8]. Moreover, prospective cohort studies have shown that increased TMAO levels could predict an elevated risk of major adverse events, such as myocardial infarction, stroke, or death [8–10]. In addition, increased levels of TMAO are strongly associated with obesity and DM [11,12]. Recent observational studies have reported TMAO levels to be elevated after bariatric surgery [13,14].

As expected, bariatric surgery changes the composition of the gut microbiome owing to the characteristics of the surgical procedures involving the reconstruction of the small intestine [15]. However, TMAO levels were reported to be increased in Norwegians after bariatric surgery [13]. Given the well-established beneficial effects of bariatric surgery on attenuating the risks of CVDs, increased level of TMAO, a molecule that has been suggested as a risk factor for CVD, after bariatric surgery is conflicting and contradictory. To the best of our knowledge, as of today, the impact of bariatric surgery on TMAO change in Asians has not been reported.

Thus, in this prospective study, we investigated the levels of TMAO and its precursors to elucidate the association between TMAO and the risk of CVD after bariatric surgery. We subdivided patients in this study according to the presence or absence of DM and the types of bariatric surgery.

2. Material and Methods

2.1. Patients and Study Design

The current study is part of a clinical trial entitled Korean Obesity Surgical Treatment Study (KOBESS), registered at www.ClinicalTrials.gov, accessed on 10 September 2021 (NCT03100292) [16]. KOBESS is a prospective, multicenter, nonrandomized, controlled study of obese Korean patients who underwent primary sleeve gastrectomy (SG) or Roux-en-Y gastric bypass (RYGB). All patients were recruited between August 2016 and April 2019. Patients with a body mass index (BMI) $\geq$ 35 kg/m^2 or a BMI 30.0–34.9 kg/m^2 and obesity-related comorbidities, such as DM, hypertension, or hyperlipidemia, were considered eligible for KOBESS. The protocol was approved by the Institutional Review Board of each clinical center (approval number for the coordinating investigator: 000000 2016-06-015), and informed written consent was obtained from all participants. Patients who had complete results for laboratory tests conducted at baseline and six months after surgery were enrolled. Patients with serum samples of less than 50 μL, which was considered insufficient volume for analysis, were excluded from the study. Of 64 KOBESS patients, 38 obese patients, 18 with and 20 without type 2 DM (T2DM), were enrolled and investigated in the current study (Supplementary Figure S1). Seventeen patients (7 with T2DM and 10 without T2DM) underwent RYGB, and 21 patients (11 with T2DM and 10 without T2DM) underwent SG.

2.2. Anthropometric and Laboratory Assessments

Patients were assessed for anthropometry and blood chemistry at baseline two weeks before surgery. Follow-up examinations were performed six months after surgery. Anthropometric data and laboratory test results were recorded for each of the 38 patients six months after bariatric surgery. Height, weight, sex, systolic and diastolic blood pressure (mmHg), and BMI (kg/m^2) were measured and recorded. Fasting blood samples were collected using a standard venipuncture and stored at –70 °C. Laboratory tests, including complete blood count, fasting plasma glucose, glycosylated hemoglobin (HbA1c), lipid profile (triglycerides, total cholesterol, high-density lipoprotein cholesterol [HDL-C], low-density lipoprotein cholesterol [LDL-C]), liver panel [aspartate aminotransferase (AST), alanine aminotransferase (ALT), γ-glutamyl transpeptidase (GTP), alkaline phosphatase (ALP)], renal panel [creatinine, blood urea nitrogen (BUN), uric acid (mg/dL)], ferritin, iron, vitamin B, and folate were performed. The diagnosis of T2DM at baseline was defined according to a previous diagnosis; HbA1c $\geq$ 6.5%, fasting serum glucose when fasting for more than 8 h $\geq$ 126 mg/dL, or serum glucose after 75 g oral glucose tolerance test $\geq$ 200 mg/dL.

2.3. Metabolomic Analysis

For targeted quantitative analysis, we performed ultra-high-performance liquid chromatography/triple quadrupole mass spectrometry (UPLC/TQ-MS) analysis. Prior to analysis, 20 μL of serum sample was extracted using 80 μL of methanol, and the aqueous supernatant was diluted with 20% acetonitrile (*v*/*v*) containing 5 ng/mL betaine-d11, an internal standard. UPLC/TQ-MS analysis was performed on an Agilent 1290 Infinity LC and an Agilent 6495 triple quadrupole MS system equipped with an Agilent Jet Stream electrospray ionization source (Agilent Technologies, USA). Chromatographic separation was carried out on an Acquity UPLC BEH amide column (2.1 mm $\times$ 50 mm, 1.7 μm; Waters) with a binary gradient system comprising 10 mM ammonium formate in water (solvent A) and acetonitrile (solvent B). The linear gradient elution was as follows: 0–1.0 min, 85% B; 1.0–2.5 min, 85–40% B; 2.5–3.0 min, 40% B; 3.0–3.1 min, 40–85% B; 3.1–5.1 min, 85% B. Quantification was performed in the multiple reaction monitoring mode using MS operation in positive ionization mode. Mass Hunter Workstation (Ver B.06.00, Agilent Technologies, USA) software was used for data acquisition and analysis. Metabolite analysis was performed on serum samples collected at baseline and six months after bariatric surgery from 37 patients. Data from one patient were excluded because of measurement failure.

2.4. Statistical Analysis

All data are expressed as the mean $\pm$ standard deviation (SD). A paired *t*-test or independent *t*-test was used to assess the difference in each variable between baseline and six months after surgery. A significance level of 0.05 was used. Statistical analyses were performed using commercial software packages (SPSS version 19; IBM, Chicago, IL, USA), and *p*-values less than 0.05 were considered to be statistically significant.

3. Results

3.1. Clinical Characteristics

As a subgroup of a prospective multicenter clinical trial, a total of 38 obese patients who underwent both bariatric surgery and laboratory tests conducted at baseline and six months after surgery were enrolled (Supplementary Figure S1). The baseline characteristics of the two groups divided by the prevalence of T2DM (18 patients with T2DM and 20 without T2DM) are presented in Table 1. At baseline, the mean age in the T2DM group was 8 years older (p = 0.034) and the HbA1c level was 2.2% higher than in the non-T2DM group (p < 0.001). In the T2DM group, BMI was slightly higher than that of non-T2DM (37.8 $\pm$ 5.9 kg/m^2 vs. 40.1 $\pm$ 6.4 kg/m^2), but there was no significant difference. There were no differences in sex, type of surgery, systolic blood pressure (SBP), diastolic blood pressure (DBP), total cholesterol, and triglyceride levels between the two groups. In the T2DM group, 7 (38.9%) patients underwent RYGB, and 11 (61.1%) underwent SG. In the non-T2DM group, 10 (50.0%) patients underwent RYGB, and 10 (50.0%) underwent SG. All surgical procedures were performed without any significant postoperative complications, and all patients received recommendations regarding dietary habits and lifestyle modifications and micronutrient supplementation (vitamin D, vitamin B_{12}, multivitamin, calcium) as required.

Table 1. Baseline characteristics of patients with type 2 diabetes mellitus (T2DM) and non-T2DM.

	T2DM (n = 18)	Non-T2DM (n = 20)	*p* Value
Gender (male: female)	13:5	14:6	0.884
Age (years)	43.8 ± 13	35.4 ± 11	0.034
BMI (kg/m^2)	37.8 ± 5.9	40.1 ± 6.4	0.271
RYGB:SG	7:11	10:10	0.505
HbA1c (%)	7.8 ± 1.6	5.6 ± 0.3	<0.001
SBP (mmHg)	131 ± 13	140 ± 20	0.123
DBP (mmHg)	80 ± 12	85 ± 18	0.324
Total cholesterol (mg/dL)	192 ± 41	183 ± 28	0.420
Triglyceride (mg/dL)	213 ± 213	152 ± 69	0.234

Data are presented as the mean ± standard deviation (SD) or number (n). T2DM, type 2 diabetes mellitus; BMI, body mass index; RYGB, Roux-en-Y gastric bypass; SG, sleeve gastrectomy, HbA1c, glycosylated hemoglobin; SBP, systolic blood pressure; DBP, diastolic blood pressure.

Table 2 shows BMI and changes in serum biochemical indices six months after surgery for two groups. After bariatric surgery, BMI decreased significantly by more than 10 kg/m^2 in both groups (both $p < 0.001$). In addition, both SBP and DBP decreased in the two groups, but the decrease was not significant. In patients with T2DM, HbA1c decreased significantly from 7.8% to 6.2% and mean value of serum glucose markedly decreased from 144 mg/dL to 105 mg/dL. Even in non-T2DM patients, mean value of serum glucose decreased from 102 mg/dL to 94 mg/dL ($p = 0.003$). AST, ALT and HDL-C were significantly improved in both groups ($p < 0.05$ for all). In addition, in non-T2DM patients, GTP, total cholesterol and triglyceride decreased significantly. Levels of BUN and uric acid of both groups remained unchanged. The level of ferritin decreased in both groups, and $VitB_{12}$ decreased in T2DM after bariatric surgery.

3.2. Changes in Metabolites

Table 3 shows the serum levels of betaine, carnitine, choline, and TMAO at baseline and six months after bariatric surgery (RYGB and SG). Betaine, carnitine, and choline are the precursors of TMAO. Serum levels of TMAO and its precursors did not change at six months after surgery. ($p > 0.05$). When stratified by the presence and absence of T2DM, serum levels of TMAO, although not statistically significant (2.2 ± 1.6 vs. 4.9 ± 5.9 μM, $p = 0.072$), appeared increased in patients with T2DM (Figure 1 and Supplementary Table S1). The levels of betaine, carnitine, and choline remained unchanged after surgery in both the T2DM and non-T2DM groups.

We stratified the patients according to the type of surgery, RYGB and SG (Table 4). We found no difference in baseline levels of TMAO and its precursors. After surgery, TMAO, betaine, and carnitine levels did not significantly change in both the T2DM and non-T2DM groups. Intriguingly, we observed significantly decreased levels of choline (3.2 ± 2.1 μM at baseline, 1.7 ± 1.4 μM after six months, $p = 0.004$) after RYBG, but not after SG ($p = 0.850$).

Based on the increased level of TMAO in patients with T2DM, we stratified patients with T2DM and non-T2DM according to the type of bariatric surgery: T2DM with RYGB (n = 7), T2DM with SG (n = 11), non-T2DM with RYGB (n = 10), and non-T2DM with SG (n = 9). We also analyzed the levels of the metabolites (Table 5). Betaine and carnitine levels were not affected by the presence of T2DM or the type of surgery. Contrary to the levels of betaine and carnitine, those of choline and TMAO appeared to be influenced by the presence of T2DM or the type of surgery. In T2DM patients who underwent RYGB, the level of TMAO increased more than twofold (2.3 ± 1.5 to 5.5 ± 3.1 μM, $p = 0.043$). In contrast, in patients with non-T2DM, TMAO levels did not change in either the RYGB or SG groups. These results suggest a possible association of TMAO with T2DM and RYGB. We also observed that the level of choline was associated with RYGB. The level of choline was attenuated in non-T2DM patients who underwent RYGB (3.2 ± 2.0 to 2.1 ± 1.5 μM, p = 0.036). The mean level of choline, although not significant, decreased from 3.3 ± 2.5 to 1.2 ± 1.2 μM (p = 0.091) in T2DM patients who underwent RYGB.

Table 2. Serum indices at baseline and six months after bariatric surgery in patients with T2DM and non-T2DM.

	T2DM (n = 18)			non-T2DM (n = 20)		
	Baseline	Six Months after Surgery	p Value	Baseline	Six Months after Surgery	p Value
Age (years)	43.8 ± 12.9			35.4 ± 10.8		
BMI (kg/m^2)	37.8 ± 5.9	27.5 ± 5.2	<0.001	40.1 ± 6.4	29.9 ± 5.2	<0.001
SBP (mmHg)	131 ± 13	124 ± 20	0.206	140 ± 20	133 ± 17	0.250
DBP (mmHg)	80 ± 12	78 ± 13	0.626	85 ± 18	80 ± 17	0.443
HbA1c (%)	7.8 ± 1.6	6.2 ± 1.1	<0.001	5.6 ± 0.3	-	-
Glucose (mg/dL)	144 ± 50	105 ± 21	0.009	102 ± 11	94 ± 6	0.003
AST (IU/L)	39.3 ± 22	22.8 ± 6.1	0.004	34.8 ± 18	20.3 ± 8.5	0.002
ALT (IU/L)	52.3 ± 37	22.5 ± 12	0.005	57.7 ± 37	19.4 ± 11.8	<0.001
GTP (IU/L)	47.1 ± 27	27.9 ± 29.8	0.086	38.4 ± 21	15.1 ± 8.7	<0.001
ALP (IU/L)	85.3 ± 22	82.1 ± 26.5	0.726	72.2 ± 17	71.4 ± 13	0.713
Total cholesterol (mg/dL)	192 ± 41	180 ± 36	0.060	183 ± 28	166 ± 26	0.012
Triglyceride (mg/dL)	213 ± 213	122 ± 54	0.079	152 ± 69	94 ± 32	<0.001
HDL-C (mg/dL)	47.1 ± 8.3	51.8 ± 10	0.030	47.5 ± 13	54.2 ± 14	0.001
LDL-C (mg/dL)	116 ± 27	109 ± 28	0.292	116 ± 30	103 ± 21	0.054
Creatinine (mg/dL)	0.79 ± 0.22	0.72 ± 0.20	0.693	0.75 ± 0.19	0.72 ± 0.15	0.287
BUN (mg/dL)	13.7 ± 7.2	13.8 ± 6.5	0.877	12.2 ± 4.0	11.3 ± 3.3	0.411
Uric acid (mg/dL)	5.5 ± 1.5	5.1 ± 1.1	0.127	6.0 ± 1.7	5.0 ± 1.3	0.004
Ferritin	165.8 ± 158.7	107.2 ± 117.8	0.011	157.8 ± 146	101.2 ± 102	0.010
Iron	101 ± 27	100 ±30	0.863	87 ± 39	105 ± 36	0.050
VitB12	621 ± 305	516 ± 218	0.040	475 ± 204	433 ± 209	0.180
Folate	9.06 ± 4.6	8.94 ± 5.3	0.921	6.61 ± 3.7	6.75 ± 4.9	0.861

Data are presented as the mean ± standard deviation. T2DM, type 2 diabetes mellitus; BMI, body mass index; SBP, systolic blood pressure; DBP, diastolic blood pressure; HbA1c, glycosylated hemoglobin; AST, aspartate aminotransferase; ALT, alanine aminotransferase; GTP, γ-glutamyl transpeptidase; ALP, alkaline phosphatase; HDL-C, high-density lipoprotein cholesterol; LDL-C, low-density lipoprotein cholesterol.

Table 3. Serum metabolites at baseline and six months after bariatric surgery.

	Baseline	Six Months after	Δ	p Value
Betaine (μM)	15.4 ± 6.1	17.2 ± 7.9	1.8 ± 6.7	0.116
Carnitine (μM)	16.0 ± 5.7	15.9 ± 5.3	−0.095 ± 4.3	0.894
Choline (μM)	4.8 ± 5.0	3.9 ± 5.3	−9.0 ± 6.4	0.396
TMAO (μM)	2.5 ± 3.0	3.5 ± 4.5	0.95 ± 5.4	0.292

Data are presented as the mean ± standard deviation. Δ, difference between baseline and six months after surgery; TMAO, trimethylamine-N-oxide.

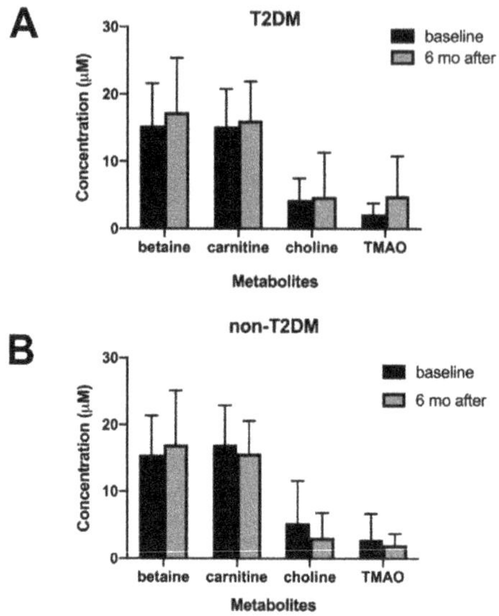

Figure 1. Serum levels of metabolites at baseline (black bars) and six months after bariatric surgery (gray bars) in (**A**) Type 2 diabetes mellitus (T2DM) and (**B**) non-T2DM patients. Abbreviation: T2DM, type 2 diabetes mellitus; TMAO. Trimethylamine-N-oxide.

Table 4. Serum indices at baseline and after six months in subjects who underwent Roux-en-Y gastric bypass (RYGB) and sleeve gastrectomy (SG).

	RYGB (n = 17)			SG (n = 21) *			
	Baseline	Six Months after	*p* value	Baseline	Six Months after	*p* Value	*p* § Value
Age (years)	41.2 ± 13.4			38.0 ± 11.7			0.444
Male: Female	6:11			5:16			0.451
T2DM: non-T2DM	7:10			11:10			0.505
BMI (kg/m^2)	39.2 ± 5.9	28.1 ± 3.8	<0.001	38.9 ± 6.5	28.4 ± 6.2	<0.001	0.865
SBP (mmHg)	128 ± 10	133 ± 23	0.450	141 ± 20	126 ± 14	0.002	0.021
DBP (mmHg)	78 ± 8	83 ± 20	0.319	86 ± 18	76 ± 8	0.060	0.125
HbA1c (%)	8.5 ± 1.1 (n = 7)	6.9 ± 1.3	0.002	7.5 ± 1.8 (n = 10)	5.8 ± 0.7	0.007	0.394
Glucose (mg/dL)	126 ± 29	105 ± 16	0.007	119 ± 48	95 ± 15	0.028	0.621
Betaine (μM)	14.5 ± 6.9	17.1 ± 8.6	0.092	16.2 ± 5.4	17.2 ± 7.6	0.529	0.411
Carnitine (μM)	14.8 ± 6.7	13.9 ± 5.9	0.405	17.0 ± 4.7	17.5 ± 4.1	0.588	0.268
Choline (μM)	3.2 ± 2.1	1.7 ± 1.4	0.004	6.2 ± 6.3	5.8 ± 6.5	0.850	0.059
TMAO (μM)	2.9 ± 3.8	3.5 ± 2.7	0.613	2.2 ± 2.0	3.5 ± 5.6	0.365	0.492

* Metabolite data from 20 patients. § Comparison of baseline values between the two groups. Data are presented as the mean ± standard deviation or number (n). RYGB, Roux-en-Y gastric bypass; SG, sleeve gastrectomy; T2DM, type 2 diabetes mellitus; BMI, body mass index; SBP, systolic blood pressure; DBP, diastolic blood pressure; HbA1c, glycosylated hemoglobin; TMAO, trimethylamine-N-oxide.

Table 5. Changes in metabolites according to diabetes and surgery type.

	T2DM with RYGB (n = 7)			T2DM with SG (n = 11)			Non-T2DM with RYGB (n = 10)			Non-T2DM with SG (n = 9)		
	Baseline	Six Months after	p Value	Baseline	Six Months after	p Value	Baseline	Six Months after	p Value	Baseline	Six Months after	p Value
Betaine (μM)	13.3 ± 7.5	15.1 ± 2.9	0.398	16.5 ± 5.5	18.8 ± 10.0	0.477	15.4 ± 6.8	18.5 ± 11.0	0.241	15.7 ± 5.5	15.3 ± 2.1	0.553
Carnitine (μM)	12.7 ± 7.1	13.1 ± 6.6	0.866	16.8 ± 4.0	18.1 ± 4.4	0.328	16.3 ± 6.3	14.6 ± 5.7	0.260	17.2 ± 5.7	16.9 ± 3.9	0.953
Choline (μM)	3.3 ± 2.5	1.2 ± 1.2	0.091	5.0 ± 3.5	7.1 ± 7.6	0.656	3.2 ± 2.0	2.1 ± 1.5	0.036	7.6 ± 8.6	4.3 ± 5.0	0.441
TMAO (μM)	2.3 ± 1.5	5.5 ± 3.1	0.043	2.2 ± 1.7	4.6 ± 7.3	0.306	3.3 ± 4.9	2.0 ± 1.1	0.878	2.2 ± 2.4	2.1 ± 2.2	0.813

Data are presented as the mean ± standard deviation or number (n). RYGB, Roux-en-Y gastric bypass; SG, sleeve gastrectomy; T2DM, type 2 diabetes mellitus; TMAO, trimethylamine-N-oxide.

4. Discussion

In our study of obese patients who underwent bariatric surgery, we observed that the serum levels of TMAO increased substantially in T2DM patients who underwent RYGB, while other precursor metabolites, betaine and carnitine, were not altered. We also observed that the level of choline decreased significantly in all patients who underwent RYGB. Meanwhile, there was no significant change in metabolites including TAMO in patients with SG regardless of diabetes.

In the current study, we observed that TMAO levels were particularly associated with T2DM and RYGB. Previous studies have reported that TMAO levels after bariatric surgery, particularly RYGB, are increased [13,14], but not after vertical banded gastroplasty [17]. Trøseid et al. reported that plasma levels of TMAO more than doubled compared to the preoperative level in 27 obese patients one year after RYGB (4.4 μM vs. 10.5 μM, $p < 0.001$) [13]. Tremaroli et al. observed increased levels of TMAO only in patients who underwent RYGB but not in those that underwent vertical-banded gastroplasty, nine years after bariatric surgery [18]. In addition, they did not observe differences in other metabolites, carnitine and betaine, between the control and surgery groups.

The mechanism underlying the increase in TMAO levels after RYGB surgery remains to be elucidated. One possibility is that this may be due to adaptive shifts in the gut microbiota. Studies have indicated that bariatric surgery produces a specific shift in the gut microbiota that persists for up to a decade after surgery and is different from the shifts related to dietary intervention for weight loss [15,18,19]. Li et al. observed a major shift in the gut phyla towards higher concentrations of Proteobacteria (52-fold), lower concentrations of Firmicutes (4.5-fold), and Bacteroidetes (twofold) in a non-obese RYGB rat model compared with sham-operated rats [20]. Tremaroli et al. suggested that the increased level of TMAO after bypass surgery might be the consequence of less anaerobic metabolism in the intestine after bypass surgery, a hypothesis that is supported by the broad increase in facultative anaerobes in the intestine after RYGB [18]. Supporting this hypothesis, a recent study indicated that Proteobacteria is the most important bacteria as it encodes the *cutC* gene that codes for choline to trimethylamine (TMA)-mediating enzyme, choline TMA-lyase [21]. Thus, adaptive shifts in the gut microbiota of RYGB surgery may be responsible for the increased level of TMAO. In the current study, however, contrary to the more than doubled level in T2DM patients who underwent RYGB, we did not observe any change in TMAO levels in non-T2DM patients who underwent RYGB. This result clearly does not support the hypothesis that adaptive shifts in the gut microbiota are responsible for the increase in TMAO levels after RYGB surgery.

Another possible explanation for the increased TMAO level after RYGB surgery is that flavin-containing monooxygenase 3 (FMO3), the hepatic enzyme that produces TMAO, might be responsible for the increase in TMAO levels. Higher levels of TMAO are associated with T2DM [11,22]. A recent meta-analysis demonstrated a positive dose-dependent association between TMAO levels and an increased risk for T2DM [23]. The study indicated that the odds ratio for DM prevalence increased by 54% per 5 μM increment in serum TMAO levels. An interesting recent study showed that FMO3 is suppressed by insulin and increases in obese/insulin-resistant humans [24]. More intriguingly, a study reported that RYGB corrects fasting hyperinsulinemia in patients with T2DM [25]. Based on the above-referenced studies, decreased production of insulin during fasting after RYGB could contribute to the increased activity of FMO3, leading to increased levels of TMAO.

In addition to the increased level of TMAO in T2DM patients who underwent RYGB, we also observed that reduced choline levels were associated with RYGB. The decreased choline level is likely due to the rearrangement of the anatomy of the intestine rather than the presence of T2DM, since choline levels were significantly reduced in all patients who underwent RYGB. In addition, we did not observe any change in choline levels in patients who underwent SG, in which the anatomy of the intestine remains intact. Adaptive shifts in gut microbiota towards higher concentrations of bacteria, such as Proteobacteria, that actively convert choline into TMA could explain the decreased choline level after RYGB.

This study is limited to the insufficient power of statistical significance. However, insufficient power of statistical significance does not exclude the possible effect of TMAO on cardiovascular disease. The aim of the study was to test the hypothesis if TMAO is associated with the reduction of cardiovascular disease in the Korean obese patients who underwent bariatric surgery. The prevalence of obesity in Korea steadily increased and the incidence of metabolic disease also concomitantly increased. Bariatric surgery has been reimbursed by National Health Insurance Service in Korea since 2019. The indication of bariatric surgery in Korea is different from that in Western countries. Bariatric surgery is indicated for Korean patients with BMI $\geq$ 35kg/m^2 or for Korean patients with BMI $\geq$ 30kg/m^2 who have comorbidities (T2DM, hypertension, dyslipidemia, obstructive sleep apnea etc.). Therefore, these data cannot be applied to the patients in Western countries. Asian people have similar characteristics and comorbidity. Based on this preliminary study, a large clinical study is underway to determine if TMAO can be a risk factor for cardiovascular disease (Clinical trials No. NCT04554758).

To the best of our knowledge, this is the first prospective study to reveal that the increase in TMAO levels after RYGB is associated with T2DM. The current study is a relatively short-term study of six months. Given the conflicting facts that high TMAO levels are implicated in CVD, while RYGB surgery reduces the risk of CVD, further prospective long-term studies are necessary to gain further insights into the relationship between TMAO levels and bariatric surgery outcomes.

Supplementary Materials: The following are available online at https://www.mdpi.com/article/10.3390/jcm10215091/s1, Figure S1: Flow chart of the KOBESS study. Table S1: The changes in metabolites at baseline and six months in subjects with T2DM and non-T2DM.

Author Contributions: Conceptualization: S.J.L., E.H. and T.K.H.; Investigation: Y.S.P., Y.-J.K., S.-U.H., Y.H. (Yeyoung Han), G.-S.H., Y.H. (Yoonseok Heo) and T.K.H.; Data Curation: Y.S.P., Y.-J.K., S.-U.H., Y.H. (Yeyoung Han), G.-S.H., Y.H. (Yoonseok Heo) and T.K.H.; Formal Analysis: S.J.L.; Validation: S.J.L.; Writing—Original Draft Preparation: S.J.L. and E.H.; Writing-Review and Editing: E.H. and T.K.H. All authors have read and agreed to the published version of the manuscript.

Funding: This research was funded by the Korean Health Technology R&D Project [HC15C1322], Ministry of Health &Welfare, Republic of Korea (for YH), and the Basic Science Research Program through the National Research Foundation of Korea (NRF) funded by the Ministry of Education [2018R1D1A1B07045737].

Institutional Review Board Statement: This study was approved by the Institutional Review Board of each participating hospital.

Informed Consent Statement: Informed consent was obtained from all subjects involved in the study.

Data Availability Statement: The data described in the manuscript, code book, and analytic code will be made available upon request pending application and approval.

Conflicts of Interest: The authors declare no conflict of interest.

References

1. Schauer, P.R.; Bhatt, D.L.; Kirwan, J.P.; Wolski, K.; Aminian, A.; Brethauer, S.A.; Navaneethan, S.D.; Singh, R.P.; Pothier, C.E.; Nissen, S.E.; et al. Bariatric surgery versus intensive medical therapy for diabetes—5-year outcomes. *N. Engl. J. Med.* **2017**, *376*, 641–651. [CrossRef] [PubMed]
2. Sjöström, L.; Lindroos, A.K.; Peltonen, M.; Torgerson, J.; Bouchard, C.; Carlsson, B.; Dahlgren, S.; Larsson, B.; Narbro, K.; Sjöström, C.D.; et al. Lifestyle, diabetes, and cardiovascular risk factors 10 years after bariatric surgery. *N. Engl. J. Med.* **2004**, *351*, 2683–2693. [CrossRef] [PubMed]
3. Koeth, R.A.; Wang, Z.; Levison, B.S.; Buffa, J.A.; Org, E.; Sheehy, B.T.; Britt, E.B.; Fu, X.; Wu, Y.; Li, L.; et al. Intestinal microbiota metabolism of L-carnitine, a nutrient in red meat, promotes atherosclerosis. *Nat. Med.* **2013**, *19*, 576–585. [CrossRef] [PubMed]
4. Brown, J.M.; Hazen, S.L. Metaorganismal nutrient metabolism as a basis of cardiovascular disease. *Curr. Opin. Lipidol.* **2014**, *25*, 48–53. [CrossRef]
5. Organ, C.L.; Otsuka, H.; Bhushan, S.; Wang, Z.; Bradley, J.; Trivedi, R.; Polhemus, D.J.; Tang, W.H.; Wu, Y.; Hazen, S.L.; et al. Choline diet and its gut microbe-derived metabolite, trimethylamine N-oxide, exacerbate pressure overload-induced heart failure. *Circ. Heart Fail.* **2016**, *9*, e002314. [CrossRef]
6. Zhu, W.; Gregory, J.C.; Org, E.; Buffa, J.A.; Gupta, N.; Wang, Z.; Li, L.; Fu, X.; Wu, Y.; Mehrabian, M.; et al. Gut microbial metabolite TMAO enhances platelet hyperreactivity and thrombosis risk. *Cell* **2016**, *165*, 111–124. [CrossRef]
7. Wang, Z.; Klipfell, E.; Bennett, B.J.; Koeth, R.; Levison, B.S.; DuGar, B.; Feldstein, A.E.; Britt, E.B.; Fu, X.; Chung, Y.M.; et al. Gut flora metabolism of phosphatidylcholine promotes cardiovascular disease. *Nature* **2011**, *472*, 57–63. [CrossRef]
8. Tang, W.H.; Wang, Z.; Levison, B.S.; Koeth, R.A.; Britt, E.B.; Fu, X.; Wu, Y.; Hazen, S.L. Intestinal microbial metabolism of phosphatidylcholine and cardiovascular risk. *N. Engl. J. Med.* **2013**, *368*, 1575–1584. [CrossRef]
9. Nie, J.; Xie, L.; Zhao, B.X.; Li, Y.; Qiu, B.; Zhu, F.; Li, G.F.; He, M.; Wang, Y.; Wang, B.; et al. Serum trimethylamine N-oxide concentration is positively associated with first stroke in hypertensive patients. *Stroke* **2018**, *49*, 2021–2028. [CrossRef]
10. Heianza, Y.; Ma, W.; DiDonato, J.A.; Sun, Q.; Rimm, E.B.; Hu, F.B.; Rexrode, K.M.; Manson, J.E.; Qi, L. Long-term changes in gut microbial metabolite trimethylamine N-oxide and coronary heart disease risk. *J. Am. Coll. Cardiol.* **2020**, *75*, 763–772. [CrossRef]
11. Dambrova, M.; Latkovskis, G.; Kuka, J.; Strele, I.; Konrade, I.; Grinberga, S.; Hartmane, D.; Pugovics, O.; Erglis, A.; Liepinsh, E. Diabetes is associated with higher trimethylamine N-oxide plasma levels. *Exp. Clin. Endocrinol. Diabetes* **2016**, *124*, 251–256. [CrossRef]
12. Dehghan, P.; Farhangi, M.A.; Nikniaz, L.; Nikniaz, Z.; Asghari-Jafarabadi, M. Gut microbiota-derived metabolite trimethylamine N-oxide (TMAO) potentially increases the risk of obesity in adults: An exploratory systematic review and dose-response meta-analysis. *Obes. Rev.* **2020**, *21*, e12993. [CrossRef]
13. Trøseid, M.; Hov, J.R.; Nestvold, T.K.; Thoresen, H.; Berge, R.K.; Svardal, A.; Lappegård, K.T. Major increase in microbiota-dependent proatherogenic metabolite TMAO one year after bariatric surgery. *Metab. Syndr. Relat. Disord.* **2016**, *14*, 197–201. [CrossRef]
14. Narath, S.H.; Mautner, S.I.; Svehlikova, E.; Schultes, B.; Pieber, T.R.; Sinner, F.M.; Gander, E.; Libiseller, G.; Schimek, M.G.; Sourij, H.; et al. An untargeted metabolomics approach to characterize short-term and long-term metabolic changes after bariatric surgery. *PLoS ONE* **2016**, *11*, e0161425. [CrossRef]
15. Palmisano, S.; Campisciano, G.; Silvestri, M.; Guerra, M.; Giuricin, M.; Casagranda, B.; Comar, M.; de Manzini, N. Changes in gut microbiota composition after bariatric surgery: A new balance to decode. *J. Gastrointest. Surg.* **2020**, *24*, 1736–1746. [CrossRef]
16. Park, Y.S.; Park, D.J.; Lee, J.H.; Lee, H.J.; Ha, T.K.; Kim, Y.J.; Ryu, S.W.; Han, S.M.; Yoo, M.W.; Park, S.; et al. Korean OBEsity Surgical Treatment Study (KOBESS): Protocol of a prospective multicentre cohort study on obese patients undergoing laparoscopic sleeve gastrectomy and Roux-en-Y gastric bypass. *BMJ Open* **2017**, *7*, e018044. [CrossRef]
17. Gralka, E.; Luchinat, C.; Tenori, L.; Ernst, B.; Thurnheer, M.; Schultes, B. Metabolomic fingerprint of severe obesity is dynamically affected by bariatric surgery in a procedure-dependent manner. *Am. J. Clin. Nutr.* **2015**, *102*, 1313–1322. [CrossRef]
18. Tremaroli, V.; Karlsson, F.; Werling, M.; Ståhlman, M.; Kovatcheva-Datchary, P.; Olbers, T.; Fändriks, L.; le Roux, C.W.; Nielsen, J.; Bäckhed, F. Roux-en-Y gastric bypass and vertical banded gastroplasty induce long-term changes on the human gut microbiome contributing to fat mass regulation. *Cell. Metab.* **2015**, *22*, 228–238. [CrossRef]
19. Ashrafian, H.; Li, J.V.; Spagou, K.; Harling, L.; Masson, P.; Darzi, A.; Nicholson, J.K.; Holmes, E.; Athanasiou, T. Bariatric surgery modulates circulating and cardiac metabolites. *J. Proteome Res.* **2014**, *13*, 570–580. [CrossRef]
20. Li, J.V.; Ashrafian, H.; Bueter, M.; Kinross, J.; Sands, C.; le Roux, C.W.; Bloom, S.R.; Darzi, A.; Athanasiou, T.; Marchesi, J.R.; et al. Metabolic surgery profoundly influences gut microbial-host metabolic cross-talk. *Gut* **2011**, *60*, 1214–1223. [CrossRef]
21. Dalla Via, A.; Gargari, G.; Taverniti, V.; Rondini, G.; Velardi, I.; Gambaro, V.; Visconti, G.L.; De Vitis, V.; Gardana, C.; Ragg, E.; et al. Urinary TMAO levels are associated with the taxonomic composition of the gut microbiota and with the choline TMA-lyase gene (cutC) harbored by *Enterobacteriaceae*. *Nutrients* **2019**, *12*, 62. [CrossRef] [PubMed]
22. Shan, Z.; Sun, T.; Huang, H.; Chen, S.; Chen, L.; Luo, C.; Yang, W.; Yang, X.; Yao, P.; Cheng, J.; et al. Association between microbiota-dependent metabolite trimethylamine-N-oxide and type 2 diabetes. *Am. J. Clin. Nutr.* **2017**, *106*, 888–894. [CrossRef] [PubMed]
23. Zhuang, R.; Ge, X.; Han, L.; Yu, P.; Gong, X.; Meng, Q.; Zhang, Y.; Fan, H.; Zheng, L.; Liu, Z.; et al. Gut microbe-generated metabolite trimethylamine N-oxide and the risk of diabetes: A systematic review and dose-response meta-analysis. *Obes. Rev.* **2019**, *20*, 883–894. [CrossRef] [PubMed]

24. Miao, J.; Ling, A.V.; Manthena, P.V.; Gearing, M.E.; Graham, M.J.; Crooke, R.M.; Croce, K.J.; Esquejo, R.M.; Clish, C.B.; Vicent, D.; et al. Flavin-containing monooxygenase 3 as a potential player in diabetes-associated atherosclerosis. *Nat. Commun.* **2015**, *6*, 6498. [CrossRef]
25. Reed, M.A.; Pories, W.J.; Chapman, W.; Pender, J.; Bowden, R.; Barakat, H.; Gavin, T.P.; Green, T.; Tapscott, E.; Zheng, D.; et al. Roux-en-Y gastric bypass corrects hyperinsulinemia implications for the remission of type 2 diabetes. *J. Clin. Endocrinol. Metab.* **2011**, *96*, 2525–2531. [CrossRef]

Journal of
Clinical Medicine

MDPI

Review

Impact of Bariatric Surgery on Adipose Tissue Biology

Óscar Osorio-Conles [1,2], Josep Vidal [1,2,3,*] and Ana de Hollanda [2,3,4,*]

1. Centro de Investigación Biomédica en Red de Diabetes y Enfermedades Metabólicas Asociadas (CIBERDEM), Instituto de Salud Carlos III (ISCIII), 28029 Madrid, Spain; oosorio@clinic.cat
2. Translational Research in Diabetes, Lipids and Obesity, Institut d'Investigacions Biomèdiques August Pi I Sunyer (IDIBAPS), 08036 Barcelona, Spain
3. Obesity Unit, Endocrinology and Nutrition Department, Hospital Clínic de Barcelona, 08036 Barcelona, Spain
4. Centro de Investigación Biomédica en Red Fisiopatologia de la Obesidad y Nutrición (CIBEROBN), Instituto de Salud Carlos III (ISCIII), 28029 Madrid, Spain

* Correspondence: jovidal@clinic.cat (J.V.); amdehol@clinic.cat (A.d.H.)

Abstract: Bariatric surgery (BS) procedures are actually the most effective intervention to help subjects with severe obesity achieve significant and sustained weight loss. White adipose tissue (WAT) is increasingly recognized as the largest endocrine organ. Unhealthy WAT expansion through adipocyte hypertrophy has pleiotropic effects on adipocyte function and promotes obesity-associated metabolic complications. WAT dysfunction in obesity encompasses an altered adipokine secretome, unresolved inflammation, dysregulated autophagy, inappropriate extracellular matrix remodeling and insufficient angiogenic potential. In the last 10 years, accumulating evidence suggests that BS can improve the WAT function beyond reducing the fat depot sizes. The causal relationships between improved WAT function and the health benefits of BS merits further investigation. This review summarizes the current knowledge on the short-, medium- and long-term outcomes of BS on the WAT composition and function.

Keywords: bariatric surgery; adipose tissue; obesity; subcutaneous adipose tissue; visceral adipose tissue; cytokines; adipokines; adipocyte

Citation: Osorio-Conles, Ó.; Vidal, J.; de Hollanda, A. Impact of Bariatric Surgery on Adipose Tissue Biology. *J. Clin. Med.* **2021**, *10*, 5516. https://doi.org/10.3390/jcm10235516

Academic Editor: David Benaiges Boix

Received: 27 September 2021
Accepted: 22 November 2021
Published: 25 November 2021

1. Introduction

White adipose tissue (WAT) has evolved to become the largest endocrine organ. Its plasticity in response to excess or deficit of nutrients is crucial to maintain metabolic health. The remodeling and expansion capacity of adipose tissue implies the orchestrated response of adipocytes, immune cells, endothelial cells, fibroblasts, the extracellular matrix, and its secretome (cytokines, hormones, microRNAs) as mediators of crosstalk between the main organs involved in metabolic health. Dysfunctional expansion of adipose tissue emerges as a key determinant of obesity-related complications. WAT expansion beyond the subcutaneous adipose tissue (SAT) capacity leads to visceral adipose tissue (VAT) expansion and ectopic fat deposition in other tissues, which are major contributors to cardiovascular disease and metabolic risk above body mass index (BMI) [1]. The precise mechanism leading to impaired adipose tissue expandability are not fully understood. Bariatric surgery (BS) currently results in weight loss and better control of comorbid obesity conditions than medical therapy. BS is also associated with a reduced risk of mortality and of some types of cancer [2]. Currently, Roux-en-Y gastric bypass (RYGBP), sleeve gastrectomy (SG), and biliopancreatic diversion (BPD) are the main surgical techniques used worldwide [3].

This review aims to delve into the biology of adipose tissue in the context of obesity and its changes after BS.

2. Obesity-Related White Adipose Tissue Dysfunction

To identify what hypothetical benefits BS has on adipose tissue biology, we need to cite first the most consensed features of obesity-related WAT dysfunction: an altered adipokine secretome [4,5], unresolved inflammation [6,7], inappropriate extracellular matrix (ECM) remodeling, and insufficient angiogenic potential [8]. The causal order in this context is not completely known; however, hypertrophic adipocytes seem more prone to this scenario as they reach the diffusional limit of oxygen, resulting in persistent hypoxia and ultimately leading to unhealthy WAT tissue expansion [8]. Given its role in WAT remodeling, some authors add autophagy dysregulation to this context [9,10]. Among these features, inflammation-related phenomena, i.e., impaired adipokine and cytokine secretion, have been undoubtedly the most exhaustively studied and tracked parameters during the postsurgical follow-up period after BS.

Obese WAT is characterized by macrophage infiltration, a condition considered as both the cause and consequence of its immune response, which leads to chronic inflammation [11,12]. Obesity-related accumulation of adipose tissue macrophages (ATMs) has been clearly demonstrated in multiple studies [13–15] and the majority of such ATMs accumulate in omental rather than subcutaneous depots [14–16]. Thus, while a small number of macrophages, preferentially localized near blood vessels and dispersed among mature adipocytes are found in lean WAT, subjects with severe obesity show a higher abundance of infiltrating macrophages forming crown-like structures (CLS) around single adipocytes [13]. Such macrophages predominantly present the M1 pro-inflammatory phenotype and promote inflammation by releasing tumor necrosis factor alpha (TNF-α) and interleukin 6 (IL-6), thus contributing to insulin resistance. Alternatively activated, M2-like macrophages play a role in WAT expansion, thermoregulation, antigen presentation, and iron homeostasis [17]. In lean humans, the number of M2 ATMs predominates, secreting anti-inflammatory cytokines and utilizing oxidative metabolism to maintain WAT homeostasis. During obesity development, their proportion compared to M1 ATMs decreases and both populations may adopt a glycolytic metabolism [18]. Once the WAT healthy growth capacity is exceeded, the production of specific adipokines and cytokines by adipocytes and ATMs is compromised and can affect other organ systems.

Although the secretome of many other pro- [19–21] and anti-inflammatory [19,22,23] mediators have been found altered in the context of obesity, those described here are the most comprehensively evaluated, and their postsurgical modulation at different follow-up times is summarized below.

2.1. *Adipose Tissue-Derived Cytokines*

Although the systemic impact of WAT cytokine production in the context of obesity and diabetes has been recently called into question [24], it has been consistently shown that BS-induced weight loss progressively decreases the infiltration of macrophages and WAT secretion of pro-inflammatory molecules [25]. Such cytokines can be both released by WAT-resident immune cells or directly from adipocytes. Below, we describe the most well-studied in the context of obesity.

2.1.1. Pro-Inflammatory

TNF-α is a 17 kDa pro-inflammatory cytokine that can be secreted from mature adipocytes but is predominantly produced within WAT stromovascular fraction, including preadipocytes, endothelial cells, smooth muscle cells, fibroblasts, leukocytes, and macrophages [26–28]. The latter is thought to be the major responsible for the elevated expression during obesity [29].

IL-1β is a major 17.5 kDa pro-inflammatory cytokine secreted mostly by macrophages [30], and its release from WAT nonfat cells is augmented during obesity [31]. With other inflammatory mediators, its production is greater in the visceral than in the subcutaneous depot [32]. Increased circulating IL-1β levels have been associated with the risk of developing type 2 diabetes [33], inasmuch as IL-1β contributes to inhibiting β-cell function and destroying β-cell mass [34,35] and impairs adipocyte insulin signaling [36].

Adipocytes, fibroblasts, and endothelial and immune cells secrete IL-6, which induces fever and liver production of the acute phase reactants, and also mediates chronic inflammatory responses [37]. Both adipocytes and macrophages are responsible for its overexpression in WAT during obesity [38,39]. Visceral rather than subcutaneous depot seems to be the main source of circulating IL-6 levels [40].

Different cell types express IL-8, such as monocytes, macrophages, fibroblasts, endothelial cells, and adipocytes [41,42]. IL-8 acts as a chemokine, attracting leukocytes [39]; as a pro-angiogenic factor [43]; and an amplifier of inflammation [44]. Secretion of IL-8 from WAT is increased [45], mainly in the visceral depot [37] during obesity, and is associated with insulin resistance [42].

IL-18 is another pro-inflammatory cytokine, produced by both hematopoietic cells and non-hematopoietic cells, which has been found to be increased in obesity [46,47] and associated with the metabolic syndrome independently of obesity and insulin resistance [48].

Chemoattractant chemokine ligand 2 (CCL2), also referred to as MCP-1, is a chemoattractant cytokine produced by, among others, myeloid cells [49] and adipocytes [50]. The latter enhances MCP-1 secretion during obesity [51], recruiting and activating macrophages through the MCP-1/IL-1β/CXCL12 signaling pathway [52]. Nevertheless, WAT expansion augmentation does not influence circulating MCP-1 levels [51].

Three isoforms of transforming growth factor-beta (TGF-β) have been identified in mammals, which are produced by all-white blood cells lineages and, to a lesser extent, by mature adipocytes [53]. Despite originally being thought to have overlapping functions, isoform-specific knockout mouse models revealed non-redundant phenotypes [54–56], TGF-1β being the predominant and most important isoform [57]. TGF-1β release from WAT is enhanced in obesity and in response to insulin and inhibitors of TNF-α and IL-β and correlates BMI and adiposity [53].

2.1.2. Anti-Inflammatory

Secreted by Th2 T-cells, M2 macrophages, and adipocytes [39,58], IL-10 is an anti-inflammatory cytokine that suppress macrophage activation [59], which has been inversely associated with BMI and body fat content [60].

Primarily secreted from mast cells and eosinophils, cytokines IL-4 and IL-13 are closely related, where the former stimulates the production of the latter [61], both sharing similar anti-inflammatory functions and receptor complexes [62]. The presence of these cytokines promotes alternative activation of macrophages into M2 cells and inhibits M1-like classical activation [63]. Both IL-4 [64] and IL-13 [65] serum concentrations are increased in obesity. Moreover, recent research showed a role for IL-4 in promoting adipocyte thermogenic capacity [66] and lipolysis [67] through hormone-sensitive lipase (HSL) modulation [68].

2.2. *Adipose Tissue-Derived Hormones*

2.2.1. Pro-Inflammatory

Mostly produced by adipocytes, leptin is a highly conserved 167 kDa peptide. It is secreted proportionally to the amount of adiposity [69,70]. Leptin acts to reduce the food intake at the level of the hypothalamus and fat stores at the level of the adipocyte [71], as well as promoting pro-inflammatory cytokine production by immune cells [38,58].

Resistin, traditionally considered a WAT-specific secretory factor, is a 12.5 kDa hormone which acts as a modulator of body cholesterol trafficking, increasing low-density lipoprotein (LDL)-cholesterol and degrading liver LDL receptors, thus contributing to atherosclerosis pathogenesis. Within WAT, resistin promotes pro-inflammatory cytokine production through the resistin receptor and is found to be increased in obesity [72]. Nevertheless, mounting evidence reveals inconsistencies between resistin's role in rodents and humans, and its relationship with insulin resistance in humans is still controversial [73], with arguments existing both for [74–76] and against [77–79] this association.

Visfatin is another proinflammatory adipokine that plays a role in insulin sensitivity and whose production is increased in obesity and correlates with visceral adiposity [80].

2.2.2. Anti-Inflammatory

Adiponectin is secreted from WAT as an oligomer of varying sizes in an inversely proportional manner to the degree of visceral adiposity [81]. Adiponectin plays an anti-inflammatory role and promotes insulin sensitivity by increasing fatty acid oxidation, thus regulating lipoprotein metabolism and inhibiting hepatic glucose production. The adiponectin-leptin ratio is considered a biomarker of inflammation in WAT [82,83].

Predominantly expressed in the visceral depot [84], omentin -34 kDa- is an anti-inflammatory adipokine with insulin-sensitizing effects whose levels are decreased in obesity and diabetes [85] and inversely correlated BMI [86]. The role of other molecules such as apelin, vaspin, and RBP4 in inflammation is less clear.

2.3. *Extracellular Matrix Remodeling and Fibrosis*

WAT is a highly dynamic organ, as it is responsible for storing and releasing energy in response to nutrient excess or shortage. As WAT expands (by adipocyte enlargement—hypertrophy; and preadipocyte recruitment—hyperplasia), ECM is remodeled to accommodate healthy WAT expansion. Like in other organs, sustained WAT inflammation can trigger aberrant ECM deposition leading to WAT fibrosis. Profibrotic mediators such as TGF-β or connective tissue growth factor (CTGF) participate in this pathway [87]. When WAT becomes fibrotic, ECM stiffness impedes healthy remodeling, causing the tissue to be metabolically dysfunctional, displaying, e.g., adipocyte death, decreased lipolysis, and disrupted cell–cell interactions [87,88]. Thus, inflammation can disarrange the tight balance between ECM composition, extracellular metalloproteinases (MMPs), and their inhibitors (TIMPs) [89]. Data from three independent studies carried out by Karine Clément's group in BS subjects identified the degree of fibrosis in SAT as a predictor for poorer weight loss response after BS [90–92]. In this context, HIF1α has been proposed to link the hypoxic milieu to fibrosis and inflammation [93]. Certainly, accumulating evidence demands further research on the relationship between multiple ECM components and adipocyte function in the context of obesity [88,94–97] and diabetes [98–100], and possible associations with BS outcomes should be explored in depth.

2.4. *Basal and Stimulated Lipolysis*

Obesity is associated with an increase in basal lipolysis and impaired insulin ability to suppress the FFA outflow [101,102]. Antagonistically, plasma catecholamines are important stimulators of lipolysis via adrenergic receptors, particularly through beta-1 (ADRB1) and beta-3 adrenergic receptors (ADRB3) in human WAT [103], and catecholamine-stimulated lipolysis has also been found to be impaired in obesity [104]. Although the classical notion of 'catecholamine resistance' in obesity seems to receive little attention today, some authors recommend its revisitation [105].

More than two decades ago, Kaartinen et al. found a good correlation between the fat cell size and response to isoproterenol in isolated SAT adipocytes from subjects with obesity undergoing BS [106]. Interestingly, after substantial BS-induced weight loss, the lipolytic effect of isoproterenol stimulation of adrenergic receptors was higher than lean controls, despite no difference in receptor density between groups. Similar results have been reported after short-term nutrition interventions [107,108]. Fasting FFA circulating levels are other relevant measures of basal lipolysis, though they are not only dependent on WAT lipolysis but also on clearance by muscle and the liver.

2.5. *Angiogenesis*

Adipogenesis and angiogenesis are tightly related processes during 'healthy' WAT expansion since adipocyte differentiation trigger blood vessel formation [109,110], and in turn, WAT endothelial cells promote preadipocyte differentiation [111]. Vascular endothelial growth factor (VEGF)-A, highly expressed in WAT, plays a capital role in angiogenesis, and its expression is raised during adipogenesis [112,113]. Besides the family of VEGF factors, the angiopoietin (ANGPT) family is also involved in vascular remodeling, maturation, and stabilization [114]. ANGPT-2, expressed in WAT endothelial cells, is considered a proangiogenic factor. Although its overexpression in mice improved the metabolic status [115], its role in the angiogenic process has not yet been elucidated. Platelet endothelial cell adhesion molecule-1 (PECAM-1/CD31) plays a role as an adhesion and signaling molecule with several roles in vascular and inflammatory processes, and its levels are increased in young men with severe obesity [116].

2.6. Autophagy

Autophagy, the cellular mechanism that promotes cell survival during nutrient depletion, may also be relevant under basal or nutrient excess conditions. During nutrient depletion, autophagy can provide essential components for energy production and biosynthesis. In circumstances of nutrient excess, autophagy plays an important role in eliminating unfolded proteins and toxic aggregates and facilitating endoplasmic reticulum homeostasis [117]. In this regard, liver autophagy has been the subject of extensive research [118], while WAT autophagy has been receiving growing attention in recent years and is now considered a key regulator of adipogenesis [9] with intricate implications in ECM remodeling and inflammation [10]. Although some authors have reported attenuated WAT autophagy in obesity [119], not all studies could confirm the sense in which obesity and/or metabolic disruption is related to WAT autophagy alterations [10], and most studies point to overactivation of WAT autophagy in obesity [120–122] and diabetes [123,124]. However, several considerations should be taken into account [10]. Since WAT autophagy can be regarded as a protective mechanism to avoid WAT maladaptation to nutritional stress, this may explain enhanced autophagy despite the increased inflammation in dysfunctional WAT. In addition, autophagy has different functions depending upon the cell type; thus, WAT cell heterogeneity should be taken into consideration. Finally, the varied technical approaches used to measure autophagy and the different depots analyzed could explain conflicting results among these studies. All of this together calls for much more research into the relationship between autophagy, obesity, and BS outcomes.

3. Bariatric Surgery—Related Changes in White Adipose Tissue Biology

Since there is no standardization and the definition of short-, mid- and long-term terminologies can vary among published reports [125], from here on, the current knowledge on this topic is summarized across five follow-up time points commonly used to report BS outcomes: $\leq$3 months (3 m), 6 m, 1 year (1 y)—all often considered to be short-term; $\geq$2 y <5 y—referred to as medium-term; and >5 y—frequently regarded as long-term post-surgery. All bariatric interventions considered in Table 1 consisted of SG, RYGB, or BPD.

Table 1. Short-, medium- and long-term outcomes of bariatric surgery on fat depot parameters, circulating and adipose tissue expression levels of cytokines, adipokines, and microRNAs.

	Short-Term			Medium-Term	Long-Term
Parameter	**≤3 m**	**≈6 m**	**1 y**	**≥2 y**	**≥5 y**
Depot size					
Subcutaneous	↓ [126]	↓ [126–129]	↓ [126,127,130]	↓ [126,131,132]	↓ [133]
Visceral	↓ [126,134]	↓ [126–129]	↓ [126,127,130,135]	↓ [126,131,132]	↓ [133]
Fat cell area					
Subcutaneous	-	↓ [136,137]	↓ [137,138]	↓ [132]	↓ [133]
Visceral	-	-	↓ [138]	-	-
Proinflammatory cytokines					
TNF-α	↑ [139,140]	↓ [141]	↓ [142–144]	↑ [145]	-
	= [146,147]	= [148–150]	= [146,148,150–152]	= 2 y [153], 3 y [154]	-
			↑ SAT [155]		
IL-1β	= [147]	-	↓ [142]	-	-
IL-6	= [147,150,156]	= [141,149,150,157]	↓ [139,142–144,150,152,156,158–160]	↓ [24]	-
	↓ [140,156,161]	↓ [139,160,162], SAT [148]	-	-	-
IL-8	= [147]	= [157]	= [152]	-	-
	↑ [156]		↓ [163]		
	↓ [161,164]				
IL-18	-	-	↓ [141]	-	-
MCP-1	↓ SAT [13]	↓ [164,165]	↓ [150,164,166]	-	-
TGF-β	= [156]	-	↓ [156]	-	-
Anti-inflammatory cytokines					
IL-4	= [140]	↑ [167]	-	-	
		↓ MNC [64]			

Table 1. *Cont.*

	Short-Term						Medium-Term		Long-Term	
Parameter	**≤3 m**		**≈6 m**		**1 y**		**≥2 y**		**≥5 y**	
IL-10	=	[147]	↑	[141,167]	↑	[168]	=	2 y [145], 4 y [169]	-	
			=	[162]	↓	[164]	-			
			↓	[164]						
IL-13	-		↑	[167]	↓	[144]	-		-	
Proinflammatory adipokines										
Leptin	↓	[140,149,162,170]	↓	[141,148–150,162,170]	↓	[144,148,150,156,158,163,168]	↓	2 y [145,153], 3 y [154], 4 y [169]	-	
Resistin	=	[150]	↓	[141]	↓	[142,158,168]	↓	[145]	-	
			↑	[150]	=	[150,171]				
Visfatin	=	[150]	=	[150]	=	[150]	-		-	
Anti-inflammatory adipokines										
Adiponectin	↑	[147,149,156]	↑	[139,141]	↑	[139,141,142,150,156,158,168]	↑	2 y [145,153], 3 y [154]	↑	[133]
	=	[146,150,156]	=	[150,162]			=	4 y [169]		
Omentin	↑	[172]	↑	[172]	↑	[172,173]	-		-	
Other adipokines										
Apelin	-		↓	[174]	-		-		-	
Vaspin	-		-		↓	[175]	-		-	
RBP-4	↓	SAT [176]	↓	[177,178]	↑	[151]	↓	[179]	-	
	=	[176]								
Fibrosis										
Subcutaneous	-		=	[180]	-		-		-	

Table 1. *Cont.*

	Short-Term			Medium-Term	Long-Term
Parameter	**≤3 m**	**≈6 m**	**1 y**	**≥2 y**	**≥5 y**
Lipolysis					
Basal	= [181]	= Isolated SAT adipocytes [181]	-	= Male [182]	= [133]
				↓ Female [133,182]	↑ SAT release [133]
Stimulated	= Isolated SAT adipocytes [181]	↓ Isolated SAT adipocytes vs. 1 m [181]		= Male [182]	-
				↓ Female [182]	
Insulin-supressed	-	↑ [137,183]		↑ [102]	-
FFA	↑ [148,181]	= [148,184,185]	↑ [101]	= [102]	-
	= [186]		= [148]		
Angiogenesis					
VEGF-A	-	-	↓ [187,188]	-	-
ANGPT-2, follistatin, HGF, PECAM-1	-	-	↓ [188]	-	-
Autophagy					
Subcutaneous	-	↑ 3–12 m post-BS [119]	-	-	-
microRNAs					
	↑↓ 7 Circulating miRNAs [189]	-	= Circulating miR-99b [190]	↑↓ 15 SAT miRNAs [191]	-
	↓ 1 VAT and 13 SAT miRNAs [192] *		↑ Circulating miR-221, miR-222 [190]	↓ SAT miR-221-3p [193]	
				↓ 12 SAT miRNAs [194]	

For cytokines, adipokines, lipolysis, and angiogenesis markers, data refer to circulating levels, unless otherwise stated. ↑, Increased; ↓, decreased; =, equal or inconclusive; -, no data; m, months; y, years; TNF-α, tumor necrosis factor-α; IL, interleukin; MCP-1, monocyte chemoattractant protein-1; TGF-β, transforming growth factor β; RBP-4, retinol binding protein 4; FFA, free fatty acids; VEGF-A, vascular endothelial growth factor A; ANGPT-2, angiopoietin-2; HGF, hepatocyte growth factor; PECAM-1, platelet endothelial cell adhesion molecule-1; SAT, subcutaneous adipose tissue; VAT, visceral adipose tissue; MNC, mononuclear cells. * after significant weight loss, collection time not reported.

3.1. Short Term

During the first year, coinciding with the rapid weight loss phase after BS, both SAT [126–130] and VAT [126–130,134,135] depots progressively reduce their size, and this is accompanied by a reduction in the area of subcutaneous [136–138] and visceral [138] adipocytes, respectively. A large adipocyte size was independently associated with a lower incidence of insulin resistance 6 months after RYGBP [136].

In the very short term after BS ($\leq$3 months), Cancello et al. showed a significant decrease of total ATMs (HAM56+ cells) in SAT after RYGB [13]. These results were confirmed in another study from the same group, wherein CD40$^+$ cells (M1-like) were also found to be decreased and CD206$^+$ and CD163$^+$ cells (M2-like) increased 3 months after RYGB [16]. This was accompanied by a reversion to the lean WAT profile, with CLS remission and ATMs again located near blood vessels [13].

Such early changes in the WAT cellular composition seem to alter the production of some cytokines, while others generate conflicting results between studies or do not seem to be modulated in the short term after BS. Thus, among the proinflammatory cytokines, MCP-1 was found to be concomitantly decreased during this period [13,150,165,166], while TGF-β or IL-1β seem to decrease only at 1 year after BS [142,147,156]. Reports on IL-6 production give conflicting results at 3 and 6 months but agree on a consistent decrease 1 year after surgery [139,142–144,146,150,152,156,158–160,168]. Similarly, reduced circulating levels of IL-18 were found 1 y post-BS [141] and after massive BS-induced weight loss, irrespective of the time elapsed since surgery [195,196].

In contrast, there is less consensus about TNF-α and IL-8, which have been found in different studies to both be increased [140,155,156,197], decreased [141–144,163,164], or unchanged [146–152,157] during this period. Similarly, BS-related outcomes on anti-inflammatory cytokine production have yielded highly contradictory results between studies during the short-term follow-up period, as is the case with IL-4 [64,140,167], IL-10 [141,147,162,164,167,168], and IL-13 [144,167]. Interestingly, circulating omentin levels decrease as early as 24 h post-BS, before any fat mass loss, and maintained for 1 y [172].

Inasmuch as surgical weight loss predominantly reduces the body fat content, it is understandable that leptin levels were found to be consistently reduced following BS [140,141,144,148–150,156,158,162,163,168,170]. The leptin levels were also reduced after the novel endovascular bariatric procedure [198]. Nevertheless, systemic leptin levels are not directly related to the amount of body weight or fat loss, since early reductions of adiposity more dramatically reduce leptin levels than later periods of weight loss [162,170]. Again, there is a lack of consensus regarding the short-term effect of BS on resistin levels, given several studies have found it to be decreased [141,142,145,158,168] or unchanged [150,171]. In the case of visfatin, Lima et al. showed unaltered levels throughout the first year after BS [150].

Despite some conflicting reports in the very short term [146,147,149,150,156], circulating adiponectin levels appear to be consistently increased 1 year after BS [139,141,142,150,152,156,158,168]. For its part, omentin was found to be increased as early as 24 h after BPD [172], and such a change is maintained for up to 1 year [172,173]. Apelin, a multifaceted biomarker [174], and vaspin, an insulin-sensitizing adipokine [175], are less investigated adipokines that showed a short-term reduction after BS. Regarding RBP-4, most studies reported a decrease in the circulating [177,178] or SAT mRNA [176] levels early after BS.

One study performed by Chabot and collaborators showed no resolution of SAT fibrosis 6 months after BS and suggested a transient association between SAT fibrosis and insulin resistance in humans with obesity [180]. Similarly, Katsogiannos et al. did not find significant differences in either the basal or stimulated lipolysis rate in SAT adipocytes at 1 and 6 months after BS but reported a decrease in isoproterenol-stimulated lipolysis at 6 versus 1 month after BS [181]. Conversely, insulin-suppressed free fatty acid (FFA) release has been found to be enhanced at 4 months [137], 7 months [183], and 1 year after

RYGBP [101]. While some authors found increased FFA levels in the early months after BS [101,148,181], others reported no differences in this period [148,184–186].

García de la Torre et al. found higher VEGF-A levels in obese women undergoing BS compared to lean controls, and such levels significantly decreased 1 y after surgery, irrespective of the surgical procedure performed [187]. At this same follow-up period, another recent study showed, in addition to VEGF-A, lower levels of several angiogenesis biomarkers such as angiopoietin 2 (ANGPT-2), follistatin, hepatocyte growth factor (HGF), and the platelet endothelial cell adhesion molecule (PECAM-1) in patients who underwent SG or laparoscopic adjustable gastric banding (LAGB) [188].

Finally, Soussi et al. found attenuated WAT autophagy in obesity, and pre- versus post-BS comparisons indicated ameliorated adipocyte autophagic clearance in all patients within 3 to 12 months after the intervention, although at different degrees because of the large time-frame in post-surgery sample collection [119].

3.2. Medium Term

Two years after surgery, both visceral and subcutaneous depots maintain reduced sizes [126,131,132] as does the abdominal subcutaneous fat cell volume [132]. There is much less data available on circulating parameters beyond 1 y after BS. While IL-6 levels are consistently found reduced 2 y [145,153], 3 y [154], and 4 y after BS [169], reports on TNF-a continue to report conflicting data [145,154]. Although reports on IL-10 also seem quite inconsistent, some authors find that, after a temporary rise in the short term, its levels return to baseline values at 2 y [145], or even continue falling at 4 y [169].

BS outcomes on leptin and adiponectin levels seem much more solid. Circulating leptin has been repeatedly found to be reduced at 2 [145,153], 3 [154], and 4 y [169], and such reductions seem to be mainly attributed to early changes in WAT. Conversely, adiponectin levels continue to progressively rise in the medium term [145,153,154]. Only one report seems to oppose this view, a contradiction that could arise from the limited number of subjects and the variety of surgical techniques included in the study [169].

Beyond the short-term inconsistencies mentioned above, a single study showed that circulating resistin, after an early decline, recovered baseline levels 2 y after gastric bypass [145]. Finally, the RBP-4 levels were found still lowered 24 months after BS. Such changes were more pronounced in the subgroup without metabolic syndrome and correlated with reductions in the waist and visceral fat diameter [179].

Despite negative results reported by Katsogiannos et al. in the short term in a mixed-sex cohort [181], Löfgren and collaborators found reduced basal and stimulated lipolysis rates at 2 y after BS exclusively in females [182], where differences in the basal rates remained only significant when lipolysis was expressed per cell surface area. In another study, the glycerol release in women who underwent RYGBP was found to be decreased postsurgically at 2 y and then increased dramatically to similar levels observed before surgery at 5 y [133]. Similarly, Manco et al. found reduced FFA levels in normoglucose-tolerant obese women 3 years after BPD [154]. Finally, insulin-mediated suppression of FFA outflow has been found to be enhanced 3 years after RYGBP [102].

3.3. Long Term

Studies on long-term outcomes after BS are restricted almost exclusively to weight-loss parameters. Thus, a recent meta-analysis at 10 or more years after all bariatric procedures reported weighted means of 56.7% excess weight loss (EWL) after GB, 45.9%EWL after LAGB, 74.1%EWL after BPD and 58.3%EWL after SG [199]. The same study reported a 48.9%EWL and 22.2%TWL 20 y after LAGB. Very similar results were previously reported by the same group at 15 y after LAGB [200]. A lower incidence [201] and greater remission [202] of T2DM have also been reported in the long term; reductions in all-cause, cardiovascular, and T2DM mortality have also been found [203]. Nevertheless, the potential impact of body fat loss on these metabolic outcomes deserves further investigation since some variables appear to be more weight-dependent, while others seem to be more adiposity-dependent from the medium-term [204].

Regarding the outcomes in WAT exclusively, we only have evidence from a single study carried out in women by Hoffstedt and collaborators at the long-term follow-up [133]. The authors reported decreased amounts of estimated SAT and VAT at 2 and 5 y and diminished SAT cell volume and increased adiponectin levels at 5 y post-BS. This study also found augmented basal glycerol release from isolated SAT adipocytes at 5 y, despite not finding changes in fasting plasma levels.

3.4. Summary of BS Outcomes on WAT

In summary, after bariatric surgery, SAT and VAT reduce their size progressively during the weight-loss phases. M1-like decrease and M2-like ATMs increase early after surgery; however, there are no data beyond the short term after BS.

Most pro-inflammatory cytokines begin to decrease early after surgery and continue to decline in the medium- and long-term. However, TGF-B or IL1B decrease only after one year of BS. There are controversial data on short-term TNFα and IL-8 levels after surgery as well as in anti-inflammatory cytokine levels in the short- and medium-term after surgery. Leptin levels drop rapidly soon after BS and then continue to decline during the follow-up; conversely, adiponectin and omentin levels rise after surgery. Resistin and visfatin dynamics show less agreement.

Regarding fibrosis, only one study reported no changes at short-term. Gender differences seem to affect basal and stimulated rates of lipolysis, which have been found decreased only in females at mid-term after BS. For its part, insulin inhibition of lipolysis was found consistently enhanced at medium- and long-term after surgery. Finally, autophagy increases and several angiogenesis-related molecules decrease at short-term, although there is a lack of reports on longer follow-up periods.

4. Other Proposed Novel Mechanisms for WAT Improvement after BS

Mitochondrial function and biogenesis have been found to be impaired in obesity, and T2DM and BS may attenuate mitochondrial damage in adipocytes. Thus, Varela-Rodríguez and colleagues reported an increased mitochondrial density and coverage, together with enhanced mitochondrial function at both the gene and protein level in abdominal SAT after RYGB- or SG-induced weight loss in a reduced cohort of patients [205]. In the very short term after RYGB, an induction of genes involved in mitochondrial biogenesis was found in SAT [206]. Similarly, increased SAT expression of transcripts related to the oxidative phosphorylation (OXPHOS) pathway has been shown 3 m [207] and 1 y after BS [137,208]. More recently, Van der Kolk et al. confirmed these findings in abdominal SAT in the short and medium term after RYGB, while opposite results were found after a low-calorie diet [209], suggesting a BS-specific effect. The authors also showed an induction of the tricarboxylic acid (TCA) cycle and fatty acid oxidation 2 y after surgery.

Beiging is the process through which WAT can change its phenotype to a brown-like adipose tissue known as beige/brite adipose tissue. Accumulating evidence from human and rodent studies in the last years suggest that RYGB predominantly enhances beige thermogenesis, while SG seems to promote brown adipose tissue thermogenesis [210]. A role for bile acids and the gut microbiome has been proposed in these mechanisms. Moreover, such thermogenic effects could depend on the fat content of the postoperative diet.

Beyond the fat mass loss and biological pathways discussed above, other mechanisms could contribute to the improvement of WAT dysfunction after BS. Thus, Frikke-Schmidt and colleagues recently summarized other potential pathways affecting the WAT function that can play a role after BS [105]. Bile acids, whose levels are persistently found to be increased after surgery [211], may improve adipocyte function acting upon the FXR receptor [212]. Another hypothesized mechanism implies gut microbiome composition. It has been found that the composition of the bacteria in the gut change after BS, and accumulating evidence shows how the bacterial composition can modulate the host immune cell population. Thus, there is the possibility that changes in the gut microbiome initiated by BS can significantly impact the WAT metabolic function by modulating immune-resident cells in WAT [213,214]. Finally, as BS has demonstrated effects on the central regulation of metabolism, potential changes in neural enervation to the WAT may mediate physiological changes after BS, as results in mice suggest [215].

Lastly, recent studies have indicated significant alterations in the expression of several putative adipose tissue-derived microRNAs (miRNAs) after BS [216]. Thus, 1 y after BS, Sangiao-Alvarellos et al. reported raised circulating levels of miR-221 and miR-222 [190], and as early as 21 days post-RYGB, Atkin et al. found modulated levels of seven miRNAs (miR-7-5p, let-7f-5p, miR-15b-5p, let-7i-5p, miR-320c, miR-205-5p, and miR-335-5p) [189], mostly related with diabetes and insulin resistance pathways. Regarding SAT expression, Ortega and collaborators identified 12 modulated miRNAs 2 y after BS, some of them previously found raised in mature adipocytes after inflammatory stimulation (such as miR-146b, miR-376c, and again miR-221) [194], while another study from the same group found significant modifications in 15 mature miRNAs, mostly related to cell cycle, metabolism, and inflammation pathways, in women who underwent RYGB [191].

5. Future Perspectives

Better understanding of the fascinating biology of WAT following BS deserves further investigation. Evaluation of the modifications of WAT biology associated not only with time elapsed after surgery but also with the amount of weight loss is a priority. Studies should help us better understand the relationship between shrinkage in WAT volume and improved WAT function with the health benefits of BS. The health burden associated with a particular BMI in subjects with a weight-reduced state following BS appears to be eased as compared to that in subjects with comparable BMI that have not undergone BS. Thus, future studies should help disentangle how BS helps restore the crosstalk between the different components of the WAT as well as the crosstalk between WAT and other organs.

Author Contributions: Conceptualization, Ó.O.-C., J.V. and A.d.H.; writing—original-draft preparation, Ó.O.-C.; writing—review and editing, Ó.O.-C., J.V. and A.d.H.; supervision, J.V. and A.d.H. All authors have read and agreed to the published version of the manuscript.

Funding: This research received no external funding.

Conflicts of Interest: The authors declare no conflict of interest.

References

1. Neeland, I.J.; Ross, R.; Després, J.-P.; Matsuzawa, Y.; Yamashita, S.; Shai, I.; Seidell, J.; Magni, P.; Santos, R.D.; Arsenault, B.; et al. Visceral and ectopic fat, atherosclerosis, and cardiometabolic disease: A position statement. *Lancet Diabetes Endocrinol.* **2019**, *7*, 715–725. [CrossRef]
2. Aminian, A.; Zajichek, A.; Arterburn, D.E.; Wolski, K.E.; Brethauer, S.A.; Schauer, P.R.; Kattan, M.W.; Nissen, S.E. Association of Metabolic Surgery with Major Adverse Cardiovascular Outcomes in Patients with Type 2 Diabetes and Obesity. *JAMA* **2019**, *322*, 1271–1282. [CrossRef] [PubMed]
3. Welbourn, R.; Hollyman, M.; Kinsman, R.; Dixon, J.; Liem, R.; Ottosson, J.; Ramos, A.; Våge, V.; Al-Sabah, S.; Brown, W.; et al. Bariatric Surgery Worldwide: Baseline Demographic Description and One-Year Outcomes from the Fourth IFSO Global Registry Report 2018. *Obes. Surg.* **2019**, *29*, 782–795. [CrossRef] [PubMed]
4. Zorena, K.; Jachimowicz-Duda, O.; Ślęzak, D.; Robakowska, M.; Mrugacz, M. Adipokines and Obesity. Potential Link to Metabolic Disorders and Chronic Complications. *Int. J. Mol. Sci.* **2020**, *21*, 3570. [CrossRef]
5. Pardo, M.; Roca-Rivada, A.; Seoane, L.M.; Casanueva, F.F. Obesidomics: Contribution of adipose tissue secretome analysis to obesity research. *Endocrine* **2012**, *41*, 374–383. [CrossRef]
6. Ellulu, M.S.; Patimah, I.; Khaza, H.; Rahmat, A.; Abed, Y.; Sci, A.M. Obesity and Inflammation: The Linking Mechanism and the Complications. *Arch. Med. Sci.* **2016**, *13*, 851–863. [CrossRef]
7. O'Rourke, R.W. Inflammation in obesity-related diseases. *Surgery* **2009**, *145*, 255–259. [CrossRef] [PubMed]
8. Crewe, C.; An, Y.A.; Scherer, P.E. The ominous triad of adipose tissue dysfunction: Inflammation, fibrosis, and impaired angiogenesis. *J. Clin. Investig.* **2017**, *127*, 74–82. [CrossRef] [PubMed]
9. Ferhat, M.; Funai, K.; Boudina, S. Autophagy in Adipose Tissue Physiology and Pathophysiology. *Antioxidants Redox Signal.* **2019**, *31*, 487–501. [CrossRef]

10. Clemente-Postigo, M.; Tinahones, A.; El Bekay, R.; Malagón, M.M.; Tinahones, F.J. The Role of Autophagy in White Adipose Tissue Function: Implications for Metabolic Health. *Metabolites* **2020**, *10*, 179. [CrossRef]
11. McNelis, J.C.; Olefsky, J.M. Macrophages, Immunity, and Metabolic Disease. *Immunity* **2014**, *41*, 36–48. [CrossRef] [PubMed]
12. Wellen, K.E.; Hotamisligil, G.S. Obesity-induced inflammatory changes in adipose tissue. *J. Clin. Investig.* **2003**, *112*, 1785–1788. [CrossRef] [PubMed]
13. Cancello, R.; Henegar, C.; Viguerie, N.; Taleb, S.; Poitou, C.; Rouault, C.; Coupaye, M.; Pelloux, V.; Hugol, D.; Bouillot, J.-L.; et al. Reduction of Macrophage Infiltration and Chemoattractant Gene Expression Changes in White Adipose Tissue of Morbidly Obese Subjects after Surgery-Induced Weight Loss. *Diabetes* **2005**, *54*, 2277–2286. [CrossRef]
14. Cancello, R.; Tordjman, J.; Poitou, C.; Guilhem, G.; Bouillot, J.L.; Hugol, D.; Coussieu, C.; Basdevant, A.; Hen, A.B.; Bedossa, P.; et al. Increased infiltration of macrophages in omental adipose tissue is associated with marked hepatic lesions in morbid human obesity. *Diabetes* **2006**, *55*, 1554–1561. [CrossRef] [PubMed]
15. Shapiro, H.; Pecht, T.; Shaco-Levy, R.; Harman-Boehm, I.; Kirshtein, B.; Kuperman, Y.; Chen, A.; Blüher, M.; Shai, I.; Rudich, A. Adipose tissue foam cells are present in human obesity. *J. Clin. Endocrinol. Metab.* **2013**, *98*, 1173–1181. [CrossRef]
16. Aron-Wisnewsky, J.; Tordjman, J.; Poitou, C.; Darakhshan, F.; Hugol, D.; Basdevant, A.; Aissat, A.; Guerre-Millo, M.; Clément, K. Human adipose tissue macrophages: M1 and M2 cell surface markers in subcutaneous and omental depots and after weight loss. *J. Clin. Endocrinol. Metab.* **2009**, *94*, 4619–4623. [CrossRef]
17. Hill, A.A.; Reid Bolus, W.; Hasty, A.H. A decade of progress in adipose tissue macrophage biology. *Immunol. Rev.* **2014**, *262*, 134–152. [CrossRef]
18. Castoldi, A.; De Souza, C.N.; Saraiva Câmara, N.O.; Moraes-Vieira, P.M. The macrophage switch in obesity development. *Front. Immunol.* **2016**, *6*, 1. [CrossRef]
19. Mancuso, P. The role of adipokines in chronic inflammation. *ImmunoTargets Ther.* **2016**, *5*, 47–56. [CrossRef]
20. Osorio-Conles, Ó.; Guitart, M.; Moreno-Navarrete, J.M.; Escoté, X.; Duran, X.; Fernandez-Real, J.M.; Gómez-Foix, A.M.; Fernández-Veledo, S.; Vendrell, J. Adipose tissue and serum CCDC80 in obesity and its association with related metabolic disease. *Mol. Med.* **2017**, *23*, 225–234. [CrossRef]
21. Caër, C.; Rouault, C.; Le Roy, T.; Poitou, C.; Aron-Wisnewsky, J.; Torcivia, A.; Bichet, J.C.; Clément, K.; Guerre-Millo, M.; André, S. Immune cell-derived cytokines contribute to obesity-related inflammation, fibrogenesis and metabolic deregulation in human adipose tissue. *Sci. Rep.* **2017**, *7*, 3000. [CrossRef]
22. Ohashi, K.; Shibata, R.; Murohara, T.; Ouchi, N. Role of anti-inflammatory adipokines in obesity-related diseases. *Trends Endocrinol. Metab.* **2014**, *25*, 348–355. [CrossRef]
23. Osorio-Conles, O.; Guitart, M.; Chacón, M.R.; Maymo-Masip, E.; Moreno-Navarrete, J.M.; Montori-Grau, M.; Näf, S.; Fernandez-Real, J.M.; Vendrell, J.; Gómez-Foix, A.M. Plasma PTX3 protein levels inversely correlate with insulin secretion and obesity, whereas visceral adipose tissue PTX3 gene expression is increased in obesity. *Am. J. Physiol. Endocrinol. Metab.* **2011**, *301*, E1254–E1261. [CrossRef] [PubMed]
24. Rakotoarivelo, V.; Lacraz, G.; Mayhue, M.; Brown, C.; Rottembourg, D.; Fradette, J.; Ilangumaran, S.; Menendez, A.; Langlois, M.-F.; Ramanathan, S. Inflammatory Cytokine Profiles in Visceral and Subcutaneous Adipose Tissues of Obese Patients Undergoing Bariatric Surgery Reveal Lack of Correlation With Obesity or Diabetes. *EBioMedicine* **2018**, *30*, 237–247. [CrossRef] [PubMed]
25. Labrecque, J.; Laforest, S.; Michaud, A.; Biertho, L.; Tchernof, A. Impact of Bariatric Surgery on White Adipose Tissue Inflammation. *Can. J. Diabetes* **2017**, *41*, 407–417. [CrossRef] [PubMed]
26. Fain, J.N.; Bahouth, S.W.; Madan, A.K. TNFα release by the nonfat cells of human adipose tissue. *Int. J. Obes.* **2004**, *28*, 616–622. [CrossRef]
27. Xu, H.; Barnes, G.T.; Yang, Q.; Tan, G.; Yang, D.; Chou, C.J.; Sole, J.; Nichols, A.; Ross, J.S.; Tartaglia, L.A.; et al. Chronic inflammation in fat plays a crucial role in the development of obesity-related insulin resistance. *J. Clin. Investig.* **2003**, *112*, 1821–1830. [CrossRef]
28. De Taeye, B.M.; Novitskaya, T.; McGuinness, O.P.; Gleaves, L.; Medda, M.; Covington, J.W.; Vaughan, D.E. Macrophage TNF-α contributes to insulin resistance and hepatic steatosis in diet-induced obesity. *Am. J. Physiol. Endocrinol. Metab.* **2007**, *293*, E713–E725. [CrossRef]
29. Weisberg, S.P.; McCann, D.; Desai, M.; Rosenbaum, M.; Leibel, R.L.; Ferrante, A.W. Obesity is associated with macrophage accumulation in adipose tissue. *J. Clin. Investig.* **2003**, *112*, 1796–1808. [CrossRef]
30. Sims, J.E.; Smith, D.E. The IL-1 family: Regulators of immunity. *Nat. Rev. Immunol.* **2010**, *10*, 89–102. [CrossRef]
31. Fain, J.N. Release of Interleukins and Other Inflammatory Cytokines by Human Adipose Tissue Is Enhanced in Obesity and Primarily due to the Nonfat Cells. *Vitam. Horm.* **2006**, *74*, 443–477.
32. Koenen, T.B.; Stienstra, R.; Van Tits, L.J.; Joosten, L.A.B.; Van Velzen, J.F.; Hijmans, A.; Pol, J.A.; Van Der Vliet, J.A.; Netea, M.G.; Tack, C.J.; et al. The inflammasome and caspase-1 activation: A new mechanism underlying increased inflammatory activity in human visceral adipose tissue. *Endocrinology* **2011**, *152*, 3769–3778. [CrossRef]
33. Spranger, J.; Kroke, A.; Möhlig, M.; Hoffmann, K.; Bergmann, M.M.; Ristow, M.; Boeing, H.; Pfeiffer, A.F.H. Inflammatory cytokines and the risk to develop type 2 diabetes: Results of the prospective population-based European Prospective Investigation into Cancer and Nutrition (EPIC)-Potsdam study. *Diabetes* **2003**, *52*, 812–817. [CrossRef]
34. Dinarello, C.A.; Donath, M.Y.; Mandrup-Poulsen, T. Role of IL-1β in type 2 diabetes. *Curr. Opin. Endocrinol. Diabetes Obes.* **2010**, *17*, 314–321. [CrossRef] [PubMed]

35. Donath, M.Y.; Dalmas, É.; Sauter, N.S.; Böni-Schnetzler, M. Inflammation in obesity and diabetes: Islet dysfunction and therapeutic opportunity. *Cell Metab.* **2013**, *17*, 860–872. [CrossRef] [PubMed]
36. Gao, D.; Madi, M.; Ding, C.; Fok, M.; Steele, T.; Ford, C.; Hunter, L.; Bing, C. Interleukin-1β mediates macrophage-induced impairment of insulin signaling in human primary adipocytes. *Am. J. Physiol. Endocrinol. Metab.* **2014**, *307*, E289–E304. [CrossRef] [PubMed]
37. Juge-Aubry, C.E.; Henrichot, E.; Meier, C.A. Adipose tissue: A regulator of inflammation. *Best Pract. Res. Clin. Endocrinol. Metab.* **2005**, *19*, 547–566. [CrossRef]
38. Rasouli, N.; Kern, P.A. Adipocytokines and the metabolic complications of obesity. *J. Clin. Endocrinol. Metab.* **2008**, *93*, s64–s73. [CrossRef]
39. Balistreri, C.R.; Caruso, C.; Candore, G. The role of adipose tissue and adipokines in obesity-related inflammatory diseases. *Mediators Inflamm.* **2020**, *2010*, 802078. [CrossRef]
40. Fontana, L.; Eagon, J.C.; Trujillo, M.E.; Scherer, P.E.; Klein, S. Visceral Fat Adipokine Secretion Is Associated With Systemic Inflammation in Obese Humans. *Diabetes* **2007**, *56*, 1010–1013. [CrossRef] [PubMed]
41. Bruun, J.M.; Pedersen, S.B.; Richelsen, B. Regulation of Interleukin 8 Production and Gene Expression in Human Adipose Tissue in Vitro1. *J. Clin. Endocrinol. Metab.* **2001**, *86*, 1267–1273. [CrossRef] [PubMed]
42. Kobashi, C.; Asamizu, S.; Ishiki, M.; Iwata, M.; Usui, I.; Yamazaki, K.; Tobe, K.; Kobayashi, M.; Urakaze, M. Inhibitory effect of IL-8 on insulin action in human adipocytes via MAP kinase pathway. *J. Inflamm.* **2009**, *6*, 25. [CrossRef] [PubMed]
43. Koch, A.E.; Polverini, P.J.; Kunkel, S.L.; Harlow, L.A.; DiPietro, L.A.; Elner, V.M.; Elner, S.G.; Strieter, R.M. Interleukin-8 as a macrophage-derived mediator of angiogenesis. *Science* **1992**, *258*, 1798–1801. [CrossRef] [PubMed]
44. Baggiolini, M.; Clark-Lewis, I. Interleukin-8, a chemotactic and inflammatory cytokine. *FEBS Lett.* **1992**, *307*, 97–101. [CrossRef]
45. Kim, C.S.; Park, H.S.; Kawada, T.; Kim, J.H.; Lim, D.; Hubbard, N.E.; Kwon, B.S.; Erickson, K.L.; Yu, R. Circulating levels of MCP-1 and IL-8 are elevated in human obese subjects and associated with obesity-related parameters. *Int. J. Obes.* **2006**, *30*, 1347–1355. [CrossRef]
46. Esposito, K.; Pontillo, A.; Di Palo, C.; Giugliano, G.; Masella, M.; Marfella, R.; Giugliano, D. Effect of Weight Loss and Lifestyle Changes on Vascular Inflammatory Markers in Obese Women: A Randomized Trial. *J. Am. Med. Assoc.* **2003**, *289*, 1799–1804. [CrossRef] [PubMed]
47. Bruun, J.M.; Stallknecht, B.; Helge, J.W.; Richelsen, B. Interleukin-18 in plasma and adipose tissue: Effects of obesity, insulin resistance, and weight loss. *Eur. J. Endocrinol.* **2007**, *157*, 465–471. [CrossRef]
48. Hung, J.; McQuillan, B.M.; Chapman, C.M.L.; Thompson, P.L.; Beilby, J.P. Elevated interleukin-18 levels are associated with the metabolic syndrome independent of obesity and insulin resistance. *Arterioscler. Thromb. Vasc. Biol.* **2005**, *25*, 1268–1273. [CrossRef] [PubMed]
49. Gschwandtner, M.; Derler, R.; Midwood, K.S. More Than Just Attractive: How CCL2 Influences Myeloid Cell Behavior Beyond Chemotaxis. *Front. Immunol.* **2019**, *10*, 2759. [CrossRef]
50. Fasshauer, M.; Blüher, M. Adipokines in health and disease. *Trends Pharmacol. Sci.* **2015**, *36*, 461–470. [CrossRef]
51. Dahlman, I.; Kaaman, M.; Olsson, T.; Tan, G.D.; Bickerton, A.S.T.; Wåhlén, K.; Andersson, J.; Nordström, E.A.; Blomqvist, L.; Sjögren, A.; et al. A unique role of monocyte chemoattractant protein 1 among chemokines in adipose tissue of obese subjects. *J. Clin. Endocrinol. Metab.* **2005**, *90*, 5834–5840. [CrossRef] [PubMed]
52. Arendt, L.M.; McCready, J.; Keller, P.J.; Baker, D.D.; Naber, S.P.; Seewaldt, V.; Kuperwasser, C. Obesity promotes breast cancer by CCL2-mediated macrophage recruitment and angiogenesis. *Cancer Res.* **2013**, *73*, 6080–6093. [CrossRef] [PubMed]
53. Fain, J.N.; Tichansky, D.S.; Madan, A.K. Transforming Growth Factor β1 release by human adipose tissue is enhanced in obesity. *Metabolism* **2005**, *54*, 1546–1551. [CrossRef]
54. Kulkarni, A.B.; Huh, C.G.; Becker, D.; Geiser, A.; Lyght, M.; Flanders, K.C.; Roberts, A.B.; Sporn, M.B.; Ward, J.M.; Karlsson, S. Transforming growth factor β1 null mutation in mice causes excessive inflammatory response and early death. *Proc. Natl. Acad. Sci. USA* **1993**, *90*, 770–774. [CrossRef] [PubMed]
55. Proetzel, G.; Pawlowski, S.A.; Wiles, M.V.; Yin, M.; Boivin, G.P.; Howles, P.N.; Ding, J.; Ferguson, M.W.J.; Doetschman, T. Transforming growth factor–β3 is required for secondary palate fusion. *Nat. Genet.* **1995**, *11*, 409–414. [CrossRef]
56. Sanford, L.P.; Ormsby, I.; Gittenberger-de Groot, A.C.; Sariola, H.; Friedman, R.; Boivin, G.P.; Lou Cardell, E.; Doetschman, T. TGFβ2 knockout mice have multiple developmental defects that are non-overlapping with other TGFβ knockout phenotypes. *Development* **1997**, *124*, 2659–2670. [CrossRef]
57. Li, M.O.; Wan, Y.Y.; Sanjabi, S.; Robertson, A.K.L.; Flavell, R.A. Transforming growth factor-β regulation of immune responses. *Annu. Rev. Immunol.* **2006**, *24*, 99–146. [CrossRef]
58. Ouchi, N.; Parker, J.L.; Lugus, J.J.; Walsh, K. Adipokines in inflammation and metabolic disease. *Nat. Rev. Immunol.* **2011**, *11*, 85–97. [CrossRef]
59. O'Farrell, A.M.; Liu, Y.; Moore, K.W.; Mui, A.L.F. IL-10 inhibits macrophage activation and proliferation by distinct signaling mechanisms: Evidence for Stat3-dependent and -independent pathways. *EMBO J.* **1998**, *17*, 1006–1018. [CrossRef]
60. Charles, B.A.; Doumatey, A.; Huang, H.; Zhou, J.; Chen, G.; Shriner, D.; Adeyemo, A.; Rotimi, C.N. The roles of IL-6, IL-10, and IL-1RA in obesity and insulin resistance in African-Americans. *J. Clin. Endocrinol. Metab.* **2011**, *96*, E2018–E2022. [CrossRef]
61. McLeod, J.J.A.; Baker, B.; Ryan, J.J. Mast cell production and response to IL-4 and IL-13. *Cytokine* **2015**, *75*, 57–61. [CrossRef]

62. Van Dyken, S.J.; Locksley, R.M. Interleukin-4-and interleukin-13-mediated alternatively activated macrophages: Roles in homeostasis and disease. *Annu. Rev. Immunol.* **2013**, *31*, 317–343. [CrossRef]
63. Benoit, M.; Desnues, B.; Mege, J.-L. Macrophage Polarization in Bacterial Infections. *J. Immunol.* **2008**, *181*, 3733–3739. [CrossRef]
64. Dandona, P.; Ghanim, H.; Monte, S.V.; Caruana, J.A.; Green, K.; Abuaysheh, S.; Lohano, T.; Schentag, J.; Dhindsa, S.; Chaudhuri, A. Increase in the mediators of asthma in obesity and obesity with type 2 diabetes: Reduction with weight loss. *Obesity* **2014**, *22*, 356–362. [CrossRef]
65. Schmidt, F.M.; Weschenfelder, J.; Sander, C.; Minkwitz, J.; Thormann, J.; Chittka, T.; Mergl, R.; Kirkby, K.C.; Faßhauer, M.; Stumvoll, M.; et al. Inflammatory cytokines in general and central obesity and modulating effects of physical Activity. *PLoS ONE* **2015**, *10*, e0121971. [CrossRef]
66. Lizcano, F.; Vargas, D.; Gómez, Á.; Torrado, A. Human ADMC-derived adipocyte thermogenic capacity is regulated by IL-4 receptor. *Stem Cells Int.* **2017**, *2017*, 2767916. [CrossRef]
67. Tsao, C.H.; Shiau, M.Y.; Chuang, P.H.; Chang, Y.H.; Hwang, J. Interleukin-4 regulates lipid metabolism by inhibiting adipogenesis and promoting lipolysis. *J. Lipid Res.* **2014**, *55*, 385–397. [CrossRef]
68. Shiau, M.Y.; Chuang, P.H.; Yang, C.P.; Hsiao, C.W.; Chang, S.W.; Chang, K.Y.; Liu, T.M.; Chen, H.W.; Chuang, C.C.; Yuan, S.Y.; et al. Mechanism of Interleukin-4 Reducing Lipid Deposit by Regulating Hormone-Sensitive Lipase. *Sci. Rep.* **2019**, *9*, 11974. [CrossRef] [PubMed]
69. Frederich, R.C.; Hamann, A.; Anderson, S.; Löllmann, B.; Lowell, B.B.; Flier, J.S. Leptin levels reflect body lipid content in mice: Evidence for diet-induced resistance to leptin action. *Nat. Med.* **1995**, *1*, 1311–1314. [CrossRef] [PubMed]
70. Maffei, M.; Halaas, J.; Ravussin, E.; Pratley, R.E.; Lee, G.H.; Zhang, Y.; Fei, H.; Kim, S.; Lallone, R.; Ranganathan, S.; et al. Leptin levels in human and rodent: Measurement of plasma leptin and ob RNA in obese and weight-reduced subjects. *Nat. Med.* **1995**, *1*, 1155–1161. [CrossRef] [PubMed]
71. Thaler, J.P.; Schwartz, M.W. Minireview: Inflammation and obesity pathogenesis: The hypothalamus heats up. *Endocrinology* **2010**, *151*, 4109–4115. [CrossRef] [PubMed]
72. Vendrell, J.; Broch, M.; Vilarrasa, N.; Molina, A.; Gómez, J.M.; Gutiérrez, C.; Simón, I.; Soler, J.; Richart, C. Resistin, adiponectin, ghrelin, leptin, and proinflammatory cytokines: Relationships in obesity. *Obes. Res.* **2004**, *12*, 962–971. [CrossRef] [PubMed]
73. Huang, X.; Yang, Z. Resistin's, obesity and insulin resistance: The continuing disconnect between rodents and humans. *J. Endocrinol. Investig.* **2016**, *39*, 607–615. [CrossRef] [PubMed]
74. Silha, J.V.; Krsek, M.; Skrha, J.V.; Sucharda, P.; Nyomba, B.L.G.; Murphy, L.J. Plasma resistin, adiponectin and leptin levels in lean and obese subjects: Correlations with insulin resistence. *Eur. J. Endocrinol.* **2003**, *149*, 331–335. [CrossRef] [PubMed]
75. Rajala, M.W.; Qi, Y.; Patel, H.R.; Takahashi, N.; Banerjee, R.; Pajvani, U.B.; Sinha, M.K.; Gingerich, R.L.; Scherer, P.E.; Ahima, R.S. Regulation of resistin expression and circulating levels in obesity, diabetes, and fasting. *Diabetes* **2004**, *53*, 1671–1679. [CrossRef]
76. Smith, S.R.; Bai, F.; Charbonneau, C.; Janderová, L.; Argyropoulos, G. A promoter genotype and oxidative stress potentially link resistin to human insulin resistance. *Diabetes* **2003**, *52*, 1611–1618. [CrossRef]
77. Savage, D.B.; Sewter, C.P.; Klenk, E.S.; Segal, D.G.; Vidal-Puig, A.; Considine, R.V.; O'Rahilly, S. Resistin/Fizz3 Expression in Relation to Obesity and Peroxisome Proliferator Activated Receptor-γ Action in Humans. *Diabetes* **2001**, *50*, 2199–2202. [CrossRef]
78. Way, J.M.; Görgün, C.Z.; Tong, Q.; Uysal, K.T.; Brown, K.K.; Harrington, W.W.; Oliver, W.R.; Willson, T.M.; Kliewer, S.A.; Hotamisligil, G.S. Adipose Tissue Resistin Expression is Severely Suppressed in Obesity and Stimulated by Peroxisome Proliferator-activated Receptor γ Agonists. *J. Biol. Chem.* **2001**, *276*, 25651–25653. [CrossRef] [PubMed]
79. Heilbronn, L.K.; Rood, J.; Janderova, L.; Albu, J.B.; Kelley, D.E.; Ravussin, E.; Smith, S.R. Relationship between serum resistin concentrations and insulin resistance in nonobese, obese, and obese diabetic subjects. *J. Clin. Endocrinol. Metab.* **2004**, *89*, 1844–1848. [CrossRef]
80. Chang, Y.H.; Chang, D.M.; Lin, K.C.; Shin, S.J.; Lee, Y.J. Visfatin in overweight/obesity, type 2 diabetes mellitus, insulin resistance, metabolic syndrome and cardiovascular diseases: A meta-analysis and systemic review. *Diabetes. Metab. Res. Rev.* **2011**, *27*, 515–527. [CrossRef]
81. Fantuzzi, G. Adiponectin and inflammation: Consensus and controversy. *J. Allergy Clin. Immunol.* **2008**, *121*, 326–330. [CrossRef]
82. Frühbeck, G.; Catalán, V.; Rodríguez, A.; Gómez-Ambrosi, J. Adiponectin-leptin ratio: A promising index to estimate adipose tissue dysfunction. Relation with obesity-associated cardiometabolic risk. *Adipocyte* **2018**, *7*, 57–62. [CrossRef]
83. Frühbeck, G.; Catalán, V.; Rodríguez, A.; Ramírez, B.; Becerril, S.; Salvador, J.; Colina, I.; Gómez-Ambrosi, J. Adiponectin-leptin ratio is a functional biomarker of adipose tissue inflammation. *Nutrients* **2019**, *11*, 454. [CrossRef]
84. Yang, R.Z.; Lee, M.J.; Hu, H.; Pray, J.; Bin Wu, H.; Hansen, B.C.; Shuldiner, A.R.; Fried, S.K.; McLenithan, J.C.; Gong, D.W. Identification of omentin as a novel depot-specific adipokine in human adipose tissue: Possible role in modulating insulin action. *Am. J. Physiol. Endocrinol. Metab.* **2006**, *290*, E1253–E1261. [CrossRef] [PubMed]
85. Tan, B.K.; Adya, R.; Randeva, H.S. Omentin: A Novel Link between Inflammation, Diabesity, and Cardiovascular Disease. *Trends Cardiovasc. Med.* **2010**, *20*, 143–148. [CrossRef] [PubMed]
86. De Souza Batista, C.M.; Yang, R.Z.; Lee, M.J.; Glynn, N.M.; Yu, D.Z.; Pray, J.; Ndubuizu, K.; Patil, S.; Schwartz, A.; Kligman, M.; et al. Omentin plasma levels and gene expression are decreased in obesity. *Diabetes* **2007**, *56*, 1655–1661. [CrossRef] [PubMed]
87. Buechler, C.; Krautbauer, S.; Eisinger, K. Adipose tissue fibrosis. *World J. Diabetes* **2015**, *6*, 548–553. [CrossRef]
88. Sun, K.; Tordjman, J.; Clément, K.; Scherer, P.E. Fibrosis and Adipose Tissue Dysfunction. *Cell Metab.* **2013**, *18*, 470–477. [CrossRef]

89. Debari, M.K.; Abbott, R.D. Adipose tissue fibrosis: Mechanisms, models, and importance. *Int. J. Mol. Sci.* **2020**, *21*, 6030. [CrossRef]
90. Divoux, A.; Tordjman, J.; Lacasa, D.; Veyrie, N.; Hugol, D.; Aissat, A.; Basdevant, A.; Guerre-Millo, M.; Poitou, C.; Zucker, J.-D.; et al. Fibrosis in human adipose tissue: Composition, distribution, and link with lipid metabolism and fat mass loss. *Diabetes* **2010**, *59*, 2817–2825. [CrossRef] [PubMed]
91. Abdennour, M.; Reggio, S.; Le Naour, G.; Liu, Y.; Poitou, C.; Aron-Wisnewsky, J.; Charlotte, F.; Bouillot, J.L.; Torcivia, A.; Sasso, M.; et al. Association of adipose tissue and liver fibrosis with tissue stiffness in morbid obesity: Links with diabetes and BMI loss after gastric bypass. *J. Clin. Endocrinol. Metab.* **2014**, *99*, 898–907. [CrossRef]
92. Bel Lassen, P.; Charlotte, F.; Liu, Y.; Bedossa, P.; Le Naour, G.; Tordjman, J.; Poitou, C.; Bouillot, J.-L.; Genser, L.; Zucker, J.-D.; et al. The FAT Score, a Fibrosis Score of Adipose Tissue: Predicting Weight-Loss Outcome after Gastric Bypass. *J. Clin. Endocrinol. Metab.* **2017**, *102*, 2443–2453. [CrossRef]
93. Marcelin, G.; Silveira, A.L.M.; Martins, L.B.; Ferreira, A.V.M.; Clément, K. Deciphering the cellular interplays underlying obesityinduced adipose tissue fibrosis. *J. Clin. Investig.* **2019**, *129*, 4032–4040. [CrossRef] [PubMed]
94. Spencer, M.; Unal, R.; Zhu, B.; Rasouli, N.; McGehee, R.E.; Peterson, C.A.; Kern, P.A. Adipose tissue extracellular matrix and vascular abnormalities in obesity and insulin resistance. *J. Clin. Endocrinol. Metab.* **2011**, *96*, E1990–E1998. [CrossRef] [PubMed]
95. Lin, D.; Chun, T.-H.; Kang, L. Adipose extracellular matrix remodelling in obesity and insulin resistance. *Biochem. Pharmacol.* **2016**, *119*, 8–16. [CrossRef]
96. Lackey, D.E.; Burk, D.H.; Ali, M.R.; Mostaedi, R.; Smith, W.H.; Park, J.; Scherer, P.E.; Seay, S.A.; McCoin, C.S.; Bonaldo, P.; et al. Contributions of adipose tissue architectural and tensile properties toward defining healthy and unhealthy obesity. *Am. J. Physiol. Endocrinol. Metab.* **2014**, *306*, E233–E246. [CrossRef] [PubMed]
97. McCulloch, L.J.; Rawling, T.J.; Sjöholm, K.; Franck, N.; Dankel, S.N.; Price, E.J.; Knight, B.; Liversedge, N.H.; Mellgren, G.; Nystrom, F.; et al. COL6A3 is regulated by leptin in human adipose tissue and reduced in obesity. *Endocrinology* **2015**, *156*, 134–146. [CrossRef] [PubMed]
98. Sun, K.; Park, J.; Gupta, O.T.; Holland, W.L.; Auerbach, P.; Zhang, N.; Goncalves Marangoni, R.; Nicoloro, S.M.; Czech, M.P.; Varga, J.; et al. Endotrophin triggers adipose tissue fibrosis and metabolic dysfunction. *Nat. Commun.* **2014**, *5*, 3485. [CrossRef]
99. Lawler, H.M.; Underkofler, C.M.; Kern, P.A.; Erickson, C.; Bredbeck, B.; Rasouli, N. Adipose Tissue Hypoxia, Inflammation, and Fibrosis in Obese Insulin-Sensitive and Obese Insulin-Resistant Subjects. *J. Clin. Endocrinol. Metab.* **2016**, *101*, 1422–1428. [CrossRef]
100. Baker, N.A.; Muir, L.A.; Washabaugh, A.R.; Neeley, C.K.; Chen, S.Y.P.; Flesher, C.G.; Vorwald, J.; Finks, J.F.; Ghaferi, A.A.; Mulholland, M.W.; et al. Diabetes-specific regulation of adipocyte metabolism by the adipose tissue extracellular matrix. *J. Clin. Endocrinol. Metab.* **2017**, *102*, 1032–1043. [CrossRef]
101. Camastra, S.; Gastaldelli, A.; Mari, A.; Bonuccelli, S.; Scartabelli, G.; Frascerra, S.; Baldi, S.; Nannipieri, M.; Rebelos, E.; Anselmino, M.; et al. Early and longer term effects of gastric bypass surgery on tissue-specific insulin sensitivity and beta cell function in morbidly obese patients with and without type 2 diabetes. *Diabetologia* **2011**, *54*, 2093–2102. [CrossRef] [PubMed]
102. Curry, T.B.; Roberts, S.K.; Basu, R.; Basu, A.; Schroeder, D.; Joyner, M.J.; Miles, J.M. Gastric bypass surgery is associated with near-normal insulin suppression of lipolysis in nondiabetic individuals. *Am. J. Physiol. Metab.* **2011**, *300*, E746–E751. [CrossRef] [PubMed]
103. Evans, B.A.; Merlin, J.; Bengtsson, T.; Hutchinson, D.S. Adrenoceptors in white, brown, and brite adipocytes. *Br. J. Pharmacol.* **2019**, *176*, 2416–2432. [CrossRef]
104. Duncan, R.E.; Ahmadian, M.; Jaworski, K.; Sarkadi-Nagy, E.; Sul, H.S. Regulation of lipolysis in adipocytes. *Annu. Rev. Nutr.* **2007**, *27*, 79–101. [CrossRef]
105. Frikke-Schmidt, H.; O'Rourke, R.W.; Lumeng, C.N.; Sandoval, D.A.; Seeley, R.J. Does bariatric surgery improve adipose tissue function? *Obes. Rev.* **2016**, *17*, 795–809. [CrossRef]
106. Kaartinen, J.M.; LaNoue, K.F.; Martin, L.F.; Vikman, H.L.; Ohisalo, J.J. β-Adrenergic responsiveness of adenylate cyclase in human adipocyte plasma membranes in obesity and after massive weight reduction. *Metabolism* **1995**, *44*, 1288–1292. [CrossRef]
107. Reynisdottir, S.; Langin, D.; Carlstrom, K.; Holm, C.; Rossner, S.; Arner, P. Effects of weight reduction on the regulation of lipolysis in adipocytes of women with upper-body obesity. *Clin. Sci.* **1995**, *89*, 421–429. [CrossRef]
108. Mauriège, P.; Imbeault, P.; Langin, D.; Lacaille, M.; Alméras, N.; Tremblay, A.; Després, J.P. Regional and gender variations in adipose tissue lipolysis in response to weight loss. *J. Lipid Res.* **1999**, *40*, 1559–1571. [CrossRef]
109. Castellot, J.J.; Karnovsky, M.J.; Spiegelman, B.M. Differentiation-dependent stimulation of neovascularization and endothelial cell chemotaxis by 3T3 adipocytes. *Proc. Natl. Acad. Sci. USA* **1982**, *79*, 5597–5601. [CrossRef]
110. Montesano, R.; Mouron, P.; Orci, L. Vascular outgrowths from tissue explants embedded in fibrin or collagen gels: A simple in vitro model of angiogenesis. *Cell Biol. Int. Rep.* **1985**, *9*, 869–875. [CrossRef]
111. Varzaneh, F.E.; Shillabeer, G.; Wong, K.L.; Lau, D.C.W. Extracellular matrix components secreted by microvascular endothelial cells stimulate preadipocyte differentiation in vitro. *Metabolism* **1994**, *43*, 906–912. [CrossRef]
112. Fukumura, D.; Ushiyama, A.; Duda, D.G.; Xu, L.; Tam, J.; Krishna, V.; Chatterjee, K.; Garkavtsev, I.; Jain, R.K. Paracrine regulation of angiogenesis and adipocyte differentiation during in vivo adipogenesis. *Circ. Res.* **2003**, *93*, e88–e97. [CrossRef] [PubMed]

113. Zhang, Q.X.; Magovern, C.J.; Mack, C.A.; Budenbender, K.T.; Wilson, K.; Rosengart, T.K. Vascular endothelial growth factor is the major angiogenic factor in omentum: Mechanism of the omentum-mediated angiogenesis. *J. Surg. Res.* **1997**, *67*, 147–154. [CrossRef] [PubMed]
114. Thomas, M.; Augustin, H.G. The role of the angiopoietins in vascular morphogenesis. *Angiogenesis* **2009**, *12*, 125–137. [CrossRef] [PubMed]
115. An, Y.A.; Sun, K.; Joffin, N.; Zhang, F.; Deng, Y.; Donzé, O.; Kusminski, C.M.; Scherer, P.E. Angiopoietin-2 in white adipose tissue improves metabolic homeostasis through enhanced angiogenesis. *eLife* **2017**, *6*, e24071. [CrossRef]
116. Montoro, J.I.M.; García, J.C.F.; Vega, M.M.; Fuentes, M.D.; Tinahones, F.J. PECAM-1 levels are increased in morbidly obese young men. *Atherosclerosis* **2020**, *315*, e59–e60. [CrossRef]
117. Kanasaki, K.; Kawakita, E.; Koya, D. Relevance of autophagy induction by gastrointestinal hormones: Focus on the incretin-based drug target and glucagon. *Front. Pharmacol.* **2019**, *10*, 476. [CrossRef]
118. Ueno, T.; Komatsu, M. Autophagy in the liver: Functions in health and disease. *Nat. Rev. Gastroenterol. Hepatol.* **2017**, *14*, 170–184. [CrossRef]
119. Soussi, H.; Reggio, S.; Alili, R.; Prado, C.; Mutel, S.; Pini, M.; Rouault, C.; Clément, K.; Dugail, I. DAPK2 Downregulation Associates With Attenuated Adipocyte Autophagic Clearance in Human Obesity. *Diabetes* **2015**, *64*, 3452–3463. [CrossRef] [PubMed]
120. Kovsan, J.; Blüher, M.; Tarnovscki, T.; Klöting, N.; Kirshtein, B.; Madar, L.; Shai, I.; Golan, R.; Harman-Boehm, I.; Schön, M.R.; et al. Altered autophagy in human adipose tissues in obesity. *J. Clin. Endocrinol. Metab.* **2011**, *96*, E268–E277. [CrossRef]
121. Jansen, H.J.; Van Essen, P.; Koenen, T.; Joosten, L.A.B.; Netea, M.G.; Tack, C.J.; Stienstra, R. Autophagy activity is up-regulated in adipose tissue of obese individuals and modulates proinflammatory cytokine expression. *Endocrinology* **2012**, *153*, 5866–5874. [CrossRef]
122. Nuñez, C.E.; Rodrigues, V.S.; Gomes, F.S.; De Moura, R.F.; Victorio, S.C.; Bombassaro, B.; Chaim, E.A.; Pareja, J.C.; Geloneze, B.; Velloso, L.A.; et al. Defective regulation of adipose tissue autophagy in obesity. *Int. J. Obes.* **2013**, *37*, 1473–1480. [CrossRef] [PubMed]
123. Öst, A.; Svensson, K.; Ruishalme, I.; Brännmark, C.; Franck, N.; Krook, H.; Sandström, P.; Kjolhede, P.; Strålfors, P. Attenuated mTOR signaling and enhanced autophagy in adipocytes from obese patients with type 2 diabetes. *Mol. Med.* **2010**, *16*, 235–246. [CrossRef] [PubMed]
124. Rodríguez, A.; Gómez-Ambrosi, J.; Catalán, V.; Rotellar, F.; Valentí, V.; Silva, C.; Mugueta, C.; Pulido, M.R.; Vázquez, R.; Salvador, J.; et al. The ghrelin O-Acyltransferase-Ghrelin system reduces TNF-α-Induced apoptosis and autophagy in human visceral adipocytes. *Diabetologia* **2012**, *55*, 3038–3050. [CrossRef]
125. Mahawar, K.K. Defining Short-term, Medium-term, Long-term, and Very Long-term Follow-up after Bariatric Surgery. *Obes. Surg.* **2018**, *28*, 1425–1426. [CrossRef]
126. Meyer-Gerspach, A.C.; Peterli, R.; Moor, M.; Madörin, P.; Schötzau, A.; Nabers, D.; Borgwardt, S.; Beglinger, C.; Bieri, O.; Wölnerhanssen, B.K. Quantification of Liver, Subcutaneous, and Visceral Adipose Tissues by MRI Before and After Bariatric Surgery. *Obes. Surg.* **2019**, *29*, 2795–2805. [CrossRef] [PubMed]
127. Keidar, A.; Appelbaum, L.; Schweiger, C.; Hershkop, K.; Matot, I.; Constantini, N.; Sosna, J.; Weiss, R. Baseline Abdominal Lipid Partitioning Is Associated with the Metabolic Response to Bariatric Surgery. *Obes. Surg.* **2014**, *24*, 1709–1716. [CrossRef]
128. Umemura, A.; Sasaki, A.; Nitta, H.; Otsuka, K.; Suto, T.; Wakabayashi, G. Effects of changes in adipocyte hormones and visceral adipose tissue and the reduction of obesity-related comorbidities after laparoscopic sleeve gastrectomy in Japanese patients with severe obesity. *Endocr. J.* **2014**, *61*, 381–391. [CrossRef]
129. Dadson, P.; Ferrannini, E.; Landini, L.; Hannukainen, J.C.; Kalliokoski, K.K.; Vaittinen, M.; Honka, H.; Karlsson, H.K.; Tuulari, J.J.; Soinio, M.; et al. Fatty acid uptake and blood flow in adipose tissue compartments of morbidly obese subjects with or without type 2 diabetes: Effects of bariatric surgery. *Am. J. Physiol. Endocrinol. Metab.* **2017**, *313*, E175–E182. [CrossRef]
130. Kim, M.K.; Jang, E.-H.; Hong, O.-K.; Chun, H.-J.; Yoo, S.-J.; Baek, K.-H.; Kim, W.; Kim, E.K.; Song, K.-H.; Kwon, H.-S. Changes in Serum Levels of Bone Morphogenic Protein 4 and Inflammatory Cytokines after Bariatric Surgery in Severely Obese Korean Patients with Type 2 Diabetes. *Int. J. Endocrinol.* **2013**, *2013*, 681205. [CrossRef]
131. Kim, M.K.; Kim, W.; Kwon, H.-S.; Baek, K.-H.; Kim, E.K.; Song, K.-H. Effects of bariatric surgery on metabolic and nutritional parameters in severely obese Korean patients with type 2 diabetes: A prospective 2-year follow up. *J. Diabetes Investig.* **2014**, *5*, 221–227. [CrossRef] [PubMed]
132. Andersson, D.P.; Hogling, D.E.; Thorell, A.; Toft, E.; Qvisth, V.; Näslund, E.; Thörne, A.; Wirén, M.; Löfgren, P.; Hoffstedt, J.; et al. Changes in subcutaneous fat cell volume and insulin sensitivity after weight loss. *Diabetes Care* **2014**, *37*, 1831–1836. [CrossRef] [PubMed]
133. Hoffstedt, J.; Andersson, D.P.; Hogling, D.E.; Theorell, J.; Näslund, E.; Thorell, A.; Ehrlund, A.; Rydén, M.; Arner, P. Long-term protective changes in adipose tissue after gastric bypass. *Diabetes Care* **2017**, *40*, 77–84. [CrossRef] [PubMed]
134. Lehmann, S.; Linder, N.; Retschlag, U.; Schaudinn, A.; Stange, R.; Garnov, N.; Dietrich, A.; Oberbach, A.; Kahn, T.; Busse, H. MRI assessment of changes in adipose tissue parameters after bariatric surgery. *PLoS ONE* **2018**, *13*, e0206735. [CrossRef]
135. Favre, L.; Marino, L.; Roth, A.; Acierno, J.; Hans, D.; Demartines, N.; Pitteloud, N.; Suter, M.; Collet, T.-H. The Reduction of Visceral Adipose Tissue after Roux-en-Y Gastric Bypass Is more Pronounced in Patients with Impaired Glucose Metabolism. *Obes. Surg.* **2018**, *28*, 4006–4013. [CrossRef] [PubMed]

136. Cotillard, A.; Poitou, C.; Torcivia, A.; Bouillot, J.-L.; Dietrich, A.; Klöting, N.; Grégoire, C.; Lolmede, K.; Blüher, M.; Clément, K. Adipocyte Size Threshold Matters: Link with Risk of Type 2 Diabetes and Improved Insulin Resistance After Gastric Bypass. *J. Clin. Endocrinol. Metab.* **2014**, *99*, E1466–E1470. [CrossRef]
137. Hansen, M.; Lund, M.T.; Gregers, E.; Kraunsøe, R.; Van Hall, G.; Helge, J.W.; Dela, F. Adipose tissue mitochondrial respiration and lipolysis before and after a weight loss by diet and RYGB. *Obesity* **2015**, *23*, 2022–2029. [CrossRef]
138. Torriani, M.; Oliveira, A.L.; Azevedo, D.C.; Bredella, M.A.; Yu, E.W. Effects of Roux-en-Y Gastric Bypass Surgery on Visceral and Subcutaneous Fat Density by Computed Tomography. *Obes. Surg.* **2015**, *25*, 381–385. [CrossRef]
139. Illán-Gómez, F.; Gonzálvez-Ortega, M.; Orea-Soler, I.; Alcaraz-Tafalla, M.S.; Aragón-Alonso, A.; Pascual-Díaz, M.; Pérez-Paredes, M.; Lozano-Almela, M.L. Obesity and inflammation: Change in adiponectin, C-reactive protein, tumour necrosis factor-alpha and interleukin-6 after bariatric surgery. *Obes. Surg.* **2012**, *22*, 950–955. [CrossRef]
140. Lips, M.A.; van Klinken, J.B.; Pijl, H.; Janssen, I.; Willems van Dijk, K.; Koning, F.; van Harmelen, V. Weight loss induced by very low calorie diet is associated with a more beneficial systemic inflammatory profile than by Roux-en-Y gastric bypass. *Metabolism* **2016**, *65*, 1614–1620. [CrossRef]
141. Vilarrasa, N.; Vendrell, J.; Sánchez-Santos, R.; Broch, M.; Megia, A.; Masdevall, C.; Gomez, N.; Soler, J.; Pujol, J.; Bettónica, C.; et al. Effect of weight loss induced by gastric bypass on proinflammatory interleukin-18, soluble tumour necrosis factor-α receptors, C-reactive protein and adiponectin in morbidly obese patients. *Clin. Endocrinol.* **2007**, *67*, 679–686. [CrossRef]
142. Schmatz, R.; Bitencourt, M.R.; Patias, L.D.; Beck, M.; Alvarez, G.D.; Zanini, D.; Gutierres, J.M.; Diehl, L.N.; Pereira, L.B.; Leal, C.A.; et al. Evaluation of the biochemical, inflammatory and oxidative profile of obese patients given clinical treatment and bariatric surgery. *Clin. Chim. Acta* **2017**, *465*, 72–79. [CrossRef]
143. Viana, E.C.; Araujo-Dasilio, K.L.; Miguel, G.P.S.; Bressan, J.; Lemos, E.M.; Moyses, M.R.; De Abreu, G.R.; De Azevedo, J.L.M.C.; Carvalho, P.S.; Passos-Bueno, M.R.S.; et al. Gastric bypass and sleeve gastrectomy: The same impact on IL-6 and TNF-α. Prospective clinical trial. *Obes. Surg.* **2013**, *23*, 1252–1261. [CrossRef] [PubMed]
144. Nestvold, T.K.; Nielsen, E.W.; Ludviksen, J.K.; Fure, H.; Landsem, A.; Lappegård, K.T. Lifestyle changes followed by bariatric surgery lower inflammatory markers and the cardiovascular risk factors C3 and C4. *Metab. Syndr. Relat. Disord.* **2015**, *13*, 29–35. [CrossRef] [PubMed]
145. Farias, G.; Netto, B.D.M.; Boritza, K.; Bettini, S.C.; Vilela, R.M.; Dâmaso, A.R. Impact of Weight Loss on Inflammation State and Endothelial Markers Among Individuals with Extreme Obesity After Gastric Bypass Surgery: A 2-Year Follow-up Study. *Obes. Surg.* **2020**, *30*, 1881–1890. [CrossRef]
146. Sdralis, E.; Argentou, M.; Mead, N.; Kehagias, I.; Alexandridis, T.; Kalfarentzos, F. A prospective randomized study comparing patients with morbid obesity submitted to sleeve gastrectomy with or without omentectomy. *Obes. Surg.* **2013**, *23*, 965–971. [CrossRef]
147. Dillard, T.H.; Purnell, J.Q.; Smith, M.D.; Raum, W.; Hong, D.; Laut, J.; Patterson, E.J. Omentectomy added to Roux-en-Y gastric bypass surgery: A randomized, controlled trial. *Surg. Obes. Relat. Dis.* **2013**, *9*, 269–275. [CrossRef]
148. Pardina, E.; Ferrer, R.; Baena-Fustegueras, J.A.; Rivero, J.; Lecube, A.; Fort, J.M.; Vargas, V.; Catalán, R.; Peinado-Onsurbe, J. Only C-reactive protein, but not TNF-α or IL6, reflects the improvement in inflammation after bariatric surgery. *Obes. Surg.* **2012**, *22*, 131–139. [CrossRef] [PubMed]
149. Miller, G.D.; Nicklas, B.J.; Fernandez, A. Serial changes in inflammatory biomarkers after Roux-en-Y gastric bypass surgery. *Surg. Obes. Relat. Dis.* **2011**, *7*, 618–624. [CrossRef] [PubMed]
150. Lima, M.M.O.; Pareja, J.C.; Alegre, S.M.; Geloneze, S.R.; Kahn, S.E.; Astiarraga, B.D.; Chaim, É.A.; Baracat, J.; Geloneze, B. Visceral fat resection in humans: Effect on insulin sensitivity, beta-cell function, adipokines, and inflammatory markers. *Obesity* **2013**, *21*, E182–E189. [CrossRef]
151. Bachmayer, C.; Lammert, A.; Hasenberg, T.; Hammes, H.P. Healthy obese and post bariatric patients—Metabolic and vascular patterns. *Exp. Clin. Endocrinol. Diabetes* **2013**, *121*, 483–487. [CrossRef]
152. Salman, M.A.; Abdallah, A.; Mikhail, H.M.S.; Abdelsalam, A.; Ibrahim, A.H.; Sultan, A.A.E.A.; El-ghobary, M.; Ismail, A.A.M.; Abouelregal, T.E.; Omar, M.G.; et al. Long-term Impact of Mini-Gastric Bypass on Inflammatory Cytokines in Cohort of Morbidly Obese Patients: A Prospective Study. *Obes. Surg.* **2020**, *30*, 2338–2344. [CrossRef] [PubMed]
153. Pérez-Romero, N.; Serra, A.; Granada, M.L.; Rull, M.; Alastrué, A.; Navarro-Díaz, M.; Romero, R.; Fernández-Llamazares, J. Effects of two variants of Roux-en-Y gastric bypass on metabolism behaviour: Focus on plasma ghrelin concentrations over a 2-year follow-up. *Obes. Surg.* **2010**, *20*, 600–609. [CrossRef]
154. Manco, M.; Fernandez-Real, J.M.; Equitani, F.; Vendrell, J.; Mora, M.E.V.; Nanni, G.; Tondolo, V.; Calvani, M.; Ricart, W.; Castagneto, M.; et al. Effect of massive weight loss on inflammatory adipocytokines and the innate immune system in morbidly obese women. *J. Clin. Endocrinol. Metab.* **2007**, *92*, 483–490. [CrossRef]
155. Jürets, A.; Itariu, B.K.; Keindl, M.; Prager, G.; Langer, F.; Grablowitz, V.; Zeyda, M.; Stulnig, T.M. Upregulated TNF Expression 1 Year After Bariatric Surgery Reflects a Cachexia-Like State in Subcutaneous Adipose Tissue. *Obes. Surg.* **2017**, *27*, 1514–1523. [CrossRef] [PubMed]
156. Lindegaard, K.K.; Jorgensen, N.B.; Just, R.; Heegaard, P.M.; Madsbad, S. Effects of Roux-en-Y gastric bypass on fasting and postprandial inflammation-related parameters in obese subjects with normal glucose tolerance and in obese subjects with type 2 diabetes. *Diabetol. Metab. Syndr.* **2015**, *7*, 12. [CrossRef] [PubMed]

157. Sajoux, I.; Lorenzo, P.M.; Gomez-Arbelaez, D.; Zulet, M.A.; Abete, I.; Castro, A.I.; Baltar, J.; Portillo, M.P.; Tinahones, F.J.; Martinez, J.A.; et al. Effect of a very-low-calorie ketogenic diet on circulating myokine levels compared with the effect of bariatric surgery or a low-calorie diet in patients with obesity. *Nutrients* **2019**, *11*, 2368. [CrossRef]
158. Marantos, G.; Daskalakis, M.; Karkavitsas, N.; Matalliotakis, I.; Papadakis, J.A.; Melissas, J. Changes in metabolic profile and adipoinsular axis in morbidly obese premenopausal females treated with restrictive bariatric surgery. *World J. Surg.* **2011**, *35*, 2022–2023. [CrossRef]
159. Rega-Kaun, G.; Kaun, C.; Ebenbauer, B.; Jaegersberger, G.; Prager, M.; Wojta, J.; Hohensinner, P.J. Bariatric surgery in morbidly obese individuals affects plasma levels of protein C and thrombomodulin. *J. Thromb. Thrombolysis* **2019**, *47*, 51–56. [CrossRef]
160. Holdstock, C.; Lind, L.; Eden Engstrom, B.; Öhrvall, M.; Sundbom, M.; Larsson, A.; Karlsson, F.A. CRP reduction following gastric bypass surgery is most pronounced in insulin-sensitive subjects. *Int. J. Obes.* **2005**, *29*, 1275–1280. [CrossRef]
161. Li, Y.; Guan, W.; Ma, S.; Lin, S.; Yang, N.; Liu, R.; Liang, H.; Zhou, H. Lipopolysaccharide and inflammatory cytokines levels decreased after sleeve gastrectomy in Chinese adults with obesity. *Endocr. J.* **2019**, *66*, 337–347. [CrossRef] [PubMed]
162. Mallipedhi, A.; Prior, S.L.; Barry, J.D.; Caplin, S.; Baxter, J.N.; Stephens, J.W. Changes in inflammatory markers after sleeve gastrectomy in patients with impaired glucose homeostasis and type 2 diabetes. *Surg. Obes. Relat. Dis.* **2014**, *10*, 1123–1128. [CrossRef] [PubMed]
163. Baltieri, L.; Cazzo, E.; de Souza, A.L.; Alegre, S.M.; de Paula Vieira, R.; Antunes, E.; de Mello, G.C.; Claudio Martins, L.; Chaim, E.A. Influence of weight loss on pulmonary function and levels of adipokines among asthmatic individuals with obesity: One-year follow-up. *Respir. Med.* **2018**, *145*, 48–56. [CrossRef] [PubMed]
164. Dalmas, E.; Rouault, C.; Abdennour, M.; Rovere, C.; Rizkalla, S.; Bar-Hen, A.; Nahon, J.L.; Bouillot, J.L.; Guerre-Millo, M.; Clément, K.; et al. Variations in circulating inflammatory factors are related to changes in calorie and carbohydrate intakes early in the course of surgery-induced weight reduction1-3. *Am. J. Clin. Nutr.* **2011**, *94*, 450–458. [CrossRef] [PubMed]
165. Monte, S.V.; Caruana, J.A.; Ghanim, H.; Sia, C.L.; Korzeniewski, K.; Schentag, J.J.; Dandona, P. Reduction in endotoxemia, oxidative and inflammatory stress, and insulin resistance after Roux-en-Y gastric bypass surgery in patients with morbid obesity and type 2 diabetes mellitus. *Surgery* **2012**, *151*, 587–593. [CrossRef] [PubMed]
166. Fenske, W.K.; Dubb, S.; Bueter, M.; Seyfried, F.; Patel, K.; Tam, F.W.K.; Frankel, A.H.; Le Roux, C.W. Effect of bariatric surgery-induced weight loss on renal and systemic inflammation and blood pressure: A 12-month prospective study. *Surg. Obes. Relat. Dis.* **2013**, *9*, 559–568. [CrossRef]
167. Wolf, R.M.; Jaffe, A.E.; Steele, K.E.; Schweitzer, M.A.; Magnuson, T.H.; Wolfe, A.; Wong, G.W. Cytokine, Chemokine, and Cytokine Receptor Changes Are Associated with Metabolic Improvements after Bariatric Surgery. *J. Clin. Endocrinol. Metab.* **2018**, *104*, 947–956. [CrossRef]
168. Jouan, Y.; Blasco, H.; Bongrani, A.; Couet, C.; Dupont, J.; Maillot, F. Preoperative Chemerin Level Is Predictive of Inflammatory Status 1 Year After Bariatric Surgery. *Obes. Surg.* **2020**, *30*, 3852–3861. [CrossRef]
169. Min, T.; Prior, S.L.; Dunseath, G.; Churm, R.; Barry, J.D.; Stephens, J.W. Temporal Effects of Bariatric Surgery on Adipokines, Inflammation and Oxidative Stress in Subjects with Impaired Glucose Homeostasis at 4 Years of Follow-up. *Obes. Surg.* **2020**, *30*, 1712–1718. [CrossRef]
170. Shimizu, H.; Hatao, F.; Imamura, K.; Takanishi, K.; Tsujino, M. Early Effects of Sleeve Gastrectomy on Obesity-Related Cytokines and Bile Acid Metabolism in Morbidly Obese Japanese Patients. *Obes. Surg.* **2017**, *27*, 3223–3229. [CrossRef]
171. De Luis, D.A.; Terroba, M.C.; Cuellar, L.; Conde, R.; Primo, D.; Aller, R.; Sagrado, M.G.; Izaola, O. Resistin levels in morbid obese patients following the biliopancreatic diversion surgery. *Horm. Metab. Res.* **2011**, *43*, 205–208. [CrossRef]
172. Lapointe, M.; Poirier, P.; Martin, J.; Bastien, M.; Auclair, A.; Cianflone, K. Omentin changes following bariatric surgery and predictive links with biomarkers for risk of cardiovascular disease. *Cardiovasc. Diabetol.* **2014**, *13*, 16. [CrossRef]
173. De Luis, D.A.; García Calvo, S.; Lopez Gomez, J.J.; Izaola, O.; Primo, D.; Pacheco, D.; Aller, R. Omentin-1 changes following biliopancreatic diversion and relationship with cardiovascular risk factors. *Ann. Nutr. Metab.* **2018**, *73*, 106–112. [CrossRef] [PubMed]
174. Soriguer, F.; Garrido-Sanchez, L.; Garcia-Serrano, S.; Garcia-Almeida, J.M.; Garcia-Arnes, J.; Tinahones, F.J.; Garcia-Fuentes, E. Apelin levels are increased in morbidly obese subjects with type 2 diabetes mellitus. *Obes. Surg.* **2009**, *19*, 1574–1580. [CrossRef] [PubMed]
175. Handisurya, A.; Riedl, M.; Vila, G.; Maier, C.; Clodi, M.; Prikoszovich, T.; Ludvik, B.; Prager, G.; Luger, A.; Kautzky-Willer, A. Serum vaspin concentrations in relation to insulin sensitivity following RYGB-induced weight loss. *Obes. Surg.* **2010**, *20*, 198–203. [CrossRef]
176. Janke, J.; Engeli, S.; Boschmann, M.; Adams, F.; Böhnke, J.; Luft, F.C.; Sharma, A.M.; Jordan, J. Retinol-binding protein 4 in human obesity. *Diabetes* **2006**, *55*, 2805–2810. [CrossRef]
177. Haider, D.G.; Schindler, K.; Prager, G.; Bohdjalian, A.; Luger, A.; Wolzt, M.; Ludvik, B. Serum retinol-binding protein 4 is reduced after weight loss in morbidly obese subjects. *J. Clin. Endocrinol. Metab.* **2007**, *92*, 1168–1171. [CrossRef] [PubMed]
178. Wang, X.; Huang, Y.; Gao, J.; Sun, H.; Jayachandran, M.; Qu, S. Changes of serum retinol-binding protein 4 associated with improved insulin resistance after laparoscopic sleeve gastrectomy in Chinese obese patients. *Diabetol. Metab. Syndr.* **2020**, *12*, 7. [CrossRef]
179. Tschoner, A.; Sturm, W.; Engl, J.; Kaser, S.; Laimer, M.; Laimer, E.; Weiss, H.; Patsch, J.R.; Ebenbichler, C.F. Retinol-binding protein 4, visceral fat, and the metabolic syndrome: Effects of weight loss. *Obesity* **2008**, *16*, 2439–2444. [CrossRef]

180. Chabot, K.; Gauthier, M.S.; Garneau, P.Y.; Rabasa-Lhoret, R. Evolution of subcutaneous adipose tissue fibrosis after bariatric surgery. *Diabetes Metab.* **2017**, *43*, 125–133. [CrossRef]
181. Katsogiannos, P.; Kamble, P.G.; Boersma, G.J.; Karlsson, F.A.; Lundkvist, P.; Sundbom, M.; Pereira, M.J.; Eriksson, J.W. Early Changes in Adipose Tissue Morphology, Gene Expression, and Metabolism after RYGB in Patients with Obesity and T2D. *J. Clin. Endocrinol. Metab.* **2019**, *104*, 2601–2613. [CrossRef]
182. Löfgren, P.; Hoffstedt, J.; Rydén, M.; Thörne, A.; Holm, C.; Wahrenberg, H.; Arner, P. Major Gender Differences in the Lipolytic Capacity of Abdominal Subcutaneous Fat Cells in Obesity Observed before and after Long-Term Weight Reduction. *J. Clin. Endocrinol. Metab.* **2002**, *87*, 764–771. [CrossRef] [PubMed]
183. Soriguer, F.; García-Serrano, S.; García-Almeida, J.M.; Garrido-Sánchez, L.; García-Arnés, J.; Tinahones, F.J.; Cardona, I.; Rivas-Marín, J.; Gallego-Perales, J.L.; García-Fuentes, E. Changes in the serum composition of free-fatty acids during an intravenous glucose tolerance test. *Obesity* **2009**, *17*, 10–15. [CrossRef]
184. Carvalho, B.M.; Oliveira, A.G.; Ueno, M.; Araújo, T.G.; Guadagnini, D.; Carvalho-Filho, M.A.; Geloneze, B.; Lima, M.M.O.; Pareja, J.C.; Carvalheira, J.B.C.; et al. Modulation of double-stranded RNA-activated protein kinase in insulin sensitive tissues of obese humans. *Obesity* **2013**, *21*, 2452–2457. [CrossRef] [PubMed]
185. Maymó-Masip, E.; Fernández-Veledo, S.; España, A.G.; Vázquez-Carballo, A.; Tinahones, F.J.; García-Fuentes, E.; Garrifo-Sanchez, L.; Del Mar Rodriguez, M.; Vendrell, J.; Chacón, M.R. The rise of soluble TWEAK levels in severely obese subjects after bariatric surgery may affect adipocyte-cytokine production induced by TNFα. *J. Clin. Endocrinol. Metab.* **2013**, *98*, E1323–E1333. [CrossRef] [PubMed]
186. Dharuri, H.; 't Hoen, P.A.C.; van Klinken, J.B.; Henneman, P.; Laros, J.F.J.; Lips, M.A.; el Bouazzaoui, F.; van Ommen, G.J.B.; Janssen, I.; van Ramshorst, B.; et al. Downregulation of the acetyl-CoA metabolic network in adipose tissue of obese diabetic individuals and recovery after weight loss. *Diabetologia* **2014**, *57*, 2384–2392. [CrossRef]
187. De La Torre, N.G.; Rubio, M.A.; Bordiú, E.; Cabrerizo, L.; Aparicio, E.; Hernández, C.; Sánchez-Pernaute, A.; Díez-Valladares, L.; Torres, A.J.; Puente, M.; et al. Effects of weight loss after bariatric surgery for morbid obesity on vascular endothelial growth factor-A, adipocytokines, and insulin. *J. Clin. Endocrinol. Metab.* **2008**, *93*, 4276–4281. [CrossRef]
188. Wiewiora, M.; Mertas, A.; Gluck, M.; Nowowiejska-Wiewiora, A.; Czuba, Z.; Piecuch, J. Effect of Weight Loss Surgery on Biomarkers of Angiogenesis in Obese Patients. *Obes. Surg.* **2020**, *30*, 3417–3425. [CrossRef]
189. Atkin, S.L.; Ramachandran, V.; Yousri, N.A.; Benurwar, M.; Simper, S.C.; McKinlay, R.; Adams, T.D.; Najafi-Shoushtari, S.H.; Hunt, S.C. Changes in blood microRNA expression and early metabolic responsiveness 21 days following bariatric surgery. *Front. Endocrinol.* **2019**, *10*, 773. [CrossRef]
190. Sangiao-Alvarellos, S.; Theofilatos, K.; Barwari, T.; Gutmann, C.; Takov, K.; Singh, B.; Juiz-Valiña, P.; Varela-Rodríguez, B.M.; Outeiriño-Blanco, E.; Duregotti, E.; et al. Metabolic recovery after weight loss surgery is reflected in serum microRNAs. *BMJ Open Diabetes Res. Care* **2020**, *8*, e001441. [CrossRef]
191. Ortega, F.J.; Mercader, J.M.; Moreno-Navarrete, J.M.; Nonell, L.; Puigdecanet, E.; Rodriquez-Hermosa, J.I.; Rovira, O.; Xifra, G.; Guerra, E.; Moreno, M.; et al. Surgery-induced weight loss is associated with the downregulation of genes targeted by MicroRNAs in adipose tissue. *J. Clin. Endocrinol. Metab.* **2015**, *100*, E1467–E1476. [CrossRef] [PubMed]
192. Macartney-Coxson, D.; Danielson, K.; Clapham, J.; Benton, M.C.; Johnston, A.; Jones, A.; Shaw, O.; Hagan, R.D.; Hoffman, E.P.; Hayes, M.; et al. MicroRNA Profiling in Adipose Before and After Weight Loss Highlights the Role of miR-223-3p and the NLRP3 Inflammasome. *Obesity* **2020**, *28*, 570–580. [CrossRef] [PubMed]
193. Mysore, R.; Ortega, F.J.; Latorre, J.; Ahonen, M.; Savolainen-Peltonen, H.; Fischer-Posovszky, P.; Wabitsch, M.; Olkkonen, V.M.; Fernández-Real, J.M.; Haridas, P.A.N. MicroRNA-221-3p regulates angiopoietin-like 8 (ANGPTL8) expression in adipocytes. *J. Clin. Endocrinol. Metab.* **2017**, *102*, 4001–4012. [CrossRef] [PubMed]
194. Ortega, F.J.; Moreno, M.; Mercader, J.M.; Moreno-Navarrete, J.M.; Fuentes-Batllevell, N.; Sabater, M.; Ricart, W.; Fernández-Real, J.M. Inflammation triggers specific microRNA profiles in human adipocytes and macrophages and in their supernatants. *Clin. Epigenetics* **2015**, *7*, 49. [CrossRef] [PubMed]
195. Botella-Carretero, J.I.; Álvarez-Blasco, F.; Ángeles Martinez-García, M.; Luque-Ramírez, M.; San Millán, J.L.; Escobar-Morreale, H.F. The decrease in serum IL-18 levels after bariatric surgery in morbidly obese women is a time-dependent event. *Obes. Surg.* **2007**, *17*, 1199–1208. [CrossRef]
196. Schernthaner, G.H.; Kopp, H.P.; Kriwanek, S.; Krzyzanowska, K.; Satler, M.; Koppensteiner, R.; Schernthaner, G. Effect of massive weight loss induced by bariatric surgery on serum levels of interleukin-18 and monocyte-chemoattractant-protein-1 in morbid obesity. *Obes. Surg.* **2006**, *16*, 709–715. [CrossRef]
197. Catalán, V.; Gómez-Ambrosi, J.; Rodríguez, A.; Ramírez, B.; Rotellar, F.; Valentí, V.; Silva, C.; Gil, M.J.; Salvador, J.; Frühbeck, G. Increased Tenascin C And Toll-Like Receptor 4 Levels in Visceral Adipose Tissue as a Link between Inflammation and Extracellular Matrix Remodeling in Obesity. *J. Clin. Endocrinol. Metab.* **2012**, *97*, E1880–E1889. [CrossRef]
198. Sangiorgi, G.M.; Cereda, A.; Porchetta, N.; Benedetto, D.; Matteucci, A.; Bonanni, M.; Chiricolo, G.; De Lorenzo, A. Endovascular Bariatric Surgery as Novel Minimally Invasive Technique for Weight Management in the Morbidly Obese: Review of the Literature. *Nutrients* **2021**, *13*, 2541. [CrossRef]
199. O'Brien, P.E.; Hindle, A.; Brennan, L.; Skinner, S.; Burton, P.; Smith, A.; Crosthwaite, G.; Brown, W. Long-Term Outcomes After Bariatric Surgery: A Systematic Review and Meta-analysis of Weight Loss at 10 or More Years for All Bariatric Procedures and a Single-Centre Review of 20-Year Outcomes After Adjustable Gastric Banding. *Obes. Surg.* **2019**, *29*, 3–14. [CrossRef]

200. O'Brien, P.E.; MacDonald, L.; Anderson, M.; Brennan, L.; Brown, W.A. Long-term outcomes after bariatric surgery: Fifteen-year follow-up of adjustable gastric banding and a systematic review of the bariatric surgical literature. *Ann. Surg.* **2013**, *257*, 87–94. [CrossRef]
201. Carlsson, L.M.S.; Peltonen, M.; Ahlin, S.; Anveden, Å.; Bouchard, C.; Carlsson, B.; Jacobson, P.; Lönroth, H.; Maglio, C.; Näslund, I.; et al. Bariatric Surgery and Prevention of Type 2 Diabetes in Swedish Obese Subjects. *N. Engl. J. Med.* **2012**, *367*, 695–704. [CrossRef]
202. Sjöström, L.; Lindroos, A.; Peltonen, M.; Torgerson, J.; Bouchard, C.; Carlsson, B.; Dahlgren, S.; Larsson, B.; Narbro, K.; Sjöström, C.D.; et al. Lifestyle, Diabetes, and Cardiovascular Risk Factors 10 Years after Bariatric Surgery. *N. Engl. J. Med.* **2004**, *351*, 2683–2693. [CrossRef] [PubMed]
203. Adams, T.D.; Gress, R.E.; Smith, S.C.; Halverson, R.C.; Simper, S.C.; Rosamond, W.D.; LaMonte, M.J.; Stroup, A.M.; Hunt, S.C. Long-Term Mortality after Gastric Bypass Surgery. *N. Engl. J. Med.* **2007**, *357*, 753–761. [CrossRef]
204. Gómez-Ambrosi, J.; Andrada, P.; Valentí, V.; Rotellar, F.; Silva, C.; Catalán, V.; Rodríguez, A.; Ramírez, B.; Moncada, R.; Escalada, J.; et al. Dissociation of body mass index, excess weight loss and body fat percentage trajectories after 3 years of gastric bypass: Relationship with metabolic outcomes. *Int. J. Obes.* **2017**, *41*, 1379–1387. [CrossRef] [PubMed]
205. Varela-Rodríguez, B.M.; Juiz-Valiña, P.; Varela, L.; Outeiriño-Blanco, E.; Bravo, S.B.; García-Brao, M.J.; Mena, E.; Noguera, J.F.; Valero-Gasalla, J.; Cordido, F.; et al. Beneficial Effects of Bariatric Surgery-Induced by Weight Loss on the Proteome of Abdominal Subcutaneous Adipose Tissue. *J. Clin. Med.* **2020**, *9*, 213. [CrossRef]
206. Jahansouz, C.; Serrot, F.J.; Frohnert, B.I.; Foncea, R.E.; Dorman, R.B.; Slusarek, B.; Leslie, D.B.; Bernlohr, D.A. Roux-en-Y Gastric Bypass Acutely Decreases Protein Carbonylation and Increases Expression of Mitochondrial Biogenesis Genes in Subcutaneous Adipose Tissue. *Obes. Surg.* **2015**, *25*, 2376–2385. [CrossRef] [PubMed]
207. Henegar, C.; Tordjman, J.; Achard, V.; Lacasa, D.; Cremer, I.; Guerre-Millo, M.; Poitou, C.; Basdevant, A.; Stich, V.; Viguerie, N.; et al. Adipose tissue transcriptomic signature highlights the pathological relevance of extracellular matrix in human obesity. *Genome Biol.* **2008**, *9*, 1–32. [CrossRef]
208. Mardinoglu, A.; Heiker, J.T.; Gärtner, D.; Björnson, E.; Schön, M.R.; Flehmig, G.; Klöting, N.; Krohn, K.; Fasshauer, M.; Stumvoll, M.; et al. Extensive weight loss reveals distinct gene expression changes in human subcutaneous and visceral adipose tissue. *Sci. Rep.* **2015**, *5*, 14841. [CrossRef]
209. van der Kolk, B.W.; Muniandy, M.; Kaminska, D.; Alvarez, M.; Ko, A.; Miao, Z.; Valsesia, A.; Langin, D.; Vaittinen, M.; Pääkkönen, M.; et al. Differential Mitochondrial Gene Expression in Adipose Tissue Following Weight Loss Induced by Diet or Bariatric Surgery. *J. Clin. Endocrinol. Metab.* **2021**, *106*, 1312–1324. [CrossRef]
210. Hankir, M.K.; Seyfried, F. Do Bariatric Surgeries Enhance Brown/Beige Adipose Tissue Thermogenesis? *Front. Endocrinol.* **2020**, *11*, 275. [CrossRef]
211. De Giorgi, S.; Campos, V.; Egli, L.; Toepel, U.; Carrel, G.; Cariou, B.; Rainteau, D.; Schneiter, P.; Tappy, L.; Giusti, V. Long-term effects of Roux-en-Y gastric bypass on postprandial plasma lipid and bile acids kinetics in female non diabetic subjects: A cross-sectional pilot study. *Clin. Nutr.* **2015**, *34*, 911–917. [CrossRef]
212. Ryan, K.K.; Tremaroli, V.; Clemmensen, C.; Kovatcheva-Datchary, P.; Myronovych, A.; Karns, R.; Wilson-Pérez, H.E.; Sandoval, D.A.; Kohli, R.; Bäckhed, F.; et al. FXR is a molecular target for the effects of vertical sleeve gastrectomy. *Nature* **2014**, *509*, 183–188. [CrossRef]
213. Magalhaes, I.; Kiaf, B.; Lehuen, A. iNKT and MAIT cell alterations in diabetes. *Front. Immunol.* **2015**, *6*, 341. [CrossRef] [PubMed]
214. Magalhaes, I.; Pingris, K.; Poitou, C.; Bessoles, S.; Venteclef, N.; Kiaf, B.; Beaudoin, L.; Da Silva, J.; Allatif, O.; Rossjohn, J.; et al. Mucosal-associated invariant T cell alterations in obese and type 2 diabetic patients. *J. Clin. Investig.* **2015**, *125*, 1752–1762. [CrossRef] [PubMed]
215. Neinast, M.D.; Frank, A.P.; Zechner, J.F.; Li, Q.; Vishvanath, L.; Palmer, B.F.; Aguirre, V.; Gupta, R.K.; Clegg, D.J. Activation of natriuretic peptides and the sympathetic nervous system following Roux-en-Y gastric bypass is associated with gonadal adipose tissues browning. *Mol. Metab.* **2015**, *4*, 427–436. [CrossRef]
216. Langi, G.; Szczerbinski, L.; Kretowski, A. Meta-Analysis of Differential miRNA Expression after Bariatric Surgery. *J. Clin. Med.* **2019**, *8*, 1220. [CrossRef] [PubMed]

Journal of
Clinical Medicine

MDPI

Communication

Managing the Unpredictable: Mechanistic Analysis and Clinical Recommendations for Lamotrigine Treatment after Bariatric Surgery

Daniel Porat [1], Carmil Azran [2], Hasan Kais [3] and Arik Dahan [1,*]

[1] Department of Clinical Pharmacology, School of Pharmacy, Faculty of Health Sciences, Ben-Gurion University of the Negev, P.O. Box 653, Beer-Sheva 8410501, Israel; poratdan@post.bgu.ac.il
[2] Clinical Pharmacy, Herzliya Medical Center, Herzliya 4685107, Israel; CarmilA@hmc.co.il
[3] Division of Surgery, Shamir (Assaf Harofeh) Medical Center, Zerifin, Beer-Yaakov 7033001, Israel; hk1966@gmail.com
* Correspondence: arikd@bgu.ac.il; Tel.: +972-8-6479483; Fax: +972-8-6479303

Abstract: Bariatric surgery may alter the absorption and overall bioavailability of oral drugs. Lamotrigine is a major antiepileptic and mood stabilizer, that its use after bariatric surgery has not yet been studied. In this article, we provide a thorough mechanistic analysis of the effects of bariatric surgery on multiple mechanisms important for the absorption, bioavailability and overall pharmacokinetics of lamotrigine. Attributable to its pharmacokinetic properties and drug characteristics, the use of lamotrigine after bariatric surgery may be challenging. The complex situation in which some mechanisms may lead to increased drug exposure (e.g., decreased metabolism, weight loss) while others to its decrease (e.g., hampered dissolution/solubility, decreased gastric volume), may result in lowered, unchanged, or enhanced lamotrigine plasma levels after the surgery. We conclude with a set of clinical recommendations for lamotrigine treatment after bariatric surgery, aiming to allow better patient care, and emphasizing the extra caution that needs to be taken with these patients.

Keywords: anticonvulsant; pharmacotherapy; oral drug absorption; epilepsy; metabolic surgery

Citation: Porat, D.; Azran, C.; Kais, H.; Dahan, A. Managing the Unpredictable: Mechanistic Analysis and Clinical Recommendations for Lamotrigine Treatment after Bariatric Surgery. *J. Clin. Med.* **2021**, *10*, 5627. https://doi.org/10.3390/jcm10235627

Academic Editors: David Benaiges Boix and Roberta Lupoli

Received: 13 October 2021
Accepted: 24 November 2021
Published: 29 November 2021

1. Introduction

Bariatric surgery is an effective long-term treatment for severe obesity and comorbidities [1]. Quite a few short- and long-term risks, though, pose a concern among clinicians and patients [2]. One of the least discussed complications of bariatric surgery involves altered oral drug absorption and bioavailability, potentially leading to efficacy/safety issues of various orally administered medications [3,4]. A few bariatric procedures are commonly available worldwide, including sleeve gastrectomy, some variations of gastric bypass surgeries, notably Roux-en-Y gastric bypass (RYGB) and the newer one-anastomosis gastric bypass (OAGB), and more; and while each procedure is unique in the gastrointestinal anatomic changes that it brings and despite the fact that literature data is mainly available on RYGB, all of these procedures may affect oral drug pharmacokinetics [5–9], with clinically significant ramifications. Until recently, the literature in this field was mainly limited to case reports and small studies. Nowadays, larger clinical trials are more common [3], however, much is still unknown regarding the different variables and mechanisms that determine the overall drug exposure following the bariatric surgery [10].

Epilepsy is a serious neurological condition requiring appropriately dosed, chronic medication treatment to allow controlled and seizure-free disease. Due to this reason, therapeutic drug monitoring is a common practice with some anticonvulsants [11]. In the context of bariatric surgery, these orally administered drugs may require extra care due to possible alterations in the mechanisms responsible for their absorption and disposition in the body [12]. In fact, some of these mechanisms are associated with increased drug exposure, while others may lead to decreased plasma drug levels [13].

Lamotrigine is a major weight neutral [14] anticonvulsant and mood stabilizer, and is among the most common medications in the US and around the world, frequently prescribed among patients with obesity, both before and after bariatric surgery. Yet, various drug characteristics make lamotrigine use challenging after these operations.

In this communication, we provide a clinically relevant analysis of the important mechanisms related to lamotrigine absorption and bioavailability after bariatric surgery. This analysis should expose clinicians and pharmacologists to the many variables involved in the complex issue of pharmacokinetics and pharmacotherapy of patients after bariatric surgery, aiming for better patient-centered care.

2. Lamotrigine Pharmacokinetics

2.1. Drug Characteristics

Lamotrigine belongs to class II of the biopharmaceutical classification system [15], as it is a low solubility and high permeability drug. Lamotrigine is a weak base (pKa = 5.7) [16], thus exhibiting pH-dependent aqueous solubility. In water at 25 °C, lamotrigine solubility is only 0.2 mg/mL. The drug is lipophilic, with logP of around 2 [17].

2.2. Absorption and Bioavailability of the Drug

Lamotrigine is rapidly and completely absorbed upon oral administration of an immediate-release dosage form, reaching maximal plasma concentration after around 3 h post-dose and systemic bioavailability of ~100%. Food has no effect on its absorption. Lamotrigine undergoes extensive metabolism to inactive glucuronide metabolites by the uridine 5′-diphospho-glucuronosyltransferase (UDP-glucuronosyltransferase, UGT) family of enzymes. It does not undergo enterohepatic recirculation. The elimination half-life of the drug after monotherapy among healthy volunteers and epileptic patients ranges widely and depends on use of concomitant antiepileptics, with glucuronidation inducing drugs, such as phenytoin, phenobarbital or carbamazepine, reducing the elimination half-life, and inhibitors such as valproic acid increasing it [18]. Lamotrigine dose varies with indication and age, and the therapeutic window is normally between 2.5 to 15 μg/mL [19].

2.3. Absorption Issues after Bariatric Surgery

Several unique drug characteristics of lamotrigine may predispose it to potential absorption issues following bariatric surgery. First of all, lamotrigine is a weak base with pH-dependent solubility. After the surgery, about 80% of the stomach is removed, including significant portion of the parietal cells, increasing the gastric pH from ~1.8 to around 6.5 after OAGB [20]. This increased gastric pH following the resection of the stomach during the bariatric procedure is expected to severely hinder the dissolution of the lamotrigine dose. Additionally, the surgery involves a great decrease in stomach volume, which means that there is less fluid available to dissolve the drug dose. Shortly after the surgery, the patient may only be able to drink a few milliliters of water upon drug administration, further limiting the dissolution of the drug dose. Additionally, after the surgery, stomach motility may be hindered [21], potentially leading to hampered disintegration of the drug product and decreased dissolution of the drug dose [20].

In cases of highly lipophilic drugs, decreased bile secretion after bypass surgeries may lead to problems with their solubilization [22]. Since lamotrigine is moderately (but not highly) lipophilic, this mechanism may or may not play a significant role in its absorption.

Importantly, since only dissolved drug is able to permeate via the enterocytes and reach the systemic circulation, hampered absorption of the drug may also be expected following the surgery. To note, the stomach pH is increased more significantly after gastric bypass than after sleeve gastrectomy (about 6.5 vs. 5, respectively), so absorption problems of lamotrigine may be especially severe after bypass procedures in particular [20]. Additionally, in bypass surgeries the duodenum and proximal jejunum are bypassed, shortening the remaining small intestine surface area and transit time available for absorption; for many drugs, and lamotrigine included, this decreased transit time throughout the small intestine may hamper the overall absorption of the drug. As for active transporter-mediated permeation, depending on the expression level of the relevant transporter in the bypassed intestinal segment, bypass surgeries may result in lower exposure of the drug to these transporters. Publications in the literature report that lamotrigine is subjected to both influx and efflux transporters, with unclear clinical impact [23,24]. It is likely that transporters have limited on lamotrigine absorption, so this mechanism does not significantly alter the overall exposure of lamotrigine.

2.4. Distribution Issues after Bariatric Surgery

Following bariatric surgery, great weight loss is often achieved shortly after the procedure. In addition, the patient loses fat tissue, and for lipophilic agents such as lamotrigine, this may lead to more drug remaining in the central compartment and not going to periphery, thus increasing the plasma levels of the drug, and making it available for central nervous system penetration, from where it exerts its therapeutic effect [25].

2.5. Metabolism Issues after Bariatric Surgery

As mentioned, lamotrigine undergoes extensive phase II metabolism to glucuronide metabolites. Importantly, it was shown that glucuronidation is enhances in obesity and decreased after bariatric surgery [26]. This phenomenon was approved in the cases of morphine and acetaminophen, both prototypical substrates for glucuronidation with decreased metabolism after surgery and high parent drug levels [27,28]. This may also be the case upon post-bariatric lamotrigine therapy. In fact, bodyweight in general, was found to be the most significant covariate on lamotrigine clearance, explained by correlation between the size of the excreting organ and bodyweight [29].

2.6. Excretion Issues after Bariatric Surgery

While lamotrigine is mainly eliminated via hepatic glucuronidation, decreased renal function was found to correlate with decreased lamotrigine clearance [29]. Meanwhile, while debatable, recent publications report potentially improved renal function shortly after bariatric surgery in patients with chronic kidney disease (CKD) [30–32]. Hence, among patients with CKD in the first year following the surgery, improved kidney function may contribute to overall decreased lamotrigine levels.

2.7. Summary of the Mechanistic Analysis

In this section, we provided several different mechanisms by which bariatric surgery may alter the disposition of lamotrigine. Notably, some of these mechanisms support increased drug levels after (vs. before) the surgery, while others may be responsible for decreased postoperative drug levels. Thus, high interpatient variability may be witnessed regarding the effect of the surgery on lamotrigine, with increased, decreased or unchanged pharmacokinetics are all possible. In addition, given the analysis above, the exact type of bariatric procedure that the patient undergoes may also play a significant role. Table 1 summarized the proposed mechanisms, dividing them to supporting increase vs. decrease in lamotrigine levels after the surgery.

Table 1. Summary of mechanisms involved in increased (↑) or decreased (↓) lamotrigine levels after gastric bypass or sleeve gastrectomy surgeries. (?) is added if mechanism effects are suspected or unknown.

The Proposed Mechanism	Gastric Bypass Surgery	Sleeve Gastrectomy
Smaller gastric volume	↓	↓
Increased stomach pH	↓↓	↓
Decreased gastric motility	↓	↓
Effects on bile secretions	↓?	-
Effects on absorption surface area	↓	-
Decreased exposure to carrier proteins	?	-
Decreased patient weight and fat tissue	↑	↑
Decreased metabolism (glucuronidation)	↑	↑
Effects on renal clearance	↓?	↓?

3. Discussion

Increased, decreased or unchanged lamotrigine levels after bariatric surgery are all possible, given the presence of factors influenced by the surgery, that promote increased drug levels, as well as factors that promote decreased levels. The overall effect of the surgery may depend on the individual patient characteristics [33,34], such as concomitant drugs taken, as well as the specific bariatric procedure undergone. In addition, when two or more altered mechanisms are involved, the magnitude and direction of changes in lamotrigine pharmacokinetics may vary [35], and while the most dominant mechanism [36] may dictate the overall trend towards increased or decreased drug levels [37], this dominant mechanism may be different from patient to patient.

Similar mechanistic analysis should be performed for more drugs [38], and in vitro, in vivo and in silico models [39] should support this mechanistic approach, producing more valuable data. The aim of this mechanistic approach is to allow prediction of the pharmacokinetic changes of a given drug before prescribing it to the post-bariatric patient and design a tailored treatment plan, hence choosing the most appropriate drug and dosing regimen.

While each drug is unique in its physicochemical and pharmacokinetic properties, various drugs share at least some common features with lamotrigine. Many newly discovered drugs have moderate-to-high lipophilicity and low-to-marginal water solubility [40], so concerns related to decreased stomach and fluid volume after the surgery apply to these drugs as well. Additionally, drugs with high maximal dose (generally over 100 mg) are more challenging in this aspect. Some therapeutic classes characterized by high dose drugs are antiepileptics, antipsychotics, antibacterials, antivirals and nonsteroidal anti-inflammatory drugs (NSAIDs). Among the drugs with basic functional group, likely to exhibit decreased solubility after gastrectomy, similarly to lamotrigine, are antipsychotics, antidepressants, antivirals, antifungals, alpha and beta-blockers, anti-anxiety medications and oral anticancer agents such as tyrosine kinase inhibitors, and more. Other drugs undergoing glucuronidation as a major metabolic pathway include (but not limited to) morphine, acetaminophen, lorazepam, mycophenolic acid, valproic acid and olanzapine, and this may support potential decreased metabolism and consequent increased drug exposure.

Realizing the need for extra care when prescribing to a patient after bariatric surgery is of importance, given the unpredictable effects of the surgery. While only older antiepileptics are routinely monitored, therapeutic drug monitoring of newer antiepileptics is also warranted after the surgery [12]. Indeed, lamotrigine should be monitored, both for potentially altered trough plasma drug levels and for clinical signs of safety issues/treatment failure. For rational management of such cases, recommendations for lamotrigine treatment after bariatric surgery are provided in the following section.

4. Clinical Recommendations

In this section we wish to summarize practical considerations for lamotrigine treatment of patients after bariatric surgery. Periodic therapeutic drug monitoring is important after the surgery. Especially in the first few months after bariatric surgery, lamotrigine levels should be checked frequently. Preferably, lamotrigine blood levels can also be measured shortly before the surgery to discern basal effective levels that should then be aimed after the operation [12]. Involvement of clinical pharmacists as advisors in the drug treatment is beneficial for both surgeons and patients.

Immediately after the surgery, the patient should be moved to dispersible tablets or liquid dosage form, or alternatively, should crush their immediate-release tablets and spread the powder in food/drink prior to ingestion (according to package insert or available company data). This is especially indicated in cases hampered drug dissolution/disintegration is likely. It is worthwhile to note that caution should be taken with extended-release dosage forms because oftentimes they should not be crushed. In case a liquid dosage form is to be used, it is important to make sure that it does not contain non-absorbable sugars, in light of the risk for dumping syndrome. In cases drug levels drop after the surgery, gradual dose increase is, of course, an option. A specific consideration regarding bariatric surgery, may be to split the daily dose; for instance, if the patient is taking lamotrigine 200 mg once daily, shifting to 100 mg twice daily may aid to prevent hampered dissolution of the drug dose. On the other hand, if drug levels are found to be high and/or the patient cannot tolerate the lamotrigine treatment, dose may have to eventually be gradually decreased. To note, some of these undesirable situations may be temporary, as adaptation mechanisms may occur in the months following the surgery, and changes in weight also take place [41].

If lamotrigine treatment is not tolerated or is ineffective, a second antiseizure medication should be added and lamotrigine may be tapered down, if appropriate, only after the new drug reaches steady state levels [42]. Importantly, some antiepileptics are glucuronidation inducers (phenytoin, phenobarbital and carbamazepine) or inhibitors (sodium valproate), so a pharmacokinetic drug-drug interaction may affect lamotrigine levels. Among the bariatric patients, over 75% are females, and the average age of the operated patient is 42, so many of these patients are of childbearing potential [43]. Therefore, while valproate (along with lamotrigine) is a first line anticonvulsant for various different epileptic disorders, in many bariatric patients, valproate treatment should not be initiated in case of unsatisfactory lamotrigine treatment following the surgery, due to being highly teratogenic [42]. Among the other antiepileptic drugs, levetiracetam and topiramate are less likely to be affected by the bariatric surgery given their physicochemical properties and pharmacokinetic profiles, and thus may seem attractive if lamotrigine treatment is not effective/tolerated after surgery [12]. Yet, an alternative/adjuvant drug should be chosen primarily based on the specific epileptic syndrome of the patient. In addition, topiramate has less favorable side-effect profile than other alternatives [42]. Alternatively, non-oral dosage forms can be used at least temporarily, immediately after the surgery. This will sidestep the unpredictable outcomes of oral drug administering after bariatric surgery.

5. Conclusions

This article shows the complexity of drug treatment after bariatric surgery [44]. Consultation with a clinical pharmacist that specializes in drug therapy after bariatric surgery is necessary to allow safe and effective drug treatment in these patients. Lamotrigine, although not routinely monitored compared to other antiepileptic drugs, should be closely monitored soon after and at least a year following the bariatric surgery.

Author Contributions: Conceptualization, D.P., C.A., H.K. and A.D.; Investigation, D.P., C.A., H.K. and A.D.; Writing—Original Draft, D.P., C.A., H.K. and A.D.; Writing—Review & Editing, D.P., C.A. and A.D.; Supervision, A.D. All authors have read and agreed to the published version of the manuscript.

Funding: This research received no external funding.

Conflicts of Interest: The authors declare no conflict of interest.

References

1. Carlsson, L.M.S.; Sjoholm, K.; Jacobson, P.; Andersson-Assarsson, J.C.; Svensson, P.A.; Taube, M.; Carlsson, B.; Peltonen, M. Life expectancy after bariatric surgery in the Swedish obese subjects study. *N. Engl. J. Med.* **2020**, *383*, 1535–1543. [CrossRef]
2. Arterburn, D.E.; Telem, D.A.; Kushner, R.F.; Courcoulas, A.P. Benefits and risks of bariatric surgery in adults: A Review. *JAMA* **2020**, *324*, 879–887. [CrossRef]
3. McLachlan, L.A.; Chaar, B.B.; Um, I.S. Pharmacokinetic changes post-bariatric surgery: A scoping review. *Obes. Rev.* **2020**, *21*, e12988. [CrossRef] [PubMed]
4. Azran, C.; Wolk, O.; Zur, M.; Fine-Shamir, N.; Shaked, G.; Czeiger, D.; Sebbag, G.; Kister, O.; Langguth, P.; Dahan, A. Oral drug therapy following bariatric surgery: An overview of fundamentals, literature and clinical recommendations. *Obes. Rev.* **2016**, *17*, 1050–1066. [CrossRef]
5. Israel, S.; Elinav, H.; Elazary, R.; Porat, D.; Gibori, R.; Dahan, A.; Azran, C.; Horwitz, E. Case report of increased exposure to antiretrovirals following sleeve gastrectomy. *Antimicrob. Agents Chemother.* **2020**, *64*, e02453-19. [CrossRef]
6. Porat, D.; Markovic, M.; Zur, M.; Fine-Shamir, N.; Azran, C.; Shaked, G.; Czeiger, D.; Vaynshtein, J.; Replyanski, I.; Sebbag, G.; et al. Increased paracetamol bioavailability after sleeve gastrectomy: A crossover pre- vs. post-operative clinical trial. *J. Clin. Med.* **2019**, *8*, 1949. [CrossRef] [PubMed]
7. Chan, G.; Hajjar, R.; Boutin, L.; Garneau, P.Y.; Pichette, V.; Lafrance, J.P.; Elftouh, N.; Michaud, J.; du Souich, P. Prospective study of the changes in pharmacokinetics of immunosuppressive medications after laparoscopic sleeve gastrectomy. *Am. J. Transplant.* **2020**, *20*, 582–588. [CrossRef] [PubMed]
8. Dahan, A.; Porat, D.; Azran, C.; Mualem, Y.; Sakran, N.; Abu-Abeid, S. Lithium toxicity with severe bradycardia post sleeve gastrectomy: A case report and review of the literature. *Obes. Surg.* **2019**, *29*, 735–738. [CrossRef]
9. Pavlovsky, C.; Egorin, M.J.; Shah, D.D.; Beumer, J.H.; Rogel, S.; Pavlovsky, S. Imatinib mesylate pharmacokinetics before and after sleeve gastrectomy in a morbidly obese patient with chronic myeloid leukemia. *Pharmacotherapy* **2009**, *29*, 1152–1156. [CrossRef]
10. Darwich, A.S.; Pade, D.; Ammori, B.J.; Jamei, M.; Ashcroft, D.M.; Rostami-Hodjegan, A. A mechanistic pharmacokinetic model to assess modified oral drug bioavailability post bariatric surgery in morbidly obese patients: Interplay between CYP3A gut wall metabolism, permeability and dissolution. *J. Pharm. Pharmacol.* **2012**, *64*, 1008–1024. [CrossRef] [PubMed]
11. Patsalos, P.N.; Spencer, E.P.; Berry, D.J. Therapeutic drug monitoring of antiepileptic drugs in epilepsy: A 2018 update. *Ther. Drug Monit.* **2018**, *40*, 526–548. [CrossRef]
12. Brown, C.S.; Rabinstein, A.A.; Nystrom, E.M.; Britton, J.W.; Singh, T.D. Antiseizure medication use in gastric bypass patients and other post-surgical malabsorptive states. *Epilepsy Behav. Rep.* **2021**, *16*, 100439. [CrossRef] [PubMed]
13. Kingma, J.S.; Burgers, D.M.T.; Monpellier, V.M.; Wiezer, M.J.; Blusse van Oud-Alblas, H.J.; Vaughns, J.D.; Sherwin, C.M.T.; Knibbe, C.A.J. Oral drug dosing following bariatric surgery: General concepts and specific dosing advice. *Br. J. Clin. Pharmacol.* **2021**. [CrossRef]
14. Ben-Menachem, E. Weight issues for people with epilepsy—A review. *Epilepsia* **2007**, *48*, 42–45. [CrossRef] [PubMed]
15. Dahan, A.; Miller, J.M.; Amidon, G.L. Prediction of solubility and permeability class membership: Provisional BCS classification of the world's top oral drugs. *AAPS J.* **2009**, *11*, 740–746. [CrossRef] [PubMed]
16. Young, R.B.; Chefetz, B.; Liu, A.; Desyaterik, Y.; Borch, T. Direct photodegradation of lamotrigine (an antiepileptic) in simulated sunlight–pH influenced rates and products. *Environ. Sci. Process. Impacts* **2014**, *16*, 848–857. [CrossRef]
17. Vaithianathan, S.; Raman, S.; Jiang, W.; Ting, T.Y.; Kane, M.A.; Polli, J.E. Biopharmaceutic risk assessment of brand and generic lamotrigine tablets. *Mol. Pharm.* **2015**, *12*, 2436–2443. [CrossRef]
18. Rambeck, B.; Wolf, P. Lamotrigine clinical pharmacokinetics. *Clin. Pharmacokinet.* **1993**, *25*, 433–443. [CrossRef]
19. Patsalos, P.N.; Berry, D.J.; Bourgeois, B.F.; Cloyd, J.C.; Glauser, T.A.; Johannessen, S.I.; Leppik, I.E.; Tomson, T.; Perucca, E. Antiepileptic drugs–best practice guidelines for therapeutic drug monitoring: A position paper by the subcommission on therapeutic drug monitoring, ILAE Commission on Therapeutic Strategies. *Epilepsia* **2008**, *49*, 1239–1276. [CrossRef]
20. Porat, D.; Vaynshtein, J.; Gibori, R.; Avramoff, O.; Shaked, G.; Dukhno, O.; Czeiger, D.; Sebbag, G.; Dahan, A. Stomach pH before vs. after different bariatric surgery procedures: Clinical implications for drug delivery. *Eur. J. Pharm. Biopharm.* **2021**, *160*, 152–157. [CrossRef] [PubMed]
21. Ferraz, A.A.; Leao, C.S.; Campos, J.M.; Coelho, A.R.; Zilbestein, B.; Ferraz, E.M. An experimental study of the electrical activity of the bypassed stomach in the Roux-en-Y gastric bypass. *Arq. Gastroenterol.* **2007**, *44*, 162–167. [CrossRef]
22. Lorico, S.; Colton, B. Medication management and pharmacokinetic changes after bariatric surgery. *Can. Fam. Physician* **2020**, *66*, 409–416.
23. Milosheska, D.; Lorber, B.; Vovk, T.; Kastelic, M.; Dolzan, V.; Grabnar, I. Pharmacokinetics of lamotrigine and its metabolite N-2-glucuronide: Influence of polymorphism of UDP-glucuronosyltransferases and drug transporters. *Br. J. Clin. Pharmacol.* **2016**, *82*, 399–411. [CrossRef] [PubMed]
24. Chan, L.N.; Lin, Y.S.; Tay-Sontheimer, J.C.; Trawick, D.; Oelschlager, B.K.; Flum, D.R.; Patton, K.K.; Shen, D.D.; Horn, J.R. Proximal Roux-en-Y gastric bypass alters drug absorption pattern but not systemic exposure of CYP3A4 and P-glycoprotein substrates. *Pharmacotherapy* **2015**, *35*, 361–369. [CrossRef] [PubMed]

25. Goto, A.; Tagawa, Y.; Moriya, Y.; Sato, S.; Furukawa, Y.; Wakabayashi, T.; Tsukamoto, T.; DeJongh, J.; van Steeg, T.J.; Moriwaki, T.; et al. Impact of acute fat mobilisation on the pharmacokinetics of the highly fat distributed compound TAK-357, investigated by physiologically based pharmacokinetic (PBPK) modeling and simulation. *Biopharm. Drug Dispos.* **2017**, *38*, 373–380. [CrossRef]
26. Palau-Rodriguez, M.; Tulipani, S.; Marco-Ramell, A.; Minarro, A.; Jauregui, O.; Gonzalez-Dominguez, R.; Sanchez-Pla, A.; Ramos-Molina, B.; Tinahones, F.J.; Andres-Lacueva, C. Characterization of metabolomic profile associated with metabolic improvement after bariatric surgery in subjects with morbid obesity. *J. Proteome Res.* **2018**, *17*, 2704–2714. [CrossRef]
27. Chen, K.F.; Chan, L.N.; Senn, T.D.; Oelschlager, B.K.; Flum, D.R.; Shen, D.D.; Horn, J.R.; Lin, Y.S. The impact of proximal Roux-en-Y gastric bypass surgery on acetaminophen absorption and metabolism. *Pharmacotherapy* **2020**, *40*, 191–203. [CrossRef] [PubMed]
28. Lloret-Linares, C.; Luo, H.; Rouquette, A.; Labat, L.; Poitou, C.; Tordjman, J.; Bouillot, J.L.; Mouly, S.; Scherrmann, J.M.; Bergmann, J.F.; et al. The effect of morbid obesity on morphine glucuronidation. *Pharmacol. Res.* **2017**, *118*, 64–70. [CrossRef] [PubMed]
29. Methaneethorn, J.; Leelakanok, N. Sources of lamotrigine pharmacokinetic variability: A systematic review of population pharmacokinetic analyses. *Seizure* **2020**, *82*, 133–147. [CrossRef]
30. Abernathy, O.L.; Okut, H.; Paull-Forney, B.G.; Schwasinger-Schmidt, T.E. Bariatric surgery improves renal function in patients with obesity. *Cureus* **2021**, *13*, e17458. [CrossRef]
31. Huang, H.; Lu, J.; Dai, X.; Li, Z.; Zhu, L.; Zhu, S.; Wu, L. Improvement of renal function after bariatric surgery: A systematic review and meta-analysis. *Obes. Surg.* **2021**, *31*, 4470–4484. [CrossRef]
32. Zhang, T.; Wang, Y.; Zhang, X.; Wang, W.; Zhao, G. The impact of bariatric surgery on renal function: A retrospective analysis of short-term outcomes. *Obes. Surg.* **2021**, *31*, 3476–3482. [CrossRef] [PubMed]
33. Ludvigsson, M.; Haenni, A. Methylphenidate toxicity after Roux-en-Y gastric bypass. *Surg. Obes. Relat. Dis.* **2016**, *12*, e55–e57. [CrossRef] [PubMed]
34. Azran, C.; Langguth, P.; Dahan, A. Impaired oral absorption of methylphenidate after Roux-en-Y gastric bypass. *Surg. Obes. Relat. Dis.* **2017**, *13*, 1245–1247. [CrossRef] [PubMed]
35. Darwich, A.S.; Henderson, K.; Burgin, A.; Ward, N.; Whittam, J.; Ammori, B.J.; Ashcroft, D.M.; Rostami-Hodjegan, A. Trends in oral drug bioavailability following bariatric surgery: Examining the variable extent of impact on exposure of different drug classes. *Br. J. Clin. Pharmacol.* **2012**, *74*, 774–787. [CrossRef]
36. Angeles, P.C.; Robertsen, I.; Seeberg, L.T.; Krogstad, V.; Skattebu, J.; Sandbu, R.; Asberg, A.; Hjelmesaeth, J. The influence of bariatric surgery on oral drug bioavailability in patients with obesity: A systematic review. *Obes. Rev.* **2019**, *20*, 1299–1311. [CrossRef] [PubMed]
37. Azran, C.; Porat, D.; Fine-Shamir, N.; Hanhan, N.; Dahan, A. Oral levothyroxine therapy postbariatric surgery: Biopharmaceutical aspects and clinical effects. *Surg. Obes. Relat. Dis.* **2019**, *15*, 333–341. [CrossRef]
38. Azran, C.; Porat, D.; Dahan, A.; Dicker, D. Treatment of COVID-19 patients post-bariatric surgery: Issues for consideration. *J. Clin. Med.* **2020**, *9*, 2827. [CrossRef] [PubMed]
39. Dahan, A.; Porat, D.; Markovic, M.; Zur, M.; Kister, O.; Langguth, P. Optimized In Silico Modeling of Drug Absorption after Gastric Bypass: The Case of Metformin. *Pharmaceutics* **2021**, *13*, 1873. [CrossRef] [PubMed]
40. Knoke, S.; Bunjes, H. Transfer investigations of lipophilic drugs from lipid nanoemulsions to lipophilic acceptors: Contributing effects of cholesteryl esters and albumin as acceptor structures. *Pharmaceuticals* **2021**, *14*, 865. [CrossRef] [PubMed]
41. Steenackers, N.; Vanuytsel, T.; Augustijns, P.; Tack, J.; Mertens, A.; Lannoo, M.; Van der Schueren, B.; Matthys, C. Adaptations in gastrointestinal physiology after sleeve gastrectomy and Roux-en-Y gastric bypass. *Lancet Gastroenterol. Hepatol.* **2021**, *6*, 225–237. [CrossRef]
42. *Epilepsies: Diagnosis and Management*; National Institute for Health and Care Excellence: London, UK, 2021. [PubMed]
43. Welbourn, R.; Hollyman, M.; Kinsman, R.; Dixon, J.; Cohen, R.; Morton, J.; Ghaferi, A.; Higa, K.; Ottosson, J.; Pattou, F.; et al. Bariatric-metabolic surgery utilisation in patients with and without diabetes: Data from the IFSO global registry 2015–2018. *Obes. Surg.* **2021**, *31*, 2391–2400. [CrossRef] [PubMed]
44. Porat, D.; Dahan, A. Medication management after bariatric surgery: Providing optimal patient care. *J. Clin. Med.* **2020**, *9*, 1511. [CrossRef] [PubMed]

Journal of
Clinical Medicine

MDPI

Article

Role of Rendezvous-Procedure in the Treatment of Complications after Laparoscopic Sleeve Gastrectomy

Dörte Wichmann [1], Veit Scheble [2], Stefano Fusco [2,*], Ulrich Schweizer [1], Felix Hönes [1], Wilfried Klingert [1], Alfred Königsrainer [1] and Rami Archid [1]

[1] Department of General and Transplant Surgery, University Hospital of Tübingen, 72076 Tübingen, Germany; doerte.wichmann@med.uni-tuebingen.de (D.W.); ulrich.schweizer@med.uni-tuebingen.de (U.S.); felix.hoenes@med.uni-tuebingen.de (F.H.); wilfried.klingert@med.uni-tuebingen.de (W.K.); alfred.koenigsrainer@med.uni-tuebingen.de (A.K.); rami.archid@med.uni-tuebingen.de (R.A.)

[2] Department of Internal Medicine 1, Division for Gastroenterology, Hepatology, Infectiology, Gastrointestinal Oncology and Geriatrics, University Hospital of Tübingen, 72076 Tübingen, Germany; veit.scheble@med.uni-tuebingen.de

* Correspondence: stefano.fusco@med.uni-tuebingen.de

Abstract: Introduction: Laparoscopic sleeve gastrectomy is one of the most commonly performed bariatric procedures worldwide with good results, high patient acceptance, and low complication rates. The most relevant perioperative complication is the staple line leak. For the treatment of this complication, endoscopic negative pressure therapy has proven particularly effective. The correct time to start endoscopic negative pressure therapy has not been the subject of studies to date. Methods: Twelve patients were included in this retrospective data analysis over three years. Endoscopic negative pressure therapy was carried out using innovative open pore suction devices. Patients were treated with simultaneous surgery and endoscopy, so called rendezvous-procedure (Group A) or solely endoscopically, or in sequence surgically and endoscopically (Group B). Therapy data of the procedures and outcome measures, including duration of therapy, therapy success, and change of treatment strategy, were collected and analysed. Results: In each group, six patients were treated (mean age 52.96 years, 4 males, 8 females). Poor initial clinical situation, time span of endoscopic negative pressure therapy (Group A 31 days vs. Group B 18 days), and mean length of hospital stay (Group A 39.5 days vs. Group B 20.17 days) were higher in patients with rendezvous procedures. One patient in Group B died during the observation time. Discussion: Rendezvous procedures for patients with staple line leaks after sleeve gastrectomy is indicated for serious ill patients with perigastric abscesses and in need of laparoscopic lavage. The one-stage complication management with the rendezvous procedure seems not to result in an obvious advantage in the further outcome in patients with staple line leaks after laparoscopic sleeve gastrectomy.

Keywords: bariatric surgery; postsurgical complication management; endoscopic negative pressure therapy

Citation: Wichmann, D.; Scheble, V.; Fusco, S.; Schweizer, U.; Hönes, F.; Klingert, W.; Königsrainer, A.; Archid, R. Role of Rendezvous-Procedure in the Treatment of Complications after Laparoscopic Sleeve Gastrectomy. *J. Clin. Med.* **2021**, *10*, 5670. https://doi.org/10.3390/jcm10235670

Academic Editor: David Benaiges Boix

Received: 11 October 2021
Accepted: 30 November 2021
Published: 30 November 2021

1. Introduction

The number of surgeries and metabolic interventions for patients with obesity have increased worldwide [1,2]. The majority of bariatric interventions are performed surgically, especially laparoscopically [3,4]. The most common surgery is the laparoscopic sleeve gastrectomy (LSG) to minimize the volume of the stomach and thus reduce food intake [5,6]. This surgical intervention is easy to implement, as it does not contain any anastomose. Surgical complications after sleeve gastrectomy remain challenging, especially the management of staple line leaks (SLL), which occur in up to 2% of LSG patients [7]. Early diagnosis of SSL is relevant for the further clinical course of the disease, but obese patients do not present the typical peritonitis picture [8]. Due to the extensive visceral fat mass, the infection is initially captured and does not spread diffusely. This aspect significantly delays the detection of SLL in obese patients [8]. The time of first diagnosis of SLL determines the further therapeutic procedure. In early SLL re-laparoscopy, lavage and super sewing of the insufficiency or endoscopic techniques for primary wound closure can be performed [9,10]. In detected SLL two days after primary surgery super sewing is not promising. Secondary wound healing techniques, such as endoscopic stent therapy or endoscopic negative pressure therapy (ENPT), are used in these cases [11].

ENPT is an effective and precious tool in the management of surgical complications after surgery of the gastrointestinal tract [12]. A drainage wrapped by an open-pore suction device (OPSD) is placed endoluminal in position of the leak or intracavitary. Via the drain a negative pressure is applied and causes wound cleansing, defect closure and tissue granulation [13]. OPSD are used as either a polyurethane sponge connected to a drain—a so called open-pore polyurethane foam drainage (OPD), or as a thin open-pore double-layered drainage film (OFD), which is hand-wrapped around a gastric tube14. An advantage of the OFD is its small outer diameter and its possible use on enteral feeding tubes for simultaneous enteral feeding and ENPT [14]. See the used OPSD in Figure 1.

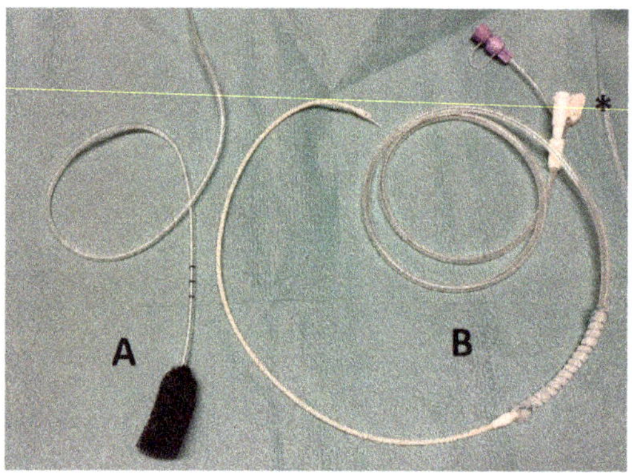

Figure 1. Two OPSD types used in this analysis: **A** = commercially available polyurethane sponge (Eso-Sponge; BBraun Melsungen, Germany); **B** = hand wrapped naso-jejunal feeding tube (Trelumina FREKA, 9 Ch intestinal tube, 16 Ch naso-gastric tube with perforations; Fresenius Kabi Deutschland GmbH, Bad Homburg, Germany) wrapping with cut to size CNP®-film (Suprasorb CNP® Drainage Film; Lohmann & Rauscher International GmbH & Co. KG, Rengsdorf, Germany), fixation with suture (Mersilene®, Polyester, 4 Ph. Eur; Ethicon—Johnson & Johnson Medical N.V., Belgium). * = closed venting tube.

The diagnostic gold standard in patients after LSG suspected for SLL is the immediate performance of sectional imaging [15]. In cases of suspected SLL with a small number of air bubbles in the position of Hiss' ankle, ENPT can lead to healing as a stand-alone therapy. When big fluid and pus collections outside the gastric lumen are visible in the CT scan, laparoscopic or radiological interventional drainage is necessary [16].

Combined surgical and endoscopic treatment, known as rendezvous procedure, is used to reduce the number of examinations under general anaesthesia for these critical ill patients. This rendezvous procedure requires increased staffing on the part of the endoscopy department. The benefits of the rendezvous procedure are currently not proven by studies.

2. Materials and Methods

2.1. Study Design

The local Institutional Review Board approved this study (IRB number: 464/2021BO2). All patients treated in the time between February 2018 and March 2021 using ENPT for SLL after LSG were considered for inclusion in this study, given the following criteria were fulfilled: confirmed diagnosis of SLL and treatment for the complication at our department. Exclusion criteria were treatment without ENPT and treatment of staple line leak outside our hospital. Informed consent was obtained from all individual participants. The focus of this analysis is postoperative complication management, so it included patients who had been operated on in another hospital.

2.2. Rendezvous Procedure

During re-laparoscopy for SLL in LSG patients, an endoscopic team consisting of a doctor and a nurse join in the operating room. During endoscopic diagnostic and placement of an OPSD, surgeons perform laparoscopy. The direct visualization of the perforation by air leakage is possible for the surgeon and the endoscopist. The application of the OPSD is carried out in the same way as described below.

2.3. One- or Two-Stage Approach

Endoscopic staff team examine the obese patient with suspected or diagnosed SLL after LSG prior or after the secondary surgery. Depending on the clinical course, patients can also be treated exclusively endoscopically. The application of the OPSD is carried out in the same way as described below.

2.4. Application of the OPSD

The first diagnostic and therapeutic endoscopy for SSL were realized in endotracheal intubation anaesthesia in all included cases. In the majority of cases an OFD was hand-made, as described elsewhere [14,16], by wrapping a very thin open-pore double-layered drainage film (Suprasorb CNP, Drainage Film; Lohmann & Rauscher International GmbH & Co. KG, Rengsdorf, Germany) on the gastric segment of a nasojejunal feeding tube (Freka Trelumina, Fresenius Kabi Deutschland GmbH, Bad Homburg Germany). Sutures (Mersilene, Polyester, 4 Ph. Eur., Ethicon, Norderstedt, Germany) were used for the fixation of drainage film around the tube. The OFD device was placed endoluminal in the gastric sleeve and was manufactured to cover the leak area with an overlap of the healthy stale line sector by 2 cm at minimum to the proximal and distal direction. The distal segment of the tube was used for enteral feeding. The OFD was guide wired pushed through the lumen.

In one case, with a perforation size of more than 2 cm, the primary OPSD was an OPD. We used the commercially available product ESO-Sponge System (BBraun Melsungen AG, Melsungen, Germany). This was positioned using the loop technique, in which a loop (Mersilene, Polyester, 4 Ph. Eur; Ethicon, Norderstedt, Germany) was fixed at the distal end of the drainage sponge, gripped with an endoscopic grasper, then placed under endoscopic view.

Drains of the OPSD were oro-nasal redirected and fixed with plasters. After placement of the OPSD drains were connected to an electric vacuum pump (KCI V.A.C. Freedom; KCI USA Inc., San Antonio, TX, USA) and a continuous vacuum of −125 mmHg was generated.

2.5. Follow-Up Procedures

According to the clinical course and the individual risk of the patients, the follow-up examinations were mostly performed under sedation and only rarely under intubation anaesthesia. A diagnostic endoscopy was performed following the removal of the OPSD. Whenever possible, re-endoscopy was performed after 5–7 days in cases treated with OFD and 3–5 days using OPD. In the case of persisting leak or in the case of uncertainty, an OPSD was reinserted, and treatment was continued.

2.6. Data Analysis

Analysis was performed using SPSS v. 24.0.0.1 (IBM, Armonk, NY, USA). Data were presented as means ± SD. Mann–Whitney U test was performed for comparing means when necessary.

3. Results

Twelve patients with SLL following LGS were included in this trial. In the observed time span, in sum, 389 patients with obesity were treated with LGS at our centre. The inhouse SSL-rate was 1.54%. Three patients were operated in other hospitals. Patients with SSL were included for the analysis and were divided into two groups:

Group A: patients treated for SSL by rendezvous procedures and

Group B: patients treated for SSL solely endoscopically or in sequence surgically and endoscopically.

The patient characteristics are shown in Table 1. In Group A, there were three patients included with complications after LGS operated in other hospitals. No patients from other hospitals were listed in Group B. The gender distribution in both groups differed, with more males in Group A. The other preoperative data were the same in both groups.

Table 1. Characteristics in patients with (Group A) or without (Group B) rendezvous procedure.

	Group A (n = 6)	Group B (n = 6)	
Number of male sexes	3	1	n.s.
Mean Age (years)	53.17	52.67	n.s.
Mean BMI (kg/m^2)	50.37	53.17	n.s.
Mean primary diagnosis of SLL (days after surgery)	8	15	n.s.
Number of detected perigastric abscesses in CT imaging	6	2	n.s.
Mean CRP (mg/dL)	27.09	24.74	n.s.
Mean White Blood Cells (µg/dL)	16,713	12,483	n.s.

Abbreviations: SLL—staple line leaks; CRP—C-reactive protein; n.s.—not significant.

On average, SLL was suspected earlier in Group A than in Group B, although there was considerable variation in both groups.

The treatment characteristics are shown in Table 2. At the time of diagnosis of staple line leaks, patients in Group A were characterized by more severe infection and, in some cases, sepsis. In six patients of Group A and two patients of Group B, peri-gastric abscesses were detected. In the intensive care unit, four patients in Group A and two patients in Group B were treated. Time span of ENPT, number of changes of the negative-pressure devices, length of hospital stays and time span of treatment on ICU differed significantly in both groups with longer therapy time in Group A.

Table 2. Treatment characteristics in patients with (Group A) or without (Group B) rendezvous procedure.

	Group A (n = 6)	Group B (n = 6)	
Mean duration on ICU (days)	6	5	n.s.
Mean number of endoscopic interventions			
-OFD	6	5	n.s.
-OPD	0	1	
Mean number of OPSD changes	5	5	n.s.
Mean duration of ENPT (days)	31	18	n.s.
Mean duration of hospital stay	39.5	20.17	0.047
Number of deceased patients	0	1	

Abbreviations: OFD—open-pore film drainage; OPD—open-pore polyurethane sponge drainage; n.s.—not significant; ENPT—endoscopic negative pressure therapy.

All patients in Group A underwent re-operation at least once. In Group B, surgery was performed in two patients. The other patients in Group B were successfully treated by ENPT solely.

In one patient of Group B OPSD dislocated, accidentally. No further therapy-associated complications occurred. No case of postoperative stricture was seen.

SLL-therapy was successful in 11/12 patients. One patient in Group B already had extensive cardiomyopathy prior to bariatric surgery and did not recover under therapeutic measures. This patient died due to septic organ failure.

All patients in Group A underwent re-operation at least once. In Group B surgery was performed in two patients. The other patients in Group B were successfully treated by ENPT solely.

In one patient of Group B, OPSD dislocated accidentally. No further therapy-associated complications occurred. No case of postoperative stricture was seen.

4. Discussion

SLL after LGS is a rare but life-threatening complication [1,2]. Patients with obesity often have pre-existing cardiovascular and pulmonary disease and undergo bariatric surgery in a compromised starting condition [3]. In cases of SLL local inflammation is often not detected early because of the high amount of visceral fat, which result in occult peritonitis without typical pain symptoms [4]. Furthermore, the longer an abdominal focus of infection persists untreated, the higher the risk for systemic inflammatory re-emergence in the sense of sepsis.

In this analysis, the time of clinical suspected SLL was in Mean on the twelfth post-operative day. Most patients presented with fever, abdominal pain, and high elevated inflammatory markers. In SLL, detection after more than 48 h after the bariatric surgery primary wound closure is not sufficient in most cases.

A CT scan is the gold standard in case of suspected SLL after LGS [5]. Depending on the imaging findings, the extent of inflammation, and the presence of an intra-abdominal abscess, the indication for re-laparoscopy for lavage and drainage is given [2].

If intra-abdominal abscesses are found, treatment with stent or clip closure of the perforation or fistula is not sufficient. The abdominal focus must be additionally drained radiologically or surgically. The drainage of secretions through an internal drainage by implantation of a double-pigtail-drainage to endoluminal can lead to a successful healing of the insufficiency in up to 78% according to the study results [6,7]. One of the reasons for the better outcome of patients in Group B is caused by the included patients without intra-abdominal abscesses in this group. Patients were less severely ill at the time point of diagnosis of SLL in Group B compared to Group A.

The ENPT is based on an OPSD (e.g., polyurethane sponge), which is either endo-luminally inserted at the stage of the leakage or intracavitary placed into the resulting insufficiency cavity. The open-pore element is fixed to a drainage with perforations, which is connected to a vacuum source. The negative pressure acts through the pores on the surrounding tissue and results in a continuous drainage of secretions, cell-detritus and bacteria, the suction induces tissue proliferation, and a decreased wound size [8–10].

ENPT is also known under the synonyms E-VAC and EVT. For ENPT as primary endoscopic procedure for leakages after bariatric surgery, possibly in combination with laparoscopy; three studies are currently available with a cumulative success rate of 90.27% in a total of 31 patients. In addition, there are numerous case reports and studies, some of which deal with the combined use of ENPT with stent procedures as first and second line therapy. An alternative closure of leakage after bariatric surgery can be successfully performed with OTSC as first or second line therapy with good results up to closure rates of 86.3% [11,12]. The most frequently performed endoscopic therapy for leakages after bariatric surgery worldwide is the stent therapy [1,13,14]. A challenge is the stent fixation in bariatric patients. Stent dislocation is the most common complication of this type of therapy [15]. Special bariatric stents with a big outer diameter and bulbs have been developed [16]. Because of a high dislocation rate and good results of the ENPT we changed our concept of stent-based treatment of SLL to ENPT in 2016.

In centres that specialize in the treatment of bariatric patients and have round-the-clock endoscopy, the rendezvous procedure is easy to implement. The concept of the rendezvous procedure is to apply a one-stage combined internal and external drainage of the abscess during one examination with endotracheal intubation to avoid reintubation and septic episodes. Especially, in patients with small leaks, a reliable identification of the leak can be made by the combined laparoscopic and endoscopic procedure.

One patient died because of septic multiorgan failure. This patient with obesity suffered pre-operatively on relevant cardiomyopathy. It must be assumed that the septic shock was so stressful for him that, despite intensive therapeutic measures, the progressive organ failure could no longer be stopped. This case impressively demonstrates that patients with bariatric surgery often suffer from significant systemic diseases and that postoperative complications quickly lead to fulminant organ failure.

The rendezvous procedure is associated with a high level of personnel effort. We wanted to use a retrospective analysis to investigate whether there is an advantage for patients who have been treated by means of a rendezvous procedure. Obese patients with SLL often require intensive care and continuation of invasive ventilation. Alternatively, to the rendezvous procedure, patients can be managed in two stages, undergoing surgery or endoscopy first and the second procedure in close interval. In summary, our analysis shows that in patients with septic complications after bariatric surgery with indication for re-laparoscopy, a simultaneous endoscopy with application of an OPSD for ENPT can be advantageous. However, a significant benefit for the rendezvous procedure is missing. The series is retrospective with a small number of cases and too time-scattered to draw any significant conclusions. A prospective series is to be preferred, given the low incidence of SLL complications.

5. Conclusions

We believe that a one- or two-step procedure with surgical and endoscopically interventions in short intervals can be applied as well. In patients without the need of re-laparoscopy, ENPT is an effective treatment tool as stand-alone interventional therapy.

Author Contributions: Conceptualization, D.W., V.S., R.A. and U.S.; methodology, D.W. and R.A.; software, D.W.; validation, D.W., W.K., A.K. and R.A.; formal analysis, D.W., U.S., A.K.; investigation, D.W., U.S.; resources, D.W., A.K., F.H. and R.A.; data curation, D.W., U.S., F.H.; writing—original draft preparation, D.W., S.F.; writing—review and editing, D.W., S.F., R.A., W.K. and A.K.; visualization, D.W., U.S.; supervision, S.F., A.K.; project administration, A.K. All authors have read and agreed to the published version of the manuscript.

Funding: This research received no external funding. The APC was funded by Open Access Fund of the University of Tübingen.

Institutional Review Board Statement: The study was conducted according to the guidelines of the Declaration of Helsinki, and approved by the Institutional Review Board of University of Tübingen (protocol code 464/2021BO2, date of approval 12 July 2021).

Informed Consent Statement: Informed consent was obtained from all subjects involved in the study.

Data Availability Statement: Data are available on request.

Conflicts of Interest: The authors declare no conflict of interest.

References

1. Chung, Y.; Park, D.G.; Kim, Y.J. Endoscopic Management of Staple Line Leak after Bariatric Surgery: Surgeon's Perspective. *Clin. Endosc.* **2021**, *54*, 805–809. [CrossRef] [PubMed]
2. Noel, P.; Nedelcu, M.; Gagner, M. Impact of the Surgical Experience on Leak Rate After Laparoscopic Sleeve Gastrectomy. *Obes. Surg.* **2016**, *26*, 1782–1787. [CrossRef]
3. Shukeri, W.; Hassan, M.H.; Hassan, W.; Zaini, R.H.M. Anastomotic Leak after Bariatric Surgery from a Critical Care Perspective: A Lesson Shared. *Malays. J. Med. Sci.* **2018**, *25*, 158–159. [CrossRef] [PubMed]
4. Montravers, P.; Guglielminotti, J.; Zappella, N.; Desmard, M.; Muller, C.; Fournier, P.; Marmuse, J.P.; Dufour, G.; Augustin, P. Clinical features and outcome of postoperative peritonitis following bariatric surgery. *Obes. Surg.* **2013**, *23*, 1536–1544. [CrossRef]
5. Hussain, A.; El-Hasani, S. Diagnostic Laparoscopy or CT Scan to Diagnose the Leak Following Bariatric Surgery. *Obes. Surg.* **2016**, *26*, 617–618. [CrossRef] [PubMed]
6. Donatelli, G.; Airinei, G.; Poupardin, E.; Tuszynski, T.; Wind, P.; Benamouzig, R.; Meduri, B. Double-pigtail stent migration invading the spleen: Rare potentially fatal complication of endoscopic internal drainage for sleeve gastrectomy leak. *Endoscopy* **2016**, *48* (Suppl. 1), E74–E75. [CrossRef]

7. Donatelli, G.; Spota, A.; Cereatti, F.; Granieri, S.; Dagher, I.; Chiche, R.; Catheline, J.M.; Pourcher, G.; Rebibo, L.; Calabrese, D.; et al. Endoscopic internal drainage for the management of leak, fistula, and collection after sleeve gastrectomy: Our experience in 617 consecutive patients. *Surg. Obes. Relat. Dis.* **2021**, *17*, 1432–1439. [CrossRef] [PubMed]
8. Kuehn, F.; Loske, G.; Schiffmann, L.; Gock, M.; Klar, E. Endoscopic vacuum therapy for various defects of the upper gastrointestinal tract. *Surg. Endosc.* **2017**, *31*, 3449–3458. [CrossRef] [PubMed]
9. Loske, G.; Liedke, M.; Schloricke, E.; Herrmann, T.; Rucktaeschel, F. Endoscopic negative-pressure therapy for duodenal leakage using new open-pore film and polyurethane foam drains with the pull-through technique. *Endoscopy* **2017**, *49*, E300–E302. [CrossRef] [PubMed]
10. Archid, R.; Wichmann, D.; Klingert, W.; Nadiradze, G.; Hones, F.; Archid, N.; Othman, A.E.; Ahmad, S.J.S.; Konigsrainer, A.; Lange, J. Endoscopic Vacuum Therapy for Staple Line Leaks after Sleeve Gastrectomy. *Obes. Surg.* **2020**, *30*, 1310–1315. [CrossRef] [PubMed]
11. Shoar, S.; Poliakin, L.; Khorgami, Z.; Rubenstein, R.; El-Matbouly, M.; Levin, J.L.; Saber, A.A. Efficacy and Safety of the Over-the-Scope Clip (OTSC) System in the Management of Leak and Fistula after Laparoscopic Sleeve Gastrectomy: A Systematic Review. *Obes. Surg.* **2017**, *27*, 2410–2418. [CrossRef]
12. Aly, A.; Lim, H.K. The use of over the scope clip (OTSC) device for sleeve gastrectomy leak. *J. Gastrointest. Surg.* **2013**, *17*, 606–608. [CrossRef]
13. de Moura, D.T.H.; de Freitas Junior, J.R.; de Souza, G.M.V.; de Oliveira, G.H.P.; McCarty, T.R.; Thompson, C.C.; de Moura, E.G.H. Endoscopic management of acute leak after sleeve gastrectomy: Principles and techniques. *Endoscopy* **2021**. [CrossRef] [PubMed]
14. Silva, L.B.; Neto, M.G.; Marchesini, J.C.; Godoy, E.S.; Campos, J. Sleeve gastrectomy leak: Endoscopic management through a customized long bariatric stent. *Gastrointest. Endosc.* **2017**, *85*, 865–866. [CrossRef] [PubMed]
15. Anastasiou, J.; Hussameddin, A.; Al Quorain, A. Mind the Gap: Successful Endoscopic Closure of a Large Gastric Sleeve Leak Using an Endoscopic Stent and Over-the-Scope Clips. *Case Rep. Gastroenterol.* **2017**, *11*, 763–768. [CrossRef] [PubMed]
16. Liu, S.Y.; Wong, S.K.; Ng, E.K. Novel oesophago-gastro-duodenal stenting for gastric leaks after laparoscopic sleeve gastrectomy. *Obes. Res. Clin. Pract.* **2015**, *9*, 214–219. [CrossRef] [PubMed]

Journal of
Clinical Medicine

MDPI

Review

Non-Alcoholic Fatty Liver Disease (NAFLD) and Bariatric/Metabolic Surgery as Its Treatment Option: A Review

Paulina Głuszyńska [1,*], Dorota Lemancewicz [2], Janusz Bogdan Dzięcioł [2] and Hady Razak Hady [1]

[1] Department of General and Endocrine Surgery, Medical University of Bialystok, 15-089 Białystok, Poland; hadyrazakh@wp.pl
[2] Department of Human Anatomy, Medical University of Bialystok, 15-089 Białystok, Poland; dorota.lemancewicz@umb.edu.pl (D.L.); anatomia@umb.edu.pl (J.B.D.)
* Correspondence: Paulina.gluszynska@gmail.com; Tel.: +48-85-831-8279

Abstract: The prevalence of non-alcoholic fatty liver disease (NAFLD) and non-alcoholic steatohepatitis (NASH) has considerably increased over the last years. NAFLD is currently the most common cause of chronic liver disease in the developing world. The diagnosis of NAFLD/NASH is often incidental, as the early-stage of disease is frequently free of symptoms. Most patients recognized with NAFLD have severe obesity and other obesity-related disease such as type 2 diabetes mellitus (T2DM), insulin-resistance, dyslipidemia and hypertension. The only proven method for NAFLD improvement and resolution is weight loss. Bariatric surgery leads to significant and long-term weight loss as well as improvement of coexisting diseases. There is a lot of evidence suggesting that metabolic/bariatric surgery is an effective method of NAFLD treatment that leads to reduction in steatosis, hepatic inflammation and fibrosis. However, there is still a need to perform long-term studies in order to determine the role of bariatric surgery as a treatment option for NAFLD and NASH. This review discusses current evidence about epidemiology, pathogenesis and treatment options for NAFLD including bariatric/metabolic surgery and its effect on improvement and resolution of NAFLD.

Keywords: non-alcoholic fatty liver disease; non-alcoholic steatohepatitis; obesity; bariatric surgery; laparoscopic sleeve gastrectomy; Roux-en-Y gastric bypass

Citation: Głuszyńska, P.; Lemancewicz, D.; Dzięcioł, J.B.; Razak Hady, H. Non-Alcoholic Fatty Liver Disease (NAFLD) and Bariatric/Metabolic Surgery as Its Treatment Option: A Review. *J. Clin. Med.* **2021**, *10*, 5721. https://doi.org/10.3390/jcm10245721

Academic Editor: David Benaiges Boix

Received: 31 October 2021
Accepted: 3 December 2021
Published: 7 December 2021

1. Introduction

Unhealthy lifestyle and dietary habits have contributed to an alarming increase in obesity and obesity-related diseases worldwide. The epidemic of obesity has led to a significant increase in the prevalence of non-alcoholic fatty liver disease (NAFLD). The prevalence of NAFLD is 25–30% of the general population and 50–90% in patients with obesity [1,2]. A recent report estimates the constant increase in the prevalence of NAFLD by the year 2030 with significant rise in hepatocellular carcinoma (HCC) and liver-related deaths [3]. NAFLD is the initial, uncomplicated medical condition that may lead to end-stage liver disease from non-alcoholic simple steatosis and steatohepatitis (NASH) to fibrosis and liver cirrhosis with its clinical consequences such as: variceal bleeding, ascites, renal failure, encephalopathy and spontaneous bacterial peritonitis [4,5]. Data from the European Liver Transplant Registry (ELTR) and United Network for Organ Sharing (UNOS) show that NAFLD and NASH have been the most rapidly growing indication for liver transplant within the last 20 years. Additionally, NAFLD is presently the most frequent non-viral hepatitis-related indication for liver transplant among adults in the United States [6,7].

NAFLD is frequently recognized as the hepatic manifestation of metabolic syndrome (MS) and remains in close association with components of MS that include increased fasting plasma glucose level and type 2 diabetes mellitus (T2DM), increased waist circumference, hypertension and dyslipidemia [8,9]. Recent studies have shown that over 80% of patients undergoing bariatric surgery have been diagnosed with NAFLD or NASH [10,11].

Bariatric/metabolic surgery is an effective treatment for morbid obesity that provides sustained and considerable weight loss with the improvement of obesity-related diseases. Reduction in body weight induced by bariatric surgery leads to potential decrease in hepatic inflammation, fat accumulation and fibrosis [12]. In the forthcoming sections of this review, we provide the information about pathogenesis, diagnosis and potential treatment options including conservative, pharmacological and bariatric surgery procedures for NAFLD according to the available literature.

2. Epidemiology

A systematic review conducted by Younossi et al. estimated the pooled, overall global prevalence of NAFLD diagnosed by imaging to be 25.24% (95% confidence interval (CI): 22.10–28.65). Their study reported the highest prevalence of NAFLD in South America (30.4%) and the Middle East (31.8%), whereas the lowest rate was reported in Africa (13.5%). The prevalences of NAFLD among patients diagnosed by blood test were 13.00% (95% CI: 4.44–32.47) for Europe, 12.89% (95% CI: 8.32–19.44) for North America, and 9.26% (95% CI: 7.07–12.05) for Asia [13]. According to Cholangitas et al., pooled NAFLD prevalence was 26.9% in the adult European population. Pooled NAFLD prevalence was higher in men than in women (32.8% vs. 19.6%). There were no differences between Mediterranean and non-Mediterranean countries. The pooled prevalence of NAFLD was higher in studies using ultrasonography and fatty liver index (FLI) for NAFLD diagnosis (27.2% and 30.1%, respectively) [14]. Current trends in dietary habits and preponderance of sedentary lifestyle contribute to the constant growth in the incidence of NAFLD worldwide. The National Health and Nutrition Examination Surveys data demonstrated a rise in the prevalence of NAFLD in the US from 5.5% (1988–1994) to 11% (2005–2008) [8], as it is estimated that the epidemic of obesity will continue to fuel the burden of NAFLD.

3. Pathogenesis of NAFLD

The pathogenesis of NAFLD is multifactorial; however, its understanding is crucial for the proper therapeutic interventions. A two-hit model of NAFLD development was proposed with the first hit consisting of hepatic steatosis, which then sensitizes the liver to injury mediated by "second hits" including: inflammatory cytokines, adipokines and oxidative stress leading to steatohepatitis and fibrosis [15]. This two-hit model has lost some favor, as it turned out too simplistic to fully describe the evolution of NAFLD, as different factors affecting disease development and progression were unveiled. Nowadays, the two-hit hypothesis was replaced with the "multiple hit" theory, which recognizes the following components in NAFLD pathophysiology: insulin resistance, obesity, gut microbiota, environmental and genetic factors. The key concept of NAFLD pathogenesis is excessive triglycerides hepatic accumulation as a result of imbalance between free fatty acids influx and efflux [16]. Excessive hepatic fat accumulation occurs in patients with obesity and T2DM, who have impaired insulin signaling. Insulin resistance leads to an uncontrolled lipolysis in adipose tissue that results in significant deposition of nonesterified free fatty acids (NFFA) in the liver [17]. Other factors contributing to excessive hepatic fat accumulation are dietary fats and de novo lipogenesis. Among dietary factors, fructose seems to have an important role, as it is both a substrate and an inducer for de novo hepatic lipogenesis [18]. The excessive inflow of triglycerides to the liver leads to inflammation, reactive oxygen species (ROS) formation, hepatocyte impaired function and lipotoxicity. Hepatocellular cells injury activates apoptotic pathways causing cellular death. This results in the progression from noninflammatory isolated steatosis to the development of nonalcoholic steatohepatitis with a risk of further evolution to fibrosis, cirrhosis and at worst to the development of hepatocellular carcinoma [19,20].

Available research shows that gut microbiota is also associated with the development of NAFLD and NASH [21,22]. The imbalance between protective and harmful bacteria, damage of intestinal barrier and disturbed immune response cause that bacterial products reach the liver through the portal vein and activate pathways responsible for proinflammatory response. Additionally, microbiota dysbiosis increases lipoprotein lipase activity and triglycerides accumulation by either decreasing choline levels or increasing methylamine level, which promotes development of NAFLD [23]. Damage of intestinal epithelial membrane leads to an impaired transport across the mucosa. Rahman et al. proved that compromised intestinal epithelial permeability contributes to development of NAFLD. The above-mentioned study showed that mice with defects or loss of junctional adhesion molecule A (JAM-A) in intestinal epithelial membrane develop more severe steatohepatitis after a diet high in saturated fat, fructose and cholesterol for 8 weeks. They also found out that colon tissue from patients with NAFLD has lower level of JAM-A and higher inflammation status as compared to patients without NAFLD [24]. Significant changes in gut microbiota are reported after bariatric surgery. Possible mechanisms for the intestinal microbiota changes include reduction in body weight, changes in food consumption, changes in ghrelin and leptin secretion and alternations in stomach pH [25,26].

Genes also have a role in the development of NAFLD. It has been discovered that genetic polymorphism can influence the NAFLD development and progression by variability in oxidative stress, inflammation and FFAs accumulation. The main genetic determinant of interindividual differences in hepatic fat content is nonsynonymous variant of patatin-like phospholipase 3 (*PNPLA3*) gene (rs738409 C/G, I148M), also known as adiponutrion [27]. The PNPLA3 variant has impaired hydrolysis activity and is less available for degradation, which leads to retention in of TG and polyunsaturated fatty acids priming accumulation of hepatic fat [28]. Another relevant genetic variant related to progressive NAFLD is the transmembrane 6 superfamily member 2 (*TM6SF2*), which is responsible for lipid retention and impairment of very low-density lipoprotein (VLDL) release by liver [29]. Loss of function in rs1260326 variant in the *GCKR* gene is also associated with increased TG concentration, steatosis and liver damage [30]. The understanding of possible nutrigenomic approaches may lead to improvement of NAFLD management and introduction of proper therapeutic strategy Figure 1.

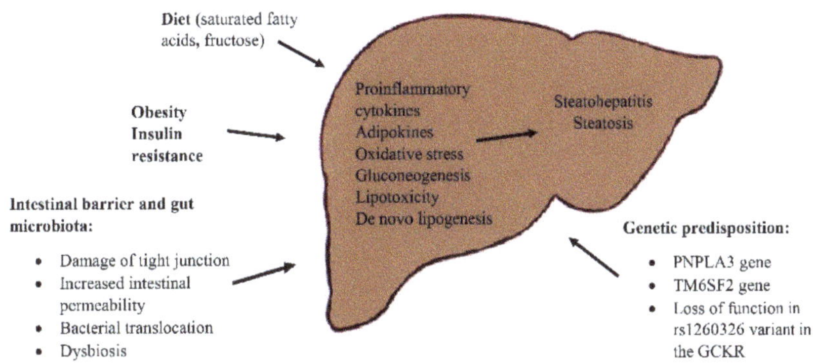

Figure 1. Pathogenesis of NAFLD.

4. Diagnosis of NAFLD

NAFLD is defined as an excessive accumulation of triglycerides in hepatocytes either by imaging or histology, simultaneously with exclusion of any significant alcohol consumption and other liver diseases [31]. Mildly elevated serum aminotransferases are the primary abnormality in NASH, although they may remain at normal level in up to 80% of patients. The alanine transaminase (ALT) level is generally higher than that of aspartate aminotransferase (AST). Other common findings in blood examination include high serum triglyceride and low HDL cholesterol level. With the development of the disease hypoalbuminemia, hyperbilirubinemia and thrombocytopenia may occur due to progression of liver injury [32]. Ultrasound is a non-invasive and widely available tool for the diagnosis of NAFLD. Characteristic sonographic findings for NAFLD include heterogeneity of liver; thick subcutaneous depth (>2 cm); quick attenuation of image 4–5 cm of depth, making deeper structures difficult to decipher, and; dispersion of echogenicity [33]. However, the use of ultrasound is very limited in patients with overweight and obesity due to excessive subcutaneous fat accumulation. The assessment of liver fibrosis without histological examination can be made by a combination of serological and imaging tests. There are several scoring systems used to estimate liver fibrosis without performing liver biopsy. NAFLD fibrosis score (NFS) is calculated based on following measurements: age, BMI, glucose blood concentration, platelet count, albumin serum level and AST/ALT ratio. Another one is the BARD score, which is composed of 3 variables: ALT/AST ratio, BMI and the presence of diabetes. BARD score of 0 or 1 are of high (96%) negative predictive value (NPV) for advanced fibrosis [34]. The AASSLD guidelines suggest the use of NFS or APRI score as non-invasive tools for clinical diagnosis. It is worth mentioning that NFS was developed as a scoring system for usage in patients with NAFLD [35]. The available ways to estimate liver fibrosis together with measured parameters are listed in Table 1 [36].

Table 1. Noninvasive assessment of liver fibrosis based on biochemical parameters.

Name of Scoring System	Used Measures
NAFLD fibrosis score (NFS)	Age, blood glucose level, BMI, platelet count, albumin, AST/ALT ratio
APRI score	aspartate aminotransferase to platelet ratio index
BAAT score	BMI, age, ALT, triglyceride level
BARD score	BMI, AST/ALT ratio, presence/absence of diabetes
Enhanced liver fibrosis (ELF) index	Plasma level of hyaluronic acid (HA), tissue inhibitor of metalloproteinase (TIMP-1), procollagen III amino terminal peptide (PIIINP)
Hepascore	Bilirubin, gamma-glutamyl transpeptidase (γ-GTP), α2-macroglobulin, hyaluronic acid levels
FIBROSpect	hyaluronic acid, TIMP-1 and α2-macroglobulin
Fibrometer	prothrombin index, platelet count, AST, urea, α2-macroglobulin, hyaluronic acid
NashTest	age, sex, height, weight, serum triglycerides, cholesterol, α2-macroglobulin, apolipoprotein A1, haptoglobin, γ-GTP, ALT, AST, total bilirubin

Magnetic resonance imaging (MRI) is a non-invasive method widely accepted by patients and doctors, and may be used as an alternative to liver biopsy in assessment of hepatic fat content [37]. Several studies have shown that magnetic resonance elastography (MRE) is a diagnostic tool for prediction of hepatic fibrosis stage in NAFLD with sensitivity of 63–87%, and specificity of 81–95% [38]. Another tool is magnetic resonance imaging-proton density fat fraction (MRI-PDFF), which has high accuracy in detecting hepatic steatosis and quantifying the degree of steatosis in NAFLD [39]. However, the gold standard for NAFLD diagnosis remains the percutaneous liver biopsy. Although liver biopsy is expensive, has increased risk of adverse events and requires professional interpretation, it should be performed in patients who benefit the most from making the right diagnosis.

According to the American Association of Liver Disease (AASLD), liver biopsy should be considered in patients with NAFLD who are at higher risk of steatohepatitis and advanced fibrosis, including those with diabetes and/or metabolic syndrome. Referral for liver biopsy should be also considered in patients who have findings of concern for cirrhosis, such as hypoalbuminemia, thrombocytopenia, AST > ALT and in patients undergoing cholecystectomy or bariatric surgery, when intraoperative biopsy is a low risk procedure [40]. The main histological characteristics of NAFLD is the accumulation of fat in the form of triglycerides within hepatocytes. The presence of >5% steatotic hepatocytes in a liver tissue is the criteria for the histological definition of NAFLD. In NAFLD, steatosis is usually macrovesicular, which means that lipid vacuole fills nearly the whole hepatocyte, and the nucleus is pushed to the side. A simple four-point scoring system that takes into account only macro- and/or mediovesicualar steatosis and estimates the percentage of hepatocytes covered with steatosis is used for steatosis grading. Normal liver (grade 0) contains fat in <5% of hepatocytes; in grade 1, 2, 3 steatotic hepatocytes are present in <33%, 33–66% and >66% of hepatocytes, respectively, [41]. In the case of NASH histological diagnosis criteria include steatosis with hepatocellular (usually in the form of ballooning) and lobular inflammation [42]. There are three scoring systems that are currently used in grading the histological features of NAFLD/NASH, which are the Brunt system, the NAFLD Activity Score (NAS) and the Steatosis-Activity-Fibrosis (SAF) System [42–45]. Scoring in individual systems together with scored histological features are presented in Tables 2–5.

Table 2. Brunt system to grade NASH activity.

Grade	Steatosis 1: ≤33% 2: 33–66% 3: ≥66%	Ballooning (Zonal Location and Severity Recorded)	Inflammation L-Lobular (0–3) 0: Absent 1: <2 foci/20× field 2: 2–4 foci/20× field 3: >4 foci/20× field	Inflammation P-Portal (0–3) 0: Absent 1: Mild 2: Moderate 3: Severe
Grade 1 (mild)	1–2	Minimal, zone 3	L = 1–2	P = 0–1
Grade 2 (moderate)	2–3	Present, zone 3	L = 2	P = 1–2
Grade 3 (severe)	2–3	Marked, predominantly zone 3	L = 3	P = 1–2

Table 3. Brunt system for staging NASH fibrosis.

Stage	Zone 3, Sinusoidal	Portal Based	Bridging	Cirrhosis
1	Focal or extensive	0	0	0
2	Focal or extensive	Focal or extensive	0	0
3	Bridging septa	Bridging septa	+	0
4	±	±	Extensive	+

Table 4. The NAFLD Activity Score.

Steatosis Grade (S)	Lobular Inflammation (L)	Hepatocyte Ballooning (B)
0: <5%	0: none	0: none
1: 5–33%	1: <2 foci/20× field	1: mild, few ballooned cells
2: 34–66%	2: 2–4 foci/20× field	2: moderate-marked, many ballooned cells
3: >66%	3: >4 foci/20× field	
	Fibrosis (evaluated with Masson trichrome stain)	
	0	None
	1a	Mild zone 3 sinusoidal fibrosis (trichrome stain to be identified)
	1b	Moderate zone 3 sinusoidal fibrosis (could be detected on H&E examination)
	1c	Portal fibrosis only
	2	Zone 3 sinusoidal fibrosis and periportal fibrosis
	3	Bridging fibrosis
	4	Cirrhosis

Table 5. Steatosis-Activity-Fibrosis (SAF) scoring system of NAFLD.

Steatosis Grade (S): 0–3 (Based on Percentage of Hepatocytes with Large and/or Medium Size Intracytoplasmic Lipid)	Lobular Inflammation: 0–2	Hepatocyte Ballooning: 0–2	Activity Grade (A): 0–4 (Sum of Score for Ballooning and Lobular Inflammation)	Fibrosis Stage (F)
S0: <5%	0: none	0: none	A1 (A = 1): mild activity	F0: no significant fibrosis
S1: 5–33%	1: ≤2 foci/20× field	1: cluster of rounded hepatocytes with pale/reticulated cytoplasm	A2 (A = 2): moderate activity	F1: 1a mild zone 3 sinusoidal fibrosis 1b moderate zone 3 sinusoidal fibrosis 1c portal fibrosis only
S2: 34–66%	2: >2 foci/20× field	2: same as 1 with enlarged hepatocytes (more than twice of normal size)	A3 and A4 (A > 2): severe activity	F2: zone 3 sinusoidal fibrosis with periportal fibrosis
S3: >66%				F3: bridging fibrosis F4: cirrhosis

5. Treatment Options of NAFLD

A considerable amount of research points out strong evidence between NASH and lifestyle modifications such as: weight loss, dietary changes and physical exercises. It has been proven that weight reduction by 5 to 10% in individuals with obesity can result with improvement in all features of NASH, including inflammation and fibrosis [46]. Dietary changes should include decrease in calorie intake, as well as changes in composition of a diet that includes reduction of carbohydrate intake (particularly simple carbohydrates, e.g., sweets, fruit juices, honey, fruits, flavored yoghurts), reduction of dietary fats with emphasis on saturated and trans fatty acids, increase in protein intake, ensuring supply of antioxidants, probiotics and prebiotics. Abstinence from alcohol is also recommended as a lifestyle intervention in NAFLD treatment [47]. However, it is very important to notice that implementing lifestyle modifications in patients with obesity can be problematic and usually does not bring the intended results. A study conducted by Dudekula et al. that aimed to find weight loss predictors in patients with obesity and NAFLD showed that 66% of research participants experienced weight reduction of less than 5% during the observation period. Weight loss between 5 to 10% was observed in 12.9% patients and reduction in body weight >10% was seen only in 6.9% of study participants [48]. Additionally, most individuals with obesity are more likely to regain weight in a short period of time [49]. The general idea of NAFLD treatment focuses on co-existing diseases such as obesity, dyslipidemia, insulin resistance and diabetes mellitus.

According to the European Association for the Study of the Liver (EASL) guidelines, pharmacological therapy should be implemented in patients with progressive NASH (bridging fibrosis and cirrhosis); early stage NASH with high risk for disease progression (increased ALT, presence of metabolic syndrome and diabetes mellitus, age >50 years) and active NASH with high necroinflammatory activities [50]. Pharmacological therapy options for NAFLD include: antidiabetic drugs, drugs modifying lipid profile, anti-obesity drugs, vitamin supplementation and novel therapeutic treatment that includes interference with inflammatory, fibrotic and apoptotic pathways. Among antidiabetics drugs pioglitazone, glucagon-like-peptide (GLP-1) analogues and liraglutide were found to be effective in NAFLD/NASH treatment. Pioglitazone was shown to significantly improve steatosis and inflammation, together with systemic and adipose- tissue resistance in one-year observation in patients with T2DM [51]. Research conducted by Bril et al. confirmed reduction of liver fibrosis and increase in adipose tissues insulin sensitivity. However, the effect was significantly greater in patients with type 2 diabetes than in patients with prediabetes [52]. Liraglutide is a long-acting GLP-1 agonist that improves key metabolic risk factors: weight, body mass index and glucose level. Besides its metabolic improvement, liraglutide was found to significantly improve liver steatosis in NAFLD patients by downregulating the expression of inflammatory mediators in the TNF-α signaling pathway [53,54]. Additionally, liraglutide affects the renin-angiotensin system (RAS), which is overactivated during NAFLD. Liraglutide was found to down regulate the ACE/Ang II/AT1R axis and antagonizes hepatocellular steatosis [55].

In the case of metformin, which is commonly used in prediabetes and diabetes treatment, no strong evidence for histological response was found in NAFLD patients [56]. Despite the fact that metformin has no specific influence on liver histology, it is recommended in NAFLD/NASH patients with T2DM due to its pleiotropic effect including reduction in body mass, and decrease in ALT activity and improvement of cardiovascular system [57]. Furthermore, a recent animal study conducted by Brandt et al. suggests that metformin has a protective effect on the development of NAFLD, which results from a protection against intestinal barrier impairment, e.g., loss of tight junction proteins. Metformin also alters intestinal microbiota composition in the proximal small intestine, which has a beneficial effect on steatosis development [58].

Vitamin supplementation has been also found to have its role in NAFLD treatment. Vitamins with antioxidant properties, such as Vitamin C and E decrease the oxidative stress that is seen in patients with NAFLD and NASH. Additionally, Vitamin E has anti-inflammatory and anti-apoptotic properties that can retard the fibrosis process and prevent from cirrhosis by modulating inflammatory response and cellular proliferation [59]. It should be mentioned that supplementation of Vitamin E is recommended for patients with NASH and stage 2 fibrosis proven in biopsy and without a family history of prostate cancer, as it was proven that high daily dose of Vitamin E (≥400 IU per day) is associated with progression of prostate cancer [60].

Data about usage of weight-loss medication in NAFLD are very scarce in the available literature. To date, only Orlistat was found to contribute to improvement in hepatic fat content, as well as the activity of ALT and AST during at least 24 weeks of therapy [61]. It is thought that Orlistat may have a potential beneficial effect on NAFLD as it stimulates weight loss, however it is not clear whether it has an independent effect on liver function. Other weight-loss medications such as naltrexone, bupropion and topiramate have no evidence of usefulness in NAFLD treatment [62].

The use of statins in NAFLD treatment is still controversial. Undoubtedly, statins decrease the level of total cholesterol, low-density lipoprotein cholesterol (LDL-C) and triglycerides, and hence limit the cardiovascular risk [63]. In the study conducted by Hyogo et al., patients were treated with 10 mg atorvastatin daily. Researchers observed significant reduction in AST, ALT and GGT concentrations as well as decrease in NAFLD Activity Score (NAS), which includes steatosis, hepatocyte ballooning and lobular inflammation [64]. The use of statins among patients with NAFLD should be implemented with co-existing dyslipidemia, as its protective effect on the cardiovascular system outweighs other adverse events and low efficacy on hepatic histopathology [47].

Among novel therapeutic perspectives, farnesoid X receptor (FXR) agonist has been investigated. Obeticholic acid (OCA or 6α-ethyl chenodeoxycholic acid, initially known as INT-747) is an FXR agonist registered for the treatment of primary biliary cholangitis due to its anticholestatic and hepatoprotective properties [65]. Data from recently performed clinical trials prove that OCA is effective in patients with biopsy-proven NASH or NAFLD [66,67]. The primary endpoint of FLINT study was histological improvement in NAFLD activity score of at least 2 points, which was achieved in 45% of patients receiving 25 mg OCA daily [66]. A study conducted by Mudaliar et al. showed that the administration of 25 or 50 mg OCA daily increases insulin sensitivity and reduces markers of hepatic inflammation and fibrosis in patient with NAFLD and T2DM [67]. Another farnesoid X receptor agonist, cilofexor (GS-9674) is under investigation as monotherapy or in combination with an acetyl-CoA carboxylase inhibitor, firsocostat (GS-0976). The combination of these two drugs showed improvement in liver steatosis and stiffness and serum markers of hepatic fibrosis [68]. Peroxisome proliferator-activated receptor (PPAR)-γ agonists such as rosiglitazone and pioglitazone have been under investigation for potential effects in NAFLD/NASH patients. The use of pioglitazone in patients with biopsy-proven NASH improves liver function and decreases liver fat content. Cusi et al. conducted a placebo-controlled RCT of 101 adults with NASH and T2DM. They documented that 58% of patients assigned to pioglitazone group (45 mg once daily) achieved the primary outcome (reduction in NAFLD activity score of at least 2 points without worsening of fibrosis) and 51% had resolution of NASH. Pioglitazone treatment was also associated with improvement in individual histological scores, including the fibrosis score, reducing hepatic triglyceride content from 19% to 7%, and improving adipose tissue, hepatic, and muscle insulin sensitivity [69]. A Fatty Liver Improvement with Rosiglitazone Therapy (FLIRT) trial showed that rosiglitazone improved steatosis and normalized transaminase levels in 47% of patients. However, no effect on other histologic lesions was documented [70].

Some experimental studies have focused on the specific inhibition of the fibrosis process in liver with the use of an inhibitory antibody to lysyl oxidase-2 (LOXL-2). LOXL-2 up-regulation was noticed in patients with NAFLD and T2DM and LOXL-2 hepatic and circulating levels correlate with histological fibrosis progression [71]. LOXL-2 inhibition paves the way for macrophage-mediated collagen degradation in liver fibrosis. However, in two phase 2b trails of patients with bonding fibrosis due to nonalcoholic steatohepatitis, simtuzumab (monoclonal LOXL-2 antibody) was found to be ineffective in decreasing hepatic collagen content [72]. Additionally, compounds interfering with apoptotic pathways have been investigated as a treatment option for NAFLD/NASH. An example is selonsertib, which is an inhibitor of the apoptosis signal-regulating kinase 1 (ASK1), and plays a significant role in hepatocyte inflammation, injury and fibrosis. In a phase 2 trial, selonsertib appeared to improve liver fibrosis in a substantial proportion of patients with NASH and stage 2 or 3 fibrosis, suggesting its potential use in NAFLD pharmacological therapy [73]. However, results from randomized phase III STELLAR trials did not show evidence that selonsertib reduces fibrosis in patients with NASH and advanced liver scarring [74].

6. Bariatric Surgery and NAFLD

Bariatric surgery aims not only to achieve considerable, long-term weight loss but also to improve the course of obesity-related diseases such as T2DM, hypertension, dyslipidemia, obstructive sleep apnea. It also reduces the risk of cardiovascular diseases such as myocardial infarction and ischemic stroke and decreases overall mortality [75–77]. A meta-analysis conducted by Sutanto et al. showed significant reduction in the incidence of major adverse cardiovascular events in bariatric surgery group as compared to the no-surgery group (OR = 0.49; 95% CI 0.40–0.60; $p < 0.00001$; I2 = 93%) [78]. Among recently available surgical methods, Roux-en-Y gastric bypass (RYGB) and laparoscopic sleeve gastrectomy (LSG) are the most commonly performed worldwide. A study conducted by Mummadi et al. summarized 15 studies with 766 paired liver biopsies. Their investigation showed the pooled proportion of patients with improvement or resolution in steatosis was 91.6% (95% confidence interval (CI), 82.4–97.6%), in steatohepatitis was 81.3% (95% CI, 61.9–94.9%), in fibrosis was 65.5% (95% CI, 38.2–88.1%), and for complete resolution of NASH was 69.5% (95% CI, 42.4–90.8%) after bariatric surgery [79]. The Swedish Obese Subjects (SOS) study showed reduction in both ALT and AST values after bariatric surgery in both short and long-term observation (2 and 10-year follow-up) [80].

NAFLD is closely associated with obesity, T2DM and other features of metabolic syndrome. All mechanisms involved in improving obesity and T2DM that appear after bariatric surgery seem to have a crucial role in amelioration or resolution of NAFLD. Weight reduction due to bariatric surgery causes inflammatory changes in patients with obesity. Klein et al. showed that gastric bypass procedure decreases the hepatic expression of factors involved in the progression of liver inflammation (macrophage chemoattractant protein 1 (MCP-1), and interleukin (IL-8)) and fibrogenesis (transforming growth factor-β1 (TGF-β1), tissue inhibitor of metalloproteinase 1 (TIMP-1), α-smooth muscle actin (α-SMA), and collagen-α1(I)) [81]. Cazzo et al. showed a significant decrease in mean NAFLD fibrosis score after RYGB and resolution rate of 55% of severe fibrosis in 12-month observation [82]. Moreover, RYGB contributes to significant reduction in NAFLD activity score, steatosis, inflammation and liver ballooning during 1-year observation [83,84].

LSG is also considered to improve the course of NAFLD. Nobili et al. showed reduced activation of local cellular compartments (hepatic progenitor cells, hepatic stellated cells, macrophages) induced by LSG, which led to the improvement in NAFLD Activity Score and liver fibrosis [85]. A study conducted by Cabré et al. proved that the histology and liver function of patients with morbid obesity significantly improved after LSG due to mechanisms involved in the reduction of oxidative stress and inflammation. They observed significant reduction in the hepatic immunochemical expression of oxidation, inflammation and fibrosis markers such as: PON-1, 4-hydroxy-2-nonenal, CD68, chemokine ligand 2 (CCL2), C-C chemokine receptor type 2 (CCR2), TNF-α, and galectin-3 between baseline liver tissue and 12 months after LSG [86]. Weight loss induced by LSG leads to the improvement in liver histology in terms of steatosis, liver fibrosis, lobular inflammation and hepatocyte ballooning. In a study conducted by Salman et al., among 81 patients undergoing LSG, 9 (11.1%) showed no steatosis at the end of 18-month follow-up, 25 (30.9%) showed no hepatocyte ballooning, 37 (45.7%) showed no lobular inflammation, and 33 (40.7%) showed complete absence of fibrosis. The above-mentioned study also showed significant improvement in postoperative liver function tests (AST, ALT, GGTP). An 18-month observation also revealed an increase in adiponectin levels and a reduction in serum levels of leptin and resistin, when compared to presurgical values. The above-mentioned data prove that both LSG and RYGB are significant surgical methods for NAFLD/NASH treatment [87].

As presented above, bariatric surgery provides proven NAFLD amelioration; however, the remaining question is whether RYGB or LSG is more effective. A systematic review and meta-analysis performed by Baldwin et al. compared RYGB and LSG using 4 separate criteria: AST and ALT concentration, NAFLD activity score and NAFLD fibrosis score. Patients undergoing both procedures showed significant reduction in AST and ALT values. Head-to-head comparison of AST mean differences trended toward LSG, but it was statistically non-significant. This study failed to show superiority between RYGB and LSG in ameliorating NAFLD [88]. Cherla et al. also proved the normalization of the liver function test by the end of the first postoperative year; however, they did not find significant differences between the SG and RYGB groups [89]. A meta-analysis performed by Silva et al. showed that RYGB patients achieve significant reduction of steatohepatitis and fibrosis, while patients undergoing LSG presented significant reduction only of steatohepatitis. According to their study, the NAFLD Activity Score significantly improved after both procedures and no differences were found between LSG and RYGB regarding histopathological changes [90]. A study conducted by Pedersen et al. showed that NAS reduced significantly in both RYGB and LSG patients 12-months after the surgery. However, RYGB patients had significantly more reduced (p = 0.007) liver steatosis (−0.91 (95% CI −1.47–−1.2) than SG patients (−0.33 (95% CI −0.54–−0.13) and greater improvement in the plasma lipid profile [83]. Luo at el. investigated liver volume and fat density in MRI in patients undergoing bariatric surgery. Their study showed that RYGB patients achieved higher weight loss and higher BMI loss when compared to the LSG group. However, the percentage decrease in liver volume and MRI-PDFF did not differ significantly between groups [91].

Despite the significant role of bariatric surgery in the treatment of NAFLD, there are some patients that will develop new or worsened features of NAFLD after bariatric procedure. The meta-analysis performed by Lee et al. showed that 12% of patients experienced development or worsening of NAFLD (95% CI, 5–20%) [92]. A 5-year prospective study performed by Mathurin et al. showed that 19.8% of patients experienced fibrosis progression 5 years after bariatric surgery for unknown reason [93]. Aggravation of NAFLD after bariatric procedure should be kept in mind when qualifying patients for bariatric surgery.

7. Conclusions

The current evidence suggests that bariatric/metabolic surgery for patients with morbid obesity leads to improvement or resolution of NAFLD/NASH in terms of steatosis, hepatic inflammation and fibrosis. Although the results of available cohort research are satisfying, they have not been proved in clinical randomized trails. Further, long-term studies are still needed to confirm the recommendation of bariatric surgery as a treatment option for NAFLD.

Author Contributions: Conceptualization, P.G. and H.R.H.; validation, P.G., D.L., H.R.H.; resources, P.G., D.L., J.B.D.; data curation, P.G., D.L., J.B.D., H.R.H.; writing—original draft preparation, P.G. and D.L.; writing—review and editing, P.G., D.L., H.R.H.; supervision, J.B.D. and H.R.H. All authors have read and agreed to the published version of the manuscript.

Funding: This research received no external funding.

Institutional Review Board Statement: Not applicable.

Informed Consent Statement: Not applicable.

Data Availability Statement: Not applicable.

Conflicts of Interest: The authors declare no conflict of interest.

References

1. Blachier, M.; Leleu, H.; Peck-Radosavljevic, M.; Valla, D.C.; Roudot-Thoraval, F. The burden of liver disease in Europe: A review of available epidemiological data. *J. Hepatol.* **2013**, *58*, 593–608. [CrossRef]
2. Divella, R.; Mazzocca, A.; Daniele, A.; Sabbà, C.; Paradiso, A. Obesity, Nonalcoholic Fatty Liver Disease and Adipocytokines Network in Promotion of Cancer. *Int. J. Biol. Sci.* **2019**, *15*, 610–616. [CrossRef] [PubMed]
3. Estes, C.; Razavi, H.; Loomba, R.; Younossi, Z.; Sanyal, A.J. Modeling the epidemic of nonalcoholic fatty liver disease demonstrates an exponential increase in burden of disease. *Hepatology* **2018**, *67*, 1231–1233. [CrossRef] [PubMed]
4. Calzadilla Bertot, L.; Adams, L.A. The Natural Course of Non-Alcoholic Fatty Liver Disease. *Int. J. Mol. Sci.* **2016**, *17*, 774. [CrossRef] [PubMed]
5. Schuppan, D.; Afdhal, N.H. Liver cirrhosis. *Lancet* **2008**, *371*, 838–851. [CrossRef]
6. Cotter, T.G.; Charlton, M. Nonalcoholic steatohepatitis after liver transplantation. *Liver Transpl.* **2020**, *26*, 141–159. [CrossRef] [PubMed]
7. Adam, R.; Karam, V.; Cailliez, V.; O Grady, J.G.; Mirza, D.; Cherqui, D.; Klempnauer, J.; Salizzoni, M.; Pratschke, J.; Jamieson, N.; et al. 2018 Annual report of the European Liver Transplant Registry (ELTR)—50-year evolution of liver transplantation. *Transpl. Int.* **2018**, *31*, 1293–1317. [CrossRef] [PubMed]
8. Younossi, Z.M.; Stepanova, M.; Afendy, M.; Fang, Y.; Younossi, Y.; Mir, H.; Srishord, M. Changes in the prevalence of the most common causes of chronic liver diseases in the United States from 1988 to 2008. *Clin. Gastroenterol. Hepatol.* **2011**, *9*, 524–530. [CrossRef] [PubMed]
9. Golabi, P.; Otgonsuren, M.; de Avila, L.; Sayiner, M.; Rafiq, N.; Younossi, Z.M. Components of metabolic syndrome increase the risk of mortality in nonalcoholic fatty liver disease (NAFLD). *Medicine* **2018**, *97*, e0214. [CrossRef] [PubMed]
10. Rheinwalt, K.P.; Drebber, U.; Schierwagen, R.; Klein, S.; Neumann, U.P.; Ulmer, T.F.; Plamper, A.; Kroh, A.; Schipper, S.; Odenthal, M.; et al. Baseline Presence of NAFLD Predicts Weight Loss after Gastric Bypass Surgery for Morbid Obesity. *J. Clin. Med.* **2020**, *9*, 3430. [CrossRef] [PubMed]
11. Soresi, M.; Cabibi, D.; Giglio, R.V.; Martorana, S.; Guercio, G.; Porcasi, R.; Terranova, A.; Lazzaro, A.L.; Emma, M.R.; Augello, G.; et al. The Prevalence of NAFLD and Fibrosis in Bariatric Surgery Patients and the Reliability of Noninvasive Diagnostic Methods. *Biomed. Res. Int.* **2020**, *2020*, 5023157. [CrossRef]
12. Madsbad, S.; Dirksen, C.; Holst, J.J. Mechanisms of changes in glucose metabolism and bodyweight after bariatric surgery. *Lancet Diabetes Endocrinol.* **2014**, *2*, 152–164. [CrossRef]
13. Younossi, Z.M.; Koenig, A.B.; Abdelatif, D.; Fazel, Y.; Henry, L.; Wymer, M. Global epidemiology of nonalcoholic fatty liver disease-Meta-analytic assessment of prevalence, incidence, and outcomes. *Hepatology* **2016**, *64*, 73–84. [CrossRef] [PubMed]
14. Cholongitas, E.; Pavlopoulou, I.; Papatheodoridi, M.; Markakis, G.E.; Bouras, E.; Haidich, A.B.; Papatheodoridis, G. Epidemiology of nonalcoholic fatty liver disease in Europe: A systematic review and meta-analysis. *Ann. Gastroenterol.* **2021**, *34*, 404–414. [CrossRef]

15. Buzzetti, E.; Pinzani, M.; Tsochatzis, E.A. The multiple-hit pathogenesis of non-alcoholic fatty liver disease (NAFLD). *Metabolism* **2016**, *65*, 1038–1048. [CrossRef] [PubMed]
16. Italian Association for the Study of the Liver (AISF). AISF position paper on nonalcoholic fatty liver disease (NAFLD): Updates and future directions. *Dig. Liver Dis.* **2017**, *49*, 471–483. [CrossRef] [PubMed]
17. Anstee, Q.M.; Targher, G.; Day, C.P. Progression of NAFLD to diabetes mellitus, cardiovascular disease or cirrhosis. *Nat. Rev. Gastroenterol. Hepatol.* **2013**, *10*, 330–344. [CrossRef]
18. Lambert, J.E.; Ramos-Roman, M.A.; Browning, J.D.; Parks, E.J. Increased de novo lipogenesis is a distinct characteristic of individuals with nonalcoholic fatty liver disease. *Gastroenterology* **2014**, *146*, 726–735. [CrossRef]
19. Hirsova, P.; Ibrabim, S.H.; Gores, G.J.; Malhi, H. Lipotoxic lethal and sublethal stress signaling in hepatocytes: Relevance to NASH pathogenesis. *J. Lipid. Res.* **2016**, *57*, 1758–1770. [CrossRef] [PubMed]
20. Hirsova, P.; Gores, G.J. Death Receptor-Mediated Cell Death and Proinflammatory Signaling in Nonalcoholic Steatohepatitis. *Cell. Mol. Gastroenterol. Hepatol.* **2015**, *1*, 17–27. [CrossRef]
21. Leung, C.; Rivera, L.; Furness, J.B.; Angus, P.W. The role of the gut microbiota in NAFLD. *Nat. Rev. Gastroenterol. Hepatol.* **2016**, *13*, 412–425. [CrossRef] [PubMed]
22. Aron-Wisnewsky, J.; Vigliotti, C.; Witjes, J.; Le, P.; Holleboom, A.G.; Verheij, J.; Nieuwdorp, M.; Clément, K. Gut microbiota and human NAFLD: Disentangling microbial signatures from metabolic disorders. *Nat. Rev. Gastroenterol. Hepatol.* **2020**, *17*, 279–297. [CrossRef] [PubMed]
23. Spencer, M.D.; Hamp, T.J.; Reid, R.W.; Fischer, L.M.; Zeisel, S.H.; Fodor, A.A. Association between composition of the human gastrointestinal microbiome and development of fatty liver with choline deficiency. *Gastroenterology* **2011**, *140*, 976–986. [CrossRef]
24. Rahman, K.; Desai, C.; Iyer, S.S.; Thorn, N.E.; Kumar, P.; Liu, Y.; Smith, T.; Neish, A.S.; Li, H.; Tan, S.; et al. Loss of Junctional Adhesion Molecule A Promotes Severe Steatohepatitis in Mice on a Diet High in Saturated Fat, Fructose, and Cholesterol. *Gastroenterology* **2016**, *151*, 733–746.e12. [CrossRef]
25. Ulker, İ.; Yildiran, H. The effects of bariatric surgery on gut microbiota in patients with obesity: A review of the literature. *Biosci. Microbiota Food Health* **2019**, *38*, 3–9. [CrossRef]
26. Ciobârcă, D.; Cătoi, A.F.; Copăescu, C.; Miere, D.; Crișan, G. Bariatric Surgery in Obesity: Effects on Gut Microbiota and Micronutrient Status. *Nutrients* **2020**, *12*, 235. [CrossRef]
27. Romeo, S.; Kozlitina, J.; Xing, C.; Pertsemlidis, A.; Cox, D.; Pennacchio, L.A.; Boerwinkle, E.; Cohen, C.C.; Hobbs, H.H. Genetic variation in PNPLA3 confers susceptibility to nonalcoholic fatty liver disease. *Nat. Genet.* **2008**, *40*, 1461–1465. [CrossRef]
28. Yuan, L.; Terrault, N.A. PNPLA3 and nonalcoholic fatty liver disease: Towards personalized medicine for fatty liver. *Hepatobiliary Surg. Nutr.* **2020**, *9*, 353–356. [CrossRef]
29. Kozlitina, J.; Smagris, E.; Stender, S.; Nordestgaard, B.G.; Zhou, H.H.; Tybjærg-Hansen, A.; Vogt, T.F.; Hobbs, H.H.; Cohen, J.C. Exome-wide association study identifies a TM6SF2 variant that confers susceptibility to nonalcoholic fatty liver disease. *Nat. Genet.* **2014**, *46*, 352–356. [CrossRef] [PubMed]
30. Beer, N.L.; Tribble, N.D.; McCulloch, L.J.; Roos, C.; Johnson, P.R.; Orho-Melander, M.; Gloyn, A.L. The P446L variant in GCKR associated with fasting plasma glucose and triglyceride levels exerts its effect through increased glucokinase activity in liver. *Hum. Mol. Genet.* **2009**, *18*, 4081–4088. [CrossRef] [PubMed]
31. Hashimoto, E.; Taniai, M.; Tokushige, K. Characteristics and diagnosis of NAFLD/NASH. *J. Gastroenterol. Hepatol.* **2013**, *28*, 64–70. [CrossRef]
32. Pujitha, K.; Savio, J. *Nonalcoholic Fatty Liver*; StatPearls Publishing: Treasure Island, FL, USA, 2021.
33. Khov, N.; Sharma, A.; Riley, T.R. Bedside ultrasound in the diagnosis of nonalcoholic fatty liver disease. *World J. Gastroenterol.* **2014**, *20*, 6821–6825. [CrossRef] [PubMed]
34. Cichoż-Lach, H.; Celiński, K.; Prozorow-Król, B.; Swatek, J.; Słomka, M.; Lach, T. The BARD score and the NAFLD fibrosis score in the assessment of advanced liver fibrosis in nonalcoholic fatty liver disease. *Med. Sci. Monit.* **2012**, *18*, CR735–CR740. [CrossRef]
35. Schmitz, S.M.; Kroh, A.; Ulmer, T.F.; Andruszkow, J.; Luedde, T.; Brozat, J.F.; Neumann, U.P.; Alizai, P.H. Evaluation of NAFLD and fibrosis in obese patients—A comparison of histological and clinical scoring systems. *BMC Gastroenterol.* **2020**, *20*, 254. [CrossRef] [PubMed]
36. Dumitrascu, D.L.; Neuman, M.G. Non-alcoholic fatty liver disease: An update on diagnosis. *Clujul Med.* **2018**, *91*, 147–150. [CrossRef]
37. Reeder, S.B.; Cruite, I.; Hamilton, G.; Sirlin, C.B. Quantitative Assessment of Liver Fat with Magnetic Resonance Imaging and Spectroscopy. *J. Magn. Reson. Imaging* **2011**, *34*, 729–749. [CrossRef]
38. Han, M.A.; Saouaf, R.; Ayoub, W.; Todo, T.; Mena, E.; Noureddin, M. Magnetic resonance imaging and transient elastography in the management of Nonalcoholic Fatty Liver Disease (NAFLD). *Expert Rev. Clin. Pharmacol.* **2017**, *10*, 379–390. [CrossRef] [PubMed]
39. Permutt, Z.; Le, T.A.; Peterson, M.R.; Seki, E.; Brenner, D.A.; Sirlin, C.; Loomba, R. Correlation between liver histology and novel magnetic resonance imaging in adult patients with non-alcoholic fatty liver disease—MRI accurately quantifies hepatic steatosis in NAFLD. *Aliment. Pharmacol. Ther.* **2012**, *36*, 22–29. [CrossRef] [PubMed]

40. Chalasani, N.; Younossi, Z.; Lavine, J.E.; Diehl, A.M.; Brunt, E.M.; Cusi, K.; Charlton, M.; Sanyal, A.J. The diagnosis and management of non-alcoholic fatty liver disease: Practice Guideline by the American Association for the Study of Liver Diseases, American College of Gastroenterology, and the American Gastroenterological Association. *Hepatology* **2012**, *55*, 2005–2023. [CrossRef] [PubMed]
41. Kleiner, D.E.; Brunt, E.M.; Van Natta, M.; Behling, C.; Contos, M.J.; Cummings, O.W.; Ferrell, L.D.; Liu, Y.C.; Torbenson, M.S.; Unalp-Arida, A.; et al. Design and validation of a histological scoring system for nonalcoholic fatty liver disease. *Hepatology* **2005**, *41*, 1313–1321. [CrossRef]
42. Brunt, E.M.; Tiniakos, D.G. Histopathology of nonalcoholic fatty liver disease. *World J. Gastroenterol.* **2010**, *16*, 5286–5296. [CrossRef] [PubMed]
43. Cataldo, I.; Sarcognato, S.; Sacchi, D.; Cacciatore, M.; Baciorri, F.; Mangia, A.; Cazzagon, N.; Guido, M. Pathology of non-alcoholic fatty liver disease. *Pathologica* **2021**, *113*, 194–202. [CrossRef] [PubMed]
44. Juluri, R.; Vuppalanchi, R.; Olson, J.; Unalp, A.; Van Natta, M.L.; Cummings, O.W.; Tonascia, J.; Chalasani, N. Generalizability of the nonalcoholic steatohepatitis Clinical Research Network histologic scoring system for nonalcoholic fatty liver disease. *J. Clin. Gastroenterol.* **2011**, *45*, 55–58. [CrossRef] [PubMed]
45. Santiago-Rolón, A.; Purcell, D.; Toro, D.H. A Comparison of Brunt's Criteria, the Non-Alcoholic Fatty Liver Disease Activity Score (NAS), and a Proposed NAS Scoring that Includes Fibrosis in Non-Alcoholic Fatty Liver Disease Staging. *Puerto Rico Health Sci. J.* **2015**, *34*, 189–194. [PubMed]
46. Chalasani, N.; Younossi, Z.; Lavine, J.E.; Diehl, A.M.; Brunt, E.M.; Cusi, K.; Charlton, M.; Sanyal, A.J. The diagnosis and management of nonalcoholic fatty liver disease: Practice guidance from the American Association for the Study of Liver Diseases. *Hepatology* **2018**, *67*, 328–357. [CrossRef]
47. Jeznach-Steinhagen, A.; Ostrowska, J.; Czerwonogrodzka-Senczyna, A.; Boniecka, I.; Shahnazaryan, U.; Kuryłowicz, A. Dietary and Pharmacological Treatment of Nonalcoholic Fatty Liver Disease. *Medicina* **2019**, *55*, 166. [CrossRef]
48. Dudekula, A.; Rachakonda, V.; Shaik, B.; Behari, J. Weight loss in nonalcoholic Fatty liver disease patients in an ambulatory care setting is largely unsuccessful but correlates with frequency of clinic visits. *PLoS ONE* **2014**, *9*, e111808. [CrossRef]
49. Sasaki, A.; Nitta, H.; Otsuka, K.; Umemura, A.; Baba, S.; Obuchi, T.; Wakabayashi, G. Bariatric surgery and non-alcoholic Fatty liver disease: Current and potential future treatments. *Front. Endocrinol.* **2014**, *5*, 164. [CrossRef] [PubMed]
50. European Association for the Study of the Liver (EASL) European Association for the Study of Diabetes (EASD); European Association for the Study of Obesity (EASO). EASL-EASD-EASO Clinical Practice Guidelines for the management of non-alcoholic fatty liver disease. *J. Hepatol.* **2016**, *64*, 1388–1402. [CrossRef] [PubMed]
51. Della Pepa, G.; Russo, M.; Vitale, M.; Carli, F.; Vetrani, C.; Masulli, M.; Riccardi, G.; Vaccaro, O.; Gastaldelli, A.; Rivellese, A.A.; et al. Pioglitazone even at low dosage improves NAFLD in type 2 diabetes: Clinical and pathophysiological insights from a subgroup of the TOSCA.IT randomised trial. *Diabetes Res. Clin. Pract.* **2021**, *178*, 108984. [CrossRef] [PubMed]
52. Bril, F.; Kalavalapalli, S.; Clark, V.C.; Lomonaco, R.; Soldevila-Pico, C.; Liu, I.C.; Orsak, B.; Tio, F.; Cusi, K. Response to Pioglitazone in Patients with Nonalcoholic Steatohepatitis with vs without Type 2 Diabetes. *Clin. Gastroenterol. Hepatol.* **2018**, *16*, 558–566.e2. [CrossRef] [PubMed]
53. Armstrong, M.J.; Gaunt, P.; Aithal, G.P.; Parker, R.; Barton, D.J.; Hull, D. Liraglutide is effective in the histological clearance of non-alcoholic steatohepatitis in a multicenter, double-blinded, randomized, placebo-controlled phase II trial. *J. Hepatol.* **2015**, *62*, S187. [CrossRef]
54. Luo, Y.; Yang, P.; Li, Z.; Luo, Y.; Shen, J.; Li, R.; Zheng, H.; Liang, Y.; Xia, N. Liraglutide Improves Non-Alcoholic Fatty Liver Disease in Diabetic Mice by Modulating Inflammatory Signaling Pathways. *Drug Des. Dev. Ther.* **2019**, *13*, 4065–4074. [CrossRef] [PubMed]
55. Yang, M.; Ma, X.; Xuan, X.; Deng, H.; Chen, Q.; Yuan, L. Liraglutide Attenuates Non-Alcoholic Fatty Liver Disease in Mice by Regulating the Local Renin-Angiotensin System. *Front. Pharmacol.* **2020**, *11*, 432. [CrossRef] [PubMed]
56. Tang, W.; Xu, Q.; Hong, T.; Tong, G.; Feng, W.; Shen, S.; Bi, Y.; Zhu, D. Comparative efficacy of anti-diabetic agents on NAFLD in patients with type 2 diabetes mellitus: A systematic review and meta-analysis of randomized and non-randomized studies. *Diabetes Metab. Res. Rev.* **2016**, *32*, 200–216. [CrossRef] [PubMed]
57. Loomba, R.; Lutchman, G.; Kleiner, D.E.; Ricks, M.; Feld, J.J.; Borg, B.B.; Modi, A.; Nagabhyru, P.; Sumner, A.E.; Liang, T.J.; et al. Clinical trial: Pilot study of metformin for the treatment of non-alcoholic steatohepatitis. *Aliment. Pharmacol. Ther.* **2009**, *29*, 172–182. [CrossRef] [PubMed]
58. Brandt, A.; Hernández-Arriaga, A.; Kehm, R.; Sánchez, V.; Jin, J.C.; Nier, A.; Baumann, A.; Camarinha-Silva, A.; Bergheim, I. Metformin attenuates the onset of non-alcoholic fatty liver disease and affects intestinal microbiota and barrier in small intestine. *Sci. Rep.* **2019**, *9*, 6668. [CrossRef]
59. Perumpail, B.J.; Li, A.A.; John, N.; Sallam, S.; Shah, N.D.; Kwong, W.; Cholankeril, G.; Kim, D.; Ahmed, A. The Role of Vitamin E in the Treatment of NAFLD. *Diseases* **2018**, *6*, 86. [CrossRef]
60. El Hadi, H.; Vettor, R.; Rossato, M. Vitamin E as a Treatment for Nonalcoholic Fatty Liver Disease: Reality or Myth? *Antioxidants* **2018**, *7*, 12. [CrossRef]
61. Zelber-Sagi, S.; Kessler, A.; Brazowsky, E.; Webb, M.; Lurie, Y.; Santo, M.; Leshno, M.; Blendis, L.; Halpern, Z.; Oren, R. A double-blind randomized placebo-controlled trial of orlistat for the treatment of nonalcoholic fatty liver disease. *Clin. Gastroenterol. Hepatol.* **2006**, *4*, 639–644. [CrossRef]

62. Pan, C.S.; Stanley, T.L. Effect of Weight Loss Medications on Hepatic Steatosis and Steatohepatitis: A Systematic Review. *Front. Endocrinol.* **2020**, *11*, 70. [CrossRef]
63. Maroni, L.; Guasti, L.; Castiglioni, L.; Marino, F.; Contini, S.; Macchi, V.; De Leo, A.; Gaudio, G.; Tozzi, M.; Grandi, A.M.; et al. Lipid targets during statin treatment in dyslipidemia patients affected by nonalcoholic fatty liver disease. *Am. J. Med. Sci.* **2011**, *342*, 383–387. [CrossRef] [PubMed]
64. Hyogo, H.; Yamagishi, S.; Maeda, S.; Kimura, Y.; Ishitobi, T.; Chayama, K. Atorvastatin improves disease activity of nonalcoholic steatohepatitis partly through its tumor necrosis factor-α-lowering property. *Dig. Liver Dis.* **2012**, *44*, 492–496. [CrossRef]
65. Venetsanaki, V.; Karabouta, Z.; Polyzos, S.A. Farnesoid X nuclear receptor agonists for the treatment of nonalcoholic steatohepatitis. *Eur. J. Pharmacol.* **2019**, *15*, 172661. [CrossRef]
66. Neuschwander-Tetri, B.A.; Loomba, R.; Sanyal, A.J.; Lavine, J.E.; Van Natta, M.L.; Abdelmalek, M.F.; Chalasani, N.; Dasarathy, S.; Diehl, A.M.; Hameed, B.; et al. Farnesoid X nuclear receptor ligand obeticholic acid for non-cirrhotic, non-alcoholic steatohepatitis (FLINT): A multicenter, randomized, placebo-controlled trial. *Lancet* **2015**, *385*, 956–965. [CrossRef]
67. Mudaliar, S.; Henry, R.R.; Sanyal, A.J.; Morrow, L.; Marschall, H.U.; Kipnes, M.; Adorini, L.; Sciacca, C.I.; Clopton, P.; Castelloe, E.; et al. Efficacy and safety of the farnesoid X receptor agonist obeticholic acid in patients with type 2 diabetes and nonalcoholic fatty liver disease. *Gastroenterology* **2013**, *145*, 574–582. [CrossRef] [PubMed]
68. Loomba, R.; Noureddin, M.; Kowdley, K.V.; Kohli, A.; Sheikh, A.; Neff, G.; Bhandari, B.R.; Gunn, N.; Caldwell, S.H.; Goodman, Z.; et al. Combination Therapies Including Cilofexor and Firsocostat for Bridging Fibrosis and Cirrhosis Attributable to NASH. *Hepatology* **2021**, *73*, 625–643. [CrossRef] [PubMed]
69. Cusi, K.; Orsak, B.; Bril, F.; Lomonaco, R.; Hecht, J.; Ortiz-Lopez, C.; Tio, F.; Hardies, J.; Darland, C.; Musi, N.; et al. Long-Term Pioglitazone Treatment for Patients with Nonalcoholic Steatohepatitis and Prediabetes or Type 2 Diabetes Mellitus. *Ann. Intern. Med.* **2016**, *165*, 305–315. [CrossRef]
70. Ratziu, V.; Giral, P.; Jacqueminet, S.; Charlotte, F.; Hartemann-Heurtier, A.; Serfaty, L.; Podevin, P.; Lacorte, J.M.; Bernhardt, C.; Bruckert, E.; et al. Rosiglitazone for nonalcoholic steatohepatitis: One-year results of the randomized placebo-controlled Fatty Liver Improvement with Rosiglitazone Therapy (FLIRT) Trial. *Gastroenterology* **2008**, *135*, 100–110. [CrossRef]
71. Dongiovanni, P.; Meroni, M.; Baselli, G.A.; Bassani, G.A.; Rametta, R.; Pietrelli, A.; Maggioni, M.; Facciotti, F.; Trunzo, V.; Badiali, S.; et al. Insulin resistance promotes Lysyl Oxidase Like 2 induction and fibrosis accumulation in non-alcoholic fatty liver disease. *Clin. Sci.* **2017**, *7*, 1301–1315. [CrossRef] [PubMed]
72. Harrison, S.A.; Abdelmalek, M.F.; Caldwell, S.; Shiffman, M.L.; Diehl, A.M.; Ghalib, R.; Lawitz, E.J.; Rockey, D.C.; Schall, R.A.; Jia, C.; et al. Simtuzumab Is Ineffective for Patients with Bridging Fibrosis or Compensated Cirrhosis Caused by Nonalcoholic Steatohepatitis. *Gastroenterology* **2018**, *155*, 1140–1153. [CrossRef] [PubMed]
73. Loomba, R.; Lawitz, E.; Mantry, P.S.; Jayakumar, S.; Caldwell, S.H.; Arnold, H.; Diehl, A.M.; Djedjos, C.S.; Han, L.; Myers, R.P.; et al. The ASK1 inhibitor selonsertib in patients with nonalcoholic steatohepatitis: A randomized, phase 2 trial. *Hepatology* **2018**, *67*, 549–559. [CrossRef] [PubMed]
74. Harrison, S.A.; Wong, V.W.; Okanoue, T.; Bzowej, N.; Vuppalanchi, R.; Younes, Z.; Kohli, A.; Sarin, S.; Caldwell, S.H.; Alkhouri, N.; et al. Selonsertib for patients with bridging fibrosis or compensated cirrhosis due to NASH: Results from randomized phase III STELLAR trials. *J. Hepatol.* **2020**, *73*, 26–39. [CrossRef]
75. Ha, J.; Jang, M.; Kwon, Y.; Park, Y.S.; Park, D.J.; Lee, J.H.; Lee, H.J.; Ha, T.K.; Kim, Y.J.; Han, S.M.; et al. Metabolomic Profiles Predict Diabetes Remission after Bariatric Surgery. *J. Clin. Med.* **2020**, *9*, 3897. [CrossRef]
76. Doumouras, A.G.; Wong, J.A.; Paterson, J.M.; Lee, Y.; Sivapathasundaram, B.; Tarride, J.E.; Thabane, L.; Hong, D.; Yusuf, S.; Anvari, M. Bariatric Surgery and Cardiovascular Outcomes in Patients with Obesity and Cardiovascular Disease: A Population-Based Retrospective Cohort Study. *Circulation* **2021**, *143*, 1468–1480. [CrossRef]
77. Diemieszczyk, I.; Woźniewska, P.; Gołaszewski, P.; Drygalski, K.; Nadolny, K.; Ładny, J.R.; Razak Hady, H. Does weight loss after laparoscopic sleeve gastrectomy contribute to reduction in blood pressure? *Pol. Arch. Intern. Med.* **2021**, *131*, 693–700. [CrossRef] [PubMed]
78. Sutanto, A.; Wungu, C.D.K.; Susilo, H.; Sutanto, H. Reduction of Major Adverse Cardiovascular Events (MACE) after Bariatric Surgery in Patients with Obesity and Cardiovascular Diseases: A Systematic Review and Meta-Analysis. *Nutrients* **2021**, *13*, 3568. [CrossRef]
79. Mummadi, R.R.; Kasturi, K.S.; Chennareddygari, S.; Sood, K.G. Effect of bariatric surgery on nonalcoholic fatty liver disease: Systematic review and meta-analysis. *Clin. Gastroenterol. Hepatol.* **2008**, *6*, 1396–1402. [CrossRef]
80. Burza, M.A.; Romeo, S.; Kotronen, A.; Svensson, P.A.; Sjöholm, K.; Torgerson, J.S.; Lindroos, A.K.; Sjöström, L.; Carlsson, L.M.; Peltonen, M. Long-term effect of bariatric surgery on liver enzymes in the Swedish Obese Subjects (SOS) study. *PLoS ONE* **2013**, *8*, e60495. [CrossRef]
81. Klein, S.; Mittendorfer, B.; Eagon, J.C.; Patterson, B.; Grant, L.; Feirt, N.; Seki, E.; Brenner, D.; Korenblat, K.; McCrea, J. Gastric bypass surgery improves metabolic and hepatic abnormalities associated with nonalcoholic fatty liver disease. *Gastroenterology* **2006**, *130*, 1564–1572. [CrossRef]
82. Cazzo, E.; Jimenez, L.S.; Pareja, J.C.; Chaim, E.A. Effect of Roux-en-y Gastric Bypass on Nonalcoholic Fatty Liver Disease Evaluated Through NAFLD Fibrosis Score: A Prospective Study. *Obes. Surg.* **2015**, *25*, 982–985. [CrossRef] [PubMed]

83. Pedersen, J.S.; Rygg, M.O.; Serizawa, R.R.; Kristiansen, V.B.; Albrechtsen, N.J.W.; Gluud, L.L.; Madsbad, S.; Bendtsen, F. Effects of Roux-en-Y Gastric Bypass and Sleeve Gastrectomy on Non-Alcoholic Fatty Liver Disease: A 12-Month Follow-Up Study with Paired Liver Biopsies. *J. Clin. Med.* **2021**, *10*, 3783. [CrossRef] [PubMed]
84. Clark, J.M.; Alkhuraishi, A.R.; Solga, S.F.; Alli, P.; Diehl, A.M.; Magnuson, T.H. Roux-en-Y gastric bypass improves liver histology in patients with non-alcoholic fatty liver disease. *Obes. Res.* **2005**, *13*, 1180–1186. [CrossRef] [PubMed]
85. Nobili, V.; Carpino, G.; De Peppo, F.; Caccamo, R.; Mosca, A.; Romito, I.; Overi, D.; Franchitto, A.; Onori, P.; Alisi, A.; et al. Laparoscopic Sleeve Gastrectomy Improves Nonalcoholic Fatty Liver Disease-Related Liver Damage in Adolescents by Reshaping Cellular Interactions and Hepatic Adipocytokine Production. *J. Pediatr.* **2018**, *194*, 100–108.e3. [CrossRef]
86. Cabré, N.; Luciano-Mateo, F.; Fernández-Arroyo, S.; Baiges-Gayà, G.; Hernández-Aguilera, A.; Fibla, M.; Fernández-Julià, R.; París, M.; Sabench, F.; Castillo, D.D.; et al. Laparoscopic sleeve gastrectomy reverses non-alcoholic fatty liver disease modulating oxidative stress and inflammation. *Metabolism* **2019**, *99*, 81–89. [CrossRef]
87. Salman, A.A.; Sultan, A.A.E.A.; Abdallah, A.; Abdelsalam, A.; Mikhail, H.M.S.; Tourky, M.; Omar, M.G.; Youssef, A.; Ahmed, R.A.; Elkassar, H.; et al. Effect of weight loss induced by laparoscopic sleeve gastrectomy on liver histology and serum adipokine levels. *J. Gastroenterol. Hepatol.* **2020**, *35*, 1769–1773. [CrossRef] [PubMed]
88. Baldwin, D.; Chennakesavalu, M.; Gangemi, A. Systematic review and meta-analysis of Roux-en-Y gastric bypass against laparoscopic sleeve gastrectomy for amelioration of NAFLD using four criteria. *Surg. Obes. Relat. Dis.* **2019**, *15*, 2123–2130. [CrossRef]
89. Cherla, D.V.; Rodriguez, N.A.; Vangoitsenhoven, R.; Singh, T.; Mehta, N.; McCullough, A.J.; Brethauer, S.A.; Schauer, P.R.; Aminian, A. Impact of sleeve gastrectomy and Roux-en-Y gastric bypass on biopsy-proven non-alcoholic fatty liver disease. *Surg. Endosc.* **2020**, *34*, 2266–2272. [CrossRef]
90. De Brito e Silva, M.B.; Tustumi, F.; de Miranda Neto, A.A.; Dantas, A.C.B.; Santo, M.A.; Cecconello, I. Gastric Bypass Compared with Sleeve Gastrectomy for Nonalcoholic Fatty Liver Disease: A Systematic Review and Meta-analysis. *Obes. Surg.* **2021**, *31*, 2762–2772. [CrossRef]
91. Luo, R.B.; Suzuki, T.; Hooker, J.C.; Covarrubias, Y.; Schlein, A.; Liu, S.; Schwimmer, J.B.; Reeder, S.B.; Funk, L.M.; Greenberg, J.A.; et al. How bariatric surgery affects liver volume and fat density in NAFLD patients. *Surg. Endosc.* **2018**, *32*, 1675–1682. [CrossRef] [PubMed]
92. Lee, Y.; Doumouras, A.G.; Yu, J.; Brar, K.; Banfield, L.; Gmora, S.; Anvari, M.; Hong, D. Complete Resolution of Nonalcoholic Fatty Liver Disease After Bariatric Surgery: A Systematic Review and Meta-analysis. *Clin. Gastroenterol. Hepatol.* **2019**, *17*, 1040–1060.e11. [CrossRef] [PubMed]
93. Mathurin, P.; Hollebecque, A.; Arnalsteen, L.; Buob, D.; Leteurtre, E.; Caiazzo, R.; Pigeyre, M.; Verkindt, H.; Dharancy, S.; Louvet, A.; et al. Prospective study of the long-term effects of bariatric surgery on liver injury in patients without advanced disease. *Gastroenterology* **2009**, *137*, 532–540. [CrossRef] [PubMed]

Journal of
Clinical Medicine

MDPI

Article

Exploring Renal Changes after Bariatric Surgery in Patients with Severe Obesity

Anna Oliveras [1,2,3,4,*], Susana Vázquez [1,2], María José Soler [5], Isabel Galceran [1,2], Xavier Duran [2], Albert Goday [2,6,7], David Benaiges [2,6,7], Marta Crespo [1,2,3,4], Julio Pascual [1,2] and Marta Riera [2,4]

1 Nephrology Department, Hospital Universitari del Mar, 08003 Barcelona, Spain; svazquez@hospitaldelmar.cat (S.V.); igalceran@hospitaldelmar.cat (I.G.); mcrespo@hospitaldelmar.cat (M.C.); julpascual@gmail.com (J.P.)
2 IMIM, Hospital del Mar Medical Research Institute, 08003 Barcelona, Spain; xduran@imim.es (X.D.); agoday@hospitaldelmar.cat (A.G.); dbenaiges@hospitaldelmar.cat (D.B.); mriera1@imim.es (M.R.)
3 Department of Experimental and Health Sciences, Area of Medicine, Universitat Pompeu Fabra, 08002 Barcelona, Spain
4 Red de Investigación Renal (REDINREN), Instituto Carlos III-FEDER, 28029 Madrid, Spain
5 Nephrology Research Group, Vall d'Hebron Research Institute (VHIR), Nephrology Department, Hospital Universitari Vall d'Hebron, Universitat Autònoma de Barcelona, 08035 Barcelona, Spain; mjsoler01@gmail.com
6 Endocrinology Department, Hospital Universitari del Mar, 08003 Barcelona, Spain
7 Medicine Department, Universitat Autònoma de Barcelona, 08193 Barcelona, Spain
* Correspondence: aoliveras@hospitaldelmar.cat; Tel.: +34-932-483-483

Abstract: Obesity-related hyperfiltration leads to an increased glomerular filtration rate (GFR) and hyperalbuminuria. These changes are reversible after bariatric surgery (BS). We aimed to explore obesity-related renal changes post-BS and to seek potential mechanisms. Sixty-two individuals with severe obesity were prospectively examined before and 3, 6 and 12 months post-BS. Anthropometric and laboratory data, 24 h-blood pressure, renin-angiotensin-aldosterone system (RAS) components, adipokines and inflammatory markers were determined. Both estimated GFR (eGFR) and albuminuria decreased from the baseline at all follow-up times (p-for-trend <0.001 for both). There was a median (IQR) of 30.5% (26.2–34.4) reduction in body weight. Plasma glucose, glycosylated hemoglobin, fasting insulin and HOMA-index decreased at 3, 6 and 12 months of follow-up (p-for-trend <0.001 for all). The plasma aldosterone concentration (median (IQR)) also decreased at 12 months (from 87.8 ng/dL (56.8; 154) to 65.4 (56.8; 84.6), $p = 0.003$). Both leptin and hs-CRP decreased ($p < 0.001$) and adiponectine levels increased at 12 months post-BS ($p = 0.017$). Linear mixed-models showed that body weight (coef. 0.62, 95% CI: 0.32 to 0.93, $p < 0.001$) and plasma aldosterone (coef. −0.07, 95% CI: −0.13 to −0.02, $p = 0.005$) were the independent variables for changes in eGFR. Conversely, glycosylated hemoglobin was the only independent variable for changes in albuminuria (coef. 0.24, 95% CI: 0.06 to 0.42, $p = 0.009$). In conclusion, body weight and aldosterone are the main factors that mediate eGFR changes in obesity and BS, while albuminuria is associated with glucose homeostasis.

Keywords: bariatric surgery; hyperfiltration; albuminuria; renin-angiotensin axis; aldosterone; glucose metabolism

Citation: Oliveras, A.; Vázquez, S.; Soler, M.J.; Galceran, I.; Duran, X.; Goday, A.; Benaiges, D.; Crespo, M.; Pascual, J.; Riera, M. Exploring Renal Changes after Bariatric Surgery in Patients with Severe Obesity. *J. Clin. Med.* **2022**, *11*, 728. https://doi.org/10.3390/jcm11030728

Academic Editor: Franco Bassetto

Received: 29 December 2021
Accepted: 27 January 2022
Published: 29 January 2022

1. Introduction

Worldwide obesity has nearly tripled since 1975 [1]. Obesity is associated with an increase in morbidity and mortality, mainly from cardiovascular disease and diabetes, among others [2]. In addition, obesity is also a major risk factor for the development of chronic kidney disease [3]. Obesity is usually characterized by an abnormally high glomerular filtration rate (GFR) and long-lasting hyperfiltration may cause renal lesions similar to secondary focal segmental glomerulosclerosis, the so-called obesity-related glomerulopathy, leading to a decrease in GFR and hyperalbuminuria [4]. In patients with severe obesity, both hyperfiltration and albuminuria are a consequence of increased intraglomerular pressure and glomerular surface area. Although the prevalence of microalbuminuria or proteinuria is higher in obese patients who have diabetes, albuminuria is still higher in non-diabetic obese patients than in the general population [5]. Finally, increased body mass index (BMI) has been linked to a loss of renal function, as well as a higher risk of end-stage renal disease [5]. In severely obese patients, lifestyle changes often fail to significantly reduce body weight. Fortunately, bariatric surgery (BS), a surgical approach that can be performed through different technical procedures, promotes weight loss so that it achieves much better results. Beyond weight loss, BS leads to the improvement of various obesity-related diseases such as hypertension, disorders of glucose and lipid metabolism, obstructive sleep apnea or non-alcoholic steatohepatitis, among others. More importantly, a recent meta-analysis [6] showed a reduction in major adverse cardiovascular events in patients with obesity and cardiovascular disease who underwent BS compared with those who did not have surgery. Recently, obesity-induced hyperfiltration and albuminuria have been shown to be reversible after bariatric surgery [4,7]. Altered renal haemodynamics as well as a deleterious adipocytokine pattern favored by obesity appear to be at the root of both obesity-related renal impairment and its improvement after BS, at least in diabetics [4,8,9].

Here we sought to assess changes in renal function at different follow-up times in patients with severe obesity undergoing BS. In addition, we explored the possible role of the renin-angiotensin aldosterone system (RAS), changes in glucose metabolism, and inflammation as potential mechanisms mediating these changes.

2. Materials and Methods

2.1. Methods

2.1.1. Study Design and Patients

The BARIHTA study is a prospective observational trial in a cohort of consecutively enrolled patients with severe obesity scheduled to undergo BS (clinicaltrials.gov identifier: NCT03115502). Details about BARIHTA trials have been previously published [10]. Thus, the BARIHTA study prospectively recruited outpatients with severe obesity who went to consultations at the Hospital del Mar (Barcelona, Catalonia, Spain) seeking surgical treatment. All individuals (both sexes, aged 18–60 years) with a medical indication for surgical intervention and who agreed to undergo the treatment with BS were invited to participate. Indications for BS included those patients with a body mass index (BMI) > 40 kg/m^2 or grade II obesity (BMI > 35 kg/m^2) plus associated comorbidities (i.e., type 2 diabetes mellitus, obesity-associated hypoventilation disorders, high blood pressure, or dyslipidemia). Patients with any endocrine disease causing obesity or severe psychiatric diseases were excluded. Detailed information on the trial was provided by qualified professionals of the Hypertension and Vascular Risk Unit (Nephrology Department, Hospital del Mar). The exclusion criteria comprised the ruling out of the BS program for any reason or the refusal to give consent. The trial was approved by the local institutional Ethic Committee in accordance with the Declaration of Helsinki, and written informed consent was obtained from all participants.

Here we evaluate and report the effects of BS on renal function and explore its possible mechanisms by analyzing its relationship with various components of the renin-angiotensin-aldosterone system (RAS), along with inflammatory markers and adipokines, as previously specified per protocol.

Demographic, anthropometric and clinical data were recorded from all participants as a baseline. Anthropometric characteristics, pharmacological treatment, office- and 24 h-ambulatory-blood pressure (BP) recordings, routine laboratory tests, including renal function as assessed by the estimated glomerular filtration rate (eGFR) and by determining albuminuria, and determinations of components of the RAS, adipokines and inflammatory markers, were obtained at baseline and 1, 3, 6 and 12 months after surgery. Changes at follow-ups are evaluated from three months on to avoid the major hemodynamic instability one month after BS. Hypertension was considered if previously diagnosed and/or if the baseline 24 h-BP was ≥130/80 mmHg. Diabetes mellitus (DM) was considered if the patient received antidiabetic treatment or had ≥2 fasting plasma glucose determinations ≥126 mg/dL or if glycosylated haemoglobin A1c was >6.5%.

About one-third of the study population was under treatment with at least one drug that interfered with the RAS. Given that these drugs could introduce a bias by interfering with renal function parameters, the main analyzes were performed separately in both the entire cohort and in the untreated patients.

2.1.2. Procedures

Blood Pressure Measurements

Brachial-BP measurements and calculation of central-BP and other arterial parameters through the oscillometric method (ARCSolver algorithm) were obtained from a Mobil-O-Graph® NG-ambulatory blood pressure (NG-ABPM) device by IEM, Stolberg, Germany. The monitor was placed on a working day between 08:00–10:00 h A.M., and after a 5 min rest, BP was consecutively determined four times at 1-min intervals. The mean was established as office BP. Brachial artery waveforms were then automatically recorded at 20-min intervals. Suitably sized cuffs were used according to the arm circumference measured in each study visit. All patients had recordings of good technical quality (≥70% valid readings). If not, a new ambulatory-BP-monitoring (ABPM) was repeated within 1 week.

Laboratory Analyses

Urinary Albumin Excretion

Urinary albumin excretion (measured by turbidimetry; lower detection limit: 0.3 mg/dl; intra-assay and inter-assay variation coefficients: 1.3% and 4.3%, respectively) was determined before BS and at the determined follow-up time-points and measured as the average of urinary albumin/creatinine ratio (ACR) from 2 fresh first-morning-void urine samples obtained on separate days. Microalbuminuria was defined as an ACR ≥ 30 mg/g.

Serum Creatinine and eGFR

Serum creatinine (SCr) was measured by an enzymatic modified Jaffe reaction (CREA; Roche Diagnostics) using the Hitachi Modular System Analyzer (Roche Diagnostics), consistent with the current National Kidney Disease Education Program recommendations for standardizing SCr measurement [11]. The intra-assay coefficient of variation was 2.3%.

There is no current agreement as to the best method to estimate the GFR in individuals with severe obesity. However, in a recently reported study [12], the modified Cockcroft-Gault (CG) equation performed best in both the overall population and the obese subgroup in terms of strength of correlation, mean bias and accuracy, as compared to both the IDMS (isotope dilution mass spectrometry) traceable simplified Modification of Diet in Renal Disease [13] and the Chronic Kidney Disease-Epidemiology Collaborative equations [14]. We obtained equivalent results to that report. Therefore, although we initially performed the analyzes by obtaining the eGFR using the three formulas separately, in the final analysis we only report data on eGFR according to the CG equation, with adjustments for body surface area.

Renin-Angiotensin-Aldosterone System (RAAS) Components

Plasma renin activity (PRA) and plasma aldosterone concentration, as well as angiotensin-converting enzyme (ACE) and angiotensin-converting enzyme-2 (ACE2) activities, were measured by validated laboratory methods [15]. Details on assay performance are reported in Appendix A.

Adipokines and Inflammatory Parameters

Leptin, adiponectin, and other cytokines and inflammatory markers, e.g., resistin, angiopoietin-2, MCP-1 and high-sensitivity C-reactive protein (hs-CRP), were also determined. See Appendix B.

Surgical Techniques

Either laparoscopic Roux-en-Y gastric bypass (LRYGB) or laparoscopic sleeve gastrectomy (LSG) were performed, and any of these two were chosen for each patient based on clinical criteria and the consensus of the Bariatric Surgery Unit. In this line, LSG was preferred in younger patients, in those with a BMI ranging from 35–40 kg/m^2, as a first-step treatment in cases with a body mass index (BMI) > 50 kg/m^2 and when drug malabsorption was to be avoided [16]. The LRYGB technique involved a 150-cm antecolic Roux limb with 25-mm circular pouch–jejunostomy and exclusion of 50 cm of the proximal jejunum. In LSG, the longitudinal resection of the stomach from the angle of His to approximately 5 cm proximal to the pylorus was performed using a 36-French bougie inserted along the lesser curvature.

2.1.3. Statistical Analyses

Elementary statistical methods were applied with statistical package SPSS for Windows version 25.0 (Cary, NC, USA). The normality assumption for continuous variables was tested through the Kolmogorov–Smirnov test. Variables fulfilling this normality assumption were summarized as the mean ± S.D. or the median (interquartile range, IQR) otherwise. Categorical data were presented as frequencies and percentages. Comparisons of analyzed variables between two observed periods were carried out by paired t tests or Wilcoxon signed rank tests. Pearson or Spearman correlation coefficients were used for testing bivariate correlations as appropriate. Separate linear mixed-models were built for both the variation of eGFR-CG and the variation of albuminuria. All variables which deviate from the normal distribution were log-transformed (ln) before being introduced into the model. In these models, data were expressed as regression coefficient, 95% confidence interval (95% CI) and *p*-value. A change was considered significant if the two-side alpha level was $\leq$0.05. We used the statistical package SPSS for Windows version 25.0 (Cary, NC, USA), and STATA package version 15 (STATA Corp., College Station, TX, USA), for statistical analysis.

About one-third of the study population received treatment with one or more drugs that interfered with RAS. Given that these drugs could introduce a bias by interfering with renal function parameters, the main analyses were performed separately in both the entire cohort and in the untreated patients.

3. Results

Sixty-two patients completed the BARIHTA study, and information on renal changes was available for all of them at the baseline and follow-ups. A flowchart is supplied (Figure S1). Baseline characteristics are shown in Table 1. Fifty-five patients (89%) had hyperfiltration, i.e., eGFR > 120 mL/min/1.73 m^2, before BS. None of the patients had chronic kidney disease based on the estimated glomerular filtration rate, nor did any of them die at follow-up.

3.1. Changes in Renal Function Parameters

The estimated GFR decreased from 155.9 ± 36.3 to 127.7 ± 27.4 mL/min/1.73 m^2 ($p < 0.001$), reflecting the hyperfiltration that characterizes patients with severe obesity. In addition, the albuminuria, as measured by the log-transformed albumin-creatinine ratio (lnACR), decreased from 1.85 ± 1.08 to 1.56 ± 0.73 ($p = 0.056$). Both the estimated GFR (Figure 1A) and the albuminuria (Figure 1B) experienced a progressive decrease from baseline to the final observation 12 months after BS at all follow-up times (*p* for trend <0.001 for both).

3.2. Changes in Body Weight, Body Mass Index, and Waist Circumference

Overall, there was a median (IQR) 30.5% (26.2–34.4) reduction in body weight 12 months after BS. Body mass index was 42.7 ± 5.6 kg/m^2 at baseline and 29.7 ± 4.8 kg/m^2 one year after BS ($p < 0.001$). Figure S2 (Supplemental Material) shows the mean (error bars

95% CI) body weight at each follow-up point. Waist circumference was 132.5 ± 12.0 cm and 105.5 ± 13.3 cm, at baseline and 12 months after BS, respectively ($p < 0.001$). A waist circumference (cm) decrease was confirmed in both men (140.2 ± 14.3 vs. 111.4 ± 16.3) and women (129.8 ± 10.1 vs. 103.4 ± 11.7), ($p < 0.001$ for both comparisons).

Table 1. The baseline clinical characteristics.

Age, Year (Mean ± S.D.)	42.1 ± 9.3
Sex, women, *n* (%)	48 (77.4)
Body weight, kg (mean ± S.D.)	117.4 ± 18.9
Waist circumference, cm (mean ± S.D.)	132.3 ± 11.5
Body mass index, Kg/m^2 (mean ± S.D.)	42.6 ± 5.5
Race, *n* (%)	
-Caucasian	56 (90.3)
-African	1 (1.6)
-Hispano-American	5 (8.1)
Current smokers, *n* (%)	17 (27.4)
Surgical procedure, *n* (%):	
-Sleeve gastrectomy	27 (43.5)
-Roux-en-Y gastric bypass	35 (56.5)
Hypertension, *n* (%)	24 (38.7)
Type 2-Diabetes Mellitus, *n* (%)	7 (11.3)
Chronic kidney disease *, *n* (%)	0 (0)
Previous major vascular event, *n* (%)	3 (4.8)

* estimated glomerular filtration rate <60 mL/min/1.73 m^2.

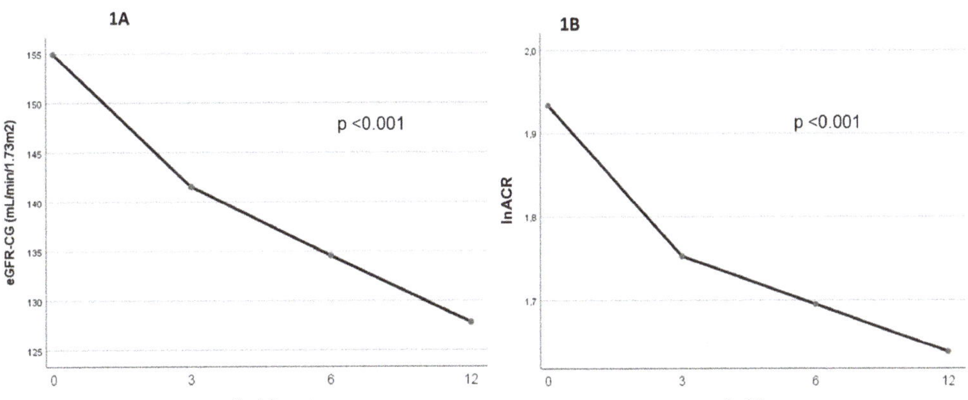

Figure 1. The changes in eGFR (**1A**) and albuminuria (**1B**) from baseline (before BS) to 12 months post-BS, with mid-points at 3 and 6 months. eGFR-CG = estimated glomerular filtration rate by the Cockcroft-Gault equation; lnACR = neperian logarithm of albumin-creatinine ratio. Values of both eGFR-CG and lnACR are given as mean ± SD.

3.3. Variation of Blood Pressure

As previously reported [10], office systolic and diastolic BP, both central and peripheral, significantly decreased at 12 months, even though more than 60% of the cohort were normotensives. In addition, central 24-h SBP decreased at 12 months, with a mean of (95% confidence interval) −3.1 mmHg (−5.5 to −0.7), $p = 0.01$ after adjustment for age and sex.

There was a statistically significant correlation between the variation at 12 months of peripheral 24-h systolic blood pressure (SBP) and the variation of both body weight (rho = 0.453, $p = 0.001$) and waist circumference (rho = 0.316, $p = 0.030$).

3.4. Changes in Glucose Metabolism Parameters and in RAS Components

Figure 2 shows the overall mean (95% CI) of fasting glucose before BS (0 months) and at 3, 6 and 12 months of follow-up. As noted, there is an initial decrease at 3 months that is maintained throughout the first year of follow-up (p for trend < 0.001).

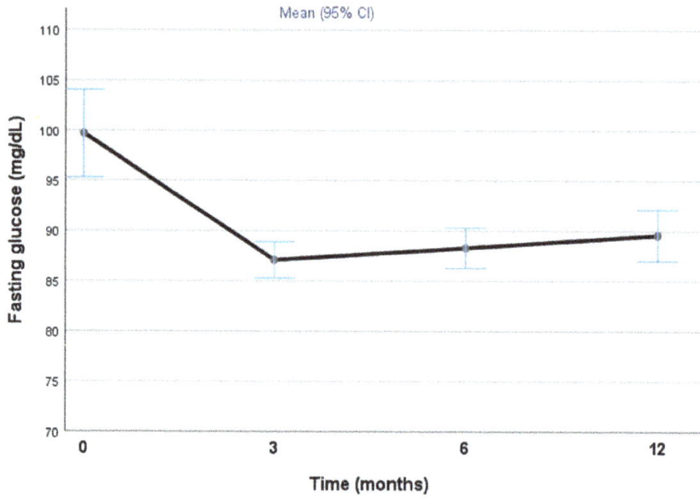

Figure 2. The changes in fasting glucose from baseline (before BS) to 12-months of follow-up, with mid-points at 3 and 6 months. Values of fasting glucose are given as the mean and corresponding 95% confidence intervals.

Figure 3 shows the overall mean of glycosylated hemoglobin, fasting insulin and HOMA-IR (homeostasis model assessment-estimated insulin resistance index) before BS (0 months) and at 3, 6 and 12 months of follow-up. There is a statistically significant decrease of these three parameters throughout the first year of follow-up (p for trend < 0.001 for all).

The changes at 12 months after BS in various components of the RAS were also assessed. As expected, there was a statistically significant decrease in plasma renin activity and aldosterone plasma concentration, as well as an increase in the ACEactivity/ACE2 activity ratio after BS (see Table 2). These changes showed a tendency to persist when the subgroup of patients without a RAS blockade treatment that could interfere with the components of the RAS was analyzed separately.

Table 2. The changes in the RAS components 12 months after bariatric surgery.

	All Patients (n = 62)			Patients without Antihypertensive Treatment (n = 42)		
	Before BS	12-Months Post-BS	p	Before BS	12-Months Post-BS	p
PRA *, ng/mL/h	0.8 (0.3; 1.3)	0.45 (0.2; 0.9)	**0.010**	0.85 (0.38; 1.3)	0.5 (0.2; 1.0)	0.074
Aldosterone *, ng/dL	87.8 (56.8; 154)	65.4 (56.8; 84.6)	**0.003**	81.6 (56.8; 110)	65.1 (56.3; 82.3)	0.090
ACE activity, RFU/µL	1244.1 ± 341.3	1287.3 ± 360.7	0.370	1272.3 ± 327.2	1295.6 ± 307.4	0.710
ACE2 activity *, RFU/µL/h	7.9 (5.8; 10.8)	6.9 (5.4; 10.8)	0.070	7.7 (5.8; 10.7)	6.9 (5.0; 11.3)	0.151
ACE act./ACE2 act.	164.5 ± 77.9	187.5 ± 78.4	**0.016**	172.7 ± 83.5	188.2 ± 74.1	0.131

(*) Data shown as median [interquartile range]. ACE = angiotensin converting enzyme; ACE2 = angiotensin converting enzyme 2; BS = bariatric surgery; PRA = plasma renin activity; RAS = renin-angiotensin system; RFU = relative fluorescence units.

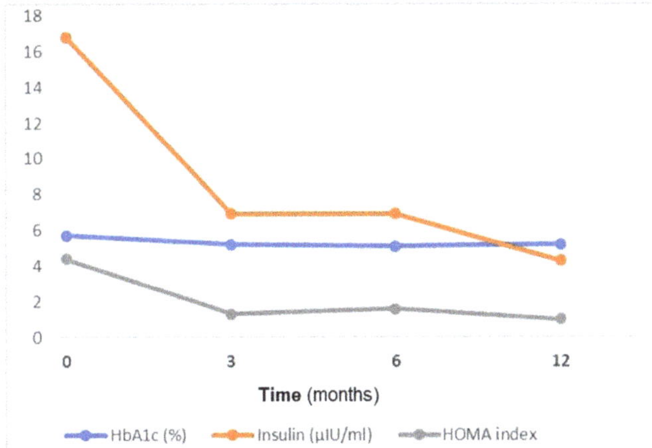

Figure 3. The changes in glycosylated hemoglobin, fasting insulin and HOMA-IR index from baseline (before BS) to 12-months of follow-up. HbA1c = glycosylated hemoglobin; HOMA = homeostasis model assessment-estimated insulin resistance.

There were statistically significant changes 12 months after BS in the explored adipokines and inflammatory markers (Table S1). As seen, leptin and hs-CRP decreased, while adiponectine and angiopoietin-2 experienced an increase 12 months after BS.

3.5. Independent Correlates of Repeated Measurements of Renal Parameters

Separate mixed-models were built for both the variation of eGFR-CG and the variation of albuminuria (Table 3). The tested independent variables were those that were clinically relevant and that showed statistically significant changes at follow-up, mainly body weight, peripheral 24h-systolic BP, several components of the RAS, various adipokines and inflammatory markers and different parameters of the glucose metabolism.

Table 3. The determinants of the variation of eGFR (3A) and of the variation of albuminuria (3B).

3A						
eGFR	**All Patients (n = 62)**			**Patients without Antihypertensive Treatment (n = 42)**		
	Coeff.	**95% CI**	***p*-value**	**Coeff.**	**95% CI**	***p*-value**
Months FU	−0.42	−1.16, 0.32	0.267	−0.69	−1.59, 0.22	0.135
Body weight, Kg	0.71	0.46, 0.96	**<0.001**	0.62	0.32, 0.93	**<0.001**
24h-systolic BP, mmHg	0.26	−0.04, 0.56	0.089	−0.03	−0. 42, 0.36	0.887
Aldosterone, ng/dL	−0.11	−0.15, −0.07	**<0.001**	−0.07	−0.13, −0.02	**0.005**
HbA1c, %	1.24	−3.84, 6.31	0.633	2.98	−2.52, 8.48	0.288
3B						
lnACR	**All Patients (n = 62)**			**Patients without Antihypertensive Treatment (n = 42)**		
	Coeff.	**95% CI**	***p*-Value**	**Coeff.**	**95% CI**	***p*-Value**
Months FU	−0.01	−0.03, 0.02	0.539	0.00	−0.02, 0.03	0.788
Body weight, Kg	−0.00	−0.01, 0.01	0.641	0.00	−0.01, 0.01	0.609
24h-systolic BP, mmHg	0.02	0.01, 0.03	**<0.001**	−0.00	−0.02, 0.01	0.582
Aldosterone, ng/dL	0.00	−0.00, 0.00	0.107	0.00	−0.00, 0.00	0.608
HbA1c, %	0.27	0.09, 0.45	**0.004**	0.24	0.06, 0.42	**0.009**

BP = blood pressure; eGFR = estimated glomerular filtration rate; FU = follow-up; HbA1c = glycosylated hemoglobin; lnACR = log-transformed albumin-creatinine ratio.

The models with a better performance show that the statistically significant independent variables for eGFR (Table 3A) were body weight and plasmatic aldosterone concentration, in both all patients and the subgroup of untreated patients. Regarding the variation of albuminuria (Table 3B), the main independent variable was the glycosylated hemoglobin. Similar results were found when the same models were tested including the HOMA insulin-resistance index instead of the glycosylated hemoglobin (see Table S2). Otherwise, the variation of leptin, adiponectin, angioietin2 and hs-CRP lost statistical significance when included in the models.

4. Discussion

The main finding of this study is that in obese patients undergoing BS the mechanisms by which the estimated glomerular filtration rate and albuminuria return to normal values are possibly different. Thus, we demonstrate that normalization of eGFR is associated with a decrease in both body weight and plasma aldosterone concentration, while a decrease in albuminuria is directly correlated with an improvement in glucose metabolism.

Weight excess is associated with an altered renal haemodynamic profile, i.e., an increased GFR relative to effective renal plasma flow, resulting in an increased filtration fraction [17]. Hyperfiltration is the hallmark of obesity-associated renal dysfunction, leading to the onset of microalbuminuria, even before major structural changes occur [18]. Characterizing the renal function of patients with severe obesity and looking for the mechanisms underlying their evolution after BS are crucial challenges, especially to prevent obesity-related kidney damage. Controlled and noncontrolled studies have shown that BS decreases eGFR [4,7,19] and albuminuria [8,19,20], suggesting that BS alleviates hyperfiltration.

Several studies have investigated the mechanisms likely to be responsible for renal changes observed in obese patients. A large number of these studies refer to hyperfiltration in general terms, focusing mainly on eGFR, especially with regard to the consequences of BS on renal function. Some of them found a relationship between the decrease in eGFR after BS and an improvement in the toxic adipokine profile observed in these patients [4,9]. In our cohort, we found a statistically significant decrease in leptin and in hs-CRP, as well as an increase in adiponectin, but these changes did not remain significant in the multivariate analyses after adjusting for other variables. On the contrary, we found that body weight and plasma aldosterone concentration decreases were the two factors that showed the strongest correlations with the restoration of eGFR to almost normal values. Some other authors have shown an association between the decrease in the percentage of high fat mass and the decrease in eGFR after BS. Of note, there is a general agreement that weight loss, but not the mechanism through with weight loss is achieved (i.e., type of surgery), is an independent predictor of restoration of renal function and prevention of chronic kidney disease [4,9,21,22]. Focusing on the role of aldosterone in the amelioration of hyperfiltration after BS in patients with obesity, it has been reported that activation of the RAS together with other mechanisms mediate increased renal sodium reabsorption in obesity-induced hypertension, high blood pressure being one of the possible causes of renal damage in these patients [23]. However, we must remark that our results are confirmed in the subgroup of untreated normotensive patients, therefore pointing to a hypertension-independent role of the RAS in renal damage in obese patients and its normalization after BS. It is suggested that the normalization of the eGFR after BS may be related to restoration in homeostasis of the RAS [24], and this is supported by experimental studies that show evidence of tubule-glomerular feedback resetting [25]. Thus, the correction of the dysregulated tubule-glomerular feedback may be the reason for those beneficial effects observed after BS.

The second relevant finding of this study is the close relationship between decreased albuminuria and improvement in all parameters of glucose metabolism. Indeed, most of the reported investigations regarding decreases in albuminuria after BS are based on cohorts of diabetic patients [20,26–28]. Podocyte dysfunction is considered of pivotal importance in the genesis of high albuminuria in both obesity and diabetes. Mechanical stress in the podocytes, secondary to glomerular hypertension, induces the differentiation and adhesion of the podocytes by reorganizing the actin cytoskeleton of the podocyte and compromising the size of the selective barrier of the slit diaphragm [8]. Here we show that improved glucose metabolism is an independent determinant of albuminuria regression, regardless of weight loss and blood pressure decrease and RAS changes, in a cohort where only 11% of patients were diabetic. Regarding the role of inflammation in decreasing albuminuria after BS, some authors have highlighted a possible role [9]. We also explored this mechanism, but although we found a correlation between changes in resistin and albuminuria, this cytokine no longer remained significant after adjusting for other variables.

We need to point out some limitations of the study. First, the GFR was estimated rather than measured directly. However, it should be noted that we determined the eGFR at various points over the 12 months and observed a significant decrease at any given time. In addition, although it has been suggested that weight loss-related changes in muscle mass influence eGFR to some extent, it is unlikely that a gradual decrease in eGFR over 12 months of follow-up will be accompanied by a continued decrease in muscle mass during this time. Second, for technical reasons, we were unable to determine interleukin-6 in most samples, so these data were excluded from the final analyses. Although it is a well-known marker of inflammation, we have complete data on hs-CRP, another hallmark of inflammation, and it was finally rejected that it played an important role in renal changes after adjustment for other variables. Finally, we cannot ignore the fact that the possible role of the RAS in changes in eGFR and glucose metabolism in changes in albuminuria are only hypotheses that should be confirmed in a randomized clinical trial.

5. Conclusions

In conclusion, our study demonstrates that weight loss and especially decreased aldosterone levels are the main factors associated to the restoration of the abnormally increased eGFR seen in obese patients after BS. This highlights the importance of the possible role of the RAS in renal hemodynamic alterations in obese patients that ultimately impair renal function. On the other hand, we show that increased albuminuria in obese patients is related to impaired glucose metabolism, regardless of blood pressure and weight loss.

Supplementary Materials: The following supporting information can be downloaded at: https://www.mdpi.com/article/10.3390/jcm11030728/s1. Figure S1. Flowchart for participants in the BAR-IHTA Study, Figure S2. Body weight change at follow-up, Table S1. Changes in adipokines and inflammatory markers 12 months after bariatric surgery. Table S2. Determinants of variation of eGFR (S2A) and of variation of albuminuria (S2B).

Author Contributions: Conceptualization, A.O., M.R. and A.G.; validation, S.V., I.G., D.B., M.C. and J.P.; formal analysis, X.D. and M.R.; investigation, I.G. and M.J.S.; methodology, X.D., resources, I.G. and S.V.; data curation, A.G. and D.B.; writing—original draft preparation, A.O.; writing—review and editing, A.O., M.R., S.V., M.C. and M.J.S.; supervision, M.J.S., M.C. and J.P.; project administration, A.O.; funding acquisition, A.O. and J.P. All authors have read and agreed to the published version of the manuscript.

Funding: The research reported in this publication was supported by the Spanish Society of Nephrology (Grant for Clinical Investigation. 2014) and by the Spanish Ministry of Health ISCIII RedinRen RD16/0009/0013.

Institutional Review Board Statement: The study was conducted according to the guidelines of the Declaration of Helsinki and approved by the Ethics Committee of Parc de Salut MAR, Barcelona, Spain (protocol code 2013/5248/I; date of approval 26 September 2013).

Informed Consent Statement: Informed consent was obtained from all subjects involved in the study.

Data Availability Statement: Not applicable.

Acknowledgments: We are indebted to Sara Alvarez, Maria Vera, Berta Xargay, Anna Faura, Tai Mooi Ho and Laia Fontdevila (Nephrology Dpt. Hospital del Mar and Hospital del Mar Medical Research Institute, Barcelona, Spain) for their effort and implication in the study. We are also indebted to David Benito (Hospital del Mar Medical Research Institute, Barcelona, Spain) for his valuable laboratory support.

Conflicts of Interest: The authors declare no conflict of interest. The funders of the study had no role in study design, data collection, data analysis, data interpretation, or the writing of the report.

Appendix A

Appendix A.1. Angiotensin-Converting Enzyme (ACE2) Enzymatic Assay

The ACE2 fluorescent enzymatic assay protocol was performed as previously described [18,19], using an ACE2-quenched fluorescent substrate (Mca-Ala-Pro-Lys(Dnp)-OH, BioMol, Hamburg, Germany; Enzo, Life Sciences, Farmingdale, NY, USA). Serum samples (2 µL) were incubated with ACE2 assay buffer [100 mM Tris·HCl, 600 mM NaCl, 10 µM ZnCl2, pH 7.5 in presence of protease inhibitors 100 µM captopril, 5 µM amastatin, 5 µM bestatin, and 10 µM Z-Pro-prolinal (from Sigma-Aldrich, St. Louis, MO, USA and Enzo Life Sciences, Farmingdale, NY, USA)] and 10 µM fluorogenic substrate in a final volume of 100 µL at 37 °C for 16 h. Serum ACE2 cleaves the substrate proportionally to the enzyme activity. Results were obtained after subtracting the background when an ACE2-especific inhibitor was added (0.6 µM DX600). Experiments were carried out in duplicate for each data point. Plates were read using a fluorescence plate reader (Tecan Infinite 200; Germany) at λex320 nm and λem400 nm. Results were expressed as RFU (relative fluorescent units)/µL serum/h.

Appendix A.2. ACE Enzymatic Assay

The ACE fluorescent enzymatic assay was performed as previously described [29,30]. For this determination, 2 µL of serum were incubated in duplicate with 73 µL of reaction buffer (0.5 M borate buffer and 5.45 M N-hippuryl-His-Leu) for 25 min at 37 °C. Finally, 15 µL of o-phthaldialdehyde (20 mg/mL) was added to the samples to form a fluorescent adduct with the enzyme-catalysed product L-histidyl-L-leucine. Fluorescence was measured at λex360 nm and λem485 nm. Results were expressed as RFU/µL serum.

Appendix B

Adipokines and Inflammatory Parameters

Cytokine and chemokine assays with Luminex kits were used. Three Milliplex MAP® kits from Millipore (Merck Millipore, Billerica, MA, USA) were used to test analytes: a 2-plex human adipokine magnetic bead panel 1 for Adiponectin and Resistin (#HADK1MAG-61K), a 3-plex human angiogenesis/growth factor magnetic bead panel 1 for Leptin (#HAGP1MAG-12K), and a 3-plex human cytokine/chemokine magnetic bead panel for MCP-1 (#HCYTOMAG-60K). According to manufacturers' instructions, all methods were performed by the same operator. All kits supplied lyophilized standards that were reconstituted and diluted at 7 serial concentrations (standard curves). Standards included all recombinant analytes tested and were considered as positive controls for the procedure. When indicated by the manufacturer, samples were diluted in assay buffer. Twenty-five µL of sample were used to capture an analyte on analyte-specific color-coded magnetic beads coated with capture antibodies. After the final wash, the beads were resuspended in sheath fluid and the median fluorescent intensity (MFI) data of 50 beads per bead set were analysed on a Luminex 200TM (Luminex Corp., Austin, TX, USA) and Bio-Plex Manager MP software (Bio-Rad, Hercules, CA, USA). Analyte concentrations were calculated by reference to an eight-point five-parameter logistic standard curve for each analyte.

References

1. WHO Organization. Obesity and Overweight. 2018. Available online: https://www.who.int/en/news-room/fact-sheets/detail/obesity-and-overweight (accessed on 19 December 2021).
2. Pi-Sunyer, X. The Medical Risks of Obesity. *Postgrad. Med.* **2009**, *121*, 21–33. [CrossRef] [PubMed]
3. Koch, V.H. Obesity Facts and Their Influence on Renal Function Across the Life Span. *Front. Med.* **2021**, *8*, 704409. [CrossRef] [PubMed]
4. Favre, G.; Anty, R.; Canivet, C.; Clément, G.; Ben-Amor, I.; Tran, A.; Gugenheim, J.; Gual, P.; Esnault, V.L.; Iannelli, A. Determinants associated with the correction of glomerular hyper-filtration one year after bariatric surgery. *Surg. Obes. Relat. Dis.* **2017**, *13*, 1760–1766. [CrossRef] [PubMed]
5. Rosenstock, J.L.; Pommier, M.; Stoffels, G.; Patel, S.; Michelis, M.F. Prevalence of Proteinuria and Albuminuria in an Obese Pop-ulation and Associated Risk Factors. *Front. Med.* **2018**, *5*, 122. [CrossRef] [PubMed]
6. Sutanto, A.; Wungu, C.D.K.; Susilo, H.; Sutanto, H. Reduction of Major Adverse Cardiovascular Events (MACE) after Bariatric Surgery in Patients with Obesity and Cardiovascular Diseases: A Systematic Review and Meta-Analysis. *Nutrients* **2021**, *13*, 3568. [CrossRef]
7. Li, K.; Zou, J.; Ye, Z.; Di, J.; Han, X.; Zhang, H.; Liu, W.; Ren, Q.; Zhang, P. Effects of Bariatric Surgery on Renal Function in Obese Patients: A Systematic Review and Meta Analysis. *PLoS ONE* **2016**, *11*, e0163907. [CrossRef]
8. Nair, M.; le Roux, C.W.; Docherty, N.G. Mechanisms underpinning remission of albuminuria following bariatric surgery. *Curr. Opin. Endocrinol. Diabetes Obes.* **2016**, *23*, 366–372. [CrossRef]
9. Fenske, W.K.; Dubb, S.; Bueter, M.; Seyfried, F.; Patel, K.; Tam, F.W.; Frankel, A.H.; Le Roux, C. Effect of bariatric surgery-induced weight loss on renal and systemic inflammation and blood pressure: A 12-month prospective study. *Surg. Obes. Relat. Dis.* **2013**, *9*, 559–568. [CrossRef]
10. Oliveras, A.; Goday, A.; Sans, L.; Arias, C.E.; Vazquez, S.; Benaiges, D.; Ramon, J.M.; Pascual, J. Changes in Central 24-h Ambu-latory Blood Pressure and Hemodynamics 12 Months After Bariatric Surgery: The Barihta Study. *Obes. Surg.* **2020**, *30*, 195–205. [CrossRef]
11. Myers, G.L.; Miller, W.G.; Coresh, J.; Fleming, J.; Greenberg, N.; Greene, T.; Hostetter, T.; Levey, A.S.; Panteghini, M.; Welch, M.; et al. Recommendations for improving SCr measurement: A report from the Laboratory Working Group of the National Kidney Disease Education Program. *Clin. Chem.* **2006**, *52*, 5–18. [CrossRef]
12. Brunetti, L.; Back, H.; Yu, S.; Jalil, U.; Kagan, L. Evaluation and enhancement of standard equations for renal function estimation in individuals with components of metabolic disease. *BMC Nephrol.* **2021**, *22*, 389. [CrossRef] [PubMed]
13. Levey, A.S.; Coresh, J.; Greene, T.; Stevens, L.A.; Zhang, Y.L.; Hendriksen, S.; Kusek, J.W.; Van Lente, F.; Chronic Kidney Disease Epidemiology Collaboration. Using Standardized Serum Creatinine Values in the Modification of Diet in Renal Disease Study Equation for Estimating Glomerular Filtration Rate. *Ann. Intern. Med.* **2006**, *145*, 247–254. [CrossRef]
14. Levey, A.S.; Stevens, L.A.; Schmid, C.H.; Zhang, Y.L.; Castro, A.F., III; Feldman, H.I.; Kusek, J.W.; Eggers, P.; Van Lente, F.; Greene, T.; et al. A new equation to estimate glomerular filtration rate. *Ann. Intern. Med.* **2009**, *150*, 604–661. [CrossRef]
15. Soler, M.J.; Riera, M.; Crespo, M.; Mir, M.; Marquez, E.; Pascual, M.J.; Puig, J.M.; Pascual, J. Circulating Angiotensin-Converting Enzyme 2 Activity in Kidney Transplantation: A Longitudinal Pilot Study. *Nephron Exp. Nephrol.* **2012**, *121*, c144–c150. [CrossRef] [PubMed]
16. Tucker, O.N.; Szomstein, S.; Rosenthal, R.J. Indications for Sleeve Gastrectomy as a Primary Procedure for Weight Loss in the Morbidly Obese. *J. Gastrointest. Surg.* **2008**, *12*, 662–667. [CrossRef] [PubMed]
17. Kwakernaak, A.J.; Toering, T.J.; Navis, G. Body mass index and body fat distribution as renal risk factors: A focus on the role of renal haemodynamics. *Nephrol. Dial. Transplant.* **2013**, *28*, iv42–iv49. [CrossRef] [PubMed]
18. Currie, A.; Chetwood, A.; Ahmed, A.R. Bariatric Surgery and Renal Function. *Obes. Surg.* **2011**, *21*, 528–539. [CrossRef] [PubMed]
19. Herman-Edelstein, M.; Weinstein, T.; Chagnac, A. Obesity-Related Glomerulopathy: Clinical Management. *Semin. Nephrol.* **2021**, *41*, 358–370. [CrossRef] [PubMed]
20. Upala, S.; Wijarnpreecha, K.; Congrete, S.; Rattanawong, P.; Sanguankeo, A. Bariatric surgery reduces urinary albumin excretion in diabetic nephropathy: A systematic review and meta-analysis. *Surg. Obes. Relat. Dis.* **2016**, *12*, 1037–1044. [CrossRef]
21. Zhang, T.; Wang, Y.; Zhang, X.; Wang, W.; Zhao, G. The Impact of Bariatric Surgery on Renal Function: A Retrospective Analysis of Short-Term Outcomes. *Obes. Surg.* **2021**, *31*, 3476–3482. [CrossRef]
22. Friedman, A.N.; Wahed, A.S.; Wang, J.; Courcoulas, A.P.; Dakin, G.; Hinojosa, M.W.; Kimmel, P.L.; Mitchell, J.E.; Pomp, A.; Pories, W.J.; et al. Effect of Bariatric Surgery on CKD Risk. *J. Am. Soc. Nephrol.* **2018**, *29*, 1289–1300. [CrossRef] [PubMed]
23. Hall, J.E.; do Carmo, J.M.; da Silva, A.A.; Wang, Z.; Hall, M.E. Obesity, kidney dysfunction and hypertension: Mechanistic links. *Nat. Rev. Nephrol.* **2019**, *15*, 367–385. [CrossRef] [PubMed]
24. Tham, J.C.; Le Roux, C.W.; Docherty, N.G. Cardiovascular, Renal and Overall Health Outcomes After Bariatric Surgery. *Curr. Cardiol. Rep.* **2015**, *17*, 34. [CrossRef] [PubMed]
25. Monu, S.R.; Maheshwari, M.; Peterson, E.L.; Carretero, O.A. Role of connecting tubule glomerular feedback in obesity related renal damage. *Am. J. Physiol. Renal. Physiol.* **2018**, *315*, F1708–F1713. [CrossRef] [PubMed]
26. Schauer, P.R.; Bhatt, D.L.; Kirwan, J.P.; Wolski, K.; Aminian, A.; Brethauer, S.A.; Navaneethan, S.D.; Singh, R.P.; Pothier, C.E.; Nissen, S.E.; et al. Bariatric Surgery versus Intensive Medical Therapy for Diabetes—5-Year Outcomes. *N. Engl. J. Med.* **2017**, *376*, 641–651. [CrossRef] [PubMed]

27. O'Brien, R.; Johnson, E.; Haneuse, S.; Coleman, K.J.; O'Connor, P.J.; Fisher, D.P.; Sidney, S.; Bogart, A.; Theis, M.K.; Anau, J.; et al. Microvascular Outcomes in Patients with Diabetes after Bariatric Surgery Versus Usual Care: A Matched Cohort Study. *Ann. Intern. Med.* **2018**, *169*, 300–310. [CrossRef] [PubMed]
28. Look AHEAD Research Group. Effect of a long-term behavioural weight loss intervention on nephropathy in overweight or obese adults with type 2 diabetes: A secondary analysis of the Look AHEAD randomised clinical trial. *Lancet Diabetes En-Docrinol.* **2014**, *2*, 801–809. [CrossRef]
29. Anguiano, L.; Riera, M.; Pascual, J.; Valdivielso, J.M.; Barrios, C.; Betriu, A.; Mojal, S.; Fernández, E.; Soler, M.J. Circulating angiotensin-converting enzyme 2 activity in patients with chronic kidney disease without previous history of cardiovascular disease. *Nephrol. Dial. Transplant.* **2015**, *30*, 1176–1185. [CrossRef]
30. Schwager, S.L.; Carmona, A.; Sturrock, E.D. A high-throughput fluorimetric assay for angiotensin I-converting enzyme. *Nat. Protoc.* **2006**, *1*, 1961–1964. [CrossRef]

Journal of
Clinical Medicine

MDPI

Review

Thyroid Function Alteration in Obesity and the Effect of Bariatric Surgery

María Cordido [1,2,3], Paula Juiz-Valiña [1,2], Paula Urones [1,2], Susana Sangiao-Alvarellos [1,2,*,†] and Fernando Cordido [1,2,4,*,†]

1 Grupo Fisiopatoloxía Endócrina, Nutricional e Médica (FENM), Facultad de Ciencias de la Salud, Universidade da Coruña, 15006 A Coruña, Spain; maria.cordido.carro@sergas.es (M.C.); paula.juiz.valina@sergas.es (P.J.-V.); paula.urones.cuesta@sergas.es (P.U.)
2 Instituto de Investigación Biomedica (INIBIC), Centro de Investigaciones Científicas Avanzadas (CICA), Universidade da Coruña, 15006 A Coruña, Spain
3 Servicio Urgencias, Hospital Universitario A Coruña, 15006 A Coruña, Spain
4 Servicio Endocrinología y Nutrición, Hospital Universitario A Coruña, 15006 A Coruña, Spain
* Correspondence: susana.sangiao@udc.gal (S.S.-A.); fernando.cordido.carballido@sergas.es (F.C.); Tel.: +34-981178127 (S.S.-A. & F.C.); Fax: +34-981178204 (S.S.-A. & F.C.)
† These authors contributed equally to this work.

Abstract: The most common endocrine disease in obesity is hypothyroidism and secondary endocrine alterations, including abnormal thyroid function, are frequent in obesity. It is unclear whether impaired thyroid function is the cause or the consequence of increased adiposity; furthermore, there are no clear data regarding the best way to dose levothyroxine for patients with both hypothyroidism and obesity, and the effect of bariatric surgery (BS). The aim of the present article is to review some controversial aspects of the relation between obesity and the thyroid: (1) Thyroid function in obesity and the effect of BS (2) Thyroid hormone treatment (THT) in obese patients with hypothyroidism and the effect of BS. In summary: In morbidly obese patients, TSH is moderately increased. Morbid obesity has a mild central resistance to the thyroid hormone, reversible with weight loss. In morbidly obese hypothyroid patients, following weight loss, the levothyroxine dose/kg of ideal weight did not change, albeit there was an increment in the levothyroxine dose/kg of actual weight. From a clinical practice perspective, in morbid obesity, diagnosing mild hypothyroidism is difficult, BS improves the altered thyroid function and THT can be adapted better if it is based on ideal weight.

Keywords: obesity; endocrine abnormalities; bariatric surgery; hypothyroidism

Citation: Cordido, M.; Juiz-Valiña, P.; Urones, P.; Sangiao-Alvarellos, S.; Cordido, F. Thyroid Function Alteration in Obesity and the Effect of Bariatric Surgery. *J. Clin. Med.* **2022**, *11*, 1340. https://doi.org/10.3390/jcm11051340

Academic Editor: David Benaiges Boix

Received: 9 February 2022
Accepted: 25 February 2022
Published: 28 February 2022

1. Introduction

The thyroid hormone (TH) controls dietary intake as well as energy expenditure, both resting and total, and consequently, obesity and different metabolic diseases can appear in patients with altered thyroid function. Furthermore, altered thyroid function is characterized by the presence of changes in total body weight and total body composition, body temperature, and metabolic expenditure [1].

Thyroid function studies are frequently indicated in the evaluation of obesity etiology [2]. It is common to find slightly increased values of thyrotropin (TSH) in obesity [3,4]. It is unclear whether the altered thyroid function present in obesity is due to the excess adiposity or, alternatively, the decreased thyroid function is the cause of the excess adiposity. The thyroid axis regulates the adipose tissue and the adipose tissue affects the activity of the thyroid axis [5].

Obesity could be considered a disease of the nervous system [6] and is a great problem to the health system at the present time, with very important consequences for health care and society [7]. In recent years, the number of obese patients has progressively augmented. In the last 40 years, obesity has reached epidemic proportions and obesity-related diseases have consistently increased in the last 30 years due, predominantly, to cardiovascular disease [8]. Spain has a prevalence of obesity of 22.9% [9] and in almost all European countries is more than 20% [2]. The age-adjusted prevalence of obesity in the USA is 40.4% in women and 35.0% in men. The corresponding values for class 3 obesity (with BMI $\geq$ 40 kg/m^2) are 9.9% for women and 5.5% for men [10]. A projection study indicates that the prevalence in the USA of obesity in adults and obesity with a BMI $\geq$ 35 kg/m^2 will increase [11]. Slightly lower results have been found all over the world [12]. As little as 5% weight loss improves the function in different organs and tissues concurrently, and progressively increased weight decrement induces changes in key adipose tissue biological pathways [13,14]. Bariatric surgery (BS), using laparoscopic banding, sleeve gastrectomy (SG), or a laparoscopic Roux-en-Y Gastric Bypass (RYGB), compared with medical treatment, has produced more marked ameliorations in diseases associated with obesity and a more marked decrease in all-cause mortality [15]. In obesity, bariatric surgery was associated with longer life duration than medical treatment, even though mortality remained elevated, in both the surgical and usual care of obese groups when compared with the general population [16]. A clear amelioration in obesity-related diseases has also been found following BS. These benefits in patients occur early, before the presence of any significant weight loss, so that benefits may be probably due to the gastrointestinal hormonal secretion modifications due to bariatric surgery [17]. In marked contrast, in patients with obesity and Type 2 diabetes treated with RYGB surgery or diet, the clinical improvement of RYGB surgery and diet were very similar and were apparently related to weight loss itself, suggesting that the benefits of BS are exclusively due to the effect of weight loss [18].

The most prevalent endocrine disease in obesity is subclinical primary hypothyroidism. It is suggested to test all patients with obesity for the presence of altered thyroid function [2]. Hypothyroidism, defined as an increased circulating TSH value, affects up to 10% of the adults, affecting more women than men [19]. Obesity is accompanied with endocrine alterations, including a decreased growth hormone (GH) response to different stimuli [20–24] and altered thyroid function [22,25]. Thyroxine values have been found to be normal, increased, and decreased in obesity; these different results are likely due to the fact that the patients were examined at various time periods, have different sexes and ages, and may differ in the severity and kind of obesity as well as in the presence of obesity comorbidities [3,4,25–28]. The disturbance of thyroid function in obese patients and the role of BS treatment on thyroid function change is unclear at the present time. There are different studies showing various results in connection with the change of thyrotropin after BS and the influence of weight decrement [28–34]. The free thyroxine (FT4) results in obese patients and the influence of BS are even more controversial [29].

As previously mentioned, the most prevalent endocrine disease in obesity is decreased thyroid function and it is recommended to measure circulating thyroid hormones in all obese patients [2]. In clinical practice, body weight is frequently used to estimate the total dose of levothyroxine (LT4) to administer in the presence of decreased thyroid function [35]. There are various reasons for increased requirements of levothyroxine in obese subjects: increased lean and fat mass [36], increased volume of distribution, or altered gastrointestinal tract absorption [37]. As such, weight loss from BS may reduce the levothyroxine needs [38,39]. Conversely, the surgical technique, by altering the anatomy and physiology of the gastrointestinal tract, could induce a decrease in the absorption of the hormone and, therefore, increase the requirements of levothyroxine [40].

The objective of the present article is to review some controversial aspects of the relation between obesity and thyroid function: (1) thyroid function in obesity and the influence of bariatric surgery; (2) thyroid hormone replacement in obese patients with hypothyroidism and the influence of bariatric surgery.

2. Thyroid Function in Obesity and the Effect of Bariatric Surgery

TH values have been found to be decreased, increased, and normal in obesity [3,4,26,28]. Our group has found increased TSH values in morbidly obese patients [34]. Rotondi et al. [4] have found augmented circulating TSH values in an ample group of severely obese subjects when compared with healthy normal weight subjects. Reinehr et al. [27] reported increased thyrotropin levels in obese children when compared with normal weight children. The degree of overweight correlated with circulating thyrotropin results. Valdes et al. [3] have found augmented circulating TSH values in severe obesity, and have suggested that reference values for thyrotropin may be unsuitable to define decreased thyroid function in persons who are severely obese.

At present, it is unclear if the slight elevation of TSH values present in obesity causes weight gain or if it is due to obesity induced activation of the hypothalamus-pituitary-thyroid (HPT) axis, causing an increase in serum TSH. In support of the latter theory, there are studies that have found that thyrotropin values decrease following surgery [34,41]. In order to clear up this question, Wang et al. [42] employed data from genome wide association studies to carry out a bidirectional mendelian randomization analysis. They found that inverse variance-weighted and mendelian randomization-Egger results indicated that genetically driven circulating thyrotropin did not lead to changes in the body mass index or increased body weight. Additionally, the inverse variance-weighted method showed that the circulating thyrotropin values could be increased by a genetically predicted high body mass index. These data clearly suggest that obesity can significantly increase TSH [42]. In addition, if increased TSH is considered a consequence of increased adiposity, our clinical practice should be modified. Slight increased thyrotropin in obese patients without any other data of decreased thyroid function should be considered normal. Nevertheless, increased thyrotropin circulating levels may elicit detrimental effects due to its actions in extra thyroidal tissues [43].

The consequences and mechanisms of increased circulating TSH in obese patients are unclear. Different mechanisms could explain the relationship of decreased thyroid function to increased adipose tissue [44]. There is a direct role of circulating thyrotropin levels in the physiological regulation of thermogenesis [45]. Thyrotropin receptors are decreased in obese patients when compared with normal subjects [46]. The elevation of circulating thyrotropin levels may be due to a compensatory activation of the HPT axis in response to increased adiposity [26]. In accordance with that hypothesis, in morbid obesity after weight loss, a positive relationship between resting energy expenditure and free thyroxine (FT4) has been found [47] and elevated FT4 has been found in obese patients [27]. This activation could be mediated by central actions of the adipose tissue hormone leptin [48]. In contrast, Marzullo [49] et al. have found that increased adiposity could trigger autoimmunity against the thyroid, suggesting that increased adiposity could be a casual mechanism for established thyroid disease.

The effect of bariatric surgery on postoperative thyroid activity evolution remains incompletely understood. Several studies have found different results regarding the variation in circulating thyrotropin values following BS and the relation of thyrotropin variation with weight decrement [28–33]. Most [29,30,32], but not all [28,33], studies have found a decrease of circulating thyrotropin values post-intervention. Our group carried out a study evaluating 129 euthyroid patients with morbid obesity before and after BS. Thyrotropin declined over time, and the thyrotropin reduction was associated with the excessive BMI loss [34]. Similar results have been found in the systematic review and meta-analysis from Guan et al. [29]. Neves et al. [32] evaluated euthyroid obese subjects and found that bariatric surgery induces a decrement of thyrotropin levels and that the decrease was associated with the weight loss following BS. In contrast, Dall'Asta et al. [33] performed an observational study evaluating healthy subjects and obese patients after gastric banding induced weight loss and found that thyrotropin values did not change. Zhang et al. [28] followed and evaluated obese subjects after RYGB surgery and found that thyrotropin values remained stable. In the study of Guan et al., free thyroxine did not change following

BS [29]. According to their data, in obese patients after BS, no variation was found in free thyroxine or free triiodothyronine values [50].

The mechanisms of the thyrotropin decrease after bariatric surgery are not yet fully understood. This fall of circulating thyrotropin levels is weight loss mediated and is not due to an effect of bariatric surgery. A decrease of circulating thyrotropin has been found in obesity after lifestyle change caused weight loss [51], and the decrement of the thyrotropin values was associated with excessive weight loss following bariatric surgery [32,34], suggesting that the decrease in thyrotropin is primarily due to the weight loss. The decrease of circulating leptin values after bariatric surgery could be the mechanism responsible for the decreased stimulation of the hypothalamus-pituitary-thyroid axis [48,52] and the decline of circulating thyrotropin values. Besides, reduced thyrotropin receptor expression and thyrotropin resistance is improved by weight loss [46]. Moreover, due to the link between the hypothalamus-pituitary-IGF-I axis and excessive adiposity [20–22,53,54] and the influence of GH on the thyroid axis [55], the relationship between the hypothalamus-pituitary-IGF-I axis and thyrotropin has been studied, but with negative results [34].

From a clinical perspective, the increased thyrotropin values in obesity stand out that it is an important clinical problem to diagnose the presence of mild hypothyroidism in obesity [25]. Hypothyroidism should be considered in obesity with marginally elevated thyrotropin values only after measuring circulating levels of TH and thyroid autoantibodies, and with data suggesting decreased TH action [25]. Marginally elevated circulating thyrotropin values could be due to a compensatory response to morbid obesity and not a real decreased thyroid hormone action [3]. Furthermore, these data do not suggest the diminution of the upper limit of thyrotropin values [56,57] to diagnose hypothyroidism in obese patients.

Elevated free thyroxine coexist with elevated thyrotropin in the clinical situation of resistance to TH, an inherited rare disease [58,59]. There are two types of resistance to thyroid hormone, hypothalamus-pituitary resistance, and decrease peripheral resistance to TH's actions. The pituitary resistance can be assessed measuring circulating TH values and TSH values or more precisely with the thyrotroph T4 Resistance Index (TT4RI) and TSH index (TSHRI) [60,61]. In extremely obese patients, TH values and thyrotropin values tend to be elevated [62]. Hence, the increased thyroxine and high thyrotropin can be conciliated if increased thyroxine and increased thyrotropin circulating values are due to a central resistance to TH. Further, the resistance could be also present at a peripheral level. An acquired mild resistance to thyroxine has been suggested by Tjorve et al. [63]. Laclaustra et al. [64] have found a clear relation between central resistance to the thyroid hormone and the prevalence of metabolic diseases like obesity and diabetes in a representative sample of the population of the United States of America.

TH action is different for each tissue, depending on TH values and on the unique mixture of cell membrane transporters, deiodinases, and thyroid hormone receptors present in each tissue [65]. The resistance to TH indices measure pituitary resistance, the thyrotropin inhibition by circulating free thyroxine values. Moreover, the presence of obesity suggests decreased thyroid function and supports that peripheral resistance to the thyroid hormone is also present [64]. Additionally, there are experimental models of reduced thyroid hormone action in excessive adiposity [65,66]. Thyroid hormone receptors are diminished on the adipose tissue of obese patients [46]. Moreover, the thyroid hormone receptor β has been found to be related with disease severity in liver tissue from morbidly obese patients with different phases of hepatic injury, following BS [67]. Furthermore, sensitivity to the thyroid hormone could be epigenetically regulated [68]. Our group has found elevated TT4RI and TSHRI in obese patients and these indices decline with weight loss [69], suggesting that the elevation of circulating thyrotropin values and free thyroxine levels could be due to a stimulation of the HPT axis [26].

The mechanisms that explain bariatric surgery induced diminution in the indices of central resistance to the thyroid hormone are unclear. The decline in the indices of central resistance to thyroid hormone has been found related to excessive weight loss following bariatric surgery [69]. This decline is likely due to weight loss itself. A diminution in circulating thyrotropin levels has been found in obesity following lifestyle induced weight loss [51] and the decline in thyrotropin levels has been found associated with excessive weight loss after bariatric surgery [32,34]. According to these data, TH resistance improves due to an increase in the reduced thyroid hormone receptor expression with weight loss [46]. The decrease in circulating leptin values [52], due to the decrease in body fat, could reduce the pituitary stimulation of the thyroid axis [48] and induce a decrease of thyrotropin. Nevertheless, leptin treatment did not modify the thyroid anatomy [70]. In the presence of extreme resistance to insulin action, the prevalence of thyroid nodules and the goiter is increased [70]. Conversely, Juiz-Valiña et al. could not find any relationship between insulin resistance and TT4RI or TSHRI [69]. Growth Hormone secretion is altered in obese patients [20–22,53,54], and circulating GH values could regulate the HPT axis. Growth hormones increased, circulating free triiodothyronine, and diminished, circulating free thyroxine values [55]. Growth hormone treatment in adult patients causes different changes in the thyroid axis, the most important is decreased free thyroxine values [71,72]. In obesity, there is a markedly decreased GH secretion, this alteration could be responsible of the increased free thyroxine values. Juiz-Valiña et al. found no relationship between the GH-IGF-1 axis and the central resistance to TH [69]. In contrast, indices of inflammation, such as c-reactive protein, highly correlate with TT4RI or TSHRI in obesity [69]. In accordance with those results, SG induces thyrotropin diminution in obesity, which correlates with an improved inflammatory state after BS [73]. In summary, the results of Juiz-Valiña et al. suggest that the decrease in TT4RI or TSHRI following bariatric surgery is primarily due to weight loss and the improved inflammatory state could be a contributory factor [69]. These data also suggest that the improvement of thyroid function is another benefit of bariatric surgery [74]. Recently reduced pituitary sensitivity to TH has been found to be associated with diabetes and hypertension in a representative group of Iranian euthyroid subjects [75]. These data reinforce the importance of the relation between reduced central sensitivity to thyroid hormone with metabolic diseases. The most important aspects of thyroid function in obesity and the effect of bariatric surgery are summarized in Table 1.

Table 1. Thyroid function in obesity and the effect of bariatric surgery.

	Thyroid Function in Obesity and the Effect of Bariatric Surgery
-	In severe obesity, thyrotropin is moderately increased. The slightly elevated thyrotropin in obese patients is due to increased adiposity.
-	Weight loss provokes a diminution of the elevated thyrotropin values. The decrease of thyrotropin after BS is dependent on the excessive weight loss.
-	BS improves the subclinical hypothyroidism of morbid obesity.
-	Morbid obesity is characterized by a mild central resistance to the thyroid hormone. Weight loss induced with BS cause a reduction in the increased pituitary resistance to thyroid hormone.

BS, Bariatric Surgery.

3. Thyroid Hormone Treatment in Obese Patients with Hypothyroidism and the Effect of Bariatric Surgery

Actually, it is not clear what happens to the dose of thyroxine in hypothyroid patients after bariatric surgery. Thus, there is a clear need of additional studies [76]. Furthermore, the effect of distinct bariatric surgery techniques on levothyroxine absorption is not clear [77]. Ojomo et al. [35] have studied thyroid hormone replacement after thyroidectomy in 122 patients and they conclude that the present standard of weight-based thyroid hormone replacement (THR) does not adequately dose underweight and overweight patients [35]. The most common starting dose of levothyroxine after a total thyroidectomy is 1.6 μg/kg [78]. This dose is adjusted based on circulating thyrotropin levels and clinical data. The dosage recommendations are often ambiguous, regarding whether the dose is based on the current total body weight (BW), estimated ideal BW (IBW) or estimated lean body weight (LBW). Obese subjects can develop hyperthyroidism if dosing is based on the same data used for non-obese subjects [79]. A more adequate thyroid hormone replacement should include the BW and body mass index of the obese patient [78].

The altered thyroxine absorption induced by bariatric surgery has been analyzed, albeit with questionable results. Since the introduction of obesity surgery in clinical practice, doubts about altered drug absorption have been featured [80,81]. Decreased thyroid function treatment mandates oral THR, and there are concerns about its adequacy after bariatric surgery [36]. The primary thyroxine absorption site is the small intestine in the jejunum and the ileum [37]. Various endogenous and exogenous factors may disturb intestinal levothyroxine absorption [82]. Bariatric surgery could probably be included in the list of factors that alter intestinal levothyroxine absorption [76]. Surgery procedures with gastric restriction (gastric banding and sleeve gastrectomy), are procedures that modify drug absorption less than procedures involving intestinal diversion [83]. Levothyroxine absorption has been found similar before and after RYGB [36]. Different studies have found an increased need for levothyroxine after jejunoileal bypass techniques [84–86]. These data are in keeping with the increased thyrotropin levels found in patients treated with the same levothyroxine dose after bariatric surgery [87,88]. Furthermore, others have found a diminution in thyroxine needs after BS [38,89]. Rudnicki et al. [90] have described that bariatric surgery improved thyroid function in hypothyroidism. Similar improvements in levothyroxine doses after bariatric surgery have been found by other authors [89,91,92]. A recent meta-analysis [41] has found that bariatric surgery promotes a decrease in the total levothyroxine requirement. In the study of Pedro et al. [77], the total levothyroxine dose before and 12 months following bariatric surgery was similar, however, the thyroxine dose/kg of actual weight was increased. Other authors have found similar results with a decrease or no change in the total levothyroxine requirement, but an increase of the weight-based levothyroxine requirement after bariatric surgery [93]. Our group has encountered that, following bariatric surgery, the total levothyroxine or the levothyroxine dose/kg of IBW did not change; however, the levothyroxine dose/body surface area, levothyroxine dose/kg of actual BW, levothyroxine dose/kg of adjusted BW and levothyroxine dose/kg of LBW increased [94].

It has been encountered that the weight-based daily levothyroxine dose increased following a Roux-en-Y Gastric Bypass, with no significant changes after sleeve gastrectomy [95]. These result highly suggest that sleeve gastrectomy and a Roux-en-Y Gastric Bypass showed different changes in levothyroxine needs. However, in agreement with Pedro et al. [77], our group study did not find the bariatric surgery technique to be a predictor of levothyroxine dose variation [94]. Similar results have been found by other authors; both sleeve gastrectomy and a Roux-en-Y Gastric Bypass improved thyroid function in the same way [90]. These data support that both procedures have similar effects on levothyroxine absorption. Altered gastric emptying modifies the levothyroxine absorption [96], and altered gastric emptying is present in the Roux-en-Y Gastric Bypass and sleeve gastrectomy [97]. This could be the mechanism that explains the similar results between the malabsorptive and restrictive techniques.

The mechanisms for bariatric surgery levothyroxine dose variations are unclear. Rubio et al. [36] have found a delay of levothyroxine absorption in the surgically-treated patients. Gkotsina et al. [40] have encountered that the pharmacokinetic data were similar following a Roux-en-Y Gastric Bypass, and that levothyroxine pharmacokinetics improve after a biliopancreatic diversion [40]. Conversely, has been found that by employing the same dose of levothyroxine before and after bariatric surgery, the serum TSH increased following bariatric surgery [88]. Levothyroxine needs are increased with malabsorptive procedures, and results about thyroxine needs with procedures combining restrictive and malabsorptive techniques are conflicting. This could be due to the different schedule of levothyroxine ingestion, the diverse effects of bariatric surgery and other endogenous and exogenous factors, like other drugs administration [97,98]. In obese, diabetic patients with primary hypothyroidism and treated with levothyroxine, metformin treatment provokes a decrease in circulating TSH [99]. Most of the studies have found that bariatric surgery induces a decrease in total levothyroxine dose [41]. Nevertheless, the different characteristics of the studies does not make it possible to draw definitive conclusions about the net effect on levothyroxine needs [100]. Furthermore, the evaluation of levothyroxine dosing is not always adjusted for weight and so does not allow for a correct comparison of the data. Lean body mass modification after bariatric surgery could also contribute to the change in levothyroxine doses [79]. Rudnicki et al. [90] have found a decrease of levothyroxine dosage after bariatric surgery in hypothyroid patients. Moreover, impaired levothyroxine pharmacokinetics in obese patients have been indicated [93]. In summary, in most of the studies, weight loss following bariatric surgery provokes a diminution in total levothyroxine needs. Juiz-Valiña et al. have found that in obese hypothyroid patients treated with BS, the absolute levothyroxine dose did not change, nor did the levothyroxine dose/kg of IBW, but the levothyroxine dose/body surface area, levothyroxine dose/kg of actual BW, or levothyroxine dose/kg of LBW significantly increased [94]. A change in the absolute levothyroxine dose and levothyroxine dose/kg of IBW was not related to excessive weight loss. On the contrary, excessive weight loss was related to an increase in the levothyroxine dose/body surface area, and levothyroxine dose/kg of present BW [94]. These data suggest that the thyroid hormone replacement change after bariatric surgery is due to a mixed mechanism, a decrease in levothyroxine needs due to weight loss and a decrease in levothyroxine absorption due to the surgical procedure. Decreased thyroid function treated patients could be metabolically different when compared with normal subjects. Accordingly, it has been found that obese hypothyroid women on levothyroxine therapy, with normal circulating thyrotropin values, have a diminished energy expenditure, suggesting that standard levothyroxine replacement does not fully correct metabolic alterations related to hypothyroidism [101]. Furthermore, other studies have encountered that hypothyroid patients treated with levothyroxine showed higher adiposity and similar insulin resistance, but healthier lipid levels compared with euthyroid obese patients [102].

The best way to titrate the levothyroxine dose for patients with decreased thyroid function and increased adiposity is not clear [78]. A weight-based dosing of the thyroid hormone inappropriately overdoses obese patients [78]. A better way for thyroid hormone dosing could consider other aspects, such as both the weight and BMI of the obese patient, and recommended using either the present weight of the obese subject with adjustment of the dose, considering the BMI or the adjusted BW [78]. Other authors have considered that the best way to titrate the levothyroxine dose is taking into account lean body mass [79]. In obese patients with a diminished thyroid function, the demand for levothyroxine is increased due to augmented fat mass and lean body mass [30]. Furthermore, in a multivariable analyses study, the levothyroxine dose was predicted by the amount of fat-free mass, hypothyroidism etiology, and the sex of the patients [102]. Juiz-Valiña et al. observed that in extreme obese patients, after bariatric surgery the levothyroxine dose/kg of IBW did not change, however, the levothyroxine dose/body surface area, levothyroxine dose/kg of actual BW, or levothyroxine dose/kg of lean BW increased [94]. In summary, thyroid hormone replacement titration in hypothyroid patients with excessive adiposity can be adjusted more correctly based on IBW. The most important aspects of thyroid hormone treatment in obese patients with hypothyroidism and the effects of bariatric surgery are summarized in Table 2.

Table 2. Thyroid hormone treatment in obese patients with hypothyroidism and the effects of bariatric surgery.

	Thyroid Hormone Treatment in Obese Patients with Hypothyroidism and the Effects of Bariatric Surgery
-	In hypothyroid severe obese patients following BS-induced weight loss, the total levothyroxine dose decreased, the levothyroxine dose/kg of IBW did not change and the levothyroxine dose/kg of actual BW increased.
-	In hypothyroid severe obese patients, after BS, the weight lost was inversely correlated with the levothyroxine dose/body surface and levothyroxine dose/kg of actual BW. The absolute levothyroxine dose and the levothyroxine dose/kg of IBW was not related with weight loss
-	The levothyroxine needs and its change after BS was similar for SG and RYGB
-	Thyroid hormone replacement in patients with obesity and hypothyroidism can be more adequately adjusted if it is based on IBW.

BW, body weight; IBW, ideal body weight; BS, Bariatric Surgery; RYGB, Roux-en-Y-Gastric Bypass; SG, Sleeve Gastrectomy.

4. Conclusions and Clinical Implications

In morbidly obese patients, TSH is moderately increased (Table 3). Weight loss provokes a diminution of the elevated thyrotropin values. This decrease of thyrotropin after BS is dependent on the excessive weight lost. These data suggest that the moderately elevated thyrotropin values present in obese patients are due to the increased adiposity of obesity. From a clinical practice point of view, diagnosing mild hypothyroidism is difficult in severe obesity, and BS improves the mild hypothyroidism of severe excessive adiposity (Table 4).

Table 3. Essential points.

	Essential Points
-	In morbid obese patients, thyrotropin is moderately increased.
-	The slightly elevated thyrotropin encountered in obese patients is reversible with weight loss and due to the increased adiposity.
-	Morbid obesity is characterized by a slight pituitary resistance to thyroid hormones that is reversible with BS-induced weight loss
-	In hypothyroid patients treated with levothyroxine and with obesity, following BS-induced weight loss, the total levothyroxine dose decrease, the levothyroxine dose/kg of actual weight increase and the levothyroxine dose/kg of IBW was stable, in most of the studies.

IBW, ideal body weight; BS, Bariatric Surgery.

Table 4. Clinical implications.

	Clinical Implications
-	Clinically, the diagnosis of subclinical hypothyroidism is difficult in severe obesity, and BS improves the mild subclinical hypothyroidism present in severe obesity.
-	The levothyroxine needs following BS were similar for SG and RYGB.
-	From a clinical practice perspective, thyroid hormone replacement in patients with obesity and hypothyroidism can be more adequately adjusted if it is based on IBW.

IBW, ideal body weight; BS, Bariatric Surgery; RYGB, Roux-en-Y-Gastric Bypass; SG, Sleeve Gastrectomy.

Morbid obesity is characterized by a mild reversible pituitary resistance to the thyroid hormone. Weight loss induced with bariatric surgery causes a reduction in the increased pituitary resistance to TH.

In morbid hypothyroid obese patients, following weight loss, the total levothyroxine dose decreased and the levothyroxine dose/kg of IBW did not change in most of the studies. However, the levothyroxine dose/kg of actual BW increased.

In morbid hypothyroid obese patients, after BS, the diminution in the percentage of weight lost was significantly inversely correlated with the levothyroxine dose/body surface and the levothyroxine dose/kg of actual BW. Additionally, the absolute levothyroxine dose and the levothyroxine dose/kg of IBW was not related with weight loss.

The levothyroxine needs and its change after bariatric surgery was similar for Sleeve Gastrectomy and Roux-en-Y-Gastric Bypass.

From a clinical practice perspective, thyroid hormone replacement in patients with obesity and hypothyroidism can be more adequately adjusted if it is based on IBW, and RYGB does not affect levothyroxine absorption differently from SG.

Author Contributions: Conceptualization: S.S.-A. and F.C.; Methodology: M.C., P.J.-V. and P.U.; Investigation, M.C., P.J.-V., S.S.-A. and F.C.; Writing manuscript: M.C. and F.C.; Writing—Review & Editing, M.C., P.J.-V., P.U., S.S.-A. and F.C.; Supervision, S.S.-A. and F.C.; Funding Acquisition, S.S.-A. and F.C. All authors have read and agreed to the published version of the manuscript.

Funding: The results of this work have been funded by the Project Nº PI16/00884 to F.C. and S.S.-A.; integrated in the National Plan for Scientific Research, Development and Technological Innovation 2013–2016, Spain, and funded by the ISCIII (Instituto de Salud Carlos III)—General Subdirection of Assessment and Promotion of the Research—European Regional Development Fund (FEDER) "A way of making Europe".

Data Availability Statement: Not applicable.

Conflicts of Interest: The authors declare no conflict of interest.

References

1. Biondi, B.; Kahaly, G.J.; Robertson, R.P. Thyroid Dysfunction and Diabetes Mellitus: Two Closely Associated Disorders. *Endocr. Rev.* **2019**, *40*, 789–824. [CrossRef] [PubMed]
2. Pasquali, R.; Casanueva, F.; Haluzik, M.; van Hulsteijn, L.; Ledoux, S.; Monteiro, M.P.; Salvador, J.; Santini, F.; Toplak, H.; Dekkers, O.M. European Society of Endocrinology Clinical Practice Guideline: Endocrine work-up in obesity. *Eur. J. Endocrinol.* **2020**, *182*, G1–G32. [CrossRef] [PubMed]
3. Valdes, S.; Maldonado-Araque, C.; Lago-Sampedro, A.; Lillo-Munoz, J.A.; Garcia-Fuentes, E.; Perez-Valero, V.; Gutierrez-Repiso, C.; Garcia-Escobar, E.; Goday, A.; Urrutia, I.; et al. Reference values for TSH may be inadequate to define hypothyroidism in persons with morbid obesity: Di@bet.es study. *Obesity* **2017**, *25*, 788–793. [CrossRef] [PubMed]
4. Rotondi, M.; Leporati, P.; La Manna, A.; Pirali, B.; Mondello, T.; Fonte, R.; Magri, F.; Chiovato, L. Raised serum TSH levels in patients with morbid obesity: Is it enough to diagnose subclinical hypothyroidism? *Eur. J. Endocrinol.* **2009**, *160*, 403–408. [CrossRef] [PubMed]
5. Walczak, K.; Sieminska, L. Obesity and Thyroid Axis. *Int. J. Environ. Res. Public. Health* **2021**, *18*, 9434. [CrossRef]
6. Caron, A.; Michael, N.J. New Horizons: Is Obesity a Disorder of Neurotransmission? *J. Clin. Endocrinol. Metab.* **2021**, *106*, e4872–e4886. [CrossRef]
7. Ballesteros Pomar, M.D.; Vilarrasa Garcia, N.; Rubio Herrera, M.A.; Barahona, M.J.; Bueno, M.; Caixas, A.; Calanas Continente, A.; Ciudin, A.; Cordido, F.; de Hollanda, A.; et al. The SEEN comprehensive clinical survey of adult obesity: Executive summary. *Endocrinol. Diabetes Nutr.* **2021**, *68*, 130–136. [CrossRef]
8. Health Effects of Overweight and Obesity in 195 Countries over 25 Years. *N. Engl. J. Med.* **2017**, *377*, 13–27. [CrossRef]
9. Gutierrez-Fisac, J.L.; Guallar-Castillon, P.; Leon-Munoz, L.M.; Graciani, A.; Banegas, J.R.; Rodriguez-Artalejo, F. Prevalence of general and abdominal obesity in the adult population of Spain, 2008-2010: The ENRICA study. *Obes. Rev.* **2012**, *13*, 388–392. [CrossRef]
10. Flegal, K.M.; Kruszon-Moran, D.; Carroll, M.D.; Fryar, C.D.; Ogden, C.L. Trends in Obesity Among Adults in the United States, 2005 to 2014. *JAMA* **2016**, *315*, 2284–2291. [CrossRef]
11. Ward, Z.J.; Bleich, S.N.; Cradock, A.L.; Barrett, J.L.; Giles, C.M.; Flax, C.; Long, M.W.; Gortmaker, S.L. Projected U.S. State-Level Prevalence of Adult Obesity and Severe Obesity. *N. Engl. J. Med.* **2019**, *381*, 2440–2450. [CrossRef] [PubMed]
12. Ng, M.; Fleming, T.; Robinson, M.; Thomson, B.; Graetz, N.; Margono, C.; Mullany, E.C.; Biryukov, S.; Abbafati, C.; Abera, S.F.; et al. Global, regional, and national prevalence of overweight and obesity in children and adults during 1980–2013: A systematic analysis for the Global Burden of Disease Study 2013. *Lancet* **2014**, *384*, 766–781. [CrossRef]
13. Magkos, F.; Fraterrigo, G.; Yoshino, J.; Luecking, C.; Kirbach, K.; Kelly, S.C.; de Las Fuentes, L.; He, S.; Okunade, A.L.; Patterson, B.W.; et al. Effects of Moderate and Subsequent Progressive Weight Loss on Metabolic Function and Adipose Tissue Biology in Humans with Obesity. *Cell Metab.* **2016**, *23*, 591–601. [CrossRef] [PubMed]
14. Varela-Rodriguez, B.M.; Juiz-Valina, P.; Varela, L.; Outeirino-Blanco, E.; Bravo, S.B.; Garcia-Brao, M.J.; Mena, E.; Noguera, J.F.; Valero-Gasalla, J.; Cordido, F.; et al. Beneficial Effects of Bariatric Surgery-Induced by Weight Loss on the Proteome of Abdominal Subcutaneous Adipose Tissue. *J. Clin. Med.* **2020**, *9*, 213. [CrossRef] [PubMed]

15. Reges, O.; Greenland, P.; Dicker, D.; Leibowitz, M.; Hoshen, M.; Gofer, I.; Rasmussen-Torvik, L.J.; Balicer, R.D. Association of Bariatric Surgery Using Laparoscopic Banding, Roux-en-Y Gastric Bypass, or Laparoscopic Sleeve Gastrectomy vs Usual Care Obesity Management With All-Cause Mortality. *JAMA* **2018**, *319*, 279–290. [CrossRef]
16. Carlsson, L.M.S.; Sjoholm, K.; Jacobson, P.; Andersson-Assarsson, J.C.; Svensson, P.A.; Taube, M.; Carlsson, B.; Peltonen, M. Life Expectancy after Bariatric Surgery in the Swedish Obese Subjects Study. *N. Engl. J. Med.* **2020**, *383*, 1535–1543. [CrossRef]
17. Tuero, C.; Valenti, V.; Rotellar, F.; Landecho, M.F.; Cienfuegos, J.A.; Fruhbeck, G. Revisiting the Ghrelin Changes Following Bariatric and Metabolic Surgery. *Obes. Surg.* **2020**, *30*, 2763–2780. [CrossRef]
18. Yoshino, M.; Kayser, B.D.; Yoshino, J.; Stein, R.I.; Reeds, D.; Eagon, J.C.; Eckhouse, S.R.; Watrous, J.D.; Jain, M.; Knight, R.; et al. Effects of Diet versus Gastric Bypass on Metabolic Function in Diabetes. *N. Engl. J. Med.* **2020**, *383*, 721–732. [CrossRef]
19. Biondi, B.; Cappola, A.R.; Cooper, D.S. Subclinical Hypothyroidism: A Review. *JAMA* **2019**, *322*, 153–160. [CrossRef]
20. Pena-Bello, L.; Seoane-Pillado, T.; Sangiao-Alvarellos, S.; Outeirino-Blanco, E.; Varela-Rodriguez, B.; Juiz-Valina, P.; Cordido, M.; Cordido, F. Oral glucose-stimulated growth hormone (GH) test in adult GH deficiency patients and controls: Potential utility of a novel test. *Eur. J. Intern. Med.* **2017**, *44*, 55–61. [CrossRef]
21. Pena-Bello, L.; Pertega-Diaz, S.; Outeirino-Blanco, E.; Garcia-Buela, J.; Tovar, S.; Sangiao-Alvarellos, S.; Dieguez, C.; Cordido, F. Effect of oral glucose administration on rebound growth hormone release in normal and obese women: The role of adiposity, insulin sensitivity and ghrelin. *PLoS ONE* **2015**, *10*, e0121087. [CrossRef] [PubMed]
22. Alvarez-Castro, P.; Sangiao-Alvarellos, S.; Brandon-Sanda, I.; Cordido, F. Endocrine function in obesity. *Endocrinol. Nutr.* **2011**, *58*, 422–432. [CrossRef] [PubMed]
23. Juiz-Valina, P.; Pena-Bello, L.; Cordido, M.; Outeirino-Blanco, E.; Pertega, S.; Varela-Rodriguez, B.; Garcia-Brao, M.J.; Mena, E.; Sangiao-Alvarellos, S.; Cordido, F. Altered GH-IGF-1 Axis in Severe Obese Subjects is Reversed after Bariatric Surgery-Induced Weight Loss and Related with Low-Grade Chronic Inflammation. *J. Clin. Med.* **2020**, *9*, 2614. [CrossRef] [PubMed]
24. Cordido, F.; Fernandez, T.; Martinez, T.; Penalva, A.; Peino, R.; Casanueva, F.F.; Dieguez, C. Effect of acute pharmacological reduction of plasma free fatty acids on growth hormone (GH) releasing hormone-induced GH secretion in obese adults with and without hypopituitarism. *J. Clin. Endocrinol. Metab.* **1998**, *83*, 4350–4354.
25. Biondi, B. Thyroid and obesity: An intriguing relationship. *J. Clin. Endocrinol. Metab.* **2010**, *95*, 3614–3617. [CrossRef]
26. Reinehr, T. Obesity and thyroid function. *Mol. Cell Endocrinol.* **2010**, *316*, 165–171. [CrossRef]
27. Reinehr, T.; Andler, W. Thyroid hormones before and after weight loss in obesity. *Arch. Dis. Child.* **2002**, *87*, 320–323. [CrossRef]
28. Zhang, H.; Liu, W.; Han, X.; Yu, H.; Zhang, P.; Jia, W. Effect of Laparoscopic Roux-en-Y Gastric Bypass Surgery on Thyroid Hormone Levels in Chinese Patients, Could It Be a Risk for Thyroid Nodules? *Obes. Surg.* **2017**, *27*, 2619–2627. [CrossRef]
29. Guan, B.; Chen, Y.; Yang, J.; Yang, W.; Wang, C. Effect of Bariatric Surgery on Thyroid Function in Obese Patients: A Systematic Review and Meta-Analysis. *Obes. Surg.* **2017**, *27*, 3292–3305. [CrossRef]
30. Yang, J.; Gao, Z.; Yang, W.; Zhou, X.; Lee, S.; Wang, C. Effect of Sleeve Gastrectomy on Thyroid Function in Chinese Euthyroid Obese Patients. *Surg. Laparosc. Endosc. Percutan. Tech.* **2017**, *27*, e66–e68. [CrossRef]
31. Liu, G.; Liang, L.; Bray, G.A.; Qi, L.; Hu, F.B.; Rood, J.; Sacks, F.M.; Sun, Q. Thyroid hormones and changes in body weight and metabolic parameters in response to weight loss diets: The POUNDS LOST trial. *Int. J. Obes.* **2017**, *41*, 878–886. [CrossRef] [PubMed]
32. Neves, J.S.; Castro Oliveira, S.; Souteiro, P.; Pedro, J.; Magalhaes, D.; Guerreiro, V.; Bettencourt-Silva, R.; Costa, M.M.; Cristina Santos, A.; Queiros, J.; et al. Effect of Weight Loss after Bariatric Surgery on Thyroid-Stimulating Hormone Levels in Patients with Morbid Obesity and Normal Thyroid Function. *Obes. Surg.* **2018**, *28*, 97–103. [CrossRef] [PubMed]
33. Dall'Asta, C.; Paganelli, M.; Morabito, A.; Vedani, P.; Barbieri, M.; Paolisso, G.; Folli, F.; Pontiroli, A.E. Weight loss through gastric banding: Effects on TSH and thyroid hormones in obese subjects with normal thyroid function. *Obesity* **2010**, *18*, 854–857. [CrossRef] [PubMed]
34. Juiz-Valina, P.; Outeirino-Blanco, E.; Pertega, S.; Varela-Rodriguez, B.M.; Garcia-Brao, M.J.; Mena, E.; Pena-Bello, L.; Cordido, M.; Sangiao-Alvarellos, S.; Cordido, F. Effect of Weight Loss after Bariatric Surgery on Thyroid-Stimulating Hormone Levels in Euthyroid Patients with Morbid Obesity. *Nutrients* **2019**, *11*, 1121. [CrossRef]
35. Ojomo, K.A.; Schneider, D.F.; Reiher, A.E.; Lai, N.; Schaefer, S.; Chen, H.; Sippel, R.S. Using body mass index to predict optimal thyroid dosing after thyroidectomy. *J. Am. Coll. Surg.* **2013**, *216*, 454–460. [CrossRef]
36. Rubio, I.G.; Galrao, A.L.; Santo, M.A.; Zanini, A.C.; Medeiros-Neto, G. Levothyroxine absorption in morbidly obese patients before and after Roux-En-Y gastric bypass (RYGB) surgery. *Obes. Surg.* **2012**, *22*, 253–258. [CrossRef]
37. Michalaki, M.A.; Gkotsina, M.I.; Mamali, I.; Markantes, G.K.; Faltaka, A.; Kalfarentzos, F.; Vagenakis, A.G.; Markou, K.B. Impaired pharmacokinetics of levothyroxine in severely obese volunteers. *Thyroid* **2011**, *21*, 477–481. [CrossRef]
38. Khan, W.F.; Singla, V.; Aggarwal, S.; Gupta, Y. Outcome of bariatric surgery on hypothyroidism: Experience from a tertiary care center in India. *Surg. Obes. Relat. Dis.* **2020**, *16*, 1297–1301. [CrossRef]
39. Richou, M.; Gilly, O.; Taillard, V.; Paul De Brauwere, D.; Donici, I.; Guedj, A.M. Levothyroxine dose adjustment in hypothyroid patients following gastric sleeve surgery. *Ann. Endocrinol.* **2020**, *81*, 500–506. [CrossRef]
40. Gkotsina, M.; Michalaki, M.; Mamali, I.; Markantes, G.; Sakellaropoulos, G.C.; Kalfarentzos, F.; Vagenakis, A.G.; Markou, K.B. Improved levothyroxine pharmacokinetics after bariatric surgery. *Thyroid* **2013**, *23*, 414–419. [CrossRef]

41. Azran, C.; Hanhan-Shamshoum, N.; Irshied, T.; Ben-Shushan, T.; Dicker, D.; Dahan, A.; Matok, I. Hypothyroidism and levothyroxine therapy following bariatric surgery: A systematic review, meta-analysis, network meta-analysis, and meta-regression. *Surg. Obes. Relat. Dis.* **2021**, *17*, 1206–1217. [CrossRef] [PubMed]
42. Wang, X.; Gao, X.; Han, Y.; Zhang, F.; Lin, Z.; Wang, H.; Teng, W.; Shan, Z. Causal Association Between Serum Thyrotropin and Obesity: A Bidirectional, Mendelian Randomization Study. *J. Clin. Endocrinol. Metab.* **2021**, *106*, e4251–e4259. [CrossRef] [PubMed]
43. Brenta, G. The Association Between Obesity and the Thyroid: Is the "Chicken or the Egg" Conundrum Finally Solved? *J. Clin. Endocrinol. Metab.* **2021**, *106*, e4281–e4283. [CrossRef] [PubMed]
44. Ylli, D.; Wartofsky, L. Can We Link Thyroid Status, Energy Expenditure, and Body Composition to Management of Subclinical Thyroid Dysfunction? *J. Clin. Endocrinol. Metab.* **2019**, *104*, 209–212. [CrossRef]
45. Endo, T.; Kobayashi, T. Thyroid-stimulating hormone receptor in brown adipose tissue is involved in the regulation of thermogenesis. *Am. J. Physiol. Endocrinol. Metab.* **2008**, *295*, E514–E518. [CrossRef]
46. Nannipieri, M.; Cecchetti, F.; Anselmino, M.; Camastra, S.; Niccolini, P.; Lamacchia, M.; Rossi, M.; Iervasi, G.; Ferrannini, E. Expression of thyrotropin and thyroid hormone receptors in adipose tissue of patients with morbid obesity and/or type 2 diabetes: Effects of weight loss. *Int. J. Obes.* **2009**, *33*, 1001–1006. [CrossRef]
47. Marzullo, P.; Minocci, A.; Mele, C.; Fessehatsion, R.; Tagliaferri, M.; Pagano, L.; Scacchi, M.; Aimaretti, G.; Sartorio, A. The relationship between resting energy expenditure and thyroid hormones in response to short-term weight loss in severe obesity. *PLoS ONE* **2018**, *13*, e0205293. [CrossRef]
48. Betry, C.; Challan-Belval, M.A.; Bernard, A.; Charrie, A.; Drai, J.; Laville, M.; Thivolet, C.; Disse, E. Increased TSH in obesity: Evidence for a BMI-independent association with leptin. *Diabetes. Metab.* **2015**, *41*, 248–251. [CrossRef]
49. Marzullo, P.; Minocci, A.; Tagliaferri, M.A.; Guzzaloni, G.; Di Blasio, A.; De Medici, C.; Aimaretti, G.; Liuzzi, A. Investigations of thyroid hormones and antibodies in obesity: Leptin levels are associated with thyroid autoimmunity independent of bioanthropometric, hormonal, and weight-related determinants. *J. Clin. Endocrinol. Metab.* **2010**, *95*, 3965–3972. [CrossRef]
50. Gokosmanoglu, F.; Aksoy, E.; Onmez, A.; Ergenc, H.; Topkaya, S. Thyroid Homeostasis After Bariatric Surgery in Obese Cases. *Obes. Surg.* **2019**, *30*, 274–278. [CrossRef]
51. Reinehr, T.; de Sousa, G.; Andler, W. Hyperthyrotropinemia in obese children is reversible after weight loss and is not related to lipids. *J. Clin. Endocrinol. Metab.* **2006**, *91*, 3088–3091. [CrossRef] [PubMed]
52. Crujeiras, A.B.; Goyenechea, E.; Abete, I.; Lage, M.; Carreira, M.C.; Martinez, J.A.; Casanueva, F.F. Weight regain after a diet-induced loss is predicted by higher baseline leptin and lower ghrelin plasma levels. *J. Clin. Endocrinol. Metab.* **2010**, *95*, 5037–5044. [CrossRef] [PubMed]
53. Hogild, M.L.; Bak, A.M.; Pedersen, S.B.; Rungby, J.; Frystyk, J.; Moller, N.; Jessen, N.; Jorgensen, J.O.L. Growth Hormone Signaling and Action in Obese versus Lean Human Subjects. *Am. J. Physiol. Endocrinol. Metab.* **2019**, *316*, E333–E344. [CrossRef] [PubMed]
54. Glad, C.A.M.; Svensson, P.A.; Nystrom, F.H.; Jacobson, P.; Carlsson, L.M.S.; Johannsson, G.; Andersson-Assarsson, J.C. Expression of GHR and downstream signaling genes in human adipose tissue-relation to obesity and weight-change. *J. Clin. Endocrinol. Metab.* **2019**, *104*, 1459–1470. [CrossRef] [PubMed]
55. Yamauchi, I.; Sakane, Y.; Yamashita, T.; Hirota, K.; Ueda, Y.; Kanai, Y.; Yamashita, Y.; Kondo, E.; Fujii, T.; Taura, D.; et al. Effects of growth hormone on thyroid function are mediated by type 2 iodothyronine deiodinase in humans. *Endocrine* **2018**, *59*, 353–363. [CrossRef]
56. Dickey, R.A.; Wartofsky, L.; Feld, S. Optimal thyrotropin level: Normal ranges and reference intervals are not equivalent. *Thyroid* **2005**, *15*, 1035–1039. [CrossRef]
57. Wartofsky, L.; Dickey, R.A. The evidence for a narrower thyrotropin reference range is compelling. *J. Clin. Endocrinol. Metab.* **2005**, *90*, 5483–5488. [CrossRef]
58. Dumitrescu, A.M.; Refetoff, S. The syndromes of reduced sensitivity to thyroid hormone. *Biochim. Biophys. Acta* **2013**, *1830*, 3987–4003. [CrossRef]
59. Ortiga-Carvalho, T.M.; Sidhaye, A.R.; Wondisford, F.E. Thyroid hormone receptors and resistance to thyroid hormone disorders. *Nat. Rev. Endocrinol.* **2014**, *10*, 582–591. [CrossRef]
60. Yagi, H.; Pohlenz, J.; Hayashi, Y.; Sakurai, A.; Refetoff, S. Resistance to thyroid hormone caused by two mutant thyroid hormone receptors beta, R243Q and R243W, with marked impairment of function that cannot be explained by altered in vitro 3,5,3′-triiodothyroinine binding affinity. *J. Clin. Endocrinol. Metab.* **1997**, *82*, 1608–1614. [CrossRef]
61. Jostel, A.; Ryder, W.D.; Shalet, S.M. The use of thyroid function tests in the diagnosis of hypopituitarism: Definition and evaluation of the TSH Index. *Clin. Endocrinol.* **2009**, *71*, 529–534. [CrossRef] [PubMed]
62. Laurberg, P.; Knudsen, N.; Andersen, S.; Carle, A.; Pedersen, I.B.; Karmisholt, J. Thyroid function and obesity. *Eur. Thyroid. J.* **2012**, *1*, 159–167. [CrossRef] [PubMed]
63. Tjorve, E.; Tjorve, K.M.; Olsen, J.O.; Senum, R.; Oftebro, H. On commonness and rarity of thyroid hormone resistance: A discussion based on mechanisms of reduced sensitivity in peripheral tissues. *Med. Hypotheses* **2007**, *69*, 913–921. [CrossRef] [PubMed]
64. Laclaustra, M.; Moreno-Franco, B.; Lou-Bonafonte, J.M.; Mateo-Gallego, R.; Casasnovas, J.A.; Guallar-Castillon, P.; Cenarro, A.; Civeira, F. Impaired Sensitivity to Thyroid Hormones Is Associated With Diabetes and Metabolic Syndrome. *Diabetes Care* **2019**, *42*, 303–310. [CrossRef] [PubMed]

65. Bianco, A.C.; Dumitrescu, A.; Gereben, B.; Ribeiro, M.O.; Fonseca, T.L.; Fernandes, G.W.; Bocco, B. Paradigms of Dynamic Control of Thyroid Hormone Signaling. *Endocr. Rev.* **2019**, *40*, 1000–1047. [CrossRef]
66. Castillo, M.; Freitas, B.C.; Rosene, M.L.; Drigo, R.A.; Grozovsky, R.; Maciel, R.M.; Patti, M.E.; Ribeiro, M.O.; Bianco, A.C. Impaired metabolic effects of a thyroid hormone receptor beta-selective agonist in a mouse model of diet-induced obesity. *Thyroid* **2010**, *20*, 545–553. [CrossRef]
67. Krause, C.; Grohs, M.; El Gammal, A.; Wolter, S.; Lehnert, H.; Mann, O.; Mittag, J.; Kirchner, H. Reduced expression of thyroid hormone receptor beta in human nonalcoholic steatohepatitis. *Endocr. Connect.* **2018**, *7*, 1448–1456. [CrossRef]
68. Anselmo, J.D.; Scherberg, N.; Dumitrescu, A.M.; Refetoff, S. Reduced Sensitivity to Thyroid Hormone as a Transgenerational Epigenetic Marker Transmitted Along Human Male Line. *Thyroid* **2019**, *29*, 778–782. [CrossRef]
69. Juiz-Valina, P.; Cordido, M.; Outeirino-Blanco, E.; Pertega, S.; Varela-Rodriguez, B.M.; Garcia-Brao, M.J.; Mena, E.; Pena-Bello, L.; Sangiao-Alvarellos, S.; Cordido, F. Central Resistance to Thyroid Hormones in Morbidly Obese Subjects Is Reversed after Bariatric Surgery-Induced Weight Loss. *J. Clin. Med.* **2020**, *9*, 359. [CrossRef]
70. Kushchayeva, Y.S.; Kushchayev, S.V.; Startzell, M.; Cochran, E.; Auh, S.; Dai, Y.; Lightbourne, M.; Skarulis, M.; Brown, R.J. Thyroid Abnormalities in Patients With Extreme Insulin Resistance Syndromes. *J. Clin. Endocrinol. Metab.* **2019**, *104*, 2216–2228. [CrossRef]
71. Fleseriu, M.; Hashim, I.A.; Karavitaki, N.; Melmed, S.; Murad, M.H.; Salvatori, R.; Samuels, M.H. Hormonal Replacement in Hypopituitarism in Adults: An Endocrine Society Clinical Practice Guideline. *J. Clin. Endocrinol. Metab.* **2016**, *101*, 3888–3921. [CrossRef] [PubMed]
72. Porretti, S.; Giavoli, C.; Ronchi, C.; Lombardi, G.; Zaccaria, M.; Valle, D.; Arosio, M.; Beck-Peccoz, P. Recombinant human GH replacement therapy and thyroid function in a large group of adult GH-deficient patients: When does L-T(4) therapy become mandatory? *J. Clin. Endocrinol. Metab.* **2002**, *87*, 2042–2045. [CrossRef] [PubMed]
73. Zhu, C.; Gao, J.; Mei, F.; Lu, L.; Zhou, D.; Qu, S. Reduction in Thyroid-Stimulating Hormone Correlated with Improved Inflammation Markers in Chinese Patients with Morbid Obesity Undergoing Laparoscopic Sleeve Gastrectomy. *Obes. Surg.* **2019**, *29*, 3954–3965. [CrossRef] [PubMed]
74. Neves, J.S.; Souteiro, P.; Oliveira, S.C.; Pedro, J.; Magalhaes, D.; Guerreiro, V.; Costa, M.M.; Bettencourt-Silva, R.; Santos, A.C.; Queiros, J.; et al. Preoperative thyroid function and weight loss after bariatric surgery. *Int. J. Obes.* **2019**, *43*, 432–436. [CrossRef]
75. Mehran, L.; Delbari, N.; Amouzegar, A.; Hasheminia, M.; Tohidi, M.; Azizi, F. Reduced Sensitivity to Thyroid Hormone Is Associated with Diabetes and Hypertension. *J. Clin. Endocrinol. Metab.* **2022**, *107*, 167–176. [CrossRef]
76. Gadiraju, S.; Lee, C.J.; Cooper, D.S. Levothyroxine Dosing Following Bariatric Surgery. *Obes. Surg.* **2016**, *26*, 2538–2542. [CrossRef]
77. Pedro, J.; Cunha, F.; Souteiro, P.; Neves, J.S.; Guerreiro, V.; Magalhaes, D.; Bettencourt-Silva, R.; Oliveira, S.C.; Costa, M.M.; Queiros, J.; et al. The Effect of the Bariatric Surgery Type on the Levothyroxine Dose of Morbidly Obese Hypothyroid Patients. *Obes. Surg.* **2018**, *28*, 3538–3543. [CrossRef]
78. Papoian, V.; Ylli, D.; Felger, E.A.; Wartofsky, L.; Rosen, J.E. Evaluation of Thyroid Hormone Replacement Dosing in Overweight and Obese Patients After a Thyroidectomy. *Thyroid* **2019**, *29*, 1558–1562. [CrossRef]
79. Santini, F.; Pinchera, A.; Marsili, A.; Ceccarini, G.; Castagna, M.G.; Valeriano, R.; Giannetti, M.; Taddei, D.; Centoni, R.; Scartabelli, G.; et al. Lean body mass is a major determinant of levothyroxine dosage in the treatment of thyroid diseases. *J. Clin. Endocrinol. Metab.* **2005**, *90*, 124–127. [CrossRef]
80. Sawaya, R.A.; Jaffe, J.; Friedenberg, L.; Friedenberg, F.K. Vitamin, mineral, and drug absorption following bariatric surgery. *Curr. Drug Metab.* **2012**, *13*, 1345–1355. [CrossRef]
81. Smith, A.; Henriksen, B.; Cohen, A. Pharmacokinetic considerations in Roux-en-Y gastric bypass patients. *Am. J. Health Syst. Pharm.* **2011**, *68*, 2241–2247. [CrossRef] [PubMed]
82. Liwanpo, L.; Hershman, J.M. Conditions and drugs interfering with thyroxine absorption. *Best Pract. Res. Clin. Endocrinol. Metab.* **2009**, *23*, 781–792. [CrossRef] [PubMed]
83. Padwal, R.; Brocks, D.; Sharma, A.M. A systematic review of drug absorption following bariatric surgery and its theoretical implications. *Obes. Rev.* **2010**, *11*, 41–50. [CrossRef]
84. Azizi, F.; Belur, R.; Albano, J. Malabsorption of thyroid hormones after jejunoileal bypass for obesity. *Ann. Intern. Med.* **1979**, *90*, 941–942. [CrossRef]
85. Bevan, J.S.; Munro, J.F. Thyroxine malabsorption following intestinal bypass surgery. *Int. J. Obes.* **1986**, *10*, 245–246.
86. Topliss, D.J.; Wright, J.A.; Volpe, R. Increased requirement for thyroid hormone after a jejunoileal bypass operation. *Can. Med. Assoc. J.* **1980**, *123*, 765–766.
87. Stone, E.; Leiter, L.A.; Lambert, J.R.; Silverberg, J.D.; Jeejeebhoy, K.N.; Burrow, G.N. L-thyroxine absorption in patients with short bowel. *J. Clin. Endocrinol. Metab.* **1984**, *59*, 139–141. [CrossRef]
88. Fallahi, P.; Ferrari, S.M.; Camastra, S.; Politti, U.; Ruffilli, I.; Vita, R.; Navarra, G.; Benvenga, S.; Antonelli, A. TSH Normalization in Bariatric Surgery Patients After the Switch from L-Thyroxine in Tablet to an Oral Liquid Formulation. *Obes. Surg.* **2017**, *27*, 78–82. [CrossRef] [PubMed]
89. Aggarwal, S.; Modi, S.; Jose, T. Laparoscopic sleeve gastrectomy leads to reduction in thyroxine requirement in morbidly obese patients with hypothyroidism. *World J. Surg.* **2014**, *38*, 2628–2631. [CrossRef]
90. Rudnicki, Y.; Slavin, M.; Keidar, A.; Kent, I.; Berkovich, L.; Tiomkin, V.; Inbar, R.; Avital, S. The effect of bariatric surgery on hypothyroidism: Sleeve gastrectomy versus gastric bypass. *Surg. Obes. Relat. Dis.* **2018**, *14*, 1297–1303. [CrossRef]

91. Zendel, A.; Abu-Ghanem, Y.; Dux, J.; Mor, E.; Zippel, D.; Goitein, D. The Impact of Bariatric Surgery on Thyroid Function and Medication Use in Patients with Hypothyroidism. *Obes. Surg.* **2017**, *27*, 2000–2004. [CrossRef] [PubMed]
92. Almunif, D.S.; Bamehriz, F.; Althuwaini, S.; Almigbal, T.H.; Batais, M.A. The Effect of Laparoscopic Sleeve Gastrectomy on Serum Thyroid-Stimulating Hormone Levels in Obese Patients with Overt and Subclinical Hypothyroidism: A 7-Year Retrospective Study. *Obes. Surg.* **2020**, *30*, 1491–1497. [CrossRef] [PubMed]
93. Fierabracci, P.; Martinelli, S.; Tamberi, A.; Piaggi, P.; Basolo, A.; Pelosini, C.; Ricco, I.; Magno, S.; Querci, G.; Ceccarini, G.; et al. Weight Loss and Variation of Levothyroxine Requirements in Hypothyroid Obese Patients After Bariatric Surgery. *Thyroid* **2016**, *26*, 499–503. [CrossRef] [PubMed]
94. Juiz-Valina, P.; Cordido, M.; Outeirino-Blanco, E.; Pertega, S.; Urones, P.; Garcia-Brao, M.J.; Mena, E.; Pena-Bello, L.; Sangiao-Alvarellos, S.; Cordido, F. Evaluation of Thyroid Hormone Replacement Dosing in Morbidly Obese Hypothyroid Patients after Bariatric Surgery-Induced Weight Loss. *J. Clin. Med.* **2021**, *10*, 3658. [CrossRef] [PubMed]
95. Julia, H.; Benaiges, D.; Molla, P.; Pedro-Botet, J.; Villatoro, M.; Fontane, L.; Ramon, J.M.; Climent, E.; Flores Le Roux, J.A.; Goday, A. Changes in Thyroid Replacement Therapy after Bariatric Surgery: Differences between Laparoscopic Roux-en-Y Gastric Bypass and Laparoscopic Sleeve Gastrectomy. *Obes. Surg.* **2019**, *29*, 2593–2599. [CrossRef]
96. Skelin, M.; Lucijanic, T.; Amidzic Klaric, D.; Resic, A.; Bakula, M.; Liberati-Cizmek, A.M.; Gharib, H.; Rahelic, D. Factors Affecting Gastrointestinal Absorption of Levothyroxine: A Review. *Clin. Ther.* **2017**, *39*, 378–403. [CrossRef]
97. Quercia, I.; Dutia, R.; Kotler, D.P.; Belsley, S.; Laferrere, B. Gastrointestinal changes after bariatric surgery. *Diabetes Metab.* **2014**, *40*, 87–94. [CrossRef]
98. Smith, C.D.; Herkes, S.B.; Behrns, K.E.; Fairbanks, V.F.; Kelly, K.A.; Sarr, M.G. Gastric acid secretion and vitamin B12 absorption after vertical Roux-en-Y gastric bypass for morbid obesity. *Ann. Surg.* **1993**, *218*, 91–96. [CrossRef]
99. Isidro, M.L.; Penin, M.A.; Nemina, R.; Cordido, F. Metformin reduces thyrotropin levels in obese, diabetic women with primary hypothyroidism on thyroxine replacement therapy. *Endocrine* **2007**, *32*, 79–82. [CrossRef]
100. Virili, C.; Antonelli, A.; Santaguida, M.G.; Benvenga, S.; Centanni, M. Gastrointestinal Malabsorption of Thyroxine. *Endocr. Rev.* **2019**, *40*, 118–136. [CrossRef]
101. Muraca, E.; Ciardullo, S.; Oltolini, A.; Zerbini, F.; Bianconi, E.; Perra, S.; Villa, M.; Cannistraci, R.; Castoldi, G.; Pizzi, P.; et al. Resting Energy Expenditure in Obese Women with Primary Hypothyroidism and Appropriate Levothyroxine Replacement Therapy. *J. Clin. Endocrinol. Metab.* **2020**, *105*, e1741–e1748. [CrossRef] [PubMed]
102. Mele, C.; Tagliaferri, M.A.; Pagano, L.; Soranna, D.; Scacchi, M.; Aimaretti, G.; Biondi, B.; Marzullo, P. Levothyroxine Replacement in Obese Adults: The Role of Metabolic Variables and Aging on Thyroid Testing Abnormalities. *J. Clin. Endocrinol. Metab.* **2019**, *104*, 6265–6274. [CrossRef] [PubMed]

Journal of
Clinical Medicine

MDPI

Article

Sarcopenia after Roux-en-Y Gastric Bypass: Detection by Skeletal Muscle Mass Index vs. Bioelectrical Impedance Analysis

Georgi Vassilev [1,*], Christian Galata [2], Alida Finze [1], Christel Weiss [3], Mirko Otto [1], Christoph Reissfelder [1] and Susanne Blank [1]

1 Department of Surgery, Medical Faculty Mannheim, Heidelberg University, 68167 Mannheim, Germany; alida.finze@umm.de (A.F.); mirko.otto@umm.de (M.O.); christoph.reissfelder@umm.de (C.R.); susanne.blank@umm.de (S.B.)
2 University Thoracic Center Mainz, Medical Faculty Mainz, 55131 Mainz, Germany; christian.galata@unimedizin-mainz.de
3 Department of Medical Statistics, Medical Faculty Mannheim, Heidelberg University, 68167 Mannheim, Germany; christel.weiss@medma.uni-heidelberg.de
* Correspondence: georgi.vassilev@umm.de; Tel.: +49-621-383-2225; Fax: +49-621-383-2166

Abstract: Background: In sarcopenic patients the skeletal muscle reduction is the primary symptom of age- or disease-related malnutrition, which is linked to postoperative morbidity and mortality. The skeletal muscle mass index (SMI) from magnet resonance imaging (MRI) is increasingly used as a prognostic factor in oncologic and surgical patients, but under-represented in the field of obesity surgery. The bioelectrical impedance analysis (BIA), on the other hand is a commonly used method for the estimation of the body composition of bariatric patients, but still believed to be inaccurate, because of patient-related and environmental factors. The aim of this study was to compare the postoperative SMI values as a direct, imaging measured indicator for muscle mass with the BIA results in patients undergoing Roux-en-Y gastric bypass (RYGB). Methods: We performed a prospective single-center trial. Patients undergoing RYGB between January 2010 and December 2011 at our institution were eligible for this study. MRI and BIA measurements were obtained 1 day before surgery and at 6, 12 and 24 weeks after surgery. Results: A total of 17 patients (four male, 13 female, average age of 41.9 years) were included. SMI values decreased significantly during the postoperative course ($p < 0.001$). Comparing preoperative and postoperative measurements at 24 weeks after surgery, increasing correlations of SMI values with body weight ($r = 0.240$ vs. $r = 0.628$), phase angle ($r = 0.225$ vs. $r = 0.720$) and body cell mass (BCM, $r = 0.388$ vs. $r = 0.764$) were observed. Conclusions: SMI decreases significantly after RYGB and is correlated to distinct parameters of body composition. These findings show the applicability of the SMI as direct imaging parameter for the measurement of the muscle mass in patients after RYGB, but also underline the important role of the BIA, as a precise tool for the estimation of patients' body composition at low costs. BIA allows a good overview of patients' status post bariatric surgery, including an estimation of sarcopenia.

Keywords: skeletal muscle mass; bioelectrical impedance analysis; Roux-Y gastric bypass

Citation: Vassilev, G.; Galata, C.; Finze, A.; Weiss, C.; Otto, M.; Reissfelder, C.; Blank, S. Sarcopenia after Roux-en-Y Gastric Bypass: Detection by Skeletal Muscle Mass Index vs. Bioelectrical Impedance Analysis. *J. Clin. Med.* **2022**, *11*, 1468. https://doi.org/10.3390/jcm11061468

Academic Editor: David Benaiges Boix

Received: 16 January 2022
Accepted: 3 March 2022
Published: 8 March 2022

1. Introduction

Obesity is a global health challenge and the main risk factor for diseases such as type 2 diabetes, cardiovascular morbidity, hypertension, sleep apnea, skeletal pain syndromes, psychological disorders, cancer and even early death [1]. Bariatric surgery has proven to be an effective strategy in treating obesity [2].

The main objective of Roux-en-Y gastric bypass (RYGB) is weight loss and improvement of metabolic comorbidities. Together with weight reduction, bariatric surgery leads to a change in body composition. Especially the fat mass decreases throughout the first months after surgery. Within this period, body cell mass (BCM), lean body mass (LBM), and absolute muscle mass and strength often also decrease [3–7]. The postoperative changes of those parameters are associated with weight loss, physical performance and risk of malnutrition and can be direct or indirect signs of a reduction in muscle mass [8,9].

Taking this into account, it is important to monitor the body composition and the skeletal muscle mass before and after bariatric surgery. There are different tools available to measure or estimate the BCM, LBM and the skeletal muscle status, such as bioelectrical impedance analysis (BIA), Dual-energy X-ray absorptiometry (DxA), handgrip dynamometry (HD) or imaging techniques including MRI and CT scan [10–12].

The analysis of single-layer images (CT scan or MRI) is used to quantify whole body muscle mass in vivo. The cross-sectional area of skeletal muscles (SMA, cm^2) at the level of the third lumbar vertebra (L3), normalized for height, can be used to calculate the skeletal muscle index (SMI, cm^2/m^2), which is linearly related to the whole-body muscle mass [13,14].

BIA is commonly performed for the evaluation of pre- and postoperative body composition delivering the parameters BCM, extracellular mass (ECM), LBM and body fat. The phase angle reflects the quality of LBM [15]. The BIA provides accurate values comparable to those obtained by dual-energy X-ray absorptiometry (DXA) at low cost [10]. It measures body component resistance and capacitance by recording a voltage drop in applied current. Capacitance causes the current to lag behind the voltage, which creates a phase shift. This shift is quantified geometrically as the angular transformation—the phase angle [5].

The general loss of muscle mass is defined as sarcopenia. The term "sarcopenic obesity" describes the co-presence of sarcopenia and obesity. SMI is a surrogate parameter for sarcopenia and thus, a reduction of SMI is related to physical disability, increased morbidity and even mortality in surgical patients. This has been investigated mostly in geriatric and oncologic patients [16–19].

In patients after bariatric surgery, the role of SMI pre- and postoperatively is rarely described in literature. The correlation between SMI- and BIA- measurements remains controversial [20].

This study aims to investigate if the BIA as a common technique for estimating the body composition is still robust in comparison with the SMI measured by MRI in a cohort of patients undergoing RYGB.

2. Materials and Methods

Patients: Between January 2010 and December 2011, an open, prospective, single center study was conducted at our institution investigating postoperative changes in body composition in bariatric patients via MRI and BIA measurements. Patients undergoing RYGB were included in the study. Further inclusion criteria were BMI 35–60 kg/m^2, body weight < 200 kg, adequate patient compliance, waist circumference < 136 cm (MRI gantry diameter) and age > 18 years. Patients with contraindications for MRI or not willing or able to give informed consent were excluded from the study. The primary analysis of this study has been published previously [12]. For this post-hoc analysis, the SMI was measured retrospectively using the MRI studies performed in the prospective trial.

Bioelectrical Impedance Analysis Bioelectrical impedance measurements were conducted according to standard protocols using a multiple frequency four-lead BIA instrument (Nutriguard-M, Data Input GmbH, Pöcking, Germany). Calculations for phase angel, body cell mass (BCM), extracellular mass (ECM), lean body mass (LBM), ECM/BCM, body fat (BF) and total body water (TBW) were made using the Nutriguard Plus software (version 5.4, Data Input GmbH, Pöcking, Germany).

Magnetic Resonance Imaging: Abdominal MRI exams were obtained using a 1.5 Tesla whole-body scanner (MAGNETOM Avanto, Siemens Healthengineers, Erlangen, Germany) following standard clinical protocols. The anatomical coverage was from the upper edge of the liver to beneath the third lumbar vertebra level.

Skeletal Muscle Mass Index: SMI was determined as published previously [20]. The SMI for each individual was calculated from MRI using two adjacent axial images within the same series. Total muscle cross-sectional area (cm^2) at L3 was determined and averaged for each patient: The lumbar vertebrae 3 was identified, and the following muscles were selected using aycan workstation pro software (version 3.12.000, aycan Digitalsysteme GmbH, Würzburg, Germany): rectus abdominis, abdominal (lateral and oblique), psoas, and paraspinal (quadratus lumborum, erector spinae). Muscle area in centimeters squared (cm^2) was calculated and then normalized for patient's height in meters squared (m^2) and reported as lumbar SMI (cm^2/m^2).

Statistical analysis: Mean and standard deviation were calculated for quantitative variables. Qualitative variables were quoted as absolute numbers and relative frequencies. With the range or interquartile range, the median was presented for skewed or ordinally scaled parameters. Changes in parameters between measurements were examined using analysis of variance for repeated measurements. Post hoc analyses for pairwise mean comparisons were performed using the Scheffé method. For correlation analyses, Pearson correlation coefficient was determined. A test result was considered statistically significant if $p < 0.05$. Statistical analyses were performed using the SAS statistical analysis software (SAS release 9.4, Cary, NC, USA).

3. Results

A total of 17 patients were included in the study; four male and 13 female. The average age of the patients was 41.9 years. Mean initial body weight was 119.34 ± 11.86 kg and mean initial BMI was 42.96 ± 4.5 kg/m^2. All patients underwent RYGB. Among other elements of the preoperative preparation like psychological, endocrinology- and nutrition expert assessment, every patient has documented at least 2.5 h of self-organized physical activity per week. When considering comorbidities, seven patients had no secondary disease, five had hypertension, four had sleep apnea, two had diabetes and one had GERD and knee arthrosis, respectively (Table 1).

Table 1. Demographic characteristics of the respondents.

Demographic Characteristics		(*n* = 17)
Age		
	Mean ± SD (Range (Max − Min))	41.9 ± 11.1 (35 (61 − 26))
Age group		
	<=35	6 (35.3)
	36–46	6 (35.3)
	>=47	5 (29.4)
Gender		
	Male	4 (23.5)
	Female	13 (76.5)
Initial body weight (kg)		
	Mean ± SD (Range (Max − Min))	119.34 ± 11.86 (47.6 (144.1 − 96.5))
Initial BMI (kg/m^2)		
	Mean ± SD (Range (Max − Min))	42.96 ± 4.5 (15.9 (52.3 − 36.4))
Initial SMI (cm^2/m^2)		
	Mean ± SD (Range (Max − Min))	52.65 ± 7.06 (28.39 (68.89 − 40.5))
Comorbidities		
	No Secondary disease	7 (50.0)
	Hypertension	5 (35.7)
	Sleep Apnea	4 (28.6)
	Diabetes	2 (14.3)
	GERD	1 (7.1)
	Knee arthrosis	1 (7.1)

Note: The value is shown as mean ± sd (range) or *n* (%). **Abbreviation:** BMI, body mass index; SMI, skeletal muscle index; GERD.

There were no postoperative surgical complications. MRI, as well as BIA, was performed one day before surgery (t1) as well as 6 weeks (t2), 12 weeks (t3) and 24 weeks (t4) after surgery. Measurements at t1 and t2 were complete for all patients while at t3 and t4 they were only complete in 11 and 7 patients, respectively.

Table 2 shows the mean values of the respective parameters measured by BIA and the SMI measured by MRI as described above. In Table 3 the *p*-values for the respective comparisons are given. Changes in body weight and BMI are significant between t1 and t2, t2 and t3, but not between t3 and t4. Overall, most pronounced changes are observed between t1 and t2 (before surgery and 6 weeks after surgery). As expected, the body fat is significantly reduced after bariatric surgery. We did not find any further significant reduction between t3 and t4. Nevertheless, the LBM as well as BCM and ECM/BCM Index changed after surgery with a significant reduction of LBM and BCM between t1 and t2 and an almost significant reduction when comparing t2 to t4. The reduction of BCM results in an increase of the ECM/BCM Index, indicating malnutrition. The muscle mass also decreased over the observed time period being displayed by SMA measurement in BIA and SMI measurement in MRI imaging. The reduction of muscle mass is significant comparing the status before and after surgery but also between t2 and t4.

Table 2. Body composition and skeletal muscle index at the different time points.

	t1	t2	t3	t4
Body weight (kg)	119.34 ± 11.86	103.67 ± 14.89	97.25 ± 10.87	92.59 ± 8.96
BMI (kg/m^2)	42.96 ± 4.5	37.31 ± 5.69	34.72 ± 5.8	34.33 ± 4.62
Basal metabolic rate (kcal)	1685.29 ± 171.36	1558.24 ± 186.76	1546.36 ± 205.97	1547.14 ± 248.98
Phase angle (°)	6.38 ± 0.88	5.56 ± 0.93	5.31 ± 1.01	5.7 ± 1.26
TBW (kg)	44.39 ± 7.58	44.14 ± 7.64	44.57 ± 6.55	43.09 ± 7.15
LBM (kg)	63.38 ± 10.34	60.31 ± 47.30	60.89 ± 8.93	58.87 ± 9.79
ECM (kg)	29.55 ± 5.74	30.5 ± 5.87	31.52 ± 4.45	29.37 ± 4.81
BCM (kg)	33.83 ± 5.45	29.81 ± 5.90	29.38 ± 6.55	29.51 ± 7.83
Index (ECM/BCM)	0.88 ± 0.13	1.04 ± 0.19	1.11 ± 0.25	1.06 ± 0.36
BF (kg)	55.96 ± 6.97	43.36 ± 8.99	36.35 ± 7.79	33.71 ± 6.45
BF (%)	47.02 ± 5.04	41.70 ± 6.01	37.28 ± 6.20	36.59 ± 6.66
SMA (cm^2)	146.73 ± 23.96	127.82 ± 24.71	124.22 ± 23.76	116.42 ± 29.37
SMI (cm^2/m^2)	52.65 ± 7.06	45.67 ± 6.62	43.84 ± 7.14	42.48 ± 7.86

Results are presented as mean ± standard deviation. t1 = before surgery, t2 = 6 weeks after surgery, t3 = 12 weeks after surgery, t4 = 24 weeks after surgery. BMI = body mass index, TBW = total body water, LBM = lean body mass, ECM = extracellular mass, BCM = body cell mass, BF = body fat, SMA = skeletal muscle area, SMI = skeletal muscle index.

Table 3. Comparison of BIA parameters between the different time points.

t	Body Weight	BMI	Basal Metabolic Rate (kcal)	Phase Angle	TBW	LBM	ECM	BCM	ECM/BCM	BF (kg)	BF (%)	SMA	SMI
1 vs. 2	<0.0001	<0.0001	<0.0001	0.0007	0.0002	0.0002	0.6115	<0.0001	0.0075	<0.0001	0.0002	<0.0001	<0.0001
1 vs. 3	<0.0001	<0.0001	<0.0001	0.0002	<0.0001	<0.0001	0.5693	<0.0001	0.0013	<0.0001	<0.0001	<0.0001	<0.0001
1 vs. 4	<0.0001	<0.0001	<0.0001	0.0052	<0.0001	<0.0001	0.9972	<0.0001	0.0079	<0.0001	<0.0001	<0.0001	<0.0001
2 vs. 3	0.0032	0.0045	0.4868	0.7336	0.7074	0.7029	0.9939	0.452	0.6751	0.0038	0.0074	0.5178	0.5735
2 vs. 4	<0.0001	<0.0001	0.0569	0.9557	0.0054	0.005	0.7076	0.0636	0.7784	0.0002	0.0015	0.0298	0.0416
3 vs. 4	0.1042	0.076	0.5251	0.9863	0.0658	0.0626	0.6024	0.5838	1	0.3965	0.7147	0.3509	0.3857

p-values for comparison between the respective time points. t1 = before surgery, t2 = 6 weeks after surgery, t3 = 12 weeks after surgery, t4 = 24 weeks after surgery. BMI = body mass index, TBW = total body water, LBM = lean body mass, ECM = extracellular mass, BCM = body cell mass, BF = body fat, SMA = skeletal muscle area, SMI = skeletal muscle index.

Figures 1–3 reveal the quartiles, interquartile range (IQR) and outliers for the variables BMI, SMI and SMA for different time points.

Table 4 summarizes the Pearson Correlation Coefficient r for comparison of SMI with the parameters of body composition measured by BIA. No relevant correlation can be observed between BMI and SMI, but we found a correlation between the phase angle, BCM,

ECM/BCM—Index and SMI. The higher the phase angle, the higher the SMI. The same applies to BCM. The higher the ratio of ECM/BCM, the lower the SMI.

Table 4. Correlation of SMI with BIA parameters.

t	Body Weight	BMI	Basal Metabolic Rate (kcal)	Phase Angle	TBW	LBM	ECM	BCM	ECM/BCM	BF (kg)	BF (%)	SMA
1	0.24085	0.38667	0.38526	0.22527	0.28819	0.28748	0.15098	0.3879	−0.24203	−0.0167	−0.18213	0.74816
2	0.42458	0.30951	0.66135	0.51569	0.476	0.4753	0.18051	0.66573	−0.50681	0.1514	−0.14671	0.82661
3	0.27591	0.2205	0.65462	0.72809	0.40136	0.40183	−0.16068	0.66083	−0.71336	−0.07564	−0.24256	0.79288
4	0.62821	0.18605	0.76101	0.71963	0.58433	0.58561	−0.05668	0.76404	−0.64093	−0.01619	−0.30592	0.87446

Pearson Correlation Coefficient r. t1 = before surgery, t2 = 6 weeks after surgery, t3 = 12 weeks after surgery, t4 = 24 weeks after surgery. BMI = body mass index, TBW = total body water, LBM = lean body mass, ECM = extracellular mass, BCM = body cell mass, BF = body fat, SMA = skeletal muscle area, SMI = skeletal muscle index.

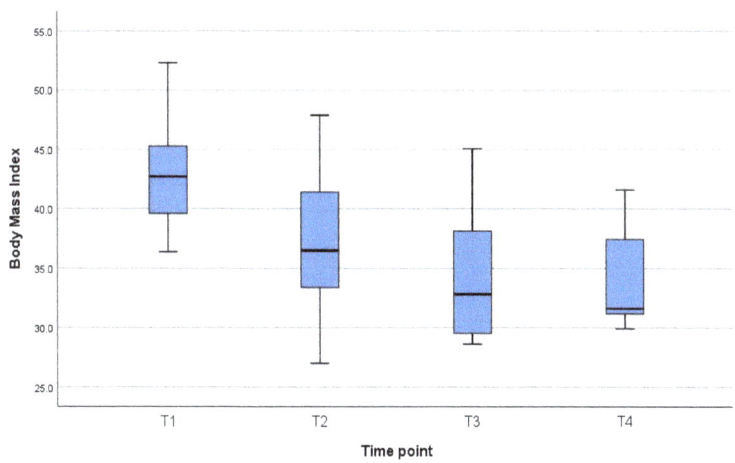

Figure 1. Box plot for BMI for different time points.

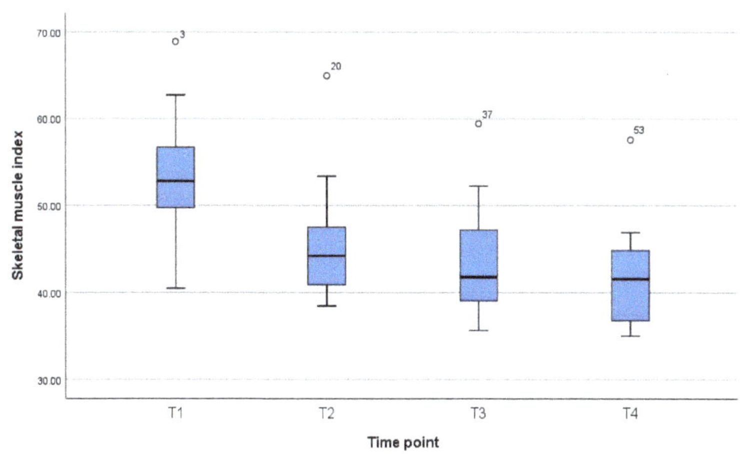

Figure 2. Box plot for SMI for different time points.

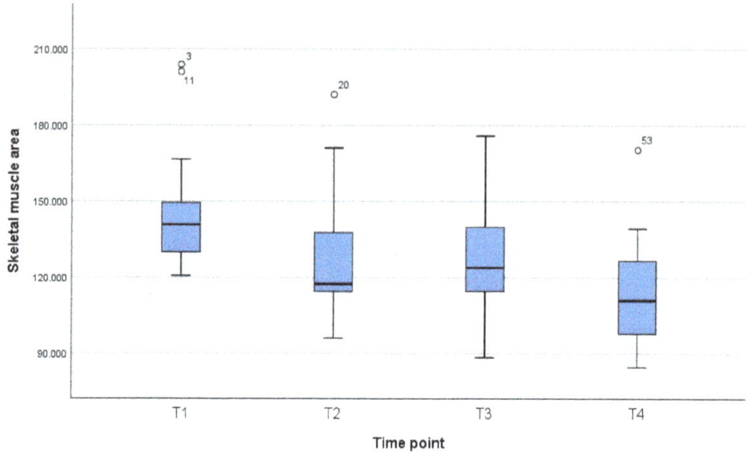

Figure 3. Box plot for SMA for different time points.

Applying the cut-offs for sarcopenia introduced by Prado et al. [21] (SMI < 52.4 cm^2/m^2 for men and <38.5 cm^2/m^2 for women), 12% of the patients were sarcopenic before surgery (one man and one woman), 17% were sarcopenic at 6 weeks after surgery, 45% at 12 weeks after surgery and 57% at 24 weeks after surgery.

4. Discussion

In the current study, we investigated the changes in the SMI measured on a single L3-MRI layer as a direct indicator for the skeletal muscle mass of obese patients undergoing a RYGB procedure compared to BIA. To our knowledge, the direct comparison of those two methods is novel. The SMI is rarely discussed in literature, concerning bariatric surgical patients, but it is widely recognized as a direct parameter of the muscle mass status, because of the high accuracy and low susceptibility to external factors, in many other fields of medicine [21]. BIA on the other side is an often-used tool, which is still not considered sufficiently reliable, because of dependence on patient related and environmental factors, such as fasting and exercise status, previously to the measurement. Our results show a strong correlation between the SMI and the main parameters of the BIA (phase angle, LBM, BCM and the ECM/BCM—Index), which indicates that both methods are comparable in terms of estimating the change in body composition after bariatric surgery. These findings are in line with a publication of Walowski et al., considering that single computed tomography or MRI layers and appendicular lean soft tissue by DXA or BIA can be used as a valid substitute for total skeletal muscle mass. All diagnostics show a high correlation concerning body composition with results from whole body imaging in cross-sectional and longitudinal analyses [22]. BIA is a very feasible and inexpensive method for determination of the body composition. The determination of SMI by MRI is a very exact method in patients with mild obesity, but still MRI is more expensive and more time consuming than BIA. Our results clearly show that BIA, performed under standardized setting, has a good applicability and precision as a direct, imaging measured method as the SMI determination. Both methods, BIA and MRI, can be used for the estimation of body composition and presence of sarcopenia in patients after RYGB. The reliability of BIA has been previously described by our study group [5,11,12]. In our center we routinely use the BIA throughout the preparation of our patients for bariatric procedure, as well as in the follow up. This technique is feasible at low costs and the present study shows, that its results are resilient in comparison to the SMI derived from MRI. We are not doing MRI exams routinely in our patients, but we determine it in case of preexisting cross- sectional imaging.

Lee et al. also described that SMI values significantly correlate to BIA parameters among RYGB- patients, but not with the percent decrease after the procedure. These findings are in principle in line to our results, even though only one CT- scan after 6 months was performed postoperatively [20].

The reduction of SMI as well as BCM, LBM and phase angle in the first six months after RYGB, detected in our study, is in line with the findings of Alba et al. The authors also describe a significant decline of total LBM and absolute muscle strength, along with weight loss and fat mass reduction during the first year after RYGB [4]. Davidson et al. also demonstrated a decrease of SMI and fat free mass (FFM) during the phase of extensive weight loss in the first year after RYGB, but subsequent changes in MRI- measured muscle mass were minimal during the further follow up of 4 years [23]. According to these results, LBM and skeletal muscle mass reduction occurs frequently after bariatric surgery and mainly during the first year after surgery. In the meantime, Alba et al. described that even during the first year after RYGB, the decline of the muscle mass does not necessarily lead to poor clinical status of the patients. Their study showed a significant improvement in physical performance tasks despite a decrease of muscle mass. This fact could be explained by changes in biomechanics, which simply make it easier for a person to move around after weight loss. Nonetheless, maintaining more muscle mass or strength leads to greater functional improvements, and future research should address a range of strategies to optimize postoperative physical performance [4].

Two of our patients (11.8%) were sarcopenic according to the Prado- definition [24] before RYGB- procedure. Both patients were still sarcopenic 6 months after surgery. At that time point 57% of the examined patients were sarcopenic. Similar findings were made by a French group, detecting 32% obese patients with sarcopenia using SMI measured by MRI, one year after laparoscopic sleeve gastrectomy. However, only 8% of this cohort was in a sarcopenic condition before surgery [25].

The combination of low muscle mass and strength with obesity can further deteriorate the health status and physical performance of bariatric patients. Still, to date, the exact clinical meaning of these findings remains unclear. Sarcopenia seems to occur frequently in combination with obesity and is deteriorated in the early phase after bariatric surgery, indicating a special need for detection prior to surgery and an intense follow-up during the postoperative period. Structured programs, including an ongoing nutritional counseling and even structured rehabilitation programs, might be necessary to prevent patients from developing further sarcopenia and malnutrition. Hansen et al. demonstrated the important role of physical activity and exercise intervention in order to improve postoperative health benefits in terms of changes in body weight and fat mass, muscle mass and strength and physical fitness [26]. In contrast to our findings, Zamboni et al. reported that the "sarcopenic obesity" seems to play an important role in elderly patients, causing age- related gain of fat tissue and loss of muscle mass and also elderly subjects having a great health risk due to sarcopenic obesity [27]. In addition, such interventions lead to a better preservation of muscle strength, muscle mass, endurance capacity, and bone mineral density as well as greater quality of life [28]. Previous BIA studies clearly explain the importance of the preoperative determination of body composition and muscle mass status among bariatric surgical patients, describing the predictive value of the phase angle (parameter of the BIA) on postoperative body composition and potential weight loss [5,15].

5. Conclusions

Sarcopenia is a major problem in patients with obesity and can deteriorate further after bariatric surgery. Our data verify the accuracy of the BIA- parameters for muscle mass in comparison to the exact measurement of the SMI in single L3 layer of the abdomen. Both methods can detect the condition of sarcopenia in bariatric patients as an important factor for body composition before and after surgery. Patients should be screened for a reduction in muscle mass preoperatively as well as during long-term follow-up. Further, prospective trials are needed to investigate the exact clinical relevance of short-term and long-term sarcopenia after surgery.

6. Limitations

Our study has some limitations, one of them being the relatively small number of participants and the number of patients lost to follow-up during the end of the study. The small sample size of this study and the heterogeneity of our patient cohort in terms of gender, BMI and age did not allow us to perform more specific or complex statistical tests as multivariate regression analysis to reinforce our statement. Still, we were able to provide sequential BIA and SMI by MRI, which allowed us to give an overview of the development of body composition and muscle mass in the first months after RYGB.

Author Contributions: Conceptualization, G.V. and S.B.; methodology, G.V. and M.O.; software, C.W.; validation, C.W., G.V. and C.G.; formal analysis, G.V., S.B. and C.G.; investigation, G.V. and M.O.; resources, C.R. and M.O.; data curation, G.V., C.W. and S.B.; writing—original draft preparation, G.V. and S.B.; writing—review and editing, G.V., S.B. and A.F.; visualization, C.W.; supervision, G.V. and M.O.; project administration, M.O. All authors have read and agreed to the published version of the manuscript.

Funding: This research received no external funding.

Institutional Review Board Statement: The study was conducted according to the guidelines of the Declaration of Helsinki, and approved by the Medical Ethics Commission II of the Medical Faculty Mannheim, Heidelberg University, Mannheim, Germany (2009-312N-MA).

Informed Consent Statement: Informed consent was obtained from all subjects involved in the study.

Data Availability Statement: The data presented in this study are available on request from the corresponding author. The data are not publicly available due tot he rules of the Medical Ethics Commission of our institution.

Conflicts of Interest: The authors declare no conflict of interest.

References

1. Feren, A.; Torheim, L.E.; Lillegaard, I.T. Development of a nutrition knowledge questionnaire for obese adults. *Food Nutr. Res.* **2011**, *55*, 7271. [CrossRef]
2. Kang, J.H.; Le, Q.A. Effectiveness of bariatric surgical procedures: A systematic review and network meta-analysis of randomized controlled trials. *Medicine* **2017**, *96*, e8632. [CrossRef]
3. Friedrich, A.E.; Damms-Machado, A.; Meile, T.; Scheuing, N.; Stingel, K.; Basrai, M.; Küper, M.A.; Kramer, K.M.; Königsrainer, A.; Bischoff, S.C. Laparoscopic sleeve gastrectomy compared to a multidisciplinary weight loss program for obesity-effects on body composition and protein status. *Obes. Surg.* **2013**, *23*, 1957–1965. [CrossRef]
4. Alba, D.L.; Wu, L.; Cawthon, P.M.; Mulligan, K.; Lang, T.; Patel, S.; King, N.J.; Carter, J.T.; Rogers, S.J.; Posselt, A.M.; et al. Changes in Lean Mass, Absolute and Relative Muscle Strength, and Physical Performance After Gastric Bypass Surgery. *J. Clin. Endocrinol. Metab.* **2019**, *104*, 711–720. [CrossRef]
5. Vassilev, G.; Hasenberg, T.; Krammer, J.; Kienle, P.; Ronellenfitsch, U.; Otto, M. The Phase Angle of the Bioelectrical Impedance Analysis as Predictor of Post-Bariatric Weight Loss Outcome. *Obes. Surg.* **2017**, *27*, 665–669. [CrossRef]
6. Ciangura, C.; Bouillot, J.-L.; Lloret-Linares, C.; Poitou, C.; Veyrie, N.; Basdevant, A.; Oppert, J.-M. Dynamics of change in total and regional body composition after gastric bypass in obese patients. *Obesity* **2010**, *18*, 760–765. [CrossRef]
7. Chaston, T.B.; Dixon, J.B.; O'Brien, P.E. Changes in fat-free mass during significant weight loss: A systematic review. *Int. J. Obes.* **2007**, *31*, 743–750. [CrossRef]
8. Hue, O.; Berrigan, F.; Simoneau, M.; Marcotte, J.; Marceau, P.; Marceau, S.; Tremblay, A.; Teasdale, N. Muscle force and force control after weight loss in obese and morbidly obese men. *Obes. Surg.* **2008**, *18*, 1112–1118. [CrossRef]
9. Steele, T.; Cuthbertson, D.J.; Wilding, J.P.H. Impact of bariatric surgery on physical functioning in obese adults. *Obes. Rev.* **2015**, *16*, 248–258. [CrossRef]
10. Madan, A.K.; Kuykendall, S.; Orth, W.S.; A Ternovits, C.; Tichansky, D.S. Does laparoscopic gastric bypass result in a healthier body composition? An affirmative answer. *Obes. Surg.* **2006**, *16*, 465–468. [CrossRef]
11. Otto, M.; Kautt, S.; Kremer, M.; Kienle, P.; Post, S.; Hasenberg, T. Handgrip strength as a predictor for post bariatric body composition. *Obes. Surg.* **2014**, *24*, 2082–2088. [CrossRef]
12. Otto, M.; Färber, J.; Haneder, S.; Michaely, H.; Kienle, P.; Hasenberg, T. Postoperative changes in body composition–comparison of bioelectrical impedance analysis and magnetic resonance imaging in bariatric patients. *Obes. Surg.* **2015**, *25*, 302–309. [CrossRef]
13. Shen, W.; Punyanitya, M.; Wang, Z.; Gallagher, D.; St.-Onge, M.-P.; Albu, J.; Heymsfield, S.B.; Heshka, S. Total body skeletal muscle and adipose tissue volumes: Estimation from a single abdominal cross-sectional image. *J. Appl. Physiol.* **2004**, *97*, 2333–2338. [CrossRef]

14. Mourtzakis, M.; Prado, C.M.; Lieffers, J.R.; Reiman, T.; McCargar, L.J.; Baracos, V.E. A practical and precise approach to quantification of body composition in cancer patients using computed tomography images acquired during routine care. *Appl. Physiol. Nutr. Metab.* **2008**, *33*, 997–1006. [CrossRef]
15. Gerken, A.L.H.; Rohr-Kräutle, K.-K.; Weiss, C.; Seyfried, S.; Reissfelder, C.; Vassilev, G.; Otto, M. Handgrip Strength and Phase Angle Predict Outcome After Bariatric Surgery. *Obes. Surg.* **2021**, *31*, 200–206. [CrossRef]
16. Lieffers, J.R.; Bathe, O.F.; Fassbender, K.; Winget, M.; Baracos, V.E. Sarcopenia is associated with postoperative infection and delayed recovery from colorectal cancer resection surgery. *Br. J. Cancer* **2012**, *107*, 931–936. [CrossRef]
17. Martin, L.; Birdsell, L.; MacDonald, N.; Reiman, T.; Clandinin, M.T.; McCargar, L.J.; Murphy, R.; Ghosh, S.; Sawyer, M.B.; Baracos, V.E. Cancer cachexia in the age of obesity: Skeletal muscle depletion is a powerful prognostic factor, independent of body mass index. *J. Clin. Oncol.* **2013**, *31*, 1539–1547. [CrossRef]
18. Cruz-Jentoft, A.J.; Baeyens, J.P.; Bauer, J.M.; Boirie, Y.; Cederholm, T.; Landi, F.; Martin, F.C.; Michel, J.-P.; Rolland, Y.; Schneider, S.M.; et al. European Working Group on Sarcopenia in Older P: Sarcopenia: European consensus on definition and diagnosis: Report of the European Working Group on Sarcopenia in Older People. *Age Ageing* **2010**, *39*, 412–423. [CrossRef]
19. Reisinger, K.W.; van Vugt, J.L.A.; Tegels, J.; Snijders, C.; Hulsewé, K.W.E.; Hoofwijk, A.G.; Stoot, J.; Von Meyenfeldt, M.F.; Beets, G.; Derikx, J.P.M.; et al. Functional compromise reflected by sarcopenia, frailty, and nutritional depletion predicts adverse postoperative outcome after colorectal cancer surgery. *Ann. Surg.* **2015**, *261*, 345–352. [CrossRef]
20. Lee, J.K.; Park, Y.S.; Kim, K.; Oh, T.J.; Chang, W. Comparison of Bioelectrical Impedance Analysis and Computed Tomography on Body Composition changes including Visceral Fat after Bariatric Surgery in Asian Patients with Obesity. *Obes. Surg.* **2021**, *31*, 4243–4250. [CrossRef]
21. Galata, C.; Hodapp, J.; Weiss, C.; Karampinis, I.; Vassilev, G.; Reissfelder, C.; Otto, M. Skeletal Muscle Mass Index Predicts Postoperative Complications in Intestinal Surgery for Crohn's Disease. *JPEN J. Parenter Enteral. Nutr.* **2020**, *44*, 714–721. [CrossRef]
22. Walowski, C.O.; Braun, W.; Maisch, M.J.; Jensen, B.; Peine, S.; Norman, K.; Müller, M.J.; Bosy-Westphal, A. Reference Values for Skeletal Muscle Mass—Current Concepts and Methodological Considerations. *Nutrients* **2020**, *12*, 755. [CrossRef]
23. Davidson, L.E.; Yu, W.; Goodpaster, B.H.; Delany, J.P.; Widen, E.; Lemos, T.; Strain, G.W.; Pomp, A.; Courcoulas, A.P.; Lin, S.; et al. Fat-Free Mass and Skeletal Muscle Mass Five Years After Bariatric Surgery. *Obesity* **2018**, *26*, 1130–1136. [CrossRef]
24. Prado, C.M.; Cushen, S.J.; Orsso, C.E.; Ryan, A. Sarcopenia and cachexia in the era of obesity: Clinical and nutritional impact. *Proc. Nutr. Soc.* **2016**, *75*, 188–198. [CrossRef]
25. Voican, C.S.; Lebrun, A.; Maître, S.; Lainas, P.; Lamouri, K.; Njiké-Nakseu, M.; Gaillard, M.; Tranchart, H.; Balian, A.; Dagher, I.; et al. Predictive score of sarcopenia occurrence one year after bariatric surgery in severely obese patients. *PLoS ONE* **2018**, *13*, e0197248. [CrossRef]
26. Hansen, D.; Decroix, L.; Devos, Y.; Nocca, D.; Cornelissen, V.; Dillemans, B.; Lannoo, M. Towards Optimized Care After Bariatric Surgery by Physical Activity and Exercise Intervention: A Review. *Obes. Surg.* **2020**, *30*, 1118–1125. [CrossRef]
27. Zamboni, M.; Mazzali, G.; Fantin, F.; Rossi, A.; Di Francesco, V. Sarcopenic obesity: A new category of obesity in the elderly. *Nutr. Metab. Cardiovasc. Dis.* **2008**, *18*, 388–395. [CrossRef]
28. Livhits, M.; Mercado, C.; Yermilov, I.; Parikh, J.A.; Dutson, E.; Mehran, A.; Ko, C.Y.; Gibbons, M.M. Exercise following bariatric surgery: Systematic review. *Obes. Surg.* **2010**, *20*, 657–665. [CrossRef]

Journal of
Clinical Medicine

MDPI

Systematic Review

Effects of Supervised Physical Exercise as Prehabilitation on Body Composition, Functional Capacity and Quality of Life in Bariatric Surgery Candidates: A Systematic Review and Meta-Analysis

Andrea Herrera-Santelices [1,2], Graciela Argüello-Florencio [3], Greice Westphal [4], Nelson Nardo Junior [4] and Antonio Roberto Zamunér [5,*]

1 Facultad de Ciencias de la Salud, Universidad Católica de Maule, Talca 3480112, Chile
2 Servicio de Medicina Física y Rehabilitación, Hospital San Juan de Dios, Curicó 3343005, Chile
3 Department of Health Sciences, Nutrition and Dietetics Career, Faculty of Medicine, Pontificia Universidad Católica de Chile, Santiago 8331150, Chile
4 Multidisciplinary Center of Obesity Studies, Department of Physical Education, Sate University of Maringa, Maringá 87020-900, Brazil
5 Laboratory of Clinical Research in Kinesiology, Department of Kinesiology, Universidad Católica del Maule, Talca 3480112, Chile
* Correspondence: beto.zam@gmail.com; Tel.: +56-71-2203100

Abstract: Background: Prehabilitation is a strategy used aiming to reduce the risk factors and complications of surgery procedures, but there is no consensus on the effectiveness of supervised physical exercise and its optimal prescription during this phase. Objectives: To determine the effects of exercise prehabilitation on body composition, functional capacity and quality of life in candidates for bariatric surgery. Search methods: A search was conducted in PubMed, Web of Science, SciELO, Scopus, MEDLINE and CINAHL. Selection criteria: Only randomized clinical trials that examined the effectiveness of supervised physical exercise were included. The main outcomes were body composition, functional capacity, quality of life and surgical outcomes. Data collection and analysis: Two researchers independently selected the literature, extracted the data and evaluated the risk of bias. A third researcher was consulted when a consensus was not reached. The risk of bias was assessed by the tool recommended by the Cochrane Collaboration, the quality of the evidence by GRADE, and to analyze the effects of prehabilitation on the primary objectives, RevMan software, version 5.3 was used. Main results: The search resulted in 4550 articles, of which 22 met the eligibility criteria, leaving 5 articles selected for this review. One article was assessed as a high bias risk and four as an uncertain risk, which included 139 candidates for bariatric surgery. Most of the studies evaluated the body composition, functional capacity and quality of life; none reported surgical outcomes. Conclusions: Supervised physical exercise has positive effects on the body composition, functional capacity and quality of life; there was no evidence for surgical outcomes, which opens up a field of study for future research of this population.

Keywords: prehabilitation; bariatric surgery; obesity; physical exercise; quality of life

Citation: Herrera-Santelices, A.; Argüello-Florencio, G.; Westphal, G.; Nardo Junior, N.; Zamunér, A.R. Effects of Supervised Physical Exercise as Prehabilitation on Body Composition, Functional Capacity and Quality of Life in Bariatric Surgery Candidates: A Systematic Review and Meta-Analysis. *J. Clin. Med.* **2022**, *11*, 5091. https://doi.org/10.3390/jcm11175091

Academic Editor: Gregory Hand

Received: 22 July 2022
Accepted: 26 August 2022
Published: 30 August 2022

1. Introduction

Obesity is a chronic disease that is progressive, recurrent and creates health problems, depending on the topographical location of excessive fat deposits. The most common health problems are metabolic syndrome, high blood pressure, sarcopenia, osteopenia, diabetes mellitus, obstructive sleep apnea syndrome, dyslipidemia, depression and anxiety disorder, among others [1]. Therefore, several treatment pharmacological, non-pharmacological and surgical strategies have been proposed [2]. In this sense, bariatric surgery (BS) has proven to be effective in solving comorbidities and promoting long-term weight loss in people with obesity [3].

When a patient undergoes major abdominal surgery, such as BS, evidence suggests that the proper preparation decreases the risks associated with the surgical procedure and promotes a recovery that includes a higher pain tolerance, fewer hospital stays, less need for rehospitalization and less surgical complications in the short and long term (e.g., venous thrombosis, surgical wound dehiscence, bowel obstruction and adhesions development, among others) [4–6].

Enhanced Recovery After Surgery (ERAS) is the current protocol used by different surgical specialties to promote post-op recovery [7]. Regarding BS, the ERAS protocol recommends several procedures and lifestyle changes, including diet control and the use of some specific pharmacological prescription [7]. In addition, patients are encouraged to participate in a preoperative weight loss program [6]. In that regard, it is well-known that exercise has multiple benefits for a person's physical and mental health, especially for those with obesity. Exercise has been used as one of the main strategies for weight control and in the treatment of different associated comorbidities, contributing to glycemic control; lowering resting blood pressure and improving body composition, cardiorespiratory fitness, sleep quality and quality of life [8,9]. Therefore, regular physical exercise could have an important role in wight loss programs during prehabilitation for BS. However, despite some randomized controlled trials (RCTs) having addressed this subject [10–12], there is currently no clarity regarding its effectiveness on surgical outcomes (e.g., hospitalization days, post-op pain tolerance, short- and long-term complications, rehospitalization, etc.); mortality and other indices to support its recommendation in the ERAS protocol for BS [13].

Therefore, the objective of this systematic review is to determine the effect of prehabilitation on the body composition, functional capacity, quality of life and surgical outcomes in patients who are candidates for BS.

2. Materials and Methods

The protocol for this systematic review was registered on PROSPERO; the registered number is: CRD42021261474 [14]. This systematic review was conducted in accordance with the PRISMA guidelines.

2.1. Search Plan and Literature Selection

The articles were searched in the following electronic databases: PubMed, Web of Science, SciELO, Scopus, MEDLINE and CINAHL between 1 and 31 July 2021 without restrictions of language or publication date. The descriptors used were: "Prehabilitation", "Physical Exercise", "Body Composition", "Functional Capacity", "Quality of Life", "Surgical Outcomes" and "Bariatric Surgery"; for the combinations of these, the Boolean operators "AND" and/or "OR" were used. All studies were exported to the 5.4 version of StArt (State of the Art through Systematic Review) software (developed by the Federal University of São Carlos).

2.2. Types of Participants/Population

Inclusion criteria

Eighteen-year-old adults or older, both sexes and candidates for a first bariatric surgery who were included in a prehabilitation program were included.

Exclusion criteria

Candidates for a second BS or reconversion surgery were excluded.

2.3. Types of Intervention/Exposition

For this review were considered randomized controlled clinical trials that applied supervised physical exercise programs described as aerobic exercise training, resistance exercise training or included both, with a duration of at least one week and performed before bariatric surgery.

2.4. Types of Comparator/Control

The control was considered as a group receiving no intervention or only the standard care, defined as advice, counseling, brochures or leaflets on various health topics or educational intervention of any kind.

2.5. Types of Outcome/Results Measurements

The studies were included if they reported the effect of the intervention on one or more of the following outcomes: (1) Body composition: evaluated through dual-energy x-energy absorptiometry or bioelectrical impedance; (2) Functional capacity: evaluated through a functional test, for example, the six-minute walk test (6MWT), the direct or indirect maximum rate of oxygen consumption (VO_2 max), the sitting to standing test or the step test among others; (3) Quality of life: evaluated through any quality of life questionnaire and (4) Surgical outcomes such as the number of hospital stay days, the need for rehospitalization within 30 days and post-op complications at 30 days were initially considered. However, they were disregarded, since these outcomes were not reported by any of the included studies.

2.6. Studies Selection

Two researchers (AH and GA) examined, independently, the studies that were identified by the search strategy using the 5.4 version of the StArt software. They were firstly identified by reading the title and the abstract. In order to be selected, the abstracts had to clearly identify the studies' design, population, intervention and outcome measurements, as previously described. In the event of a disagreement, a third researcher (GW) was consulted who determined whether the article was included or not. Then, both researchers moved on to reading the entirety of the potentially eligible articles and examined their eligibility according to the inclusion criteria. Again, if there was a disagreement, a third researcher was consulted. Conference reports and letters to the editor were excluded.

2.7. Data Extraction

After selecting the studies, two researchers (AH and GA) independently extracted the data according to a "standard data extraction form" created by two researchers from the team (AZ and AH). In the event of a disagreement between the reviewers, the data was subjected to consensus or arbitration by a third reviewer (GW). Both reviewers conducted a pilot test of data extraction using the standard data extraction form on two randomized controlled clinical trials that were related to exercise and its effect on cardiovascular risk factors.

2.8. Risk of Bias Assessment

The studies' risk of bias was independently evaluated by two researchers (AH and GA) through the "Cochrane Risk of Bias Tool", with 6 bias domains: selection, realization, detection, attrition, report and others. Each domain is qualified as a high, low or uncertain risk of bias (https://www.bmj.com/content/343/bmj.d5928, accessed on 25 October 2021). Punctuation disagreements were discussed between them until a consensus was reached; in case there was no agreement, a third researcher (GW) was consulted.

2.9. Evaluation of the Quality of Scientific Evidence

The quality of evidence in the studies was evaluated under GRADE (Grading of Recommendations Assessment, Development and Evaluation) criteria, including the study's limitations, the consistency of the effect, the inaccuracy, the evidence, and the publication bias. The webpage www.gradepro.org was used.

2.10. Statistical Analysis

A meta-analysis was carried out using Review Manager software (RevMan, version 5.3). Continuous outcomes were meta-analyzed using a random effects model and standard mean differences (SMDs). Heterogeneity was quantified by the I-squared (I^2) test and classified as low: $I^2 < 25\%$, moderate: $I^2 = 25.1–50\%$ and high: $I^2 > 50.1\%$.

3. Results

3.1. Article Selection

Figure 1 shows the flow chart pertaining to the identification of the studies and the selection process of these. The results from searching the database were 4550 articles, of which 626 were extracted while screening, because they were duplicates. Thus, 3924 were analyzed by reading the title and its abstract, excluding 3902; then, 22 met the eligibility criteria, 17 were excluded when the entire article was read and, finally, 5 studies were included in this review.

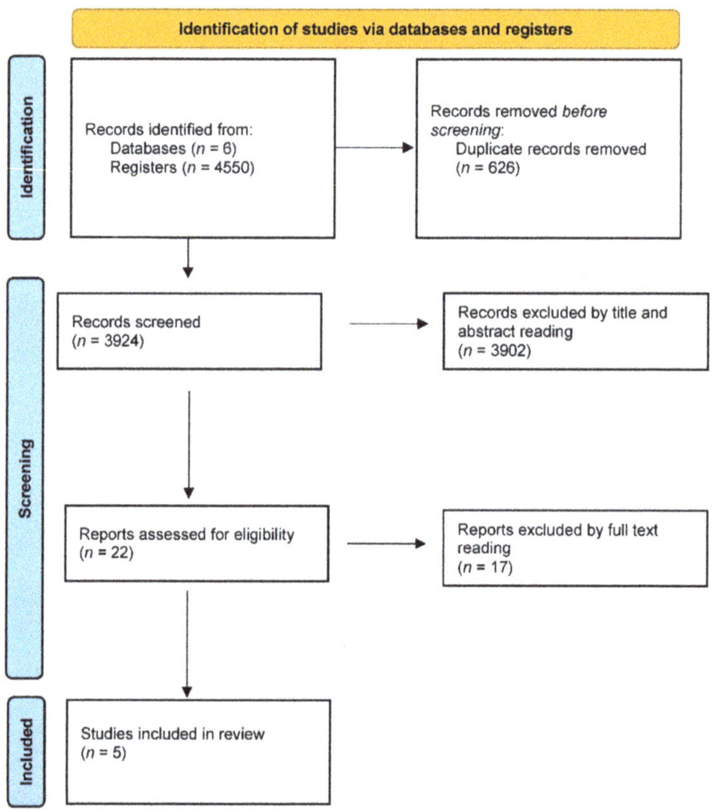

Figure 1. Article identification PRISMA flow chart.

3.2. Articles' Descriptions

Table 1 shows, in detail, the description of each article. The five articles selected for review and meta-analysis were published between 2010 and 2021 in English; four of them were performed on the American continent [11,15–17] and one in Europe [18].

Table 1. Description of each article.

[18] Arman et al. (2021)	
Randomization	**Software Stratified by Sex and Age Was Used.**
Participants	21 participants: 1 man—20 women. **Institution:** Rehabilitation and Physical Therapy Department, Health Sciences Department, Istanbul University-Cerrahpasa. **Country:** Turkey. **Inclusion criteria:** candidates to a BS, 18 years or older, both sexes. **Exclusion criteria:** participants with comorbidities that prevent their participation in the prehabilitation program like the existence of acute pain, cardiac pain or a previous dolor heart attack, cardiac failure, diabetes, or uncompensated hypertension.
Intervention	**Program of the institution:** 1. Warm-up (10–15 min): walk was performed on a treadmill; heart rate was monitored with a pulse oximeter and as a goal it was set at 50 to 60 heartbeats. 2. Load (30–45 min): exercises for core stabilization were progressively performed in supine position, long sitting position, knee position, crawling position, foot over one leg position and sitting on a ball as exercise. Involved a combination of strengthening, resistance, and balance exercises, along with breathing. Exercises for each main muscle group were performed during 2 cycles of 7 and 10 repetitions at a moderate intensity of 50% of maximum repetition. As sessions progressed the number and intensity of exercises were gradually increased. 3. Cool down (10 min): stretching large muscle groups like hamstrings, hip flexors, shoulder muscles, etc. **Total days of training:** 16. **Duration of intervention:** 8 weeks. **Frequency per week:** 2 times. **Load adjustment:** not detailed in the text.
Outcome measurements	**1. Body composition:** BMI, fat mass in kg, fat mass in %, free fat mass in kg. (Bioelectrical impedance analysis). **2. Functional capacity:** 6MWT, chair stand test, postural stability test, abdominal strength, core flexor strength, modified push up test. **3. Quality of life:** OSQOL. **4. Surgical objectives:** not studied in the research.
Global risk bias	**Uncertain.**
[11] Baillot et al. (2016)	
Randomization	Used software stratified by sex and maximum aerobic capacity (> o ≤ 7 MET).
Participants	29 participants: 7 men—22 women. **Institution:** Centre hospitalier universitaire de Sherbrooke (CHUS), Quebec. **Country:** Canada. **Inclusion criteria:** candidates to BS, 18 years old or older, both sexes. **Exclusion criteria:** participants with comorbidities that prevent their participation in the prehabilitation program like a medical contraindication to practice physical activity, functional limitations that do not allow them to perform the 6MWT, not understanding the French language, or decompensated neuro-psychiatric pathology.
Intervention	**Gym program:** 1. Warm-up (10 min). 2. Aerobic phase: 30 min of exercise (treadmill, walking circuit, arm ergometer, elliptical machine) 3. Resistance phase: 20 to 30 min. 4. Cool down: 10 min. **Total days of training:** 24. **Intervention duration:** 12 weeks. **Frequency per week:** 2 times. **Load adjustment:** Aerobic: according to HRR from 55 to 75/80%. 8 levels were determined: A: 55%, B: 55%, C: 55%, D: 55%/65%, E: 65%, F: 65%/75%, G: 75% and H: 75%/85%. The duration was of 24 min at an A level and 30 min during rest. Resistance: increased from 2 to 3 sets, from 12 to 15 repetitions and at a weight of 5 to 12 lbs. for men, and 2 to 10 lbs. for women.

Table 1. *Cont.*

Outcome measurements	**1. Body composition:** BMI, fat mass in %. (Bioelectrical impedance analysis). **2. Functional capacity:** 6MWT, chair stand test, half squat test, arm curl test. **3. Quality of life:** WRQOL. **4. Surgical objectives:** not studied in the research.
Global risk bias	**High.**
[15] **Baillot et al. (2018)**	
Randomization	Used software stratified by sex and maximum aerobic capacity (> o ≤ 7 MET).
Participants	25 participants: 5 men—20 women. **Institution:** Centre hospitalier universitaire de Sherbrooke (CHUS), Quebec. **Country:** Canada. **Inclusion criteria:** candidates to a BS, 18-year-old or older, both sexes. **Exclusion criteria:** participants with comorbidities that prevent their participation in the prehabilitation program like a medical contraindication to practice physical activity, functional limitations that do not allow them to perform the 6MWT, not understanding the French language, or decompensated neuro-psychiatric pathology.
Intervention	**Gym program:** 1. Warm up: 10 min. 2. Aerobic phase: 30 min of exercise on the treadmill, walking circuit, arm ergometer, elliptical machine, aerobic dance. 3. Resistance phase: 20 to 30 min with small equipment, elastic bands, medicine balls, dumbbells, sticks. 4. Cool down: 10 min. **Total days of training:** 36. **Intervention duration:** 12 weeks. **Frequency per week:** 3 times. **Load adjustment:** Aerobic: according to a HRR from 55 to 75/80% (there are no more details in the article).
Outcome measurements	**1. Body composition:** BMI, free fat mass in %. (Bioelectrical impedance analysis). **2. Functional capacity:** 6MWT, half squat test. **3. Quality of life:** WRQOL. **4. Surgical objectives:** not studied in the research.
Global risk bias	**Uncertain.**
[16] **Funderburk et al. (2010)**	
Randomization	Unexplained.
Participants	7 participants: 1 man, 6 women. **Institution:** Hospital Pitt County Memorial, Rehabilitation center, Greenville. **Country:** United States of America. **Inclusion criteria:** candidates to a BS, 18 years old or older, both sexes. **Exclusion criteria:** no reports in the article.
Intervention	**Program of the institution:** The program included a warmup with exercises (walking in the water), strength and resistance exercises, and Ai Chi exercises for balance, core strengthening, and relaxation. Ai Chi is an aquatic exercise that was designed to increase relaxation, range of motion, and mobility. It is performed standing with the water at shoulder level using a combination of deep breathing and complete slow movements of the lower and superior extremities, as well as the torso. (There are no more details in the article). **Total days of training:** 24. **Intervention duration:** 12 weeks. **Frequency per week:** 2 times. **Load adjustment:** not detailed in the article.

Table 1. *Cont.*

Outcome measurements	**1. Body composition:** not studied in the article. **2. Functional capacity:** 6MWT, chair stand test, postural stability test, abdominal strength, core flexor strength, modified push up test. **3. Quality of life:** SF 36. **4. Surgical objectives:** not studied in the research.
Global risk bias	**Uncertain.**
[17] **Marcon et al. (2017)**	
Randomization	In blocks of 12 participants.
Participants	57 participants: 6 men—51 women. **Institution:** Hospital de Clinicas de Porto Alegre, Porto Alegre. **Country:** Brazil. **Inclusion criteria:** candidates to a BS, 18 years old or older, both sexes. **Exclusion criteria:** participants with comorbidities that prevent their participation in the prehabilitation program, participating in another supervised exercise program, patients with a class III or IV of heart functional capacity, orthopedic problems, severe retinopathy, severe neuropathy, drug addiction, severe mental illness, severe metabolic decompensation (250 mg/DI of blood glucose, systolic pressure over 200 mmHg, diastolic pressure over 100 mmHG).
Intervention	**Gym program:** Included aerobic exercise and stretching, intensity was measured by Borg's scale, using a range between 2 to 4, considering it low to moderate intensity respectively. Arm and leg movements were alternated, moving to simulate walking. Stretching included: arms, legs, torso, and neck for 6 min after the aerobic phase in each session. (There are no more details in the article). **Total days of training:** 32. **Intervention duration:** 16 weeks. **Frequency per week:** 2 times. **Load adjustment:** not detailed in the article.
Outcome measurements	**1.- Body composition:** BMI. (Bioelectrical impedance analysis) **2.- Functional capacity:** 6MWT, VO_2 max from equations after the test. **3.- Quality of life:** not studied in the research. **4.- Surgical objectives:** not studied in the research.
Global risk bias	**Uncertain.**

BS: bariatric surgery, BMI: body mass index, 6MWT: 6-min walk test, OSQOL: Obesity-Specific Quality of life, HRR: heart rate reserve, WRQOL: Weight-Related Quality of Life, SF 36: quality of life questionnaire related to health.

3.3. Participants

A total of 139 participants were enrolled in the five selected studies. The data from 115 participants were used for the meta-analysis on the body composition (BMI) [11,15,17,18], 75 participants for the fat mass percentage (FM%) [11,15,18], 46 for the free fat mass (FFM Kg) [15,18], 61 participants for the meta-analysis of the 6MWT [17,18] and 53 participants for the meta-analysis of the quality of life total score [15,16,18]. Regarding the demographics characteristics of the included studies, the sample size varied between 7 and 57 participants, the age ranged between 28 and 54 years old, 116 participants were women and all the studies included men.

3.4. Types of Intervention/Exposition

The duration of the intervention programs in the included studies ranged from 8 to 16 weeks. Twelve weeks of intervention were used in three out of the five articles [11,15,16]. One study had an intervention session frequency of three times a week [15] and twice a week. The duration of each session varied between 25 and 80 min, and the location was either a hospital gym or an educational institution where the researchers belonged [11,15–18].

In regards to the type of training, the combination of aerobic and resistance exercise was used in three studies; the other two used aerobic [11] and resistance [18] training separately. The average amount of sessions was 26.4, with a range between 16 and 32 sessions.

3.5. Types of Comparator/Control

Only one study did not use any kind of intervention as a control [16]. Standard care was used for the rest of the studies, counseling being the one used most. One study added cognitive–behavioral therapy to the standard care [17].

3.6. Risk of Bias Evaluation

Figures 2 and 3 show detailed results of the general risk of bias evaluation and the evaluation per study, respectively. The randomization generation sequence (selection bias) was judged as a low risk in all the included studies. On the other hand, the selective reporting data (report bias) was classified as an uncertain risk in all the studies. A high risk of bias can be noted in 20% of the included articles for the following items: incomplete results data (attrition bias), blinding of the participants and personnel (performance bias) and for other biases.

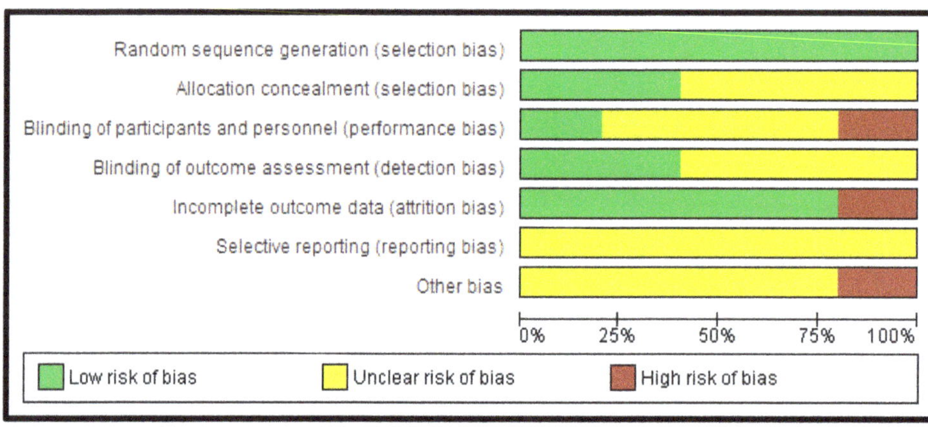

Figure 2. Evaluation of the general risk of bias.

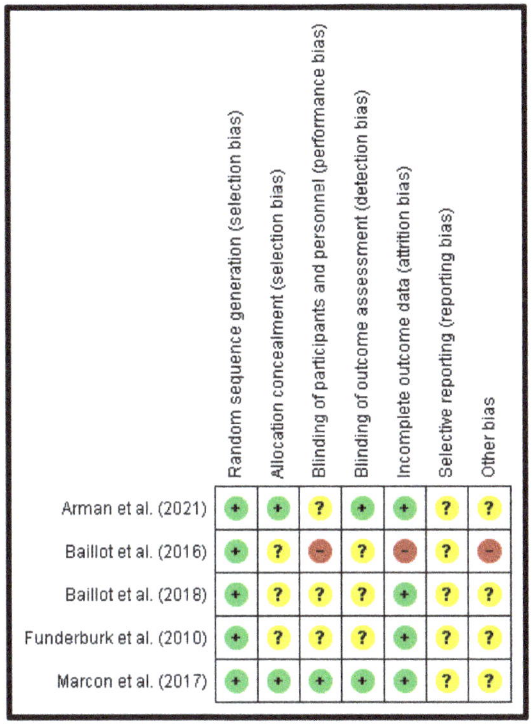

Figure 3. Risk of bias evaluation per study [11,15–18]. Red (-) = high risk of bias; Yellow (?) = unknown risk of bias; Green (+) = low risk of bias.

3.7. Prehabilitation Effects on the Outcome Measurements

3.7.1. Body Composition

Four studies measured the body composition and reported the BMI [11,15,17,18], FM% [11,15,18] or FFM, expressed in kilograms [15,18]. Other indexes were reported, such as abdominal fat in percentage, abdominal muscular mass in kilograms and fat mass in kilograms. However, they were not used for the meta-analysis, since it was only one study [18]. Overall, the results indicated no significant effect of prehabilitation in favor of the experiment or controls for body composition indexes ($p > 0.05$). Figure 4 shows the forest plot for BMI using the random effects model to compare the experimental versus control groups. The results showed a pooled effect of −0.71 ($IC_{95\%}$: −1.55 to 0.1; $p = 0.09$). The heterogeneity was 76%, and the quality of evidence was very low (Table 2).

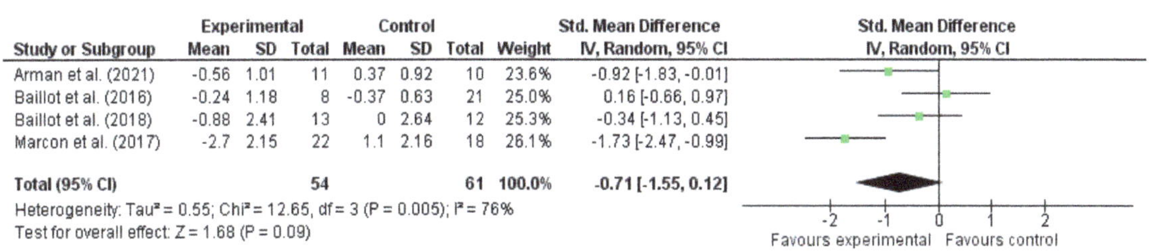

Figure 4. Forest plot of the body composition and the BMI subgroup [11,15,17,18].

Table 2. Quality of evidence for the body composition, BMI, FM% and FFM Kg.

Certainty Assessment						No. of Patients		Effect		Certainty
No. of Studies	Study Design	Risk of Bias	Inconsistency	Indirectness	Imprecision	Other Considerations	Aerobic Physical Exercise, Resistance or Both	Standard Care (no Exercise)	Relative (95% CI)	Absolute (95% CI)	
4	randomised trials	Serious [a]	Serious [b]	not serious	Serious [c]	none	54	61	-	SMD 0.71 SD **fewer** (1.55 fewer to 0.12 more)	⊕○○○ Very low
3	randomised trials	Serious [d]	not serious	not serious	not serious	none	39	36	-	SMD 0.38 SD **more** (0.47 fewer to 1.85 more)	⊕⊕⊕○ Moderate
2	randomised trials	Serious [e]	not serious	not serious	not serious	none	24	22	-	SMD 0.41 SD **fewer** (1 fewer to 0.18 more)	⊕⊕⊕○ Moderate

[a] Downgraded one level due to risk of bias (>25% of the participants were from studies with a high risk of bias). [b] Downgraded one level due to clear inconsistency of results. [c] Downgraded one level due to imprecision. [d] Downgraded one level due to risk of bias (>25% of the participants were from studies with a high risk of bias). [e] Downgraded one level due to risk of bias (both studies with uclear risk of bias).

Regarding the effect of an intervention on the FM% (Figure 5), the three studies included in the analysis resulted in a pooled effect of 0.38 ($CI_{95\%}$: −0.08 to 0.84; $p = 0.11$). The heterogeneity was 0%, and the quality of the evidence was moderate (Table 2).

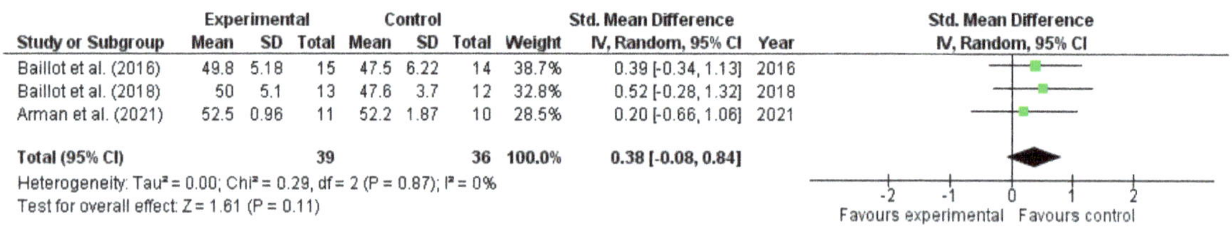

Figure 5. Forest plot of the body composition for the FM% subgroup [11,15,18].

Figure 6 shows the analysis of the FFM kg subgroup. The pooled effect size was −0.41 (IC95%: −1.00 to 0.18; $p = 0.17$) and a heterogeneity of 0%, with a moderate quality of evidence (Table 2).

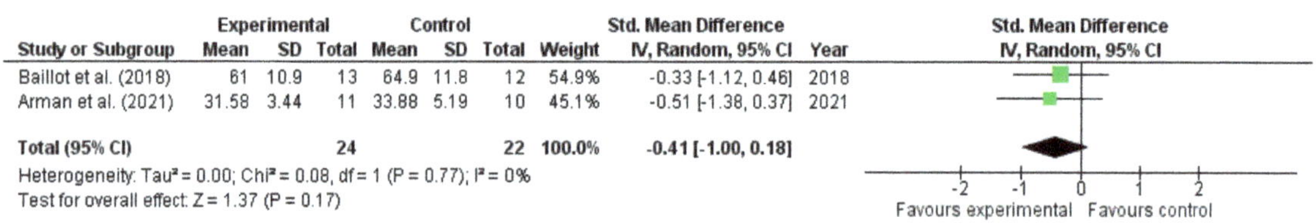

Figure 6. Forest plot of the body composition for the FFM Kg subgroup [11,18].

3.7.2. Functional Capacity

All studies evaluated the functional capacity. The 6MWT was the most used test. Two studies reported the results as the distance traveled in meters [17,18] and one in the number of total steps [16]. Baillot studies [11,15] did not show the values for the test results, which is why they were not included in the meta-analysis.

The VO_2 max was an outcome reported for only one study, which was estimated from a 6MWT equation [17]. Other indicators were used for the outcome report: the chair stand test [11,15,17,18], postural stability test, abdominal strength, core flexor strength and the modified push-up test were not analyzed statistically.

Figure 7 and Table 3 show the random effect analysis of the functional capacity for the 6MWT and the quality of evidence, respectively. The pooled effect was 2.59 ($IC_{95\%}$:1.89–3.30;

$p < 0.0001$) in favor of exercise, showing a low heterogeneity ($I^2 = 0\%$) and high quality of evidence.

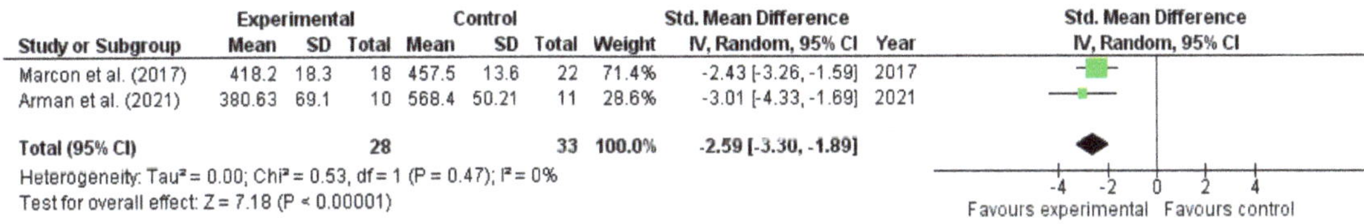

Figure 7. Forest plot of the functional capacity for the 6MWT [17,18].

Table 3. Quality of evidence for the functional capacity of the 6MWT.

Certainty Assessment							No. of Patients		Effect		Certainty
No. of Studies	Study Design	Risk of Bias	Inconsistency	Indirectness	Imprecision	Other Considerations	Aerobic Physical Exercise, Resistance or Both	Standard Care (no Exercise)	Relative (95% CI)	Absolute (95% CI)	
2	randomised trials	not serious	not serious	not serious	not serious	none	33	28	-	SMD **2.59 SD more** (1.89 more to 3.3 more)	⊕⊕⊕⊕ High

3.7.3. Quality of Life

Four studies evaluated the quality of life [11,15,16,18]: the SF-36 questionnaire, Weight-Related Quality of Life (WRQOL) and Obesity Specific Quality of Life (OSQOL) were used. Baillot et al. (2016) [11] did not report the post-intervention values, so it was not included in the meta-analysis. The SMD was used to combine the results of the three included studies. The random effect model resulted in a pooled effect size of 0.88 ($CI_{95\%}$: 0.23–1.99; $p = 0.12$; Figure 8), and the quality of evidence was moderate (Table 4).

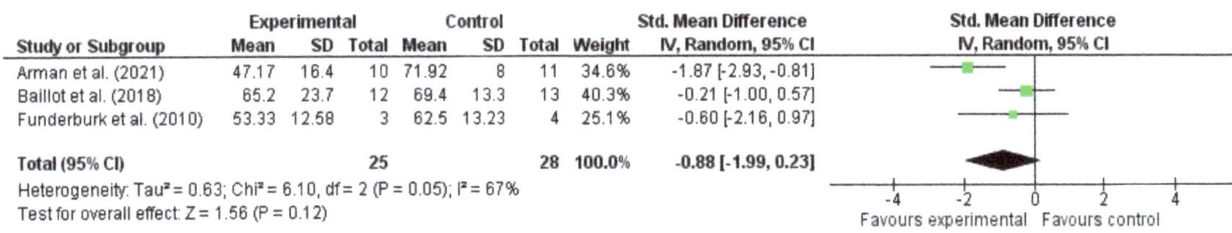

Figure 8. Forest plot of the quality of life total score [15,16,18].

Table 4. Quality of evidence for the quality of life total score.

Certainty Assessment							No. of Patients		Effect		Certainty
No. of Studies	Study Design	Risk of Bias	Inconsistency	Indirectness	Imprecision	Other Considerations	Aerobic Physical Exercise, Resistance or Both	Standard Care (no Exercise	Relative (95% CI)	Absolute (95% CI)	
3	randomised trials	serious[a]	not serious	not serious	not serious	none	28	25	-	SMD **0.88 SD more** (0.23 fewer to 1.99 more)	⊕⊕⊕◯ Moderate

3.7.4. Surgical Outcomes

No study reported the results for this outcome measurement.

4. Discussion

This systematic review's objective was to determine the effect of prehabilitation on the body composition, functional capacity, quality of life and surgical outcomes in patients who are candidates for bariatric surgery. In the last 10 years, a series of studies have evaluated the effects of physical training programs in the context of BS; most of which were done after the surgery. To the best of our knowledge, only two reviews [19,20] reported the effects of exercise on BS candidates in some variables considered in this study, but they did not perform a meta-analysis. Moreover, only two studies included in the previous reviews were RCTs, strengthening the relevance of the present study.

The results of this systematic review of RCTs showed that supervised exercise as prehabilitation before BS has positive effects on the body composition (i.e., BMI, FM% and FFM Kg); functional capacity (6MWT) and quality of life. In this sense, our results corroborate the findings of previous systematic reviews on this subject [19,20], who reported, in a descriptive manner, similar results.

The international guidelines for the current treatment recommend that exercise programs for weight loss in obesity prioritize continuous aerobic exercise with a moderate intensity and complement this approach, whenever possible, with resistance training [21]. Although these recommendations are for people who are in nonsurgical treatment for obesity, aerobic exercise was the mostly used intervention modality in the included studies. Three studies combined aerobic and resistance training [11,15,16], one study used only resistance training [18] and the other one used only aerobic exercise [17]. On the other hand, the intensity was heterogenous among the included studies. Regarding the intensity of aerobic exercise, two studies prescribed intensities ranging from 55% to 75/80% of the reserve heart rate [11,15], one study prescribed the exercise intensity ranging from 2 to 4 on the Borg CR10 scale [17] and one did not present details on the exercise intensity [16]. For resistance training, one study prescribed exercise at 50% of one maximal repetition [18], two studies prescribed the resistance intensity according to sex [11,15] and one study did not report details on the intensity prescription [16]. The study that found the greatest improvement on the BMI prior to BS was Marcon et al. (2017) [17], while the greatest improvement in the quality of life was that reported by Arman et al. (2021) [18]. In addition, both studies [17,18] reported significant improvements on the functional capacity. Therefore, considering the protocols are mostly heterogenous among the included studies, it is not possible to conclude what type of training and intensity are the most suitable and effective for BS candidates. Future RCT studies should address this subject to better guide clinicians during prehabilitation.

Regular physical exercise has several effects on metabolism [22]. It is documented that, on obese people, aerobic training at a moderate intensity improves many comorbidity markers associated with it, such as glucose metabolic alteration, dyslipidemia and hypertension, as well as those indicating cardiovascular disease risk factors (e.g., systematic inflammation, oxidative stress and diabetes) [22,23]. Moreover, it also increases free fatty acids oxidation and reduces the total fat and visceral fat [24]. At a muscular level, the increase of the mitochondrial content as an effect from aerobic training at a moderate intensity has a series of metabolic effects (e.g., a higher rate of fatty acid oxidation, a higher breakdown of carbohydrates and a better glucose uptake in the cells, among others), contributing to improving their performance during exercise and, therefore, functional capacity [25]. Those factors could explain the results found in this systematic review.

Regarding the quality of life, the current results corroborated the findings of Carraça et al. (2021) [26]. The authors conducted a systematic review and meta-analysis on the effects of exercise on the quality of life and other psychosocial variables in participants overweight and obese. The results showed that exercise has a positive effect on the quality of life. Regular physical exercise helps in treating depression and anxiety; reduces stress levels, improves sleep quality and has positive effects on the performance of daily life activities, which translates to a better quality of life for people with obesity [26].

5. Study Limitations

Although this systematic review and meta-analysis has methodological strengths, some limitations must be mentioned. First, the search for information was performed by only one researcher (AH); however, the terms and search strings were defined by the researchers in collaboration with a university-based librarian with experience in systematic reviews. Second, the fact that there are a limited number of studies that evaluate preoperative interventions can influence the meta-analysis results. Consequently, the results are not conclusive yet. Finally, these results show evidence of the need for studies that include a greater number of participants and other relevant variables such as postoperative complications, days of hospital stay, the need for rehospitalization within 30 days after the surgery, pain tolerance, etc.

6. Conclusions

Prehabilitation has positive effects on the body composition, functional capacity and quality of life in patients who are candidates for bariatric surgery. Apparently, supervised aerobic training at a frequency of two times a week and a duration of 45–60 min per session for 12 weeks is the most preferred protocol used for this population. However, there is still a lack of research studying the effects of exercise as a prehabilitation on surgical outcomes.

Author Contributions: Conceptualization: A.H.-S., A.R.Z., G.A.-F.; methodology development: A.H.-S., G.W., G.A.-F.; Risk of Bias Assessment: A.H.-S., G.A.-F., G.W.; Evaluation of the Quality of Scientific Evidence: A.H.-S., A.R.Z.; Meta-analysis: A.H.-S., A.R.Z.; Data interpretation: A.H.-S., G.A.-F., G.W., N.N.J., A.R.Z.; Writing—original draft preparation: A.H.-S., G.A.-F., G.W., N.N.J., A.R.Z.; Writing—review and editing: A.H.-S., G.A.-F., G.W., N.N.J., A.R.Z. All authors have read and agreed to the published version of the manuscript.

Funding: This research received no external funding.

Institutional Review Board Statement: Not applicable.

Informed Consent Statement: Not applicable.

Data Availability Statement: All data are available upon request to the corresponding author.

Conflicts of Interest: The authors declare no conflict of interest.

Abbreviations

BS	Bariatric surgery.
ERAS	Enhanced recovery after surgery.
6MWT	Six-minute walking test.
VO_2 max	Maximal oxygen uptake.
GRADE	Grading of recommendations assessment, development, and evaluation.
SMD	Standard mean differences.
CORE	Core muscles of the body.
BMI	Body mass index.
OSQOL	Obesity Specific Quality of life.
HRR	Heart rate reserve.
WRQOL	Weight-Related Quality of Life.
SF 36	Health-related quality of life questionnaire.
FM%	Fat mass in percent.
FFM Kg	Fat free mass in kilograms.
CI	Confidence interval.
RCTs	Randomized control trials

References

1. Schroeder, R.; Garrison, J.M., Jr.; Johnson, M.S. Treatment of adult obesity with bariatric surgery. *Am. Fam. Physician* **2011**, *84*, 805–814.
2. Wharton, S.; Lau, D.C.; Vallis, M.; Sharma, A.M.; Biertho, L.; Campbell-Scherer, D.; Adamo, K.; Alberga, A.; Bell, R.; Boulé, N.; et al. Obesity in adults: A clinical practice guideline. *CMAJ* **2020**, *192*, E875–E891. [CrossRef]

3. O'Brien, P.E.; Hindle, A.; Brennan, L.; Skinner, S.; Burton, P.; Smith, A.; Crosthwaite, G.; Brown, W. Long-Term Outcomes After Bariatric Surgery: A Systematic Review and Meta-analysis of Weight Loss at 10 or More Years for All Bariatric Procedures and a Single-Centre Review of 20-Year Outcomes After Adjustable Gastric Banding. *Obes. Surg.* **2019**, *29*, 3–14. [CrossRef]
4. Segelman, J.; Nygren, J. Evidence or eminence in abdominal surgery: Recent improvements in perioperative care. *World J. Gastroenterol.* **2014**, *20*, 16615–16619. [CrossRef]
5. Senturk, J.C.; Kristo, G.; Gold, J.; Bleday, R.; Whang, E. The Development of Enhanced Recovery After Surgery Across Surgical Specialties. *J. Laparoendosc. Adv. Surg. Tech.* **2017**, *27*, 863–870. [CrossRef]
6. Dang, J.T.; Szeto, V.G.; Elnahas, A.; Ellsmere, J.; Okrainec, A.; Neville, A.; Malik, S.; Yorke, E.; Hong, D.; Biertho, L.; et al. Canadian consensus statement: Enhanced recovery after surgery in bariatric surgery. *Surg. Endosc.* **2020**, *34*, 1366–1375. [CrossRef]
7. Stenberg, E.; Falcão, L.F.D.R.; O'Kane, M.; Liem, R.; Pournaras, D.J.; Salminen, P.; Urman, R.D.; Wadhwa, A.; Gustafsson, U.O.; Thorell, A. Guidelines for Perioperative Care in Bariatric Surgery: Enhanced Recovery After Surgery (ERAS) Society Recommendations: A 2021 Update. *World J. Surg.* **2022**, *46*, 729–751. [CrossRef]
8. Delgado Floody, P.; Jerez Mayorga, D.; Caamaño Navarrete, F.; Osorio Poblete, A.; Thuillier Lepeley, N.; Alarcón Hormazábal, M. Doce semanas de ejercicio físico intervalado con sobrecarga mejora las variables antropométricas de obesos mórbidos y obesos con comorbilidades postulantes a cirugía bariátrica. *Nutr. Hosp.* **2015**, *32*, 2007–2011.
9. Carbone, S.; Del Buono, M.G.; Ozemek, C.; Lavie, C.J. Obesity, risk of diabetes and role of physical activity, exercise training and cardiorespiratory fitness. *Prog. Cardiovasc. Dis.* **2019**, *62*, 327–333. [CrossRef]
10. Marc-Hernández, A.; Ruiz-Tovar, J.; Aracil, A.; Guillén, S.; Moya-Ramón, M. Impact of Exercise on Body Composition and Cardiometabolic Risk Factors in Patients Awaiting Bariatric Surgery. *Obes. Surg.* **2019**, *29*, 3891–3900. [CrossRef] [PubMed]
11. Baillot, A.; Mampuya, W.M.; Dionne, I.J.; Comeau, E.; Méziat-Burdin, A.; Langlois, M.-F. Impacts of Supervised Exercise Training in Addition to Interdisciplinary Lifestyle Management in Subjects Awaiting Bariatric Surgery: A Randomized Controlled Study. *Obes. Surg.* **2016**, *26*, 2602–2610. [CrossRef]
12. Lloréns, J.; Rovira, L.; Ballester, M.; Moreno, J.; Hernández-Laforet, J.; Santonja, F.-J.; Cassinello, N.; Ortega, J. Preoperative Inspiratory Muscular Training to Prevent Postoperative Hypoxemia in Morbidly Obese Patients Undergoing Laparoscopic Bariatric Surgery. A Randomized Clinical Trial. *Obes. Surg.* **2015**, *25*, 1003–1009. [CrossRef] [PubMed]
13. Whittle, J.; Wischmeyer, P.E.; Grocott, M.P.W.; Miller, T.E. Surgical Prehabilitation: Nutrition and Exercise. *Anesthesiol. Clin.* **2018**, *36*, 567–580. [CrossRef]
14. Andrea Herrera, A.Z.; Nardo, N. Prehabilitation Effects on Body Composition, Functional Capacity, Quality of Life and Surgical Outcomes in Bariatric Surgery Candidates. PROSPERO, 2021, CRD42021261474. Available online: https://www.crd.york.ac.uk/prospero/display_record.php?ID=CRD42021261474 (accessed on 25 October 2021).
15. Baillot, A.; Vallée, C.-A.; Mampuya, W.M.; Dionne, I.J.; Comeau, E.; Méziat-Burdin, A.; Langlois, M.-F. Effects of a Pre-surgery Supervised Exercise Training 1 Year After Bariatric Surgery: A Randomized Controlled Study. *Obes. Surg.* **2018**, *28*, 955–962. [CrossRef] [PubMed]
16. Funderburk, J.; Callis, S. Aquatic intervention effect on quality of life prior to obesity surgery: A pilot study. *Annu. Recreat.* **2010**, *18*, 66–78.
17. Marcon, E.R.; Baglioni, S.; Bittencourt, L.; Lopes, C.L.N.; Neumann, C.R.; Trindade, M.R.M. What Is the Best Treatment before Bariatric Surgery? Exercise, Exercise and Group Therapy, or Conventional Waiting: A Randomized Controlled Trial. *Obes. Surg.* **2017**, *27*, 763–773. [CrossRef] [PubMed]
18. Arman, N.; Tokgoz, G.; Seyit, H.; Karabulut, M. The effects of core stabilization exercise program in obese people awaiting bariatric surgery: A randomized controlled study. Complement. *Ther. Clin. Pract.* **2021**, *43*, 101342. [CrossRef]
19. Bellicha, A.; van Baak, M.A.; Battista, F.; Beaulieu, K.; Blundell, J.E.; Busetto, L.; Carraça, E.V.; Dicker, D.; Encantado, J.; Ermolao, A.; et al. Effect of exercise training before and after bariatric surgery: A systematic review and meta-analysis. *Obes. Rev.* **2021**, *22* (Suppl. 4), e13296. [CrossRef]
20. Pouwels, S.; Wit, M.; Teijink, J.A.; Nienhuijs, S.W. Aspects of Exercise before or after Bariatric Surgery: A Systematic Review. *Obes. Facts* **2015**, *8*, 132–146. [CrossRef]
21. O'Donoghue, G.; Blake, C.; Cunningham, C.; Lennon, O.; Perrotta, C. What exercise prescription is optimal to improve body composition and cardiorespiratory fitness in adults living with obesity? A network meta-analysis. *Obes. Rev.* **2021**, *22*, e13137. [CrossRef]
22. Golbidi, S.; Mesdaghinia, A.; Laher, I. Exercise in the metabolic syndrome. *Oxid. Med. Cell. Longev.* **2012**, *2012*, 349710. [CrossRef] [PubMed]
23. Morrison, M.C.; Kleemann, R. Role of Macrophage Migration Inhibitory Factor in Obesity, Insulin Resistance, Type 2 Diabetes, and Associated Hepatic Co-Morbidities: A Comprehensive Review of Human and Rodent Studies. *Front. Immunol.* **2015**, *6*, 308. [CrossRef] [PubMed]
24. Liñán, Á.C.; Sánchez-Oliver, A.J.; Reina, I.G.; Carmona, W.S.; González-Jurado, J.A. Erddef. Ejercicio físico, obesidad e inflamación. *EmásF Rev. Digit. Educ. Física* **2016**, *41*, 65–82.

25. Lundby, C.; Jacobs, R.A. Adaptations of skeletal muscle mitochondria to exercise training. *Exp. Physiol.* **2016**, *101*, 17–22. [CrossRef]
26. Carraça, E.V.; Encantado, J.; Battista, F.; Beaulieu, K.; Blundell, J.E.; Busetto, L.; van Baak, M.; Dicker, D.; Ermolao, A.; Farpour-Lambert, N.; et al. Effect of exercise training on psychological outcomes in adults with overweight or obesity: A systematic review and meta-analysis. *Obes. Rev.* **2021**, *22* (Suppl. 4), e13261. [CrossRef]

Journal of
Clinical Medicine

MDPI

Systematic Review

Effect of Bariatric Surgery on Intima Media Thickness: A Systematic Review and Meta-Analysis

Tannaz Jamialahmadi [1,2], Željko Reiner [3], Mona Alidadi [1], Wael Almahmeed [4], Prashant Kesharwani [5], Khalid Al-Rasadi [6], Ali H. Eid [7], Manfredi Rizzo [8] and Amirhossein Sahebkar [1,9,10,*]

1 Applied Biomedical Research Center, Pharmaceutical Technology Institute, Mashhad University of Medical Sciences, Mashhad 9177948564, Iran
2 Department of Nutrition, Faculty of Medicine, Mashhad University of Medical Sciences, Mashhad 9177918564, Iran
3 Department of Internal Medicine, University Hospital Center Zagreb, 10000 Zagreb, Croatia
4 Heart and Vascular Institute, Cleveland Clinic Abu Dhabi, Abu Dhabi P.O. Box 124140, United Arab Emirates
5 Department of Pharmaceutics, School of Pharmaceutical Education and Research, Jamia Hamdard, New Delhi 110062, India
6 Medical Research Centre, Sultan Qaboos University, Muscat P.O. Box 373, Oman
7 Department of Basic Medical Sciences, QU Health, Qatar University, Doha P.O. Box 2713, Qatar
8 Department of Health Promotion, Mother and Child Care, Internal Medicine and Medical Specialties, School of Medicine, University of Palermo, 90133 Palermo, Italy
9 Biotechnology Research Center, Pharmaceutical Technology Institute, Mashhad University of Medical Sciences, Mashhad 9177948954, Iran
10 Department of Biotechnology, School of Pharmacy, Mashhad University of Medical Sciences, Mashhad 9177948954, Iran
* Correspondence: sahebkara@mums.ac.ir or amir_saheb2000@yahoo.com

Citation: Jamialahmadi, T.; Reiner, Ž.; Alidadi, M.; Almahmeed, W.; Kesharwani, P.; Al-Rasadi, K.; Eid, A.H.; Rizzo, M.; Sahebkar, A. Effect of Bariatric Surgery on Intima Media Thickness: A Systematic Review and Meta-Analysis. *J. Clin. Med.* **2022**, *11*, 6056. https://doi.org/10.3390/jcm11206056

Academic Editor: David Benaiges Boix

Received: 22 August 2022
Accepted: 10 October 2022
Published: 13 October 2022

Abstract: Background: Obesity, and in particular extreme obesity, as a global health problem is an important risk factor for many diseases, including atherosclerotic cardiovascular disease (ACVD). Bariatric surgery might stop or slow atherogenesis by decreasing excessive weight in the early stages of atherogenesis, by suppressing low-grade systemic inflammation as well as by inhibiting oxidative stress and endothelial dysfunction. The aim of this meta-analysis was to provide an answer to whether bariatric surgery has a significant effect on intima-media thickness (IMT) which is a surrogate marker of early atherosclerosis and has a good correlation with atherosclerotic coronary heart disease. Methods: A systematic literature search in PubMed, Scopus, Embase, and Web of Science as well as grey literature was performed from inception to 1 July 2022. The meta-analysis was performed using Comprehensive Meta-Analysis (CMA) V3 software. Overall, the estimate of effect size was measured by a random effects meta-analysis. To account for the heterogeneity of studies regarding study design, characteristics of the populations, and treatment duration, a random-effects model (using the DerSimonian–Laird method) and the generic inverse variance weighting approach were used. To assess the existence of publication bias in the meta-analysis, the funnel plot, Begg's rank correlation, and Egger's weighted regression tests were used. Results: The meta-analysis of 30 trials, including 1488 subjects, demonstrated a significant decrease in IMT after bariatric surgery. The reduction in IMT was also robust in the leave-one-out sensitivity analysis. It must be stressed that the results of the random-effects meta-regression did not suggest any relationship between the changes in IMT and delta body mass index (BMI) or duration of follow-up after the bariatric surgery. However, the subgroup analyses showed a better IMT reduction after laparoscopic sleeve gastrectomy (LSG) when compared to Roux-en-Y gastric bypass (RYGB). Within a year, the IMT follow-up values showed a further improvement. Conclusions: Bariatric surgery significantly reduced IMT. Significant associations were found between the surgery type and IMT changes, as well as a significant effect of follow-up duration on the changes of IMT after bariatric surgery.

Keywords: obesity; bariatric surgery; intima-media thickness; atherosclerosis; meta-analysis; coronary heart disease

1. Introduction

Almost all countries are witnessing a pandemic of overweight and obesity with a devastating trend, which is best illustrated by the fact that obesity has nearly tripled since 1975. In 2016, more than 1.9 billion adults aged 18 years and older were overweight and 3% of the world's population, or more than 650 million people, were obese with an increasing prevalence [1]. In most developed countries, the rates of obesity are much higher so that, for example, in the USA more than 40% of adults are obese [2]. It is well known that obesity as a global health issue is also an important risk factor for many diseases, including atherosclerotic cardiovascular disease (ACVD), and it is associated with an increased ACVD morbidity and mortality [3]. This is primarily explained by a systemic low-grade inflammatory state in obesity which is not only a risk for ACVD but also for metabolic syndrome (MetSy), type 2 diabetes mellitus (T2DM), nonalcoholic fatty liver disease (NAFLD), nonalcoholic steatohepatitis (NASH), chronic kidney disease, different types of cancers, and other inflammatory diseases, including pancreatitis, psoriasis, atopic dermatitis, and autoimmune arthritis [4–8]. Obesity is also associated with oxidative stress which may promote the development of vascular wall lesions causing endothelial dysfunction; thus, predisposing the arterial wall to morphological and functional damages leading to atherogenesis.

No matter how it is achieved, weight reduction decreases the risk of ACVD, cardiovascular events, as well as cardiovascular and total mortality. Bariatric surgery is a surgical treatment, which is used primarily for patients who are severely obese to decrease their excessive weight. The types of bariatric surgery are sleeve gastrectomy (SG), laparoscopic adjustable gastric band (LAGB), Roux-en-Y gastric bypass (RYGB), biliopancreatic diversion/duodenal switch (BPD/DS), and one anastomosis gastric bypass/mini gastric bypass (OAGB/MGB) [9]. There are data suggesting the positive impact of bariatric surgery on several cardiometabolic indicators [10–15]. There have been reports indicating that bariatric surgery might prevent or slow down atherogenesis in the early stages by breaking the vicious circle between inflammation and endothelial dysfunction [16].

Measuring intima-media thickness (IMT), particularly carotid IMT (CIMT), by ultrasonography is considered to be a surrogate marker of early atherosclerotic changes in the arteries. This could help to improve the prediction of cardiovascular events in different arterial territories because of the positive correlation between increased IMT and atherosclerotic changes in coronary arteries, i.e., with coronary heart disease (CHD) [17–20]. Therefore, IMT is used in predicting CHD and improving the cardiovascular risk prediction models. Although some studies have suggested that bariatric surgery has a beneficial effect and might decrease IMT, other studies could not find any change in IMT in obese patients after bariatric surgery.

Following bariatric surgery, several cardiovascular-related risk factors can be improved, including insulin resistance, type 2 diabetes, hypertension, and hyperlipidemia; however, it is worth mentioning that these improvements are not the only effect of weight loss [21,22]. Since obesity provokes an inflammation-prone environment, bariatric surgery seems to decrease cytokines involved in this process, especially CRP and IL-6, as shown in a recent meta-analysis [23–25].

Since the data concerning the effects of bariatric surgery on IMT are conflicting, the aim of this systematic review and meta-analysis is to provide a clear answer as to whether bariatric surgery can decrease IMT or not.

2. Methods

2.1. Search Strategy

The 2009 preferred reporting items for systematic reviews and meta-analysis (PRISMA) guidelines were used to prepare this systematic review and meta-analysis [26]. PubMed, Scopus, Embase, Web of Science, as well as grey literature (CareSearch, Google, and the Grey Literature Report), and all reference lists of retrieved articles were searched from inception to 1 July 2022 using the following keywords in titles and abstracts: ("intima media thickness" OR "intima-media thickness" OR "carotid intima media thickness" OR "carotid intima media" OR "artery intima media thickness" OR "intima media thickness measurement" OR "intima media thickness cardiovascular" OR "carotid intima media thickness measurement" OR "intima-media thickness measurements" OR "carotid intima media thickness cardiovascular" OR "intima-media thickness" OR CIMT OR IMT OR "carotid intima-media thickness" OR "carotid intima media" OR "Carotid atherosclerosis" OR "intima-media") AND ("bariatric surgery" OR gastroplast* OR "gastric bypass" OR "Roux-en-Y" OR "gastric band" OR "biliopancreatic diversion" OR gastrectom* OR "duodenal switch" OR "weight loss surgery" OR "gastrointestinal diversion" OR gastroenterostom* OR "jejunoileal bypass" OR "obesity surgery" OR "weight-loss surgery" OR "bariatric procedure" OR "sleeve surgery" OR "metabolic surgery").

2.2. Study Selection

All studies investigating the effects of bariatric surgery on carotid intima media thickness (CIMT) were included, based upon our pre-determined inclusion criteria. Case studies, non-English studies, reviews, and animal studies were not considered. A study had to provide documented CIMT data before surgery and after a post-operative observation period to be included in this meta-analysis. This systematic review and meta-analysis was not registered in any registry.

2.3. Data Extraction

All titles and abstracts were separately screened by two authors (TJ and MA). When there was a disagreement concerning the eligibility of a study, the paper was examined collaboratively, and a decision was reached. Study characteristics (the name of the primary author, the year of publication, study design, type of surgery, length of follow-up, health status of the participants, major clinical and demographic variables, values of IMT, and sample size) were extracted from each study.

2.4. Quality Assessment

The Newcastle–Ottawa Scale (NOS) was used to estimate the quality of the studies included in this meta-analysis [27,28]. This scale considers three features of each qualified study: (1) study patient selection (4 elements); (2) study population comparability (one item); and (3) exposure determination (3 items) in case-control studies or result of interest in cohort studies.

2.5. Quantitative Data Synthesis

The meta-analysis was performed using Comprehensive Meta-Analysis (CMA) V3 software (Biostat Inc., Englewood, NJ, USA) [29]. The weighted mean difference (WMD) with relevant CIs was determined for continuous outcomes. From each group, sample sizes, means, and standard deviations were obtained for each relevant outcome to calculate WMD. Overall, the estimate of effect size was measured by a random effects meta-analysis. To account for the heterogeneity of studies with regard to study design, characteristics of the populations, and treatment duration, the random-effects model (using the DerSimonian–Laird method) and the generic inverse variance weighting approach were used [26]. Sensitivity analysis using the leave-one-out approach (i.e., deleting one study each time and repeating the analysis) was applied to analyze the effect of each study on the overall effect size [30].

2.6. Meta-Regression

To investigate the association between BMI change and follow-up duration after surgery with the estimated effect size, these parameters were included into a random-effect meta-regression model.

2.7. Subgroup Analysis

A subgroup analysis was completed to describe heterogeneity, and to further characterize outcomes for the type of surgery and follow-up period.

2.8. Publication Bias

The funnel plot, Egger's weighted regression, as well as Begg's rank correlation tests were used to examine the presence of publication bias in the meta-analysis. The "trim and fill" approach was used to insert potentially missing studies when there were indications of funnel plot asymmetry. In the case of a significant result, the number of potentially missing studies needed to make the *p*-value non-significant was determined using the "fail-safe N" approach as another evidence of publication bias [31].

3. Results

Among 356 published studies identified by a systematic databases search, 173 were directly related to the topic of this study. In total, 143 studies were excluded after careful evaluation (43 studies were reviews, 38 studies were excluded because they did not match the inclusion criteria, 34 studies did not report sufficient data, and 8 were non-English papers). Therefore, 30 studies which evaluated IMT after bariatric surgery were included (Table 1). Figure 1 shows the process of study selection.

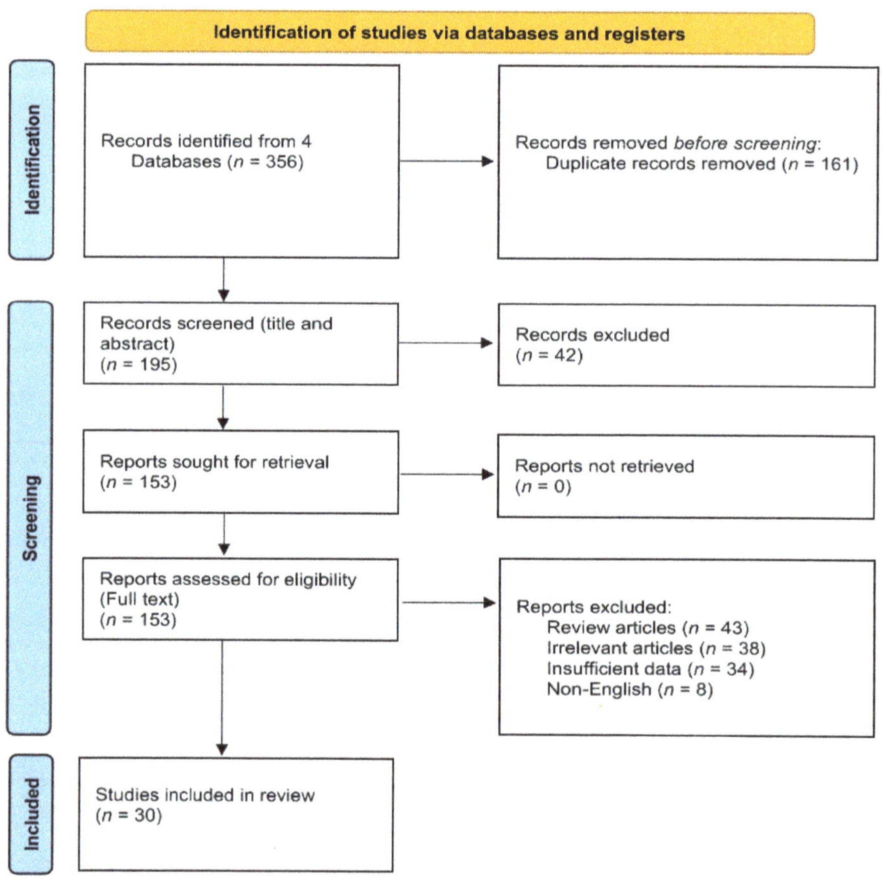

Figure 1. Flowchart of the included studie.

Table 1. Characteristics of studies measuring IMT.

Study, Year	Study Design	Follow-up	Treatment	Control	Clinical Outcome C-IMT	Patients	No. of Patients
Yavuz et al., 2021 [32]	Observational study	6 months 12 months	LSG or RYGB	-	Significant reduction was observed after 6 months	Patients with Class 3 obesity mean age of 42.3 ± 10.1 years.	41
Salman et al., 2021 [33]	Prospective study	6 months 12 months	LSG	-	Significant reduction was observed after 12 months	Patients with obesity and high cardiovascular risk M/F (63/57) mean age of 43.7 ± 8.5 years.	120
Melchor-López et al., 2021 [34]	Case–control study	9 months	LSG or RYGB	-	Significant reduction was observed No change	Patients with morbid obesity ≥ 10% reduction in CIMT Patients with morbid obesity <10% reduction in CIMT 75% F mean age 44.5 years.	28 12
Kaul et al., 2021 [35]	Prospective study	6 months 12 months	LSG or RYGB or OAGB	-	Significant reduction was observed after 6 months	Patients with obesity 70% F mean age of 40.8 ± 10.7 years.	40
Cekici et al., 2021 [36]	Prospective study	6 months	LSG	-	Significant reduction was observed	Patients with severe obesity 35F/12M mean age of 38 ± 10.48 years.	47
Ministrini et al., 2020 [37]	Single arm, open labeled, prospective pilot study	10–12 months	LSG	-	Significant reduction was observed	Patients with severe obesity 77.2% F, average age of 44.0 ± 10.1 years.	54
Kaya and Elkan, 2020 [38]	Prospective cohort study	6 months	LSG	-	Significant reduction was observed	Patients with morbid obesity 67.6% M mean age of 37.6 ± 11.2 years.	71
Gómez-Martin et al., 2020 [39]	Prospective study	12 months	LSG RYGB	diet and lifestyle modification	Significant reduction was observed in both groups compared with baseline and control group	Women with severe obesity mean age of 48 ± 9 years.	20 20
Elitok et al., 2020 [40]	Observational study	3 months 6 months 9 months 12 months	RYGB	-	Significant reduction was observed after 9 months	Patients with morbid obesity 13 F Mean age of 40.4 ± 5.6 years.	23
Domenech-Ximenos et al., 2020 [41]	Prospective observational study	3 years	RYGB	1. nonsurgical approaches 2. without any intervention (healthy controls)	Significant reduction was observed compared with nonsurgical approaches	Patients with class 3 obesity 17 F 46 (38–54) age	21
Cobeta et al., 2020 [42]	Observational study	6 months	LSG RYGB	diet and lifestyle modification	Significant reduction was observed in both groups compared with baseline and control group	Men with severe obesity and high cardiovascular risk 48 ± 8 age	20 20
Carmona-Maurici et al., 2020 [16]	Observational study	6 months 12 months	RYGB or LSG	-	No change	Patients with obesity and plaque Patients with obesity without plaque F (56%) mean age of 51.8 ± 1.8 years.	32 34

Table 1. *Cont.*

Study, Year	Study Design	Follow-up	Treatment	Control	Clinical Outcome C-IMT	Patients	No. of Patients
Borzi et al., 2020 [43]	Observational study	6–24 months (mean:16 ± 8)	Adjustable GB or GBP or BPD	Medical nutrition treatment	No change	Patients with obesity F/M 13/4 Mean age of 39.8 ± 10.4 years.	17
Yang et al., 2019 [44]	Retrospective study	12 months	RYGB or LSG	-	Significant reduction was observed	Patients with obesity and T2D Patients with obesity without T2D	28 62
Solini et al., 2019 [45]	Prospective observational study	12 months	RYGB	-	Significant reduction was observed	Nondiabetic subjects with severe obesity F/M 19/6 Mean age of 46.7 ± 12.9 years.	25
Gluszewska et al., 2019 [46]	Prospective cohort study	10 days 6 months	RYGB or LSG	-	Significant reduction was observed after 6 months	Patients with extreme obesity 45% M Mean age of 45.6 (±10.9) years.	71
Rius et al., 2019 [47]	Case-control study	12 months	RYGB or LSG	-	No change	Patients with morbid obesity 77.5% F Mean age of 45.0 ± 11.7 years.	33
Jonker et al., 2018 [48]	Prospective study	6 months 12 months	LSG or RYGB	-	Significant reduction was observed after 12 months	Women with obesity Men with obesity F 83.1% Mean age of 42.5 (19.4–62.1) years.	111 35
Altin et al., 2018 [49]	Prospective study	6 months	LSG	-	Significant reduction was observed	Patients with severe obesity (79F/26M) Mean age of 43.61 12.42 years.	105
Tromba et al., 2017 [50]	Observational study	3 months 6 months	LSG	-	Significant reduction was observed after 6 months	Patients with obesity 27 F Mean age of 38.7 ± 9 years	45
Chen et al., 2017 [51]	Retrospective study	12 months	RYGB	-	Significant reduction was observed	Patients with obesity and T2D F/M 17/16 Mean age of 47.7 ± 11.6 years	33
Marchesi et al., 2017 [52]	Prospective study	1 month 12 months	RYGB	-	Significant reduction was observed after 12 months	Women with morbid obesity Mean age of 42.68	22
Yorulmaz et al., 2016 [53]	Prospective study	4–5 months (average: 4.6 months)	LSG	-	Significant reduction was observed	Patients with minimum BMI of 40, who did not have any known chronic diseases 14F/2M, Average age of 39.12 ± 10.63 years.	16
Solmaz et al., 2016 [54]	Prospective study	3 months 6 months	LSG LGP	-	Significant reduction was observed after 3 months	Patients with obesity F/M 31/17 42.96 ± 7.87 (LSG) 38.3 ± 9.88 (LGP)	25 23
Graziani et al., 2014 [55]	Observational study	252 ± 108 days	bariatric surgery	-	No change	Patients with obesity Mean age of 39.8 ± 8.0	48

Table 1. *Cont.*

Study, Year	Study Design	Follow-up	Treatment	Control	Clinical Outcome C-IMT	Patients	No. of Patients
Tschoner et al., 2013 [56]	Prospective study	5 years	SAGB or GBP	-	Significant reduction was observed	Patients with morbid obesity 40F/12M Mean age of 35.3 years.	52
Bravo et al., 2013 [57]	Prospective study	354 ± 92.1 days	LSG or RYGB	-	Significant reduction was observed	Patients with obesity Mean age of 43.6 ± 8.1 years.	27
Lundby-Christensen et al., 2012 [58]	Observational prospective study	6 months 12 months	RYGB	-	Significant reduction was observed 12 months after RYGB in patients with T2D/IGT	Patients with obesity and normal glucose tolerance 31.3% M Mean age of 44.8 ± 10.4 Patients with obesity and type 2 diabetes or impaired glucose tolerance (T2D/IGT) 33.3% M Mean age of 47.4 ± 6.7	16 18
Geloneze et al., 2012 [59]	Observational study	1 month 6 months 12 months	RYGB	-	Significant reduction was observed	Patients with obesity without Gly482Ser polymorphism 24F/2M Mean age of 37.2 ± 10.7 Patients with obesity and Gly482Ser polymorphism of the ppargc1a gene 23F/6M Mean age of 37.2 ± 9.4	26 29
Sarmento et al., 2009 [60]	Observational study	3 months 6 months 12 months	RYGB	-	Significant reduction was observed after 6 months	Women with morbid obesity Mean age of 44.1 ± 9.8 years.	18

RYGB, Roux-en-Y Gastric Bypass; LSG, Laparoscopic Sleeve Gastrectomy; OAGB, One Anastomosis Gastric Bypass; GB, gastric banding; GBP, Gastric bypass; BPD, Biliopancreatic diversion; LGP, Laparoscopic Gastric Plication; SAGB, Single-anastomosis gastric bypass.

3.1. *Quality Assessment of the Included Studies*

In cohort studies, although most of the selected studies [16,32,33,35–46,48–60] showed representativeness of the cases, the majority of them were distinguished by a lack of nonexposed group definition information. Since most of the studies did not include a control group, they were not assessed for comparability. In case-control studies [34,47], the included studies met the selection and exposure criteria. Quality assessment of the selected studies is presented in Tables 2 and 3.

3.2. *Effect of Bariatric Surgery on IMT*

The meta-analysis of 30 trials, including 1488 subjects, demonstrated a significant decrease in IMT after bariatric surgery (WMD: −0.081, 95% CI: −0.101, −0.061, $p < 0.001$) (Figure 2A). The reduction in IMT was robust in the leave-one-out sensitivity analysis (Figure 2B). In other words, the iterative removal of each included trial from the meta-analysis did not cause a significant change in the pooled estimate of effect size.

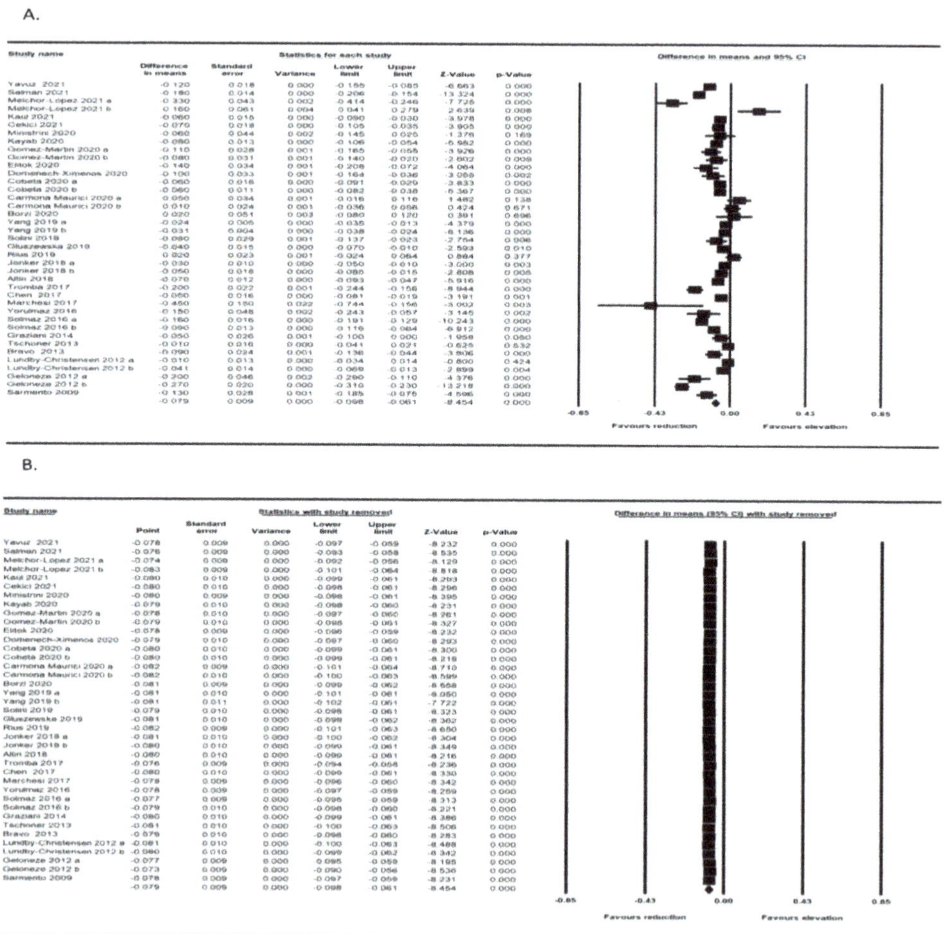

Figure 2. (**A**) Forest plot displaying standardized mean difference and 95% confidence intervals showing the consequence of bariatric surgery on IMT [16,32–60]; (**B**) Leave-one-out sensitivity analyses indicating the effect of bariatric surgery on IMT [16,32–60].

Table 2. Quality of bias assessment of the included publication in accordance with the Newcastle–Ottawa scale (cohort studies).

Study	Selection				Comparability	Outcome		
	Representativeness of the Exposed Cohort	Selection of the Nonexposed Cohort	Ascertainment of Exposure	Demonstration that Outcome of Interest Was not Present at the Beginning of the Study	Comparability of Cohorts on the Basis of the Design or Analysis	Assessment of Outcome	Follow-up Was Not Long Enough for Outcomes to Occur	Adequacy of Follow-up of Cohorts
Yavuz et al., 2021 [32]	*	-	*	*	-	*	*	-
Salman et al., 2021 [33]	*	-	*	*	-	*	*	*
Kaul et al., 2021 [35]	*	-	*	*	-	*	*	*
Cekici et al., 2021 [36]	*	-	*	*	-	*	*	*
Ministrini et al., 2020 [37]	*	-	*	*	-	*	*	*
Kaya et al., 2020 [38]	*	-	*	*	-	*	*	*
Gómez-Martin et al., 2020 [39]	*	*	*	*	*	*	*	*
Elitok et al., 2020 [40]	*	-	*	*	-	*	*	*
Domenech-Ximenos et al., 2020 [41]	*	*	*	*	*	*	*	*
Cobeta et al., 2020 [42]	*	*	*	*	*	*	*	*
Carmona-Maurici et al., 2020 [16]	*	-	*	*	-	*	*	-
Borzi et al. 2020 [43]	*	-	*	*	-	*	*	*
Yang et al., 2019 [44]	*	-	-	-	-	*	*	-
Solini et al., 2019 [45]	*	-	*	*	-	*	*	*
Gluszewska et al., 2019 [46]	*	-	*	*	-	*	*	*
Jonker et al., 2018 [48]	*	-	*	*	-	*	*	-
Altin et al., 2018 [49]	*	-	*	*	-	*	*	*
Tromba et al., 2017 [50]	*	-	*	*	-	*	*	*
Chen et al., 2017 [51]	-	*	*	-	*	*	*	*
Marchesi et al., 2017 [52]	*	-	*	*	-	*	*	*
Yorulmaz et al., 2016 [53]	*	-	*	*	-	*	*	*
Solmaz et al., 2016 [54]	*	-	*	*	-	*	*	*
Graziani et al., 2014 [55]	*	-	*	*	-	*	*	*
Tschoner et al., 2013 [56]	*	-	*	*	-	*	*	*
Bravo et al., 2013 [57]	*	-	*	*	-	*	*	*
Lundby-Christensen et al., 2012 [58]	*	*	*	*	-	*	*	*
Geloneze et al., 2012 [59]	*	-	*	*	-	*	*	*
Sarmento et al., 2009 [60]	*	-	*	*	-	*	*	*

Table 3. Quality of bias assessment of the included publication in accordance with the Newcastle–Ottawa scale (case-control studies).

Study	Selection				Comparability	Exposure		
	The Definition Was Adequate	Representativeness of the Cases	Selection of Controls	Definition of Controls	Comparability of Cases and Controls on the Basis of the Design or Analysis	Ascertainment of Exposure	The Same Method of Ascertainment for Cases and Controls	Non-Response Rate
Melchor-López et al., 2021 [34]	*	*	*	*	-	*	*	*
Rius et al., 2019 [47]	*	*	*	*	*	*	*	*

3.3. Meta-Regression

The impact of potential confounders on the IMT reducing the effect of bariatric surgery was assessed by random-effects meta-regression. The findings did not suggest any relationship between the changes in IMT and delta body mass index (BMI) (slope: 0.002; 95% CI: −0.005, 0.010; $p = 0.670$) or duration of follow-up (slope: 0.001; 95% CI: −0.0008, 0.0034; $p = 0.227$) (Figure 3A,B).

A.

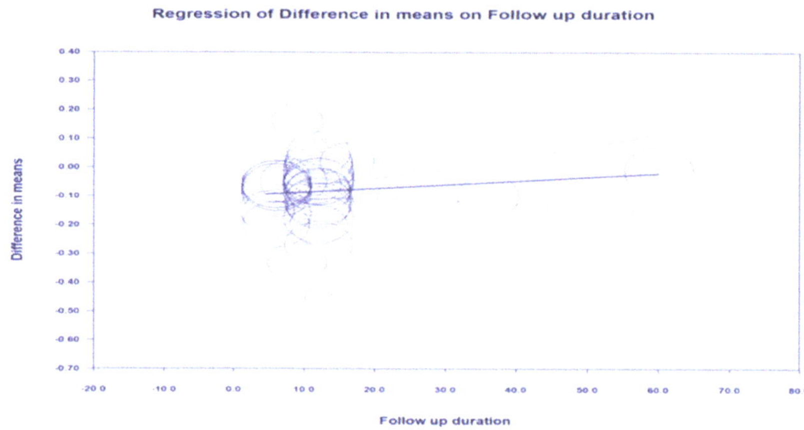

B.

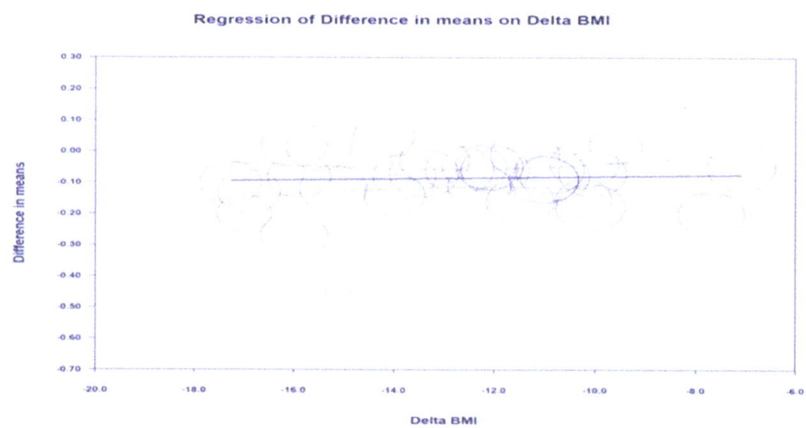

Figure 3. Random-effects meta-regression for evaluating the effect of: (**A**) delta BMI; (**B**) follow-up duration.

3.4. Subgroup Analysis

A subgroup analysis was also performed based on surgery type and treatment duration (<12 months and ≥12 months). The subgroup analyses demonstrated significant associations between surgery types and IMT changes ($p < 0.001$). The improvement of IMT in patients who had laparoscopic sleeve gastrectomy (LSG) surgery was better than in those who had Roux-en-Y gastric bypass (RYGB). Furthermore, a significant effect of follow-up duration on the changes of IMT after bariatric surgery was observed with further improvement in IMT in the follow-up period of less than 12 months (Figure 4A,B).

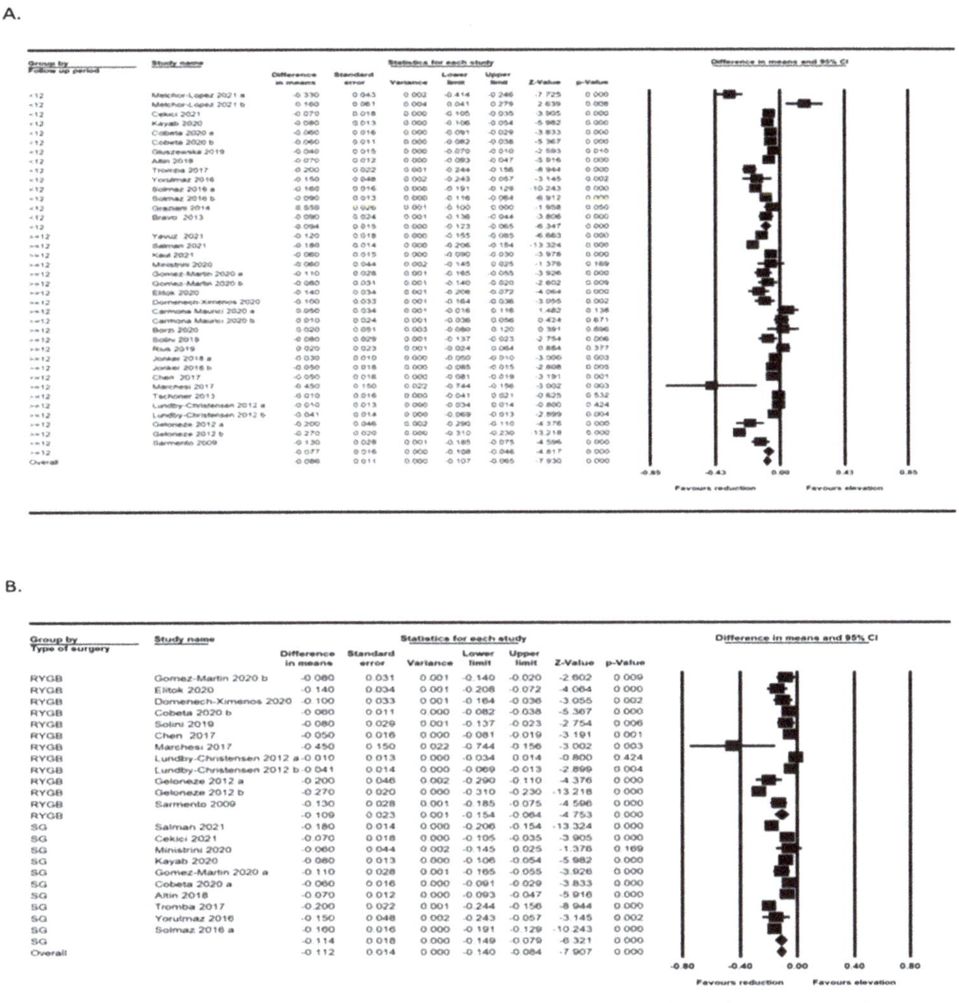

Figure 4. Subgroup analysis based on the follow-up period [32–37,39–43,45–60] (**A**) and type of surgery [33,37–42,45,49,50,52–54,58–60] (**B**).

3.5. Publication Bias

Although the results of Egger's linear regression test (intercept = −2.685, standard error = 0.892; 95% CI = −4.493, −0.877, t = 3.009, df = 37, two-tailed $p = 0.004$) suggested that publication bias existed in the meta-analysis concerning the effect of bariatric surgery on IMT, Begg's rank correlation test (Kendall's Tau with continuity correction = −0.143, z = 1.282, two-tailed p-value = 0.199) did not indicate the presence of publication bias. The trim and fill test showed three "missing" studies in order to adjust publication bias. The "fail-safe N" test showed that 39 missing studies would be needed to reduce the effect size to a non-significant ($p < 0.001$) level (Figure 5).

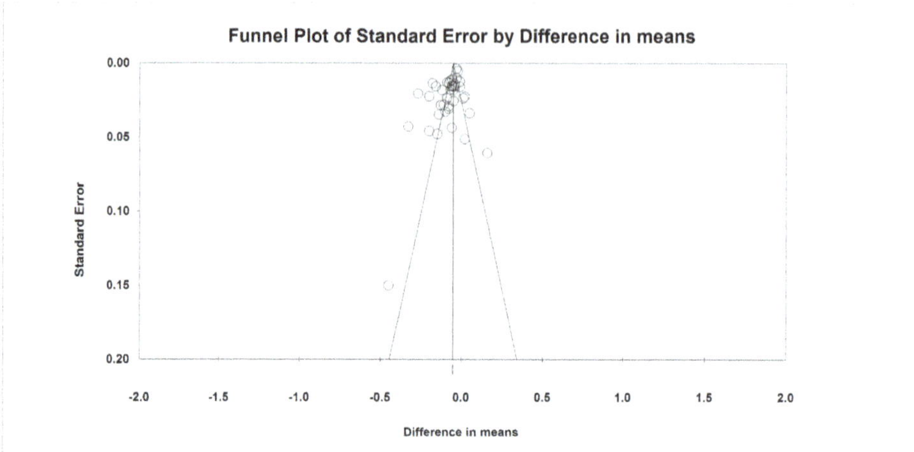

Figure 5. Funnel plot of standard error by difference in means.

4. Discussion

The results of this meta-analysis of 30 trials, including 1488 subjects, showed a significant decrease in IMT after bariatric surgery, and the reduction in IMT was also robust in the leave-one-out sensitivity analysis. It must be stressed that the results of the random-effects meta-regression did not suggest any relationship between the changes in IMT and delta BMI or duration of follow-up after the bariatric surgery. However, the subgroup analyses showed significant associations between the surgery types and IMT changes and a significant effect of follow-up duration on the changes of IMT after bariatric surgery.

One important question which might theoretically influence the results of this meta-analysis is a sex difference in obese subjects concerning IMT. However, this issue was clarified in a recent study showing that IMT was significantly higher in men than in women but this difference disappeared after adjustment for covariables, such as waist circumference, age, HDL-cholesterol, and mean arterial blood pressure [61]. It has also been shown that bariatric surgery caused a significant IMT decrease in subjects with obesity in all age categories; however, the beneficial effects were more pronounced in younger individuals, which is quite understandable and easily explicable [48].

As already mentioned, it has been previously shown that obesity is associated with thicker arterial walls, i.e., increased IMT which seems to be independent of other cardiovascular risk factors [62,63]. It has been also shown that obesity is associated with T2DM and other risk factors for CHD such as dyslipidemia [64]. On the other hand, patients with severe dyslipidemia, such as familial hypercholesterolemia (FH), have increased IMT when compared with controls [65]. This is true not only for adult patients with FH but also for children with FH [66]. However, bariatric surgery in patients who had severe obesity caused a decrease in extremely atherogenic oxidized LDL particles in the blood and this phenomenon seemed to be dependent on BMI changes [10]. An earlier study showed that bariatric surgery caused a decrease in total cholesterol, triglycerides, oxidized LDL particles, and apolipoprotein B, and an increase in HDL-cholesterol and apolipoprotein A concentrations that occurred regardless of the type of surgical procedure; however, LDL-cholesterol only decreased after RYGB [67]. However, these authors could not find any correlation between the changes in serum lipid concentrations and those in IMT. A recent meta-analysis showed that pulse wave velocity (PWV) as a measure of arterial stiffness decreased significantly after bariatric surgery. This is important because atherosclerosis causes arteries to lose their elasticity and become more stiff; thereby resulting in increased PWV which predicts subsequent ACVD events [11].

Similar to our meta-analysis, a previously published small meta-analysis showed a significant reduction in IMT after bariatric surgery and indicated that the percentage of changes in BMI were associated with changes in IMT [68]. The results of the present meta-analysis also fit well with the results of another most recently published meta-analysis of 21 population-based cohort studies, involving 2,857,016 participants, which compared the effects of bariatric surgery and nonsurgical approaches on cardiovascular outcomes in patients with obesity [69]. This meta-analysis showed that bariatric surgery reduced major adverse cardiovascular events, including the risk of myocardial infarction, stroke, cardiovascular death, and all-cause death.

The present study has some limitations. Perhaps the most important one is the fact that until relatively recently there was a lack of IMT measurement standardization (method, mean/maximal thickness, carotid segment, including or excluding plaque) which could influence the predictive value in CHD risk estimation in different studies; therefore, this might also have an impact on the results of this meta-analysis [70]. In addition, according to the observational design of the included studies, we could not perform a comparative evaluation of the effects of bariatric surgery and medical treatment on IMT.

5. Conclusions

The results of this meta-analysis suggest that bariatric surgery significantly reduced IMT. Since increased IMT reflecting early structural atherosclerotic changes in patients with severe obesity seems to be independently associated with ACVD, the results of this study may have clinical implications for individuals with severe obesity and high cardiovascular risk. This suggests a beneficial antiatherosclerotic effect of bariatric surgery. Future prospective studies with a precise follow-up, bigger sample size, and different markers that could predict the outcomes of bariatric surgery regarding elimination of co-morbidities should add more objective data to the spectrum of benefits of weight loss surgery.

Funding: This research received no external funding.

Institutional Review Board Statement: Not applicable.

Informed Consent Statement: Not applicable.

Data Availability Statement: Not applicable.

Acknowledgments: Tannaz Jamialahmadi was supported by the Wael-Almahmeed and IAS research training grant.

Conflicts of Interest: The authors declare no conflict of interest.

References

1. WHO (World Health Organisation). *Obesity and Overweight*; WHO: Geneva, Switzerland, 2021.
2. Centers for Disease Control and Prevention. *Adult Obesity Facts*; CDC: Atlanta, GA, USA, 2021.
3. Kim, M.S.; Kim, W.J.; Khera, A.V.; Kim, J.Y.; Yon, D.K.; Lee, S.W.; Shin, J.I.; Won, H.-H. Association between adiposity and cardiovascular outcomes: An umbrella review and meta-analysis of observational and Mendelian randomization studies. *Eur. Heart J.* **2021**, *42*, 3388–3403. [CrossRef] [PubMed]
4. Theel, W.; Boxma-de Klerk, B.M.; Dirksmeier-Harinck, F.; van Rossum, E.F.; Kanhai, D.A.; Apers, J.; van Dalen, B.M.; de Knegt, R.J.; Holleboom, A.G.; Tushuizen, M.E. Evaluation of nonalcoholic fatty liver disease (NAFLD) in severe obesity using noninvasive tests and imaging techniques. *Obes. Rev.* **2022**, *23*, e13481. [CrossRef] [PubMed]
5. Stasi, A.; Cosola, C.; Caggiano, G.; Cimmarusti, M.T.; Palieri, R.; Acquaviva, P.M.; Rana, G.; Gesualdo, L. Obesity-Related Chronic Kidney Disease: Principal Mechanisms and New Approaches in Nutritional Management. *Front. Nutr.* **2022**, *9*, 925619. [CrossRef]
6. Cottam, D.R.; Mattar, S.G.; Barinas-Mitchell, E.; Eid, G.; Kuller, L.; Kelley, D.E.; Schauer, P.R. The chronic inflammatory hypothesis for the morbidity associated with morbid obesity: Implications and effects of weight loss. *Obes. Surg.* **2004**, *14*, 589–600. [CrossRef]
7. Guo, Z.; Yang, Y.; Liao, Y.; Shi, Y.; Zhang, L.-J. Emerging Roles of Adipose Tissue in the Pathogenesis of Psoriasis and Atopic Dermatitis in Obesity. *JID Innov.* **2022**, *2*, 100064. [CrossRef] [PubMed]
8. Van Raemdonck, K.; Umar, S.; Szekanecz, Z.; Zomorrodi, R.K.; Shahrara, S. Impact of obesity on autoimmune arthritis and its cardiovascular complications. *Autoimmun. Rev.* **2018**, *17*, 821–835. [CrossRef]

9. Coelho, C.; Crane, J.; Agius, R.; McGowan, B. The bariatric-metabolic physician's role in managing clinically severe obesity. *Curr. Obes. Rep.* **2021**, *10*, 263–273. [CrossRef]
10. Jamialahmadi, T.; Reiner, Ž.; Alidadi, M.; Kroh, M.; Cardenia, V.; Xu, S.; Al-Rasadi, K.; Santos, R.D.; Sahebkar, A. The Effect of Bariatric Surgery on Circulating Levels of Oxidized Low-Density Lipoproteins Is Apparently Independent of Changes in Body Mass Index: A Systematic Review and Meta-Analysis. *Oxidative Med. Cell. Longev.* **2021**, *2021*, 4136071. [CrossRef]
11. Jamialahmadi, T.; Reiner, Ž.; Alidadi, M.; Kroh, M.; Simental-Mendia, L.E.; Pirro, M.; Sahebkar, A. Impact of Bariatric Surgery on Pulse Wave Velocity as a Measure of Arterial Stiffness: A Systematic Review and Meta-analysis. *Obes. Surg.* **2021**, *31*, 4461–4469. [CrossRef]
12. Jamialahmadi, T.; Alidadi, M.; Atkin, S.L.; Kroh, M.; Almahmeed, W.; Moallem, S.A.; Al-Rasadi, K.; Rodriguez, J.H.; Santos, R.D.; Ruscica, M.; et al. Effect of Bariatric Surgery on Flow-Mediated Vasodilation as a Measure of Endothelial Function: A Systematic Review and Meta-Analysis. *J. Clin. Med.* **2022**, *11*, 4054. [CrossRef]
13. Jamialahmadi, T.; Jangjoo, A.; Rezvani, R.; Goshayeshi, L.; Tasbandi, A.; Nooghabi, M.J.; Rajabzadeh, F.; Ghaffarzadegan, K.; Mishamandani, Z.J.; Nematy, M. Hepatic Function and Fibrosis Assessment Via 2D-Shear Wave Elastography and Related Biochemical Markers Pre- and Post-Gastric Bypass Surgery. *Obes. Surg.* **2020**, *30*, 2251–2258. [CrossRef]
14. Nabavi, N.; Ghodsi, A.; Rostami, R.; Torshizian, A.; Jamialahmadi, T.; Jangjoo, A.; Nematy, M.; Bahari, A.; Ebrahimzadeh, F.; Mahmoudabadi, E.; et al. Impact of Bariatric Surgery on Carotid Intima-Media Thickness in Patients with Morbid Obesity: A Prospective Study and Review of the Literature. *Obes. Surg.* **2022**, *32*, 1563–1569. [CrossRef]
15. van Veldhuisen, S.L.; Gorter, T.M.; van Woerden, G.; de Boer, R.A.; Rienstra, M.; Hazebroek, E.J.; van Veldhuisen, D.J. Bariatric surgery and cardiovascular disease: A systematic review and meta-analysis. *Eur. Heart J.* **2022**, *43*, 1955–1969. [CrossRef] [PubMed]
16. Carmona-Maurici, J.; Cuello, E.; Sánchez, E.; Miñarro, A.; Rius, F.; Bueno, M.; de la Fuente, M.C.; Olsina Kissler, J.J.; Vidal, T.; Maria, V.; et al. Impact of bariatric surgery on subclinical atherosclerosis in patients with morbid obesity. *Surg. Obes. Relat. Dis.* **2020**, *16*, 1419–1428. [CrossRef] [PubMed]
17. Roumeliotis, A.; Roumeliotis, S.; Panagoutsos, S.; Theodoridis, M.; Argyriou, C.; Tavridou, A.; Georgiadis, G.S. Carotid intima-media thickness is an independent predictor of all-cause mortality and cardiovascular morbidity in patients with diabetes mellitus type 2 and chronic kidney disease. *Ren. Fail.* **2019**, *41*, 131–138. [CrossRef]
18. Zhang, Y.; Fang, X.; Hua, Y.; Tang, Z.; Guan, S.; Wu, X.; Liu, H.; Liu, B.; Wang, C.; Zhang, Z. Carotid artery plaques, carotid intima–media thickness, and risk of cardiovascular events and all-cause death in older adults: A 5-year prospective, community-based study. *Angiology* **2018**, *69*, 120–129. [CrossRef]
19. Saba, L.; Antignani, P.L.; Gupta, A.; Cau, R.; Paraskevas, K.I.; Poredos, P.; Wasserman, B.; Kamel, H.; Avgerinos, E.D.; Salgado, R. International Union of Angiology (IUA) consensus paper on imaging strategies in atherosclerotic carotid artery imaging: From basic strategies to advanced approaches. *Atherosclerosis* **2022**, *354*, 23–40. [CrossRef]
20. Abeysuriya, V.; Perera, B.; Wickremasinghe, A. Regional and demographic variations of Carotid artery Intima and Media Thickness (CIMT): A Systematic review and meta-analysis. *PLoS ONE* **2022**, *17*, e0268716. [CrossRef]
21. Gloy, V.L.; Briel, M.; Bhatt, D.L.; Kashyap, S.R.; Schauer, P.R.; Mingrone, G.; Bucher, H.C.; Nordmann, A.J. Bariatric surgery versus non-surgical treatment for obesity: A systematic review and meta-analysis of randomised controlled trials. *BMJ* **2013**, *347*, f5934. [CrossRef]
22. Vest, A.R.; Heneghan, H.M.; Agarwal, S.; Schauer, P.R.; Young, J.B. Bariatric surgery and cardiovascular outcomes: A systematic review. *Heart* **2012**, *98*, 1763–1777. [CrossRef]
23. Zagorski, S.M.; Papa, N.N.; Chung, M.H. The effect of weight loss after gastric bypass on Creactive protein levels. *Surg. Obes. Relat. Dis.* **2005**, *1*, 81–85. [CrossRef] [PubMed]
24. Yudkin, J.S.; Stehouwer, C.D.A.; Emeis, J.J.; Coppack, S.W. C-reactive protein in healthy subjects: Associations with obesity, insulin resistance, and endothelial dysfunction: A potential role for cytokines originating from adipose tissue? *Arterioscler. Thromb. Vasc. Biol.* **1999**, *19*, 972–978. [CrossRef] [PubMed]
25. Rao, S.R. Inflammatory markers and bariatric surgery: A meta-analysis. *Inflamm. Res.* **2012**, *61*, 789–807. [CrossRef]
26. Sutton, A.J.; Abrams, K.R.; Jones, D.R.; Jones, D.R.; Sheldon, T.A.; Song, F. *Methods for Meta-Analysis in Medical Research*; Wiley Chichester: Chichester, UK, 2000; Volume 348.
27. Higgins, J.P. *Cochrane Handbook for Systematic Reviews of Interventions*; Version 5.0.1; The Cochrane Collaboration: London, UK, 2008. Available online: http://www.cochrane-handbook.org (accessed on 25 April 2022).
28. Wells, G.A.; Shea, B.; O'Connell, D.A.; Peterson, J.; Welch, V.; Losos, M.; Tugwell, P. *The Newcastle-Ottawa Scale (NOS) for Assessing the Quality of Nonrandomised Studies in Meta-Analyses*; Oxford: Oxford, UK, 2000.
29. Borenstein, M.; Hedges, L.; Higgins, J.; Rothstein, H. *Comprehensive Meta-Analysis*; Version 2 Biostat; Meta-Analysis: Englewood, NJ, USA, 2005.
30. Banach, M.; Serban, C.; Ursoniu, S.; Rysz, J.; Muntner, P.; Toth, P.P.; Jones, S.R.; Rizzo, M.; Glasser, S.P.; Watts, G.F. Statin therapy and plasma coenzyme Q10 concentrations—A systematic review and meta-analysis of placebo-controlled trials. *Pharmacol. Res.* **2015**, *99*, 329–336. [CrossRef]
31. Duval, S.; Tweedie, R. Trim and fill: A simple funnel-plot–based method of testing and adjusting for publication bias in meta-analysis. *Biometrics* **2000**, *56*, 455–463. [CrossRef]

32. Yavuz, D.G.; Apaydin, T.; Imre, E.; Uygur, M.M.; Yazici, D. Skin Autofluorescence and Carotid Intima-Media Thickness Evaluation Following Bariatric Surgery in Patients with Severe Obesity. *Obes. Surg.* **2021**, *31*, 1055–1061. [CrossRef] [PubMed]
33. Salman, M.A.; Salman, A.A.; El Sherbiny, M.; Elkholy, S.; Youssef, A.; Labib, S.; El-Din, M.T.; Monazea, K.A.; Tourky, M.S.; Mikhail, H.M.S.; et al. Changes of Carotid Intima-Media Thickness After Sleeve Gastrectomy in High Cardiovascular Risk Patients: A Prospective Study. *Obes. Surg.* **2021**, *31*, 3541–3547. [CrossRef]
34. Melchor-López, A.; Suárez-Cuenca, J.A.; Banderas-Lares, D.Z.; Peña-Sosa, G.D.L.; Salamanca-García, M.; Vera-Gómez, E.; Hernández-Patricio, A.; Gutiérrez-Buendía, J.A.; Zamora-Alemán, C.R.; Alcaráz-Estrada, S.L.; et al. Identification of adipose tissue-related predictors of the reduction in cardiovascular risk induced by metabolic surgery. *J. Int. Med. Res.* **2021**, *49*, 03000605211012569. [CrossRef]
35. Kaul, A.; Kumar, A.; Baksi, A.; Singla, V.; Aggarwal, S.; Gulati, G.; Narang, R.; Kashyap, L. Impact of bariatric surgery on carotid intima-medial thickness and cardiovascular risk: Results of a prospective study. *Surg. Endosc. Other Interv. Tech.* **2021**, *35*, 6006–6012. [CrossRef]
36. Cekici, Y.; Kaya, B.C.; Elkan, H. The Effect of Laparoscopic Sleeve Gastrectomy on Subclinical Atherosclerosis in Patients with Severe Obesity. *Obes. Surg.* **2021**, *31*, 738–745. [CrossRef]
37. Ministrini, S.; Ricci, M.A.; Nulli Migliola, E.; De Vuono, S.; D'Abbondanza, M.; Paganelli, M.T.; Vaudo, G.; Siepi, D.; Lupattelli, G. Chemerin predicts carotid intima-media thickening in severe obesity. *Eur. J. Clin. Investig.* **2020**, *50*, e13256. [CrossRef] [PubMed]
38. Kaya, B.C.; Elkan, H. The impact of weight loss after laparoscopic sleeve gastrectomy on early markers of atherosclerotic vascular disease: A prospective study. *Kardiol. Pol.* **2020**, *78*, 674–680. [CrossRef] [PubMed]
39. Gómez-Martin, J.M.; Aracil, E.; Insenser, M.; de la Peña, G.; Lasunción, M.A.; Galindo, J.; Escobar-Morreale, H.F.; Balsa, J.A.; Botella-Carretero, J.I. Changes in Soluble TWEAK Concentrations, but Not Those in Amyloid-β(1–40), Are Associated with a Decrease in Carotid Intima-Media Thickness after Bariatric Surgery in Obese Women. *Obes. Facts* **2020**, *13*, 321–330. [CrossRef] [PubMed]
40. Elitok, A.; Emet, S.; Bayramov, F.; Karaayvaz, E.; Türker, F.; Barbaros, U.; Özcan, M. Effect of bariatric surgery on flow-mediated dilation and carotid intima-media thickness in patients with morbid obesity: 1-year follow-up study. *Anatol. J. Cardiol.* **2020**, *23*, 218–222. [CrossRef] [PubMed]
41. Domenech-Ximenos, B.; Cuba, V.; Daunis-i-Estadella, P.; Thio-Henestrosa, S.; Jaldo, F.; Biarnes, C.; Molina, X.; Xifra, G.; Ricart, W.; Bardera, A.; et al. Bariatric Surgery-Induced Changes in Intima-Media Thickness and Cardiovascular Risk Factors in Class 3 Obesity: A 3-Year Follow-Up Study. *Obesity* **2020**, *28*, 1663–1670. [CrossRef]
42. Cobeta, P.; Osorio, A.; Cuadrado-Ayuso, M.; Garcia-Moreno, F.; Pestana, D.; Galindo, J.; Botella-Carretero, J.I. Sleeve Gastrectomy and Gastric Bypass Decrease the Carotid Intima-Media Thickness in Obese Men: Association with Weight Loss, Cardiovascular Risk Factors, and Circulating Testosterone. *Obes. Surg.* **2020**, *30*, 851–859. [CrossRef]
43. Borzi, A.M.; Buscemi, C.; Corleo, D.; Randazzo, C.; Rosafio, G.; Pantuso, G.; Buscemi, S. Endothelial Function in Obese Patients Treated with Bariatric Surgery. *Diabetes Metab. Syndr. Obes.-Targets Ther.* **2020**, *13*, 247–256. [CrossRef]
44. Yang, W.; Jiang, S.; Cheung, P.N.; Wang, C. Effects and predictive factors of bariatric surgery on carotid intima-media thickness in patients with obesity Cardiovascular risk and bariatric surgery. *Obes. Surg.* **2019**, *29*, 140.
45. Solini, A.; Seghieri, M.; Santini, E.; Giannini, L.; Biancalana, E.; Taddei, S.; Volterrani, D.; Bruno, R.M. Renal Resistive Index Predicts Post-Bariatric Surgery Renal Outcome in Nondiabetic Individuals with Severe Obesity. *Obesity* **2019**, *27*, 68–74. [CrossRef]
46. Gluszewska, A.; Gryglewska, B.; Rewiuk, K.; Zarzycki, B.; Dzieza-Grudnik, A.; Kwater, A.; Major, P.; Budzynski, A.; Gasowski, J.; Grodzicki, T. Arterial structure and function and its short- and long-term changes after bariatric surgery. *J. Physiol. Pharmacol.* **2019**, *70*, 909–916. [CrossRef]
47. Rius, F.; Sanchez, E.; Betriu, A.; Baena-Fustegueras, J.A.; Yeramian, A.; Vidal, T.; Hernandez, M.; Lopez-Cano, C.; Bueno, M.; Gutierrez-Carrasquilla, L.; et al. Influence of Morbid Obesity and Bariatric Surgery Impact on the Carotid Adventitial Vasa Vasorum Signal. *Obes. Surg.* **2018**, *28*, 3935–3942. [CrossRef] [PubMed]
48. Jonker, F.H.W.; van Houten, V.A.A.; Wijngaarden, L.H.; Klaassen, R.A.; de Smet, A.A.E.A.; Niezen, A.; Schelfhout, L.J.D.M.; Bruning, T.A.; van der Harst, E. Age-Related Effects of Bariatric Surgery on Early Atherosclerosis and Cardiovascular Risk Reduction. *Obes. Surg.* **2018**, *28*, 1040–1046. [CrossRef] [PubMed]
49. Altin, C.; Erol, V.; Aydin, E.; Yilmaz, M.; Tekindal, M.A.; Sade, L.E.; Gulay, H.; Muderrisoglu, H. Impact of weight loss on epicardial fat and carotid intima media thickness after laparoscopic sleeve gastrectomy: A prospective study. *Nutr. Metab. Cardiovasc. Dis.* **2018**, *28*, 501–509. [CrossRef] [PubMed]
50. Tromba, L.; Tartaglia, F.; Carbotta, S.; Sforza, N.; Pelle, F.; Colagiovanni, V.; Carbotta, G.; Cavaiola, S.; Casella, G. The Role of Sleeve Gastrectomy in Reducing Cardiovascular Risk. *Obes. Surg.* **2017**, *27*, 1145–1151. [CrossRef]
51. Chen, J.; Yu, H.Y.; Chen, L.; Wu, L.; Hu, B.; Bao, Y.Q.; Jiang, L.X. Effect of Roux-en-Y gastric bypass on carotid intima-media thickness in Chinese obese patients with type 2 diabetes. *Surg. Obes. Relat. Dis.* **2017**, *13*, 1530–1535. [CrossRef]
52. Marchesi, F.; Giacosa, R.; Reggiani, V.; De Sario, G.; Tartamella, F.; Melani, E.; Mita, M.T.; Cinieri, F.G.; Cecchini, S.; Ricco, M.; et al. Morphological Changes in the Carotid Artery Intima after Gastric Bypass for Morbid Obesity. *Obes. Surg.* **2017**, *27*, 357–363. [CrossRef]
53. Yorulmaz, G.; Cilekar, M.; Bilge, U.; Akcan, E.; Akalin, A. Carotid intima-media thickness and insulin resistance changes in patients who underwent sleeve gastrectomy: A prospective study. *Niger. J. Clin. Pract.* **2016**, *19*, 344–348. [CrossRef]

54. Solmaz, A.; Arlcl, S.; Gülçiçek, O.B.; Yavuz, E.; Yiğitbaş, H.; Erçetin, C.; Öncü, M.; Çelebi, F.; Çelik, A.; Kutaniş, R. Influence of Bariatric Surgery on Carotid Intima-Media Thickness. *Bariatr. Surg. Pract. Patient Care* **2016**, *11*, 56–60. [CrossRef]
55. Graziani, F.; Leone, A.M.; Basile, E.; Cialdella, P.; Tritarelli, A.; Della Bona, R.; Liuzzo, G.; Nanni, G.; Iaconelli, A.; Iaconelli, A.; et al. Endothelial Progenitor Cells in Morbid Obesity-Pathogenetic Implications. *Circ. J.* **2014**, *78*, 977–985. [CrossRef]
56. Tschoner, A.; Sturm, W.; Gelsinger, C.; Ress, C.; Laimer, M.; Engl, J.; Laimer, E.; Muhlmann, G.; Mittermair, R.; Kaser, S.; et al. Long-term Effects of Weight Loss after Bariatric Surgery on Functional and Structural Markers of Atherosclerosis. *Obesity* **2013**, *21*, 1960–1965. [CrossRef]
57. Bravo, G.G.; Bunout, D.; Mella, J.; Quiroga, E.; de la Maza, M.P.; Cavada, G.; Hirsch, S. Bariatric surgery decreases carotid intima-media thickness in obese subjects. *Nutr. Hosp.* **2013**, *28*, 1102–1108. [CrossRef]
58. Lundby-Christensen, L.; Tarnow, L.; Vaag, A.; Wiinberg, N.; Hansen, D.; Worm, D.; Hvolris, L.; Naver, L.; Almdal, T. Carotid intima-media thickness is reduced 12 months after gastric bypass surgery in patients with type 2 diabetes. *Diabetologia* **2012**, *55*, S505.
59. Geloneze, S.R.; Geloneze, B.; Morari, J.; Matos-Souza, J.R.; Lima, M.M.; Chaim, E.A.; Pareja, J.C.; Velloso, L.A. PGC1α gene Gly482Ser polymorphism predicts improved metabolic, inflammatory and vascular outcomes following bariatric surgery. *Int. J. Obes.* **2012**, *36*, 363–368. [CrossRef] [PubMed]
60. Sarmento, P.L.F.A.; Plavnik, F.L.; Zanella, M.T.; Pinto, P.E.; Miranda, R.B.; Ajzen, S.A. Association of carotid intima-media thickness and cardiovascular risk factors in women pre- and post-bariatric surgery. *Obes. Surg.* **2009**, *19*, 339–344. [CrossRef] [PubMed]
61. van Mil, S.R.; Biter, L.U.; van de Geijn, G.J.M.; Birnie, E.; Dunkelgrun, M.; Ijzermans, J.N.; van der Meulen, N.; Mannaerts, G.H.; Castro Cabezas, M. The effect of sex and menopause on carotid intima-media thickness and pulse wave velocity in morbid obesity. *Eur. J. Clin. Investig.* **2019**, *49*, e13118.
62. Dalmas, E.; Kahn, J.-F.; Giral, P.; Abdennour, M.; Bouillot, J.-L.; Fellahi, S.; Oppert, J.-M.; Clément, K.; Guerre-Millo, M.; Poitou, C. Intima-media thickness in severe obesity: Links with BMI and metabolic status but not with systemic or adipose tissue inflammation. *Diabetes Care* **2013**, *36*, 3793–3802. [CrossRef]
63. Sandgren, T.; Sonesson, B.; Ahlgren, Å.R.; Länne, T. The diameter of the common femoral artery in healthy human: Influence of sex, age, and body size. *J. Vasc. Surg.* **1999**, *29*, 503–510. [CrossRef]
64. Boras, J.; Ljubic, S.; Car, N.; Metelko, Z.; Petrovecki, M.; Lovrencic, M.V.; Reiner, Z. Lipoprotein (a) predicts progression of carotid artery intima-media thickening in patients with type 2 diabetes: A four-year follow-up. *Wien. Klin. Wochenschr.* **2010**, *122*, 159–164. [CrossRef]
65. Reiner, Ž.; Simental-Mendía, L.; Ruscica, M.; Katsiki, N.; Banach, M.; Rasadi, K.; Jamialahmadi, T.; Sahebkar, A. Pulse wave velocity as a measure of arterial stiffness in patients with familial hypercholesterolemia: A systematic review and meta-analysis. *Arch. Med. Sci.* **2019**, *15*, 1365–1374. [CrossRef]
66. Reiner, Ž. *Impact of Early Evidence of Atherosclerotic Changes on Early Treatment in Children with Familial Hypercholesterolemia*; American Heart Association: Dallas, TX, USA, 2014; Volume 114, pp. 233–235.
67. Gómez-Martin, J.M.; Balsa, J.; Aracil, E.; Cuadrado-Ayuso, M.; Rosillo, M.; De la Peña, G.; Lasunción, M.; Escobar-Morreale, H.F.; Botella-Carretero, J.I. Beneficial changes on plasma apolipoproteins A and B, high density lipoproteins and oxidized low density lipoproteins in obese women after bariatric surgery: Comparison between gastric bypass and sleeve gastrectomy. *Lipids Health Dis.* **2018**, *17*, 145. [CrossRef]
68. Lupoli, R.; Di Minno, M.; Guidone, C.; Cefalo, C.; Capaldo, B.; Riccardi, G.; Mingrone, G. Effects of bariatric surgery on markers of subclinical atherosclerosis and endothelial function: A meta-analysis of literature studies. *Int. J. Obes.* **2016**, *40*, 395–402. [CrossRef] [PubMed]
69. Borui, T.; Zhang, Y.; Wang, Y.; Wang, X.; An, Z.; Yu, X. Effect of Bariatric Surgery on Long-Term Cardiovascular Outcomes: A Systematic Review and Meta-analysis of Population-Based Cohort Studies. *Surg. Obes. Relat. Dis.* **2022**, *18*, 1074–1086.
70. Poredoš, P.; Cífková, R.; Maier, J.A.M.; Nemcsik, J.; Šabovič, M.; Jug, B.; Ježovnik, M.K.; Schernthaner, G.H.; Antignani, P.L.; Catalano, M. Preclinical atherosclerosis and cardiovascular events: Do we have a consensus about the role of preclinical atherosclerosis in the prediction of cardiovascular events? *Atherosclerosis* **2022**, *348*, 25–35. [CrossRef] [PubMed]

Journal of
Clinical Medicine

MDPI

Article

Body Weight Reduction by Bariatric Surgery Reduces the Plasma Levels of the Novel Orexigenic Gut Hormone Insulin-like Peptide 5 in Patients with Severe Obesity

Angelo Di Vincenzo [1], Marika Crescenzi [1], Marnie Granzotto [1], Sara Zancaner [1], Roberto Fabris [1], Mirto Foletto [2], Luca Prevedello [2], Federico Capone [1], Roberto Vettor [1] and Marco Rossato [1,*]

[1] Department of Medicine—DIMED, University Hospital of Padova, 35128 Padova, Italy; angelo.divincenzo@unipd.it (A.D.V.); marikacrescenzi@hotmail.com (M.C.); roberto.fabris@aopd.veneto.it (R.F.); roberto.vettor@unipd.it (R.V.)

[2] Department of Surgical, Oncological and Gastroenterological Sciences—DISCOG, University Hospital of Padova, 35128 Padova, Italy; mirto.foletto@unipd.it (M.F.)

* Correspondence: marco.rossato@unipd.it

Abstract: Insulin-like factor 5 (INSL5), a novel hormone secreted by the enteroendocrine cells of the distal colon, has been implicated in appetite and body weight regulation in animals given its orexigenic properties. We investigated basal INSL5 plasma levels in a group of morbidly obese subjects before and after laparoscopic sleeve gastrectomy. Furthermore, we analyzed the expression of *INSL5* in human adipose tissue. Before bariatric surgery, obese subjects showed basal INSL5 plasma levels that were positively correlated with BMI, fat mass, and leptin plasma levels. After weight loss by laparoscopic sleeve gastrectomy, INSL5 plasma levels in obese subjects were significantly lower than those observed before surgery. Finally, we did not detect any expression of the *INSL5* gene in human adipose tissue, both at the mRNA and protein levels. The present data show that subjects with obesity have INSL5 plasma levels positively correlating with adiposity markers. After bariatric surgery, INSL5 plasma levels decreased significantly, and this decrease was not directly due to the loss of adipose tissue since this tissue does not express *INSL5*. Considering the orexigenic properties of INSL5, the reduction of its plasma levels after bariatric surgery in obese subjects could participate in the still unclear mechanisms leading to appetite reduction that characterize bariatric surgery procedures.

Keywords: obesity; adipose tissue; INSL5; leptin; BMI; bariatric surgery; sleeve gastrectomy

Citation: Di Vincenzo, A.; Crescenzi, M.; Granzotto, M.; Zancaner, S.; Fabris, R.; Foletto, M.; Prevedello, L.; Capone, F.; Vettor, R.; Rossato, M. Body Weight Reduction by Bariatric Surgery Reduces the Plasma Levels of the Novel Orexigenic Gut Hormone Insulin-like Peptide 5 in Patients with Severe Obesity. *J. Clin. Med.* **2023**, *12*, 3752. https://doi.org/10.3390/jcm12113752

Academic Editor: David Benaiges Boix

Received: 19 March 2023
Revised: 26 April 2023
Accepted: 10 May 2023
Published: 29 May 2023

1. Introduction

Obesity is a chronic disease with a continuously increasing prevalence [1], with important systemic complications including heart disease, diabetes mellitus, hypertension, dyslipidemia, stroke, atherosclerosis, and specific types of cancer [2]. Since obesity is due mainly to an unbalance between energy intake and expenditure, the first-line interventions for overweight and obese subjects are diet and physical exercise that promote calorie restriction and increase energy expenditure. Although these interventions often result in initial weight reduction, the majority of patients with obesity fail to maintain the weight loss in the long term, probably due to many different compensatory changes, above all in appetite regulatory mechanisms [3,4]. On the contrary, bariatric surgery causes substantial long-term weight loss and is an effective intervention for the morbidly obese to achieve marked and long-term weight loss and improve obesity-related comorbidities. For these reasons, bariatric surgery is now considered the most successful method for treating morbid obesity and its associated diseases, such as type 2 diabetes [5].

Bariatric surgery has now quite well-defined beneficial effects on hunger, not only due to gastric restriction but also to the modulation of appetite-regulatory hormones coming mainly from the gut, such as ghrelin, PYY, CKK, and GLP-1 [6,7].

Insulin-like factor 5 (INSL5) is a novel hormone secreted primarily by the enteroendocrine cells of the colon and rectum that has been implicated in both mealtime hunger and the regulation of body weight in animals given its orexigenic properties [8–10]. INSL5 belongs to the relaxin/insulin superfamily of peptides consisting of insulin, insulin-like growth factors 1 and 2 (IGF–1 and IGF–2), relaxins 1 and 2, and insulin-like peptides 3, 4, 5, 6, and 7 (INSL 3–7) [11]. Relaxins have many different roles, such as regulation of female and male reproductive tract functions, signaling in the central nervous system, vasodilation and heart stimulation in the cardiovascular system, regulation of fibrotic processes, and wound healing [12].

INSL5, one of the latest identified members of the relaxin superfamily, has been shown to be expressed mainly in the terminal part of the gastrointestinal tract, particularly in the colon and rectum, but it is also expressed in many other tissues as well, including the brain, pituitary, thyroid, kidney, and uterus [13].

Although they are structurally related to insulin, the relaxin family peptides produce their physiological effects by activating a group of four G protein-coupled receptors (GPCRs), named relaxin family peptide receptors 1–4 (RXFP1–4) [11,12].

While it is clear that the relaxin family of peptides has important physiological roles, there are still many unanswered questions about the precise roles of many of them.

In the present study, we evaluated INSL5 plasma levels in a group of patients with obesity before and one year after significant weight and adipose tissue loss obtained by laparoscopic sleeve gastrectomy. Furthermore we investigated the relationship of INSL5 plasma levels with classic obesity related parameters such as BMI, waist circumference, fat mass and with leptin plasma levels. Finally we explored the hypothesis that adipose tissue can be the source of INSL5 production.

2. Materials and Methods

2.1. Patients

We retrieved stored blood samples from forty morbidly obese patients (29 females and 11 males) previously recruited from the Bariatric Unit of the University Hospital of Padova. Each patient was evaluated before and 12 months after laparoscopic sleeve gastrectomy (LSG) with general clinical parameters (body temperature, blood pressure, heart rate, breath frequency, blood oxygen saturation) and with anthropometric measurements (weight, height, BMI, waist circumference). In all 40 patients, we evaluated glucose and insulin plasma levels together with leptin and INSL5 plasma levels. Blood samples were drawn in the morning (between 8 and 9 a.m.) after an overnight fast. Before and after one year of LSG, twenty-nine out of the forty patients with obesity who underwent bariatric surgery also performed body composition analysis using bioimpedenzometry, as previously described [14].

In our Center LSG is performed as the first-choice bariatric surgery procedure. All patients were operated by the same bariatric surgery team when indicated, according with the NIH consensus criteria for bariatric surgery (BMI higher than 35 kg/m^2 in the presence of co-morbidities or with a BMI higher than 40 kg/m^2) [14]. Absolute exclusion criteria included alcohol addiction and severe psychiatric disorders. Full details of the surgical technique have been published recently by our group [15].

2.2. Measurement of INSL5 Plasma Levels

Blood samples have been collected into vacutainer tubes containing EDTA. After gentle rocking of the tubes several times immediately after the collection of blood for anticoagulation, the blood is then transferred from the lavender vacutainer tubes to centrifuge tubes containing aprotinin (0.6 TIU/mL of blood) and gently rocked several times to inhibit the activity of proteinases. Tubes were then centrifuged at 1600× g for 15 min at 4 °C, and plasma was collected and kept at −80 °C until INSL5 determination using a commercial EIA kit from Phoenix Pharmaceuticals (#EK-035-70, Burlingame, CA, USA) according to the manufacturer's instructions. The minimum detection level was 80 pg/mL. The cross-reactivity of the antibody raised against human INSL5 was 0% to human insulin, INSL3, INSL4, INSL6, INSL7 (Relaxin 3), and Relaxin 2. Intra- and inter-assay variations were <10% and <15%, respectively.

Leptin was measured in the same blood samples utilizing an ELISA kit (#E04649H, Cusabio, Houston, TX, USA) with a 0.156 ng/mL–10 ng/mL detection range and a sensitivity of 0.060 ng/mL.

2.3. Isolation of Human Adipose Tissue

Subcutaneous adipose tissue (SAT) was obtained from nine subjects undergoing elective surgery for minor abdominal diseases who were otherwise healthy and not taking any drugs. Each SAT sample was processed as previously described [15]. Briefly, all adipose tissue samples were collected during laparoscopic surgery in the abdominal region. In particular, 1 cm^3 SAT was obtained excising subcutaneous fat at trocar site and then it was gently rinsed in PBS buffer, immediately frozen in liquid nitrogen and stored at $-80°$ C for further analyses.

2.4. RNA Isolation and Reverse Transcription PCR (RT-PCR) in Adipose Tissue

RNA isolation from SAT was performed using an affinity column-based method (RNEasy Kit, Qiagen GmbH, Hilden, Germany). After homogenization of 100 mg of tissue in QIAzol Lysis Reagent with TissueLyser, chloroform was added and mixed by vortexing for subsequent phase separation through centrifugation. In the upper aqueous phase, the RNA was added to 1 volume of 70% ethanol and mixed thoroughly by inverting the tube up and down several times. Each sample was then loaded on the RNEasy spin column, and from this step on, the manufacturer's protocol was followed. At the end, the RNA was eluted in 50 µL of RNAse-free water. Quantity and quality of the RNA were evaluated by a DeNovix DS-11 spectrophotometer (Resnova, Ariccia, Italy) using OD 260 for calculation of the concentration and the ratios 260/280 and 260/230 for assessing the purity of the samples. First-strand cDNAs were accomplished in a 60 min incubation at 37 °C using 2 µg RNA, 200 U/µL M-MLV reverse transcriptase, and 0.5 µg/µL random primers (Promega Corp., Madison, WI, USA). A quantity of 10 ng of cDNA was used to detect Insulin-like 5 (INSL5) gene expression on the Veriti 96-Well Thermal Cycler (ABI Applied Biosystems, Waltham, MA, USA) using Pfu DNA Polymerase (Promega Corp., Madison, WI, USA). The ribosomal protein lateral stalk subunit P0 (RPLP0) housekeeping gene was used to avoid deviations from the process of measurement.

2.5. Western Blotting Analysis for INSL5 in Human Adipose Tissue

For protein analysis, SAT samples, colon tissue and HeLa cells (as positive controls) were homogenized in RIPA Lysis Buffer with phosphatase and protease inhibitors cocktail. Total protein concentration was determined using a colorimetric assay (Pierce ™BCA Protein Assay kit, #23225, Thermo Fisher Scientific, Waltham, MA, USA). Samples of 30 µg protein were subjected to SDS PAGE using 4-12% polyacrylamide precast gel at a voltage of 160V. Proteins were then transferred to a Hybond ECL nitrocellulose membrane and blocked with 5% (*w*/*v*) dried non-fat milk in Tris buffered saline (TBS)/Tween 20. For INSL5 protein detection, we utilized a 1:1000 diluted rabbit primary antibody (#105325, Abcam, Cambridge, MA, USA), a 1:2500 diluted antibody for leptin (#PA1-052, Invitrogen, Waltham, MA, USA), and a 1:5000 diluted mouse primary antibody for ß-actin (#A5441, Sigma Aldrich, Milan, Italy), used as a reference protein. An IgG-HRP-conjugated secondary antibody was used for protein detection. Immunoreactive bands have been visualized with the ECL plus reagent kit (GE Healthcare Italy, Milan, Italy).

2.6. Statistical Analysis

The results were expressed as means ± SD. Data obtained before and after weight loss were compared using the Student's *t*-test. Correlations were performed by simple linear regression analysis, and Spearman's correlation coefficients were used to evaluate the correlations between INSL5 plasma levels and other clinical and hormonal parameters. A p value < 0.05 was considered statistically significant. The statistical analysis was carried out using GraphPad PRISM software (version 9.5.1; GraphPad Software Inc., San Diego, CA, USA).

3. Results

3.1. Clinical, Anthropometric, and Metabolic Characteristics of the Obese Patients before and after LSG

Table 1 reports the anthropometric parameters before and one year after LSG in obese patients. As expected, LSG induced a significant body weight reduction along with a significant loss in fat mass and waist circumference. Furthermore, as expected, leptin plasma levels showed a significant reduction one year after LSG, along with fat mass reduction.

Table 1. Body weight parameters and leptin plasma levels before and one year after Laparoscopic Sleeve Gastrectomy (LSG) in obese patients. Data for weight, BMI, waist circumference, and leptin plasma levels have been obtained in all patients (n = 40). Data for fat mass have been obtained in 29 patients (N.A., not applicable).

	Before-LSG	After-LSG	p
Weight (Kg)	133.2 ± 27.4	95.3 ± 23.1	<0.0001
BMI (Kg/m^2)	47.4 ± 7.0	33.8 ± 6.1	<0.0001
%Total body weight loss	-	28.5 ± 8.8	N.A.
Waist circumference (cm)	131.4 ± 15.5	104.0 ± 14.6	<0.0001
Fat mass (Kg)	59.4 ± 17.5	32.1 ± 13.4	<0.0001
Leptin (μg/L)	38.0 ± 16.9	16.1 ± 13.5	<0.0001

3.2. Plasma Levels of INSL5 before and after Laparoscopic Sleeve Gastrectomy

We did not observe any significant gender difference in plasma INSL5 levels (0.88 ± 0.42 vs. 0.70 ± 0.21, for women and men, respectively, p = 0.173), even after adjustment for BMI. Thus, data from men and women were considered as a whole. As shown in Figure 1, INSL5 plasma levels in obese patients before LSG showed a strong positive correlation with BMI and with fat mass. In agreement with these relationships, INSL5 plasma levels were positively and significantly correlated with plasma levels of leptin, the main secretory product of adipose tissue directly related to fat mass. We did not observe any significant correlation between INSL5 plasma levels and both waist circumference and free fat mass (Figure 1). After one year of bariatric surgery and a significant reduction of BMI, waist circumference, and fat mass (see Table 1), we did not observe any significant correlation of these parameters with INSL5 plasma levels (Figure 2).

Interestingly, one year after laparoscopic sleeve gastrectomy, obese subjects showed a markedly reduced body weight and fat mass, together with a significant reduction of INSL5 plasma levels that were 23% lower than those observed before weight loss (Figure 2).

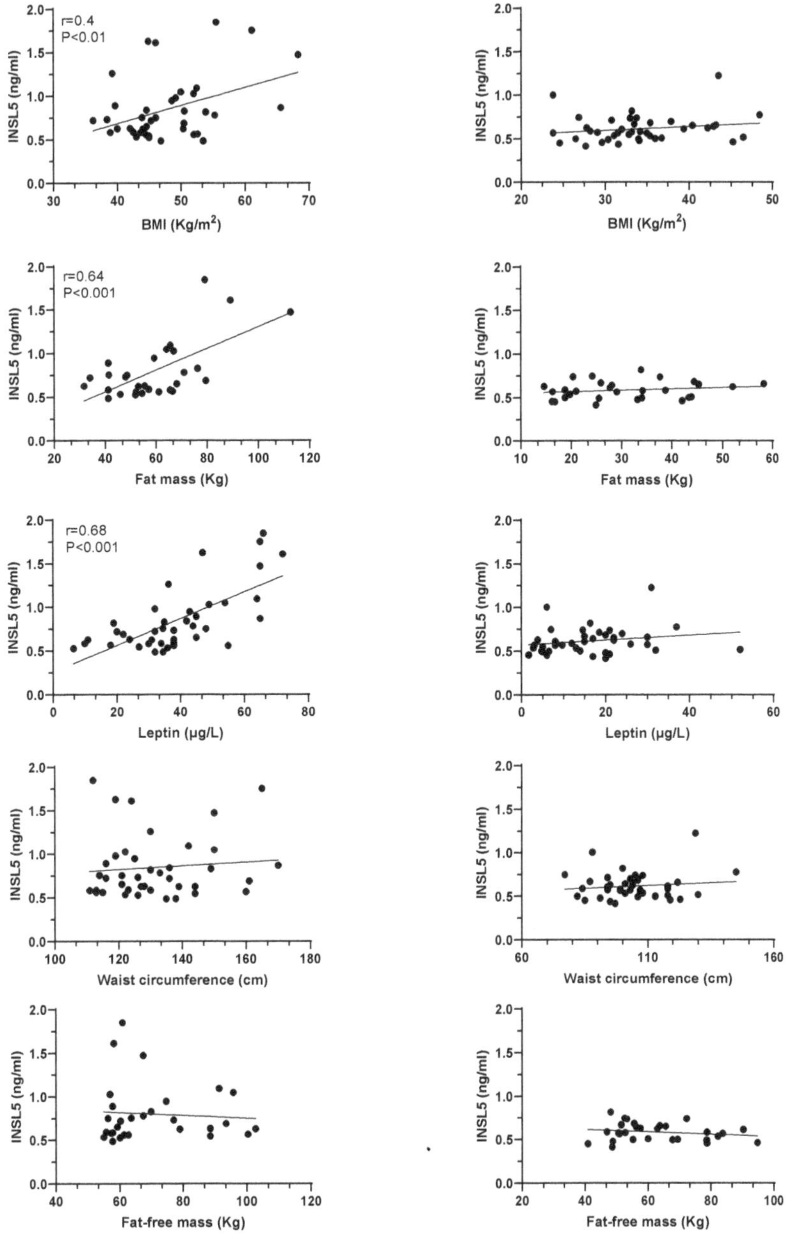

Figure 1. Correlations between INSL5 plasma levels and BMI, fat mass, fat free mass and leptin plasma levels in obese subjects before (left columns) and after (right columns) bariatric surgery. Data for BMI and leptin plasma levels have been obtained in all patients (n = 40). Data for fat mass and fat-free mass have been obtained in 29 patients (see Materials and Methods Section).

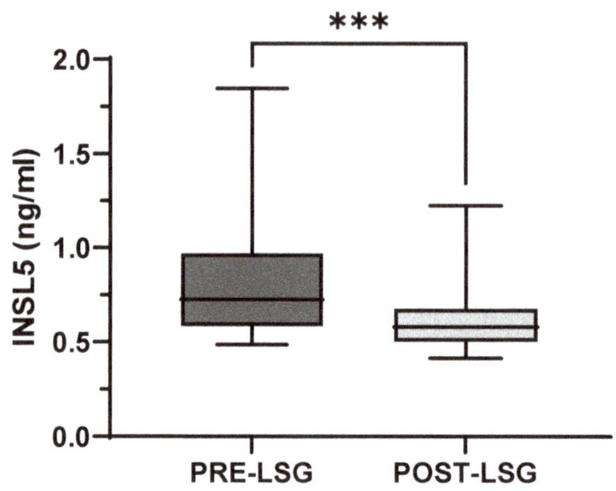

Figure 2. INSL5 plasma levels in obese subjects before (PRE-LSG) and after (POST-LSG) Laparoscopic Sleeve Gastrectomy (LSG). *** $p < 0.0001$.

3.3. INSL5 mRNA and Protein Expression in Human White Adipose Tissue

Gene expression data showed the presence of *INSL5* mRNA in the human colon and in HeLa cells used as positive controls, while no amplification plot was obtained from subcutaneous adipose tissue (Figure 3A). The expression of the RpLp0 housekeeping gene was the same in each sample (Figure 3A). The specificity of the real-time PCR for *INSL5* gene expression was determined on an electrophoresis agarose gel, and a single band of 81 bp was obtained only in control samples (Figure 3A).

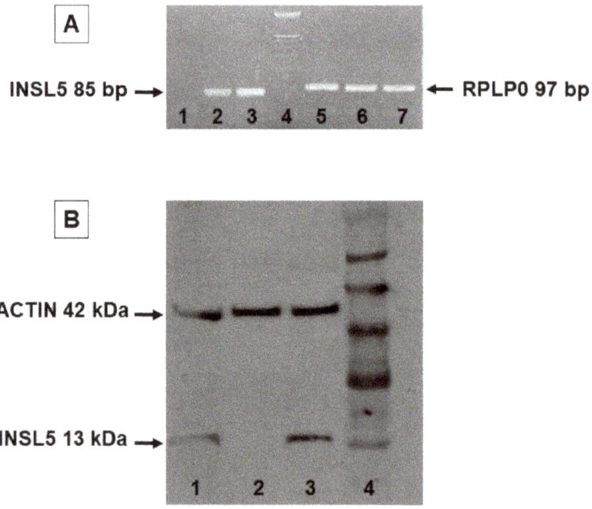

Figure 3. INSL5 is not expressed in human adipose tissue. (**A**): Qualitative RT-PCR analysis of *INSL5* mRNA expression in ex vivo adipose tissue (lane 1), HeLa cells, and colon tissue (positive controls, lane 2 and 3, respectively), 100 bp DNA ladder (lane 4), and RPLP0 housekeeping gene detection (lanes 5–7). (**B**): Western blot analysis of INSL5 protein expression in HeLa cells (lane 1), human subcutaneous adipose tissue (lane 2), and colon tissue (lane 3). Lane 4 reports the Seeblue pre-stained protein standard.

Similarly, the results from traditional Western blotting provided a main band of 13 KD for INSL5 only in colon tissue and HeLa cells used as positive controls, while no signal was obtained in subcutaneous adipose tissue. The 42 KD b-actin bands were used as a reference control for all samples (Figure 3B).

4. Discussion

INSL5 is a novel hormone of the relaxin superfamily that has been first identified as a secretory product of the enteroendocrine L cells of the distal gut (mainly colon and rectum), although it is also expressed in a number of different tissues such as the brain, pituitary, thyroid, kidney, and uterus [16]. In previous animal studies, given its orexigenic properties, INSL5 has been implicated in both mealtime hunger and the regulation of body weight [8–10].

Here we show that in humans, the novel orexigenic hormone INSL5 is detectable at significant concentrations in the plasma of obese subjects, with no differences between males and females. In obese patients, we observed that INSL5 plasma levels showed a strong positive correlation between classic markers of obesity such as BMI, fat mass, and leptin plasma levels. Since INSL5 is an orexigenic hormone, positive correlations between INSL5 plasma levels and BMI, fat mass, and leptin levels were expected. These direct and significant correlations were not observed after one year of bariatric surgery and significant reductions in body weight, BMI, fat mass, and leptin plasma levels. Interestingly, after significant weight loss due to LSG, we observed a significant reduction of INSL5 plasma levels. The close direct correlation between obesity markers and INSL5 plasma levels, together with the decrease in INSL5 concentration after fat mass reduction, pointed to adipose tissue as a possible source of INSL5. However, the molecular studies performed in the present study did not show any expression of INSL5 both at the mRNA and protein levels, thus excluding the possibility that the loss of adipose mass after LSG could be responsible for the decrease in INSL5 plasma levels. The lack of any correlation of INSL5 plasma levels with waist circumference would not be surprising since the mechanisms regulating INSL5 secretion are still unclear, and as shown here, the adipose tissue does not seem to have any role in INSL5 secretion. On the other hand, all the studies published so far have pointed to enteroendocrine-L cells as the main (if not unique) source of INSL5 in humans.

The pathophysiological meaning of the present observations is still unclear. It has been recently shown that Insl5$^{-/-}$ mice display alterations in glucose homeostasis and impaired fertility [9]. Furthermore, the expression of INSL5 in the gut of the mouse and the orexigenic effects induced by its administration that are blunted by its blockade suggest that INSL5 might be involved in food intake regulation, as shown for other gut hormones that are secreted by the enteroendocrine cells widely distributed along the gastrointestinal tract. These cells are deputed to sense gut content and to release hormones, such as ghrelin, cholecystokinin, and glucagon, like peptide 1 and peptide YY, that, after entering the circulation or interacting with the gut nervous system, can signal to distant target cells within the brain or act locally on neighboring gut cells and neuronal networks to regulate food intake and thus energy balance and body weight. In this respect, it has been shown that obesity and diabetes mellitus can be associated with alterations of enteroendocrine cell hormonal secretion [8,17]. Indeed, recent studies have demonstrated that only the peripheral and not the intracerebroventricular administration of INSL5 induces an increase in appetite leading to obesity in mice, although data published so far on the expression of the INSL5 receptor RXFP4 in the hypothalamus have shown contrasting results [8,9].

Nevertheless, INSL5 represents the second so far identified gut hormone, after ghrelin, with orexigenic properties [8,9]. In this respect, the reduction of INSL5 plasma levels observed after bariatric surgery-induced weight and fat mass loss could participate in the still unclear mechanisms leading to appetite reduction characterized by these surgical procedures [18]. While it has been recently reported that the signaling pathway activated by INSL5 is activated in target cells expressing its receptor [19,20], the specific signals regulating INSL5 secretion in humans are still unknown. It is possible that energetic substrate intake can regulate its secretion by adipose tissue. In this regard, in mice, INSL5 secretion is reduced by food intake, further underlying the role of this hormone in the regulation of energetic homeostasis. Furthermore, it has been recently reported that in mice, INSL5 influences glucose homeostasis by stimulating insulin secretion from pancreatic islet cells that have been shown to express the INSL5 receptor RXFP4 [9]. Those authors suggested a potential role for INSL5 signaling in the regulation of insulin secretion and pancreatic beta-cell homeostasis [9]. Finally, although there is a strong direct relationship between INSL5 and leptin plasma levels, the role of leptin as a possible mediator of INSL5 secretion needs further study.

5. Conclusions

In conclusion, the present study demonstrates that the orexigenic hormone INSL5 is detectable in humans and that its plasma concentrations show a positive correlation with BMI, fat mass, and leptin plasma levels in obese subjects and are significantly reduced after weight loss. These observations could contribute to extending our knowledge of the well-known modulation of the gut orexigenic signals induced after bariatric surgery in obese subjects. Finally, these observations suggest that the modulation of the INSL5/RXFP4 axis might represent a target for the treatment of obesity in humans.

Author Contributions: Conceptualization and design, M.R., A.D.V. and M.G.; experimental M.R., M.G., S.Z., R.F., M.C. and F.C.; laparoscopic sleeve gastrectomy, M.F. and L.P.; data analysis, M.R., M.G., M.C., S.Z. and R.V.; data interpretation of experimental results, M.R., A.D.V., S.Z. and R.V.; preparation of figures and manuscript—draft, M.R., S.Z., M.G., M.C. and A.D.V.; manuscript—edit and revision for relevant intellectual content, M.R., A.D.V., M.G., M.C., M.F., R.F., S.Z. and R.V. All authors contributed to the article and approved the submitted version. M.R. is the guarantor of this work. All authors have read and agreed to the published version of the manuscript.

Funding: The study has been supported by grant no. ROSS_PRIV20_01 from the University of Padova, Italy.

Institutional Review Board Statement: The study was conducted according to the guidelines of the Declaration of Helsinki and approved by the Ethics Committee of the University Hospital of Padova (approval no. RF-2016-02363566).

Informed Consent Statement: Informed written consent was obtained from all subjects involved in the study.

Data Availability Statement: The raw data supporting the conclusions of this article will be made available by the authors upon justified request, without undue reservation.

Acknowledgments: The authors wish to thank Sonia Leandri for her technical support.

Conflicts of Interest: The authors declare no conflict of interest.

References

1. Bray, G.A.; Frühbeck, G.; Ryan, D.H.; Wilding, J.P. Management of obesity. *Lancet* **2016**, *387*, 1947–1956. [CrossRef] [PubMed]
2. Whitlock, G.; Lewington, S.; Sherliker, P.; Clarke, R.; Emberson, J.; Halsey, J.; Qizilbash, N.; Collins, R.; Peto, R. Body-mass index and cause-specific mortality in 900,000 adults: Collaborative analyses of 57 prospective studies. *Lancet* **2009**, *373*, 1083–1096. [CrossRef] [PubMed]
3. Sumithran, P.; Prendergast, L.A.; Delbridge, E.; Purcell, K.; Shulkes, A.; Kriketos, A.; Proietto, J. Long–term persistence of hormonal adaptation to weight loss. *N. Engl. J. Med.* **2011**, *365*, 1597–1604. [CrossRef] [PubMed]
4. Anderson, J.W.; Konz, E.C.; Frederich, R.C.; Wood, C.L. Long–term weight–loss mainteinance: A meta–analysis of US studies. *Am. J. Clin. Nutr.* **2001**, *74*, 579–584. [CrossRef] [PubMed]
5. Sjöström, L.; Peltonen, M.; Jacobson, P.; Sjöström, C.D.; Karason, K.; Wedel, H.; Ahlin, S.; Anveden, Å.; Bengtsson, C.; Bergmark, G.; et al. Bariatric surgery and long-term cardiovascular events. *JAMA* **2012**, *307*, 56–65. [CrossRef] [PubMed]
6. Goldstone, A.P.; Miras, A.D.; Scholtz, S.; Jackson, S.; Neff, K.J.; Pénicaud, L.; Geoghegan, J.; Chhina, N.; Durighel, G.; Bell, J.D.; et al. Link between increased satiety gut hormones and reduced food reward after gastric bypass surgery for obesity. *J. Clin. Endocrinol. Metab.* **2016**, *101*, 599–609. [CrossRef] [PubMed]

7. Benaiges, D.; Más-Lorenzo, A.; Goday, A.; Ramon, J.M.; Chillarón, J.J.; Pedro-Botet, J.; Flores-Le Roux, J.A. Laparoscopic sleeve gastrectomy: More than a restrictive bariatric surgery procedure? *World J. Gastroenterol.* **2015**, *21*, 11804–11814. [CrossRef] [PubMed]
8. Grosse, J.; Heffron, H.; Burling, K.; Akhter-Hossain, M.; Habib, A.M.; Rogers, G.J.; Richards, P.; Larder, R.; Rimmington, D.; Adriaenssens, A.A.; et al. Insulin-like peptide 5 is an orexigenic gastrointestinal hormone. *Proc. Natl. Acad. Sci. USA* **2014**, *111*, 11133–11138. [CrossRef] [PubMed]
9. Burnicka-Turek, O.; Mohamed, B.A.; Shirneshan, K.; Thanasupawat, T.; Hombach-Klonisch, S.; Klonisch, T.; Adham, I.M. INSL5-deficient mice display an alteration in glucose homeostasis and an impaired fertility. *Endocrinology* **2012**, *153*, 4655–4665. [CrossRef] [PubMed]
10. Mashima, H.; Ohno, H.; Yamada, Y.; Sakai, T.; Ohnishi, H. INSL5 may be a unique marker of colorectal endocrine cells and neuroendocrine tumors. *Biochem. Biophys. Res. Commun.* **2013**, *432*, 586–592. [CrossRef] [PubMed]
11. Halls, M.L.; Bathgate, R.A.; Sutton, S.W.; Dschietzig, T.B.; Summers, R.J. International Union of Basic and Clinical Pharmacology. XCV. Recent advances in the understanding of the pharmacology and biological roles of relaxin family peptide receptors 1-4, the receptors for relaxin family peptides. *Pharmacol. Rev.* **2015**, *67*, 389–440. [CrossRef] [PubMed]
12. Bathgate, R.A.D.; Halls, M.L.; Van der Westhuizen, E.T.; Callander, G.E.; Kocan, M.; Summers, R.J. Relaxin family peptides and their receptors. *Physiol. Rev.* **2013**, *93*, 405–480. [CrossRef] [PubMed]
13. Rossato, M.; Granzotto, M.; Macchi, V.; Porzionato, A.; Petrelli, L.; Calcagno, A.; Vencato, J.; De Stefani, D.; Silvestrin, V.; Rizzuto, R.; et al. Human white adipocytes express the cold receptor TRPM8 which activation induces UCP1 expression, mitochondrial activation and heat production. *Mol. Cell. Endocrinol.* **2014**, *383*, 137–146. [CrossRef] [PubMed]
14. Editorial Office. Gastrointestinal Surgery for Severe Obesity. *Obes. Surg.* **1991**, *1*, 257–266.
15. Belligoli, A.; Sanna, M.; Serra, R.; Fabris, R.; Dal Prà, C.; Conci, S.; Fioretto, P.; Prevedello, L.; Foletto, M.; Vettor, R.; et al. Incidence and predictors of hypoglycemia 1 year after laparoscopic sleeve gastrectomy. *Obes. Surg.* **2017**, *27*, 3179–3186. [CrossRef] [PubMed]
16. Liu, C.; Kuei, C.; Sutton, S.; Chen, J.; Bonaventure, P.; Wu, J.; Nepomuceno, D.; Kamme, F.; Tran, D.T.; Zhu, J.; et al. INSL5 is a high affinity specific agonist for GPCR142 (GPR100). *J. Biol. Chem.* **2005**, *280*, 292–300. [CrossRef] [PubMed]
17. Ricardo-Silgado, M.L.; McRae, A.; Acosta, A. Role of enteroendocrine hormones in appetite and glycemia. *Obes. Med.* **2021**, *346*, 100332. [CrossRef] [PubMed]
18. Cummings, D.E.; Weigle, D.S.; Frayo, R.S.; Breen, P.A.; Ma, M.K.; Dellinger, E.P.; Purnell, J.Q. Plasma ghrelin levels after diet-induced weight loss or gastric bypass surgery. *N. Engl. J. Med.* **2002**, *346*, 1623–1630. [CrossRef] [PubMed]
19. Ang, S.Y.; Hutchinson, D.S.; Evans, B.A.; Hossain, M.A.; Patil, N.; Bathgate, R.A.; Kocan, M.; Summers, R.J. The actions of relaxin family peptides on signal transduction pathways activated by the relaxin family peptide receptor RXFP4. *Naunyn. Schmiedebergs. Arch. Pharmacol.* **2017**, *390*, 105–111. [CrossRef] [PubMed]
20. Patil, N.A.; Rosengren, K.J.; Separovic, F.; Wade, J.D.; Bathgate, R.A.D.; Hossain, M.A. Relaxin family peptides: Structure-activity relationship studies. *Br. J. Pharmacol.* **2017**, *174*, 950–961. [CrossRef] [PubMed]

Journal of
Clinical Medicine

MDPI

Article

The Effect of Laparoscopic Sleeve Gastrectomy on the Course of Non-Alcoholic Fatty Liver Disease in Morbidly Obese Patients during One Year of Follow Up

Paulina Głuszyńska [1,*], Aleksander Łukaszewicz [1], Inna Diemieszczyk [2], Jan Chilmończyk [1], Joanna Reszeć [3], Anna Citko [4], Łukasz Szczerbiński [4,5], Adam Krętowski [4,5] and Hady Razak Hady [1]

1 Department of General and Endocrine Surgery, Medical University of Bialystok, 15-276 Bialystok, Poland; alexander.luk6@gmail.com (A.Ł.); janchilmonczyk@gmail.com (J.C.); hadyrazakh@wp.pl (H.R.H.)
2 Department of Surgery, Independent Public Health Care Center in Lapy, 18-100 Lapy, Poland; demeschik.inna@gmail.com
3 Department of Medical Pathomorphology, Medical University of Bialystok, 15-269 Bialystok, Poland; joasia@umb.edu.pl
4 Clinical Research Centre, Medical University of Bialystok, 15-276 Bialystok, Poland; anna.citko@umb.edu.pl (A.C.); lukasz.szczerbinski@umb.edu.pl (Ł.S.); adam.kretowski@umb.edu.pl (A.K.)
5 Department of Endocrinology, Diabetology and Internal Diseases, Medical University of Bialystok, 15-276 Bialystok, Poland
* Correspondence: paulina.gluszynska@gmail.com; Tel.: +48-85-831-8279

Abstract: Background: Morbid obesity co-exists with non-alcoholic fatty liver disease in up to 90% of cases. Laparoscopic sleeve gastrectomy leads to a reduction in body mass and thus may improve the course of non-alcoholic fatty liver disease. The aim of this study was to evaluate the effect of laparoscopic sleeve gastrectomy on the resolution of non-alcoholic fatty liver disease. Methods: The study included 55 patients with non-alcoholic fatty liver disease who underwent laparoscopic sleeve gastrectomy at a tertiary institution. The analysis consisted of preoperative liver biopsy, abdominal ultrasound, weight loss parameters, Non-Alcoholic Fatty Liver Fibrosis Score and selected laboratory parameters. Results: Before the surgery, 6 patients were diagnosed with grade 1 liver steatosis, 33 patients with grade 2 and 16 patients with grade 3. One year after the surgery, only 21 patients had features of liver steatosis at ultrasound. All weight loss parameters showed statistically significant changes during the observation; the median percentage of total weight loss was 31.0% (IQR: 27.5; 34.5) with $p = 0.0003$, the median percentage of excess weight loss was 61.8% (IQR: 52.4; 72.3) with $p = 0.0013$ and the median percentage of excess body mass index loss was 71.0% (IQR: 61.3; 86.9) with $p = 0.0036$ 12 months after laparoscopic sleeve gastrectomy. The median Non-Alcoholic Fatty Liver Fibrosis Score at baseline was 0.2 (IQR: −0.8; 1.0) and decreased to −1.6 (IQR: −2.4; −0.4) ($p < 0.0001$). Moderate negative correlations between Non-Alcoholic Fatty Liver Fibrosis Score and percentage of total weight loss ($r = -0.434$, $p < 0.0001$), percentage of excess weight loss ($r = -0.456$, $p < 0.0001$) and percentage of excess body mass index loss ($r = -0.512$, $p < 0.0001$) were found. Conclusions: The study supports the thesis that laparoscopic sleeve gastrectomy is an effective method for treatment of non-alcoholic fatty liver disease in patients with morbid obesity.

Keywords: bariatric/metabolic surgery; laparoscopic sleeve gastrectomy; non-alcoholic fatty liver disease; morbid obesity

Citation: Głuszyńska, P.; Łukaszewicz, A.; Diemieszczyk, I.; Chilmończyk, J.; Reszeć, J.; Citko, A.; Szczerbiński, Ł.; Krętowski, A.; Razak Hady, H. The Effect of Laparoscopic Sleeve Gastrectomy on the Course of Non-Alcoholic Fatty Liver Disease in Morbidly Obese Patients during One Year of Follow Up. *J. Clin. Med.* **2023**, *12*, 4122. https://doi.org/10.3390/jcm12124122

Academic Editor: David Benaiges Boix

Received: 28 April 2023
Revised: 15 June 2023
Accepted: 16 June 2023
Published: 18 June 2023

1. Introduction

The pandemic of obesity has become a serious issue of public health worldwide as the size of the obese population has almost tripled over the last four decades and continues to rise [1]. This HAS resulted in a significant increase in the prevalence of non-alcoholic fatty liver disease (NAFLD). NAFLD is currently the most common chronic liver disease, with an estimated global prevalence at 25–30%, rising up to 90% in morbidly obese patients [2].

According to US guidelines, NAFLD is recognized when there is $\geq$ 5% steatotic hepatocytes in imaging or histology with no alcohol-, drug- or viral-induced steatosis [3]. The spectrum of NAFLD ranges from benign hepatocellular steatosis to non-alcoholic steatohepatitis (NASH), fibrosis and eventually cirrhosis and may lead to the development of hepatocellular carcinoma (HCC). It is believed that one third of patients at an early stage of NASH will progress to fibrosis within 5 to 10 years after the diagnosis. Considering indications for liver transplant, NAFLD/NASH is currently the most rapidly growing cause of HCC among patients on the waiting list in the United States, increasing from 2.1% in 2002 to 16.2% in 2016 ($p < 0.0001$) [4]. According to the US National Liver Transplantation Registry from 2018, 34.6% of liver transplant recipients had a BMI >3 0 kg/m^2, and almost 14% had a BMI > 35 kg/m^2 [5]. The main management option for obesity-related NAFLD is weight reduction by 7–10% with lifestyle modifications including dietary changes and physical activity. However, this goal may be difficult to achieve in obese patients and even more problematic to maintain. Studies have shown that more than 90% of obese patients cannot achieve this target during one year of observation [6,7]. Bariatric surgery is an option for obese individuals who fail to achieve suitable weight loss with lifestyle changes and pharmacological methods. Bariatric surgery can help obese individuals achieve recommended weight reduction and thus improve the course of NAFLD. The additional benefits of bariatric surgery include resolution or amelioration of hypertension, hyperlipidemia and type 2 diabetes and reduction of cardiovascular risk and mortality [8,9]. One of the most commonly performed bariatric procedures worldwide is laparoscopic sleeve gastrectomy (LSG). The IFSO Global Registry 2018 Report provided data from 51 different countries; data were reported on 87,467 sleeve gastrectomy operations (46.0%), 72,645 Roux-en-Y gastric bypass operations (38.2%), 14,516 one-anastomosis gastric bypass procedures (7.6%) and 9534 gastric banding operations (5.0%) [10]. LSG reduces stomach volume and also causes a decrease in ghrelin level, which is also called "a hormone of appetite" [11,12]. The following study aims to show changes in the course of NAFLD in morbidly obese patients undergoing laparoscopic sleeve gastrectomy in one year of observation and support the thesis that the above-mentioned bariatric procedure is an effective method for treating the liver manifestation of metabolic syndrome.

2. Materials and Methods

This is a retrospective study of patients who underwent laparoscopic sleeve gastrectomy and were diagnosed with liver steatosis in abdominal ultrasound prior to the surgery. The procedures were performed in the University Hospital at a tertiary institution between 2019 and 2021. Patients were qualified for surgical treatment of morbid obesity according to the Polish Guidelines on Metabolic and Bariatric Surgery [13]. The inclusion criteria for the surgical procedure comprised inability to achieve sustained weight loss with conservative management and BMI $\geq$ 40.0 kg/m^2 or 35–40 kg/m^2 with the presence of at least one obesity-related co-morbidity such as type 2 diabetes mellitus or insulin resistance, hypertension, dyslipidemia, obstructive sleep apnea, non-alcoholic fatty liver disease and non-alcoholic steatohepatitis, osteoarthritis, coronary artery disease and infertility in women resulting from polycystic ovary syndrome. Patients with obesity-related endocrine diseases, clinically significant or unstable mental health concerns and addiction to alcohol or psychostimulants and women planning on pregnancy within two years after a potential surgery were excluded from the surgical procedure. Study inclusion criteria: patients who underwent LSG as a primary obesity surgery, patients with diagnosed NAFLD based on abdominal ultrasound and no additional procedures during laparoscopic sleeve gastrectomy. The approximate time between diagnosis of NAFLD and bariatric procedure was 6 months. Exclusion criteria were viral hepatitis, autoimmune hepatitis, hemochromatosis, alcoholic liver cirrhosis and complications during the surgery or observation period. Patients were also excluded from the study when there was a lack of necessary data. Figure 1 presents the explanation of the ultimate definition of the study group.

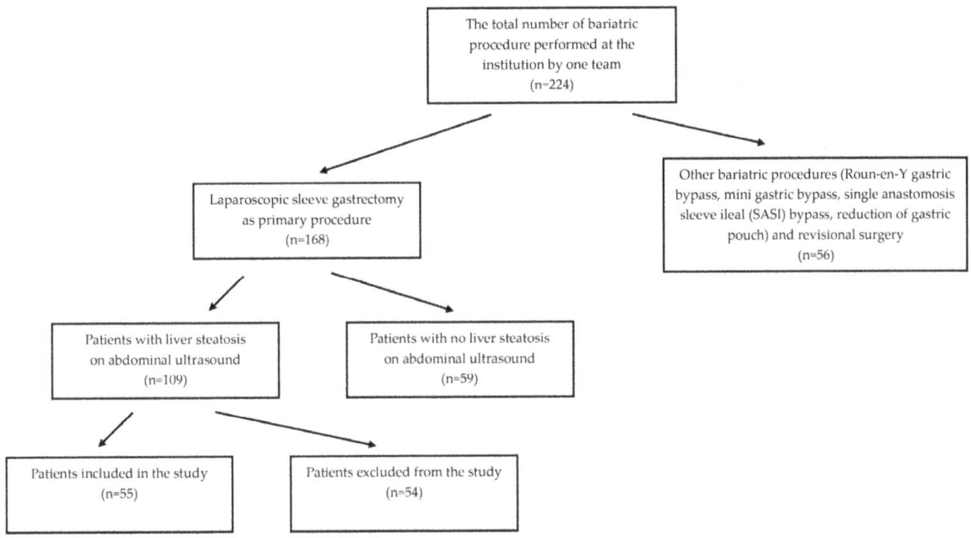

Figure 1. Graphical guidelines for study group selection.

Demographic and clinical data were gathered before the surgery, as well as 6 and 12 months after the bariatric procedure. Postoperative weight loss was expressed in terms of percent total weight loss (%TWL), percent excess weight loss (%EWL) and percent excess BMI loss (%EBMIL). The following equations were used:

- Percent total weight loss: %TWL = (initial weight-current weight)/(initial weight) × 100;
- Percent excess BMI loss: %EBMIL = (initial BMI-postoperative BMI)/(initial BMI-25) × 100;
- Percent excess weight loss: %EWL = (initial weight-postoperative weight)/(initial weight-ideal weight) × 100, where ideal weight is defined by the weight corresponding to a BMI of 25 kg/m^2.

Biochemical analysis included aspartate aminotransferase (AST), alanine aminotransferase, (ALT), gamma-glutamyl transpeptidase (GGT), lactate dehydrogenase (LDH), bilirubin, serum albumin, fasting glucose level, platelet count, total cholesterol, triglyceride, HDL cholesterol and LDL cholesterol levels.

Advanced hepatic fibrosis was assessed by the Non-Alcoholic Fatty Liver Disease Fibrosis Score (NAFLD Fibrosis Score). The calculation was performed according to the following formula:

NAFLD Fibrosis Score = $-1.675 + 0.037 \times$ age (years) $+ 0.094 \times$ BMI (kg/m^2) $+ 1.13 \times$ hyperglycemia/diabetes (yes = 1, no = 0) $+ 0.99 \times$ AST/ALT ratio $- 0.013 \times$ platelets ($\times 10^9/L - 0.66 \times$ albumin, g/dL). Values below -1.455 were considered as the absence of liver fibrosis and those above 0.676 as the presence of advanced hepatic fibrosis. Values between -1.455 and 0.676 were considered as indeterminate hepatic fibrosis [14].

Abdominal ultrasound was performed before the surgical procedure and 6 and 12 months after the surgery. Liver steatosis in abdominal ultrasound was graded as follow:

- Score 0 (absent)—normal echotexture of the liver;
- Score 1 (mild)—a slight and diffuse increase in liver echogenicity with normal visualization of the diaphragm and of the portal vein wall;
- Score 2 (moderate)—a moderate increase in liver echogenicity with slightly impaired appearance of the portal vein wall and the diaphragm;

- Score 3 (severe)—marked increase in liver echogenicity with poor or no visualization of portal vein wall, diaphragm and posterior part of the right liver lobe.

The hepatic biopsy was performed during the laparoscopic sleeve gastrectomy. Histopathological examination included the assessment of the presence or absence of steatosis, fibrosis and lobular inflammation.

2.1. Surgical Technique

The greater curvature of the stomach was dissected starting by 6 cm to the pylorus up to the His angle. The reduction in stomach volume was performed using a 36-Fr bougie and 60 mm linear staplers. At the end, the leak test was performed with the use of methylthioninium chloride solution and air. The gastric specimen was sent to pathology examination. Patients were discharged home a day after the surgery if no complications occurred.

2.2. Data Analysis

Data were analyzed using GraphPad Prism 9.0.0 software (GraphPad Software, San Diego, CA, USA). Normality of distribution was checked by the W Shapiro–Wilk test. The Wilcoxon matched-pairs signed-rank test was used for comparison between the two groups. The ANOVA Friedmann test was applied to comparisons between more than two groups and the paired Dunn's test for post hoc analysis. Continuous values are presented as medians with interquartile ranges. The correlation between examined parameters and the strength of that relationship was measured with the nonparametric Spearman rank-order correlation coefficient. The significance level was set at $p < 0.05$.

3. Results

The study group included 55 patients, 32 men (58%) and 23 women (42%). The median age of patients at the time of surgery was 43.5 years (22–54 years). The median preoperative BMI was 45.6 (IQR: 42.5; 50.2) kg/m^2. Of the patients, 62% (n = 34) had hypertension, 27% insulin resistance or type 2 diabetes (n = 15) and 41% hypercholesterolemia (n = 23). Preoperatively, 6 patients were diagnosed with grade 1 liver steatosis, 33 patients with grade 2 and 16 patients with grade 3. One year after the surgery, only 21 patients had features of liver steatosis in abdominal ultrasound—grade 1 was observed in 19 patients and grade 2 in 2 patients. The assessment of liver steatosis and its changes in abdominal ultrasound during one year of observation is presented in Table 1 and Figure 2. The analysis of preoperative liver specimens revealed hepatic steatosis in all patients, inflammatory features in 32 patients (58.2%) and liver fibrosis in 12 patients (21.8%).

Table 1. The assessment of liver steatosis in abdominal ultrasound during one year of observation.

Liver Steatosis Status \ Follow Up		0	6 Months	12 Months
Steatosis	Grade 0	N/A	20 (37%)	34 (62%)
	Grade 1	6 (11%)	20 (37%)	19 (35%)
	Grade 2	33 (60%)	13 (24%)	2 (4%)
	Grade 3	16 (29%)	2 (4%)	0
Partial remission		N/A	27 (49%)	16 (29%)
Total remission		N/A	20 (37%)	34 (62%)

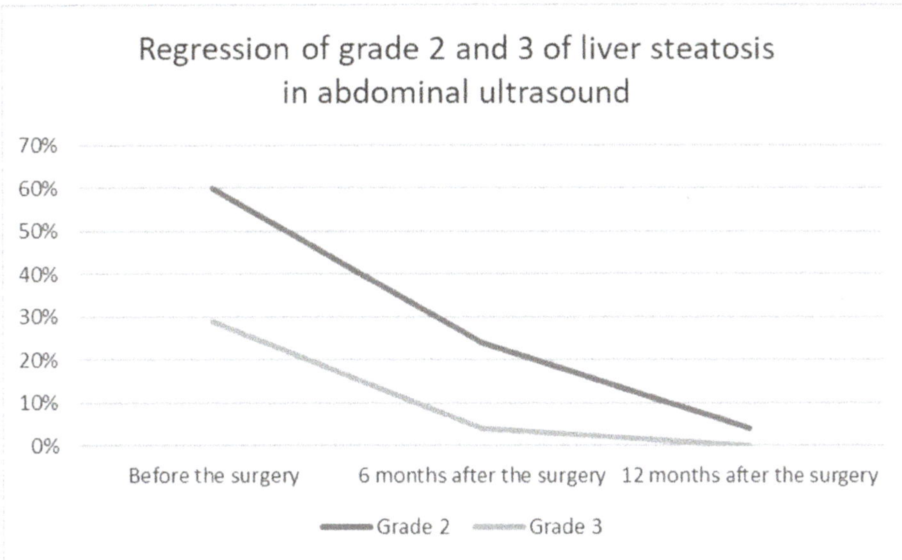

Figure 2. Graphical presentation of liver steatosis regression in abdominal ultrasound.

All parameters representing postoperative weight loss showed a statistically significant increase in one year of observation. The median %EBMIL rose from 61.8% (IQR: 53.6; 74.4) 6 months after the surgery to 71.0% (IQR: 61.3; 86.9) 12 months after the bariatric procedure ($p = 0.0036$). The median %EWL increased to 61.8% (IQR: 52.4; 72.3) with $p = 0.0013$ and median %TWL to 32.5% (IQR: 28.2; 36.9) with $p = 0.0003$ one year after the bariatric procedure. The results of bariatric effect in the study group are presented in Table 2 and Figure 3.

The amelioration in liver enzymes profile was observed in one year of follow up, including AST (25.5 (IQR: 19.0; 37.0) vs. 20.0 (IQR: 17.0; 26.0)), ALT (41.10 (IQR: 21.0; 53.9) vs. 19.0 (IQR: 16.0; 24.0)), GGT (28.5 (IQR: 21.6; 56.5) vs. 18.0 (IQR: 13.7; 35.0)) and LDH (235.0 (IQR: 186.0; 271.0) vs. 176.0 (IQR: 152.0; 184.0)). Table 3 presents changes in selected laboratory parameters and NAFLD Fibrosis Score during the observation.

Table 2. Results of bariatric effects in study group.

Variables	0	6 Months	12 Months	*p*-Value
BMI (kg/m^2)	45.6 (42.5–50.2)	33.5 (29.4–35.8)	31.0 (27.5–34.5)	**<0.0001**
%TWL	N/A	29.2 (25.2–32.4)	32.5 (28.2–36.9)	**0.0003**
%EWL	N/A	53.5 (46.3–62.4)	61.8 (52.4–72.3)	**0.0013**
%EBMIL	N/A	61.8 (53.6–74.4)	71.0 (61.3–86.9)	**0.0036**

Values are expressed as median (IQR). BMI, body mass index; %EBMIL, percentage of excess BMI loss; %EWL, percentage of excess weight loss; %TWL, percentage of total weight loss; N/A, not applicable.

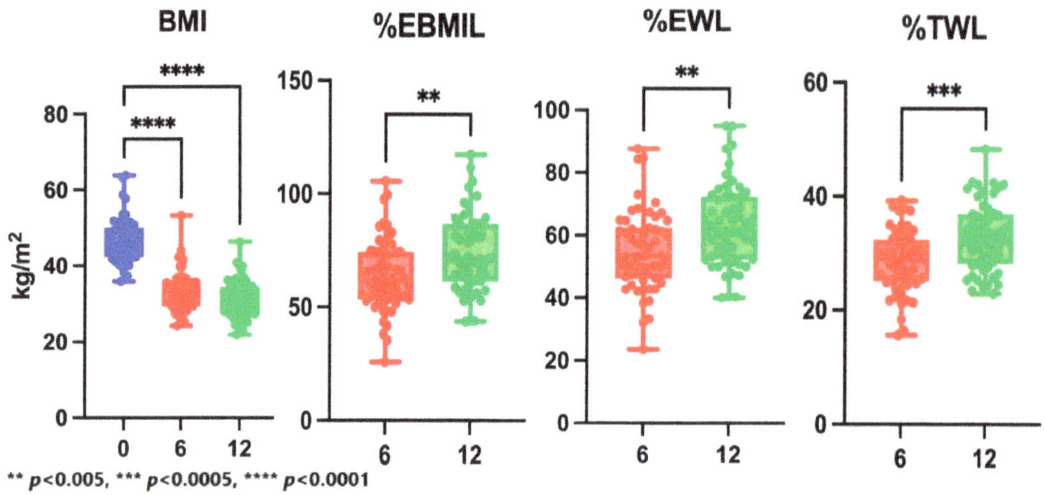

Figure 3. Changes in weight loss parameters during the observation. BMI, body mass index; %EBMIL, percentage of excess BMI loss; %EWL, percentage of excess weight loss; %TWL, percentage of total weight loss. Blue color refers to the preoperative examination, red—6 months after the surgery and green—12 months after the surgery.

Table 3. Results of selected laboratory parameters during one year of follow up.

Variables	0	6 Months	12 Months	*p*-Value
ALB (g/dL)	3.8 (3.7–3.9)	4.0 (3.9–4.2)	4.0 (3.9–4.1)	**<0.0001**
PLT ($\times 10^9$/L)	234.0 (20.5–274.0)	218.0 (190.0–276.0)	233.0 (200.0–268.0)	0.5600
FPG (mg/dL)	110.0 (94.0–130.0)	94.0 (89.0–99.0)	89.0 (83.0–96.0)	**<0.0001**
Bilirubin (mg/dL)	0.6 (0.4–0.7)	0.8(0.5–0.9)	0.9 (0.6–1.1)	**0.0002**
GGT (IU/L)	28.5 (21.6–56.5)	18.0 (12.5–27.0)	18.0 (13.7–35.0)	**0.0003**
LDH (IU/L)	235.0 (186.0–271.0)	179.0 (154.0–203.0)	176.0 (152.0–184.0)	**<0.0001**
ALT (IU/L)	41.1 (21.0–53.9)	21.0 (14.7–26.0)	19.0 (16.0–24.0)	**<0.0001**
AST (IU/L)	25.5 (19.0–37.0)	18.1 (14.0–24.0)	20.0 (17.0–26.0)	**0.0002**
Total cholesterol (mg/dL)	178.0 (148.0–193.0)	178.0 (144.0–201.0)	180.0 (153.0–180.0)	0.8285
LDL (mg/dL)	114.4 (96.3–129.0)	106.4 (82.0–133.0)	113.5 (76.0–132.6)	0.6769
HDL (mg/dL)	45.8 (37.1–50.4)	47.5 (39.8–57.6)	54.0 (46.8–65.0)	**<0.0001**
TG (mg/dL)	156.1 (112.0–215.0)	109.0 (76.0–139.0)	86.0 (61.0–134.0)	**<0.0001**
NAFLD Fibrosis Score	0.2 (−0.8–1.0)	−1.1 (−2.3–−0.2)	−1.6 (−2.4–−0.4)	**<0.0001**

Values are expressed as median (IQR). ALB, serum albumin; PLT, platelet count; FPG, fasting plasma glucose; GGT, gamma-glutamyl transpeptidase; LDH, lactate dehydrogenase (LDH); ALT, alanine transaminase; AST, aspartate transaminase; LDL, low-density lipoprotein; TG, triglyceride; HDL, high-density lipoprotein.

The median NAFLD Fibrosis Score at baseline was 0.2 (IQR: −0.8; 1.0) and decreased to −1.6 (IQR: −2.4; −0.4) one year after the surgery ($p < 0.0001$). There was a negative moderate correlation between NAFLD Fibrosis Score and mean %TWL (r = −0.434, $p < 0.0001$), %EWL (r = −0.456, $p < 0.0001$) and %EBMIL (r = −0.512, $p < 0.0001$). The assessment of the risk of advanced liver fibrosis and its changes during the observation is presented in Figure 4.

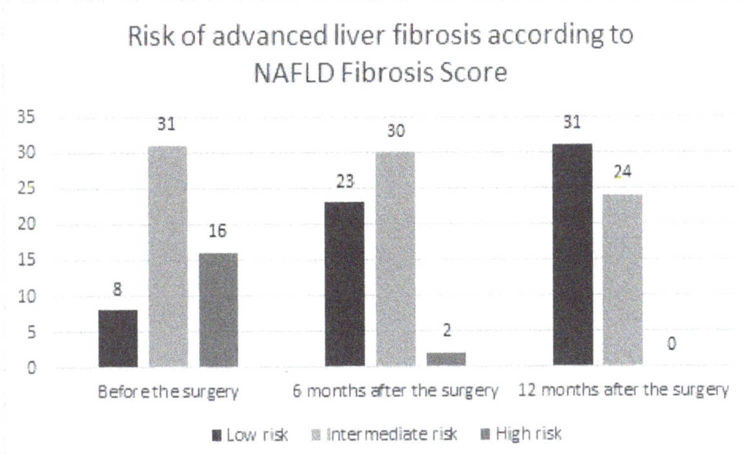

Figure 4. Risk of advanced hepatic fibrosis based on NAFLD Fibrosis Score.

4. Discussion

This study investigated the impact of one of the bariatric procedures, laparoscopic sleeve gastrectomy, on the course of non-alcoholic fatty liver disease during one year of observation.

Despite a number of promising treatment options for NAFLD, including antidiabetic and anti-obesity drugs, drugs modifying the lipid profile, vitamin E supplementation and novel therapeutic treatments inclusive of medication that interfere with inflammatory, fibrotic and apoptotic pathways, healthy lifestyle modification combined with a decrease in body mass remains at the core of management of NAFLD and NASH [15]. Dietary recommendations for individuals with obesity and non-alcoholic fatty liver disease include: reduction in energy intake, reduction in fructose consumption and a well-balanced diet comprising 40–50% energy from carbohydrates, ≤30% fat (saturated fatty acids >7% and <10% total energy) and about 20% protein [16]. However, very often, the above recommendations are difficult to fulfill, and obese patients fail to achieve the expected weight loss. Several studies have shown that laparoscopic sleeve gastrectomy causes significant weight loss over both short- and long-term observation periods [17–19]. Kraljević et al. analyzed 307 patients who underwent LSG as a primary bariatric procedure. The mean %EBMIL was 62.8 ± 23.1% after 5 years, 53.6 ± 24.6% after 10 years and 51.2 ± 20.3% after 13 years [20]. Our study also proved that laparoscopic sleeve gastrectomy contributes to considerable body mass reduction in patients with morbid obesity, reaching a median %EBMIL of 71.0% (IQR: 61.3; 86.9) after 12 months. Algooneh et al. analyzed the impact of %EWL on the resolution of NAFLD. A significant resolution of NAFLD was seen in patients achieving a mean %EWL > 50% (OR 10.1; $p < 0.001$). However, resolution of NAFLD was observed even in patients with a mean %EWL of 30% (OR 7.0, $p = 0.024$) [21]. In this study, the median percentage of excess weight loss reached 61.8% (IQR: 52.4; 72.3) one year after laparoscopic sleeve gastrectomy.

In a study conducted by Mattar et al., it was observed that weight loss induced by bariatric surgery (Roux-en-Y gastric bypass (RYGB) or LSG) causes significant improvement or resolution of NAFLD and NASH in liver histology, including steatosis, inflammation and fibrosis [22]. Fakhry et al. conducted a wide metanalysis that included 21 studies with a total number of 2374 patients who had undergone bariatric surgery (vertical-banded gastroplasty (VGB), laparoscopic adjustable gastric banding (LAGB), RYGB or LSG). They provided strong evidence that bariatric surgery not only improves biochemical and histological features of NAFLD but also terminates the progression of the disease and resolves it in up to 30% of patients [23]. In our study, the total resolution rate for liver steatosis in abdominal ultrasound was 62% (34 patients) one year after laparoscopic sleeve gastrectomy.

Bower et al. conducted a systematic review and proved that bariatric surgery is associated with improvement of the histological features of NAFLD, including steatosis (50.2 and 95%CI of 35.5–65.0), fibrosis (11.9 and 95% CI of 7.4–16.3%) and lobular inflammation (50.7 and 95% CI, 26.6–74.8%) [24]. Another metanalysis that included 32 cohort studies comprising 3093 biopsy specimens showed that bariatric surgery is an effective method for the treatment of NAFLD, resulting in biopsy-confirmed resolution of steatosis in 66% patients (95% CI, 56–75%), inflammation in 50% (95% CI, 35–64%), ballooning degeneration in 76% (95% CI, 64–86%) and fibrosis in 40% (95% CI, 29–51%). However, this metanalysis showed new features or worsening of NAFLD in 12% (95% CI, 5–20%) of patients [25]. Moretto et al. analyzed 78 morbidly obese patients who had undergone gastric bypass and had undergone liver biopsy during the surgery and after weight loss. They found that the prevalence of liver fibrosis was 44.9% (CI 95% 33.6–56.6%) at the first biopsy and 30.8% (CI 95% 20.8–42.2%) after weight loss ($p = 0.027$) [26]. However, it is also known that rapid weight loss may increase the risk of hepatic fibrosis. Weight loss of more than 1.6 kg per week results in a rapid reduction in hepatic fat and a subsequent increase in visceral free fatty acids and proinflammatory cytokines, which may worsen the course of the histological features of NAFLD [27]. An interesting observation was made by Mathurin et al. Their research showed that the improvement of steatosis and ballooning occurred mainly during the first year after bariatric surgery and persisted up to 5 years postoperatively. However, they noticed that liver fibrosis worsened at 5 years even though more than 95% of patients had a Fibrosis Score $\leq$ F1 [28]. The research conducted by Mottin et al. showed that 16 out of 90 patients (17.8%) who underwent bariatric surgery had the same degree of liver steatosis at the second biopsy as during the operation [29].

A study conducted by Ruiz-Tover et al. showed that liver steatosis measured by abdominal ultrasound improves after sleeve gastrectomy. A complete resolution in liver steatosis was observed in 90% of patients included in their study [30]. Complete resolution measured by ultrasonography in our study was seen in 62% of all patients. Another study conducted by Elyasinia et al. proved that both laparoscopic sleeve gastrectomy and gastric bypass significantly enhance hepatic status in ultrasonography. Preoperatively, 81.8% of patients were diagnosed with grade I or II liver steatosis. One year after the surgery, 72.7% of patients presented no NASH signs in ultrasonography [31]. According to our study, 19 patients (34.5%) had grade 1 liver steatosis in abdominal ultrasonography after one year of observation.

The previously mentioned research conducted by Bower et al. also confirmed an amelioration in liver enzymes profile, including ALT (11.36 u/L, 95%CI 8.36–14.39), AST (3.91 u/L, 95%CI 2.23–5.59), ALP (10.55 u/L, 95%CI 4.40–16.70) and gamma-GT (18.39 u/L, 95%CI 12.62–24.16) [19]. A study conducted by Kirkpatrick et al. revealed a reduction in liver enzymes including ALT (66.21 vs. 28.58) and AST (46.28 vs. 24.69) during 12 months of observation [32]. Groth et al. also observed an amelioration in the liver enzymes profile in patients undergoing laparoscopic sleeve gastrectomy during 6 months of follow up (AST 22.0 (19.0–28.0) vs. 16.0 (13.0–22.0), $p < 0.001$, and ALT 27.5 (20.5–41.0) vs. 19.0 (15.0–27.0), $p < 0.001$) with no statistical differences regarding gender ($p = 0.840$) [33]. Similar results were observed in our study. We noted a statistically significant reduction in AST, ALT, GGT and LDH serum activity. A reduction of transaminase levels decreases the risk of progression to fibrosis and the end stage of liver disease. Additionally, Lee et al. proved that patients with elevated serum aminotransferase levels are at a higher risk not only of liver disease but also of all-cause mortality [34].

Nascimento et al. analyzed changes in NAFLD Fibrosis Score before and after bariatric surgery. The NAFLD Fibrosis Score changed from -0.6845 before the surgery to -1.6898 12 months after the procedure ($p < 0.0002$), indicating an absence of advanced liver fibrosis in any patient 12 months after the surgery [35]. An intermediate degree of fibrosis was identified in 12 patients (46.2%) one year after the bariatric procedure. The research conducted by Yang et al. also revealed statistically significant changes in the NAFLD score (−1.636 vs. −2.123, $p < 0.001$) over a two-year observation period [36]. Sandvik et al. observed a significant overall shift towards lower risk categories of advanced hepatic fibrosis based on NAFLD Fibrosis Score in 11.6 years of observation (NAFLD Fibrosis Score −1.32 (IQR −2.33; −0.39) vs. −1.71 (IQR −2.49; −0.95, $p < 0.001$) 11.6 years after surgery). In the above-mentioned study, a weak negative correlation between the decrease in NAFLD Fibrosis Score and weight loss parameters (%EWL (r = −0.251, $p < 0.0001$) and %TWL (r = −0.280, $p < 0.0001$)) was observed [37]. In our study, a statistically significant decrease in NAFLD Fibrosis Score was also seen. Additionally, we found a moderate negative correlation between NAFLD Fibrosis Score and weight loss parameters, including the percentage of total and excess weight loss and the percentage of excess BMI loss. Salman et al. analyzed patients with NASH-related liver cirrhosis of Child class A scheduled for laparoscopic sleeve gastrectomy due to morbid obesity. In their observation, the fibrosis score regressed to F2 in 19 patients (26.8%) and F3 in 29 (40.8%) during 30 months of follow up. Additionally, patients with improved Fibrosis Score had significantly higher weight loss ($p <0.001$). Thirty months after surgical treatment, 53.8% of cases with borderline NASH and 36.8% of those with probable NASH showed complete resolution. This study proved that bariatric surgery may be an option in patients with NASH-related hepatic fibrosis and morbid obesity [38]. In a study conducted by Murakami et al., the NAFLD activity score was reduced in 10 of the 11 patients (90.9%), and there was a significant difference between before and 1 year after laparoscopic sleeve gastrectomy ($p < 0.05$). Non-alcoholic steatohepatitis was no longer demonstrated in 81.8% patients in liver biopsy 1 year after the surgery; however, the fibrosis stage did not significantly ameliorate 1 year after laparoscopic sleeve gastrectomy [39].

The main limitation of our study is the fact that postoperative liver steatosis was evaluated with ultrasonography and not by hepatic biopsy to examine histological features of NAFLD. Some researchers may question ultrasonography as an imaging tool to predict the presence and severity of liver steatosis based on the fact that it is a performer-dependent and subjective imaging method. Generalizability of our results could be also impaired by the low number of participants, and therefore it is important to remember that some patients undergoing laparoscopic sleeve gastrectomy will not experience the amelioration of liver steatosis during observation. The surgical procedure may not always improve the grade of hepatic steatosis, or, in rare cases, it may even worsen the condition of the liver. Additionally, longer observation could be performed in order to achieve strong evidence that LSG improves the course of NAFLD.

5. Conclusions

In conclusion, our study confirms the thesis that laparoscopic sleeve gastrectomy is an effective method for the treatment of NAFLD in morbidly obese patients. Weight loss induced by LSG resolved NAFLD in more than 50% of patients according to ultrasound features of steatosis in one year of observation. Laparoscopic sleeve gastrectomy led to significant decrease in liver enzymes concentration and a reduction in NAFLD Fibrosis Score. Considering the increasing global prevalence of NAFLD, laparoscopic sleeve gastrectomy may be a crucial method of treatment in patients with morbid obesity and hepatic steatosis.

Author Contributions: Conceptualization, P.G. and A.Ł.; methodology, P.G. and I.D.; software, A.Ł. and J.C.; formal analysis, P.G., I.D. and J.C.; investigation, P.G., H.R.H., J.R. and A.C.; writing—original draft preparation, P.G. and I.D.; writing—review and editing, all authors; supervision, Ł.S., H.R.H. and A.K. All authors have read and agreed to the published version of the manuscript.

Funding: This research received no external funding.

Institutional Review Board Statement: The study was conducted according to the guidelines of the Declaration of Helsinki and approved by the Bioethics Committee of the Medical University of Bialystok (the reference numbers of the consent: R-I-002/248/2018 and R-I-002/386/2018).

Informed Consent Statement: Written informed consent was obtained from all individual participants included in the study.

Data Availability Statement: Not applicable.

Conflicts of Interest: The authors declare no conflict of interest.

References

1. Chauhan, M.; Singh, K.; Thuluvath, P.J. Bariatric Surgery in NAFLD. *Dig. Dis. Sci.* **2022**, *67*, 408–422. [CrossRef] [PubMed]
2. Fazel, Y.; Koenig, A.B.; Sayiner, M.; Goodman, Z.D.; Younossi, Z.M. Epidemiology and natural history of nonalcoholic fatty liver disease. *Metabolism* **2016**, *65*, 1017–1025. [CrossRef]
3. Chalasani, N.; Younossi, Z.; Lavine, J.E.; Diehl, A.M.; Brunt, M.E.; Cusi, K.; Charlton, M.; Sanyal, J.A. The diagnosis and management of non-alcoholic fatty liver disease: Practice guideline by the American Gastroenterological Association, American Association for the Study of Liver Diseases, and American College of Gastroenterology. *Gastroenterology* **2012**, *142*, 1592–1609.
4. Younossi, Z.; Stepanova, M.; Ong, J.P.; Jacobson, I.M.; Bugianesi, E.; Duseja, A.; Eguchi, Y.; Wong, V.W.; Negro, F.; Yilmaz, Y.; et al. Nonalcoholic steatohepatitis is the fastest growing cause of hepatocellular carcinoma in liver transplant candidates. *Clin. Gastroenterol. Hepatol.* **2019**, *17*, 748–755.e3. [CrossRef]
5. Kwong, A.; Kim, W.R.; Lake, J.R.; Smith, J.M.; Schladt, D.P.; Skeans, M.A.; Noreen, S.M.; Foutz, J.; Miller, E.; Snyder, J.J.; et al. OPTN/SRTR 2018 annual data report: Liver. *Am. J. Transpl.* **2020**, *20*, 193–299. [CrossRef] [PubMed]
6. Chalasani, N.; Younossi, Z.; Lavine, J.E.; Diehl, A.M.; Brunt, E.M.; Cusi, K.; Charlton, M.; Sanyal, A.J. The diagnosis and management of nonalcoholic fatty liver disease: Practice Guideline by the American Association for the Study of Liver Diseases, American College of Gastroenterology, and the American Gastroenterological Association. *Hepatology* **2012**, *55*, 2005–2023. [CrossRef]
7. Vilar-Gomez, E.; Martinez-Perez, Y.; Calzadilla-Bertot, L.; Torres-Gonzalez, A.; Gra-Oramas, B.; Gonzalez-Fabian, L.; Friedman, S.L.; Diago, M.; Romero-Gomez, M. Weight loss through lifestyle modification significantly reduces features of nonalcoholic steatohepatitis. *Gastroenterology* **2015**, *149*, 367–378.e15. [CrossRef] [PubMed]
8. Diemieszczyk, I.; Woźniewska, P.; Gołaszewski, P.; Drygalski, K.; Nadolny, K.; Ładny, J.R.; Hady, H.R. Does weight loss after laparoscopic sleeve gastrectomy contribute to reduction in blood pressure? *Pol. Arch. Intern. Med.* **2021**, *131*, 693–700. [CrossRef]
9. Doumouras, A.G.; Wong, J.A.; Paterson, J.M.; Lee, Y.; Sivapathasundaram, B.; Tarride, J.E.; Thabane, L.; Hong, D.; Yusuf, S.; Anvari, M. Bariatric Surgery and Cardiovascular Outcomes in Patients with Obesity and Cardiovascular Disease: A Population-Based Retrospective Cohort Study. *Circulation* **2021**, *143*, 1468–1480. [CrossRef]
10. Welbourn, R.; Hollyman, M.; Kinsman, R.; Dixon, J.; Liem, R.; Ottosson, J.; Ramos, A.; Våge, V.; Al-Sabah, S.; Brown, W.; et al. Bariatric Surgery Worldwide: Baseline Demographic Description and One-Year Outcomes from the Fourth IFSO Global Registry Report 2018. *Obes. Surg.* **2019**, *29*, 782–795.
11. Ali, M.; Khan, S.A.; Mushtaq, M.; Haider, S.A. Comparison of Laparoscopic Sleeve Gastrectomy (LSG) with Laparoscopic Gastric Bypass (LRYGB) in Bariatric Surgery. *Cureus* **2021**, *13*, e14022. [CrossRef]
12. Wang, Y.; Guo, X.; Lu, X.; Mattar, S.; Kassab, G. Mechanisms of Weight Loss After Sleeve Gastrectomy and Adjustable Gastric Banding: Far More Than Just Restriction. *Obesity* **2019**, *27*, 1776–1783. [CrossRef]
13. Budzyński, A.; Major, P. Polskie rekomendacje w zakresie chirurgii bariatrycznej i metabolicznej. *Med. Prakt.–Chir.* **2016**, *6*, 13–25.
14. Schmitz, S.M.; Kroh, A.; Ulmer, T.F.; Andruszkow, J.; Luedde, T.; Brozat, J.F.; Neumann, U.P.; Alizai, P.H. Evaluation of NAFLD and fibrosis in obese patients—A comparison of histological and clinical scoring systems. *BMC Gastroenterol.* **2020**, *20*, 254. [CrossRef]
15. Głuszyńska, P.; Lemancewicz, D.; Dzięcioł, J.B.; Razak Hady, H. Non-Alcoholic Fatty Liver Disease (NAFLD) and Bariatric/Metabolic Surgery as Its Treatment Option: A Review. *J. Clin. Med.* **2021**, *10*, 5721. [CrossRef] [PubMed]
16. Kargulewicz, A.; Stankowiak-Kulpa, H.; Grzymisławski, M. Dietary recommendations for patients with nonalcoholic fatty liver disease. *Prz. Gastroenterol.* **2014**, *9*, 18–23. [CrossRef] [PubMed]
17. Murshid, K.R.; Alsisi, G.H.; Almansouri, F.A.; Zahid, M.M.; Boghdadi, A.A.; Mahmoud, E.H. Laparoscopic sleeve gastrectomy for weight loss and treatment of type 2 diabetes mellitus. *J. Taibah Univ. Med. Sci.* **2021**, *16*, 387–394. [CrossRef]
18. Diamantis, T.; Apostolou, K.G.; Alexandrou, A.; Griniatsos, J.; Felekouras, E.; Tsigris, C. Review of long-term weight loss results after laparoscopic sleeve gastrectomy. *Surg. Obes. Relat. Dis.* **2014**, *10*, 177–183. [CrossRef]
19. Hirth, D.A.; Jones, E.L.; Rothchild, K.B.; Mitchell, B.C.; Schoen, J.A. Laparoscopic sleeve gastrectomy: Long-term weight loss outcomes. *Surg. Obes. Relat. Dis.* **2015**, *11*, 1004–1007. [CrossRef]
20. Kraljević, M.; Cordasco, V.; Schneider, R.; Peters, T.; Slawik, M.; Wölnerhanssen, B.; Peterli, R. Long-term Effects of Laparoscopic Sleeve Gastrectomy: What Are the Results Beyond 10 Years? *Obes. Surg.* **2021**, *31*, 3427–3433. [CrossRef]
21. Algooneh, A.; Almazeedi, S.; Al-Sabah, S.; Ahmed, M.; Othman, F. Non-alcoholic fatty liver disease resolution following sleeve gastrectomy. *Surg. Endosc.* **2016**, *30*, 1983–1987. [CrossRef] [PubMed]
22. Mattar, S.G.; Velcu, L.M.; Rabinovitz, M.; Demetris, A.J.; Krasinskas, A.M.; Barinas-Mitchell, E.; Eid, G.M.; Ramanathan, R.; Taylor, D.S.; Schauer, P.R. Surgically-induced weight loss significantly improves nonalcoholic fatty liver disease and the metabolic syndrome. *Ann. Surg.* **2005**, *242*, 610–617. [CrossRef]

23. Fakhry, T.K.; Mhaskar, R.; Schwitalla, T.; Muradova, E.; Gonzalvo, J.P.; Murr, M.M. Bariatric surgery improves nonalcoholic fatty liver disease: A contemporary systematic review and meta-analysis. *Surg. Obes. Relat. Dis.* **2019**, *15*, 502–511. [CrossRef]
24. Bower, G.; Toma, T.; Harling, L.; Jiao, L.R.; Efthimiou, E.; Darzi, A.; Athanasiou, T.; Ashrafian, H. Bariatric Surgery and Non-Alcoholic Fatty Liver Dis-ease: A Systematic Review of Liver Biochemistry and Histology. *Obes. Surg.* **2015**, *25*, 2280–2289. [CrossRef]
25. Lee, Y.; Doumouras, A.G.; Yu, J.; Brar, K.; Banfield, L.; Gmora, S.; Anvari, M.; Hong, D. Complete Resolution of Nonalcoholic Fatty Liver Disease After Bariatric Surgery: A Systematic Review and Meta-analysis. *Clin. Gastroenterol. Hepatol.* **2019**, *17*, 1040–1060.e11. [CrossRef]
26. Moretto, M.; Kupski, C.; da Silva, V.D.; Padoin, A.V.; Mottin, C.C. Effect of bariatric surgery on liver fibrosis. *Obes. Surg.* **2012**, *22*, 1044–1049. [CrossRef] [PubMed]
27. Gasteyger, C.; Larsen, T.M.; Vercruysse, F.; Astrup, A. Effect of a dietary-induced weight loss on liver enzymes in obese subjects. *Am. J. Clin. Nutr.* **2008**, *87*, 1141–1147. [CrossRef] [PubMed]
28. Mathurin, P.; Hollebecque, A.; Arnalsteen, L.; Buob, D.; Leteurtre, E.; Caiazzo, R.; Pigeyre, M.; Verkindt, H.; Dharancy, S.; Louvet, A.; et al. Prospective study of the long-term effects of bariatric surgery on liver injury in patients without advanced disease. *Gastroenterology* **2009**, *137*, 532–540. [CrossRef] [PubMed]
29. Mottin, C.C.; Moretto, M.; Padoin, A.V.; Kupski, C.; Swarowsky, A.M.; Glock, L.; Duval, V.; Braga da Silva, J. Histological behavior of hepatic steatosis in morbidly obese patients after weight loss induced by bariatric surgery. *Obes. Surg.* **2005**, *15*, 788–793. [CrossRef] [PubMed]
30. Ruiz-Tovar, J.; Alsina, M.E.; Alpera, M.R.; OBELCHE Group. Improvement of nonalcoholic fatty liver disease in morbidly obese patients after sleeve gastrectomy: Association of ultrasonographic findings with lipid profile and liver enzymes. *Acta Chir. Belg.* **2017**, *117*, 363–369. [CrossRef]
31. Elyasinia, F.; Jalali, S.M.; Zarini, S.; Sadeghian, E.; Sorush, A.; Pirouz, A. The Effect of Laparoscopic Sleeve Gastrectomy and Gastric Bypass Surgery on Non-Alcoholic Steatohepatitis in Iranian Patients with Obesity. *Middle East J. Dig. Dis.* **2021**, *13*, 200–207. [CrossRef] [PubMed]
32. Kirkpatrick, K.; Paull-Forney, B.; Okut, H.; Schwasinger-Schmidt, T. Bariatric Metabolic Surgery Reduced Liver Enzyme Levels in Patients with Non-Alcohol Fatty Liver Disease. *Kans. J. Med.* **2021**, *14*, 209–214. [CrossRef]
33. Groth, D.; Woźniewska, P.; Olszewska, M.; Zabielski, P.; Ładny, J.R.; Dadan, J.; Zalewska, A.; Błachnio-Zabielska, A.; Diemieszczyk, I.; Krętowski, A.; et al. Gender-related metabolic outcomes of laparoscopic sleeve gastrectomy in 6-month follow-up. *Wideochir. Inne Tech. Maloinwazyjne* **2020**, *15*, 148–156. [CrossRef]
34. Lee, H.; Shin, D.W.; Lee, T.H.; Yang, H.K.; Ahn, E.; Yoon, J.M.; Lee, H.K.; Suh, B.; Son, K.Y.; Kim, J.S.; et al. Association Between Change in Serum Aminotransferase and Mortality: A Nationwide Cohort Study in Korea. *Medicine* **2016**, *95*, e3158. [CrossRef] [PubMed]
35. Nascimento, T.M.; Alves-Júnior, A.; Nunes, M.A.; de Freitas, T.R.; da Silva, M.A.; Alves, M.R. Comparison of hepatic profile in pre and postoperative of bariatric surgery: Private vs. public network. *Arq. Bras. Cir. Dig.* **2015**, *28*, 274–277. [CrossRef] [PubMed]
36. Yang, A.; Nguyen, M.; Ju, I.; Brancatisano, A.; Ryan, B.; van der Poorten, D. Utility of Fibroscan XL to assess the severity of non-alcoholic fatty liver disease in patients undergoing bariatric surgery. *Sci. Rep.* **2021**, *11*, 14006. [CrossRef] [PubMed]
37. Sandvik, E.C.S.; Aasarød, K.M.; Johnsen, G.; Hoff, D.A.L.; Kulseng, B.; Hyldmo, Å.A.; Græslie, H.; Nymo, S.; Sandvik, J.; Fossmark, R. The Effect of Roux-en-Y Gastric Bypass on Non-Alcoholic Fatty Liver Disease Fibrosis Assessed by FIB-4 and NFS Scores-An 11.6-Year Follow-Up Study. *J. Clin. Med.* **2022**, *11*, 4910. [CrossRef] [PubMed]
38. Salman, M.A.; Mikhail, H.M.S.; Nafea, M.A.; Sultan, A.A.E.A.; Elshafey, H.E.; Tourky, M.; Awad, A.; Abouelregal, T.E.; Ahmed, R.A.; Ashoush, O.; et al. Impact of laparoscopic sleeve gastrectomy on fibrosis stage in patients with child-A NASH-related cirrhosis. *Surg. Endosc.* **2021**, *35*, 1269–1277. [CrossRef] [PubMed]
39. Murakami, E.; Nakahara, T.; Hiramatsu, A.; Morio, K.; Fujino, H.; Yamauchi, M.; Kawaoka, T.; Tsuge, M.; Imamura, M.; Aikata, H.; et al. Therapeutic effects of sleeve gastrectomy for non-alcoholic steatohepatitis estimated by paired liver biopsy in morbidly obese Japanese patients. *Medicine* **2021**, *100*, e26436. [CrossRef] [PubMed]

Journal of
Clinical Medicine

MDPI

Article

Combined Effect of Genetic Variants on Long-Term Weight Response after Bariatric Surgery

Macarena Torrego-Ellacuría [1], Ana Barabash [1,2,3], Pilar Matía-Martín [1,2], Andrés Sánchez-Pernaute [2,4], Antonio J. Torres [2,4], Alfonso L. Calle-Pascual [1,2,3] and Miguel A. Rubio-Herrera [1,2,*]

1 Department of Endocrinology and Nutrition, Hospital Clínico San Carlos, IdISSC, 28040 Madrid, Spain; macarena.torrego@gmail.com (M.T.-E.)
2 Faculty of Medicine, Department of Medicine, Universidad Complutense, 28040 Madrid, Spain
3 Centro de Investigación Biomédica en Red de Diabetes y Enfermedades Metabólicas Asociadas (CIBERDEM), 28040 Madrid, Spain
4 Department of Surgery, Hospital Clínico San Carlos, IdISSC, 28040 Madrid, Spain
* Correspondence: marubioh@gmail.com

Abstract: The pathophysiology of body weight control involves complex interactions between hormonal, environmental, behavioral and genetic factors. The purpose of this study was to analyze the association between single nucleotide polymorphisms (SNPs) of 13 genes encoding gastrointestinal peptides, their receptors or the proteins involved in their expression, with long-term weight response in a cohort of 375 patients undergoing bariatric surgery (BS). To evaluate weight response, we combined several variables to define specific response phenotypes six years after surgery. The study protocol was registered in ISRCTN (ID80961259). The analysis of the selected SNPs was performed via allelic discrimination using Taqman® probes (Applied Biosystems, Foster City, CA, USA). The genotype association study was performed using the SNPstat program, with comparisons adjusted for sex, age, initial body mass index, type 2 diabetes, hypertension diagnosis and the type of surgery. We identified eight genetic variants associated with the weight response to BS, independently of the presurgery patient profile and the type of surgical technique, from which we calculated the unweighted risk score (RS) for each phenotype. The highest scoring category in each RS was significantly associated with lower weight loss ($p = 0.0001$) and greater weight regain ($p = 0.0012$) at the end of the follow-up.

Keywords: risk score; SNP; bariatric surgery; weight regain; weight loss

Citation: Torrego-Ellacuría, M.; Barabash, A.; Matía-Martín, P.; Sánchez-Pernaute, A.; Torres, A.J.; Calle-Pascual, A.L.; Rubio-Herrera, M.A. Combined Effect of Genetic Variants on Long-Term Weight Response after Bariatric Surgery. *J. Clin. Med.* **2023**, *12*, 4288. https://doi.org/10.3390/jcm12134288

Academic Editors: David Benaiges Boix and Akira Tsuburaya

Received: 16 May 2023
Revised: 21 June 2023
Accepted: 23 June 2023
Published: 26 June 2023

1. Introduction

Bariatric surgery (BS) achieves substantial and persistent effects on weight loss in patients with morbid obesity (MO) and improves the management of obesity-associated comorbidities [1–4]. However, there is inter-individual variability in terms of the maximum weight loss achieved [5,6] and long-term weight regain [7,8]. Genetic variation among individuals underlies the variety of physiological responses in the context of BS, caloric restriction and altered gastrointestinal hormones [9], with a lower degree of variability in weight loss observed in genetically related subjects compared to genetically unrelated matched individuals in the medium to long term after the intervention [10].

Genome-wide association studies (GWAS) have identified more than 300 single nucleotide polymorphism (SNP) involved in eating behavior and energy expenditure, associated with body mass index (BMI) and adiposity traits [11–13]; however, in BS intervention, studies are very limited [14]. Since 2003, Genetic Risk Score (GRS) studies have been conducted to study weight loss and BMI evolution after BS, based on groups of SNPs in loci identified in previous GWASs and replicated in various populations [12,15–17]. Depending on the study, the SNPs included Vary. The results of the GRS studies suggest that some variants may modulate differences in weight response to BS, but there is little evidence generated on the subject.

The primary objective of our work was to identify genetic markers associated with weight loss and its long-term maintenance after different BS surgical techniques. Considering the physiological mechanisms involving gastrointestinal peptides and their signaling in the appetite-regulating brain nuclei involved in body weight control at gastrointestinal and hypothalamic level [18,19], the genetic variants selected encode for peptides, their receptors or the proteins involved in their expression that are implicated in the control of energy intake and expenditure.

2. Materials and Methods

This is a single-center retrospective study based on a prospective database from the Hospital Clinico San Carlos, Madrid (HCSC). The cohort included 375 patients aged between 18 and 65 years (BMI > 40 kg/m^2 or BMI $\geq$ 35 kg/m^2 associated with comorbidity) that were selected from a cohort of 510 subjects who underwent a first bariatric surgical procedure between 2009 and 2014, after applying the exclusion criteria previously reported [20] together with the exclusion of subjects of Latin ethnicity and without genotyping. The project was approved by the HCSC Clinical Research Ethics Committee (16 February 2009). The study protocol was registered at https://www.isrctn.com/ (accessed on 1 January 2023) (ID ISRCTN80961259). Demographic, clinical and anthropometric information was collected in the electronic health records prior to surgery. Type 2 diabetes (T2D) and hypertension (HTN) were diagnosed and categorized. The different surgical techniques (STs) were sleeve gastrectomy (SG), Roux-en-Y gastric bypass (RYGB), biliopancreatic diversion with or without duodenal switch (BPD-DS) and single anastomosis duodeno-ileal bypass with sleeve gastrectomy (SADI-S), as malabsorptive procedures. The type of surgical technique was chosen according to clinical practice criteria of hospital protocol based on age, BMI and comorbidities.

The 375 cases were followed up after surgery, with annual appointments up to 8 years with weight measurements [20]. The main variables for assessing weight response include the percentage of total weight lost (%TWL), the percentage of excess weight loss (%EWL), with ideal weight calculated for a BMI of 25 kg/m^2 and WR as a percentage of maximum weight loss (%WR_MWL) [21]. Nadir weight was determined based on all the postoperative weight measures available, considering the lowest value. The end of clinical follow-up was established in year 6 since it was the common period of follow-up of the entire sample according to the inclusion dates.

2.1. Selection of Candidate SNPs

The genetic variants included in the association study with weight response were 48 SNP-like variants of 13 genes: GHSR, WFS1, BDNF, MC4R, GIPR, DPPIV, NPYR, CLOCK, GLP1R, TCF7L2, KCNJ11, FTO and PYY. Table 1 lists the genes and SNPs included, with the reference allele in each category. The genetic variants of the CLOCK gene (rs3749474, rs1801260 and rs4580704) were analyzed in a previous work undertaken by our group [22].

The genetic variants included were chosen following the candidate gene selection strategy. On the one hand, the SNPs of genes, which have been previously described as being associated with obesity or weight response phenotypes, or which have functional repercussions (modification of protein expression or structure), were studied directly (MC4R, FTO, BDNF, GHSR, WFS1, GIPR, TCF7L2, KCNJ11 and CLOCK genes). For candidate genes where no associated phenotype has yet been described (GLP1R, DPPIV, NPYR and PYY genes), a haplotype study was performed using a tagSNP approach. The selection of the tag SNPs (minimum allele frequency MAF—greater than 5%) was carried out by consulting public-domain specialized databases for each candidate gene (HapMap International public project [23], dbSNP [24] and Ensembl project [25]). To identify the tag SNPs, the Haploview 4.1 program was used, which handles the data from the aforementioned databases. We included tag SNPs that allow for the detection of haplotypes with a frequency higher than 10% in the Caucasian population.

Table 1. Genes and SNP included in the association study.

Candidate Gen	SNP	Reference Allele	Assay ID
GHSR	rs572169	C	C___1079489_20
WFS1	rs10010131	A	C__30473796_10
BDNF	rs6265	C	C__11592758_10
MC4R	rs17782313	T	C__32667060_10
GIPR	rs10423928	T	C__30103605_10
DPPIV	rs17759529	C	C__34245343_10
DPPIV	rs2389643	C	C__15784426_10
DPPIV	rs2268889	C	C__15875589_10
DPPIV	rs12995983	T	C___2789708_20
DPPIV	rs3788979	C	C___2789710_10
DPPIV	rs741529	G	C___2789719_10
DPPIV	rs12469968	G	C___2789726_10
DPPIV	rs1861975	A	C___2789730_10
NPY2R	rs6849115	T	C__30852111_10
NPY2R	rs11099992	A	C_____44829_10
NPY2R	rs6857715	C	C__29013142_10
NPY2R	rs1047214	C	C___7427258_20
NPY2R	rs17304901	G	C__32705343_10
NPY2R	rs11728843	G	C__30852113_10
NPY1R	rs9764	T	C___8788046_10
NPY1R	rs7687423	A	C___8066900_10
NPY1R	rs11100489	T	C__31208177_10
NPY5R	rs11100493	T	C_____74249_10
NPY5R	rs4632602	C	C__29684077_20
NPY5R	rs11724320	T	C_____74248_10
NPY5R	rs7678265	C	C_____74246_30
CLOCK	rs3749474	C	C__26405955_10
CLOCK	rs1801260	A	C___8746719_20
CLOCK	rs4580704	G	C__28028791_10
GLP1R	rs10305439	C	C___2491169_10
GLP1R	rs2143734	A	C__16072581_20
GLP1R	rs877446	A	C__11607361_10
GLP1R	rs6923761	G	C__25615272_20
GLP1R	rs932443	T	C___2491141_10
GLP1R	rs2300612	T	C__15755173_10
GLP1R	rs2268640	G	C___2491124_10
TCF7L2	rs7903146	C	C__29347861_10
TCF7L2	rs12255372	G	C____291484_20
KCNJ11	rs5215	C	C___2991148_10
KCNJ11	rs5218	G	C___2991149_20
KCNJ11	rs5219	T	C__11654065_10
KCNJ11	rs886288	A	C___9686373_10
FTO	rs9939609	T	C__30090620_10
FTO	rs9939973	G	C__11776771_10
PYY	rs2700831	T	C___2964503_10
PYY	rs9890045	G	C__30502516_20
PYY	rs1684668	T	C__11887233_10
PYY	rs1618809	A	C__27061985_10

2.2. DNA Extraction and Genotyping of Samples

Two peripheral blood tubes (EDTA) of 10 mL each were collected from each patient. DNA was extracted from peripheral leukocytes after a series of washes with red cell lysis buffer and further treated with the DNAzol®—Genomic DNA Isolation Reagent extraction kit, following the manufacturer's protocol. The concentration and purity were determined using a NanoDrop™ 2000/2000C spectrophotometer. Genotyping was performed using predesigned TaqMan assays for each SNP (Assay ID included in Table 1) using a 7500 Fast Real-Time PCR System (Applied Biosystems, Foster City, CA, USA). A genotyping call rate over 95% per plate, negative sample controls and three well-differentiated genotyping clusters were required to validate results.

2.3. Statistical Analyses

The data were expressed as the mean and standard deviation or median and interquartile range for continuous variables and absolute and relative frequencies for categorical variables. SNPStats software was used to evaluate Hardy–Weinberg equilibrium and the genotype association study with weight response at nadir and at year 6, under multiple inheritance models with respect to allele reference homozygotes [24]: co-dominant, dominant, recessive, over-dominant and log-additive [26]. To evaluate the best model, the Akaike Information Criterion (AIC) was used, choosing the model with the lowest AIC value. A linear regression analysis was performed for quantitative response variables (%TWL, %EWL and %WR_MWL), expressing the results with the mean, standard error and mean differences (95%CI). For response variables coded as a binary variable (%WR_MWL > 20% [21], %EWL > 50% [27]), a logistic regression analysis was performed, expressing the results including genotype frequencies, proportions and OR (95%CI).

The association study of SNPs and weight loss and regain after BS was performed on the overall sample. With the results of the association of each individual variant with the weight response to BS, an unweighted risk score (RS) was calculated for each associated phenotype: RS_%TWL_nadir, RS_%TWL_6y, and RS-%WR_MWL. Each SNP was assigned a value of 2 for the homozygote of the risk allele, a value of 1 for the heterozygote of the risk allele, and a value of 0 for all other combinations. We refer to the risk allele for each SNP as the one that was significantly associated with lower weight loss or higher weight regain in the association study in our cohort. The sum of the genetic variant scores was calculated to obtain the RS-associated phenotype (RS-phenotype) scoring per patient. The RS- phenotype scoring was coded as a categorical variable around the 75th percentile (score P > 75 vs ≤P75). The association of the RS-phenotype codified scoring categories with the weight response variables was studied by means of logistic or linear regression analyses, replicating the SNPS-weight response association analysis. All of the comparisons were adjusted for sex, age, initial BMI, pre-surgery T2D and HTN diagnosis and the type of surgery. All p-values lower than 0.05 were deemed statistically significant.

3. Results

3.1. Association Study with Weight Response

The percentage of surgical techniques performed in these cases were as follows, 16% SG, 54.66% RYGB, and 29.3% malabsorptive (77% SADI-S, 23% BPD-DS), with a median follow-up of six years (IQR = 5–8) after BS. At the time of the surgery, the mean BMI was 44.87 ± 6.59 kg/m^2, and the prevalence of T2D and HTN was 35.7% and 49%, respectively. Table 2 shows the description of the demographic profile and the weight loss and weight regain variables included as phenotypes in the association study.

Table 2. Demographic profile and weight response variables at the follow-up. (N = 375).

Variable	Value
Age, in years	44.79 ± 11.99
Female gender, n (%)	259 (69)
%TWL_nadir,	38.79 ± 9.84
%EWL_nadir,	91.19 ± 23.69
%TWL_6y	31.67 ± 11.62
%EWL_6y	74.08 ± 26.89
%EWL6y > 50%, n (%)	311 (82.93)
%WR_MWL, median (IQR)	15.76 (7.99–28.69)
%WR_MWL > 20%, n (%)	154 (41.1)

Mean (SD) unless otherwise stated. TWL, total weight loss; EWL, excess weight loss; nadir, maximum weight loss achieved; 6y, at 6 years of follow-up; WR_MWL, percentage of weight regain from the maximum weight loss.

From the 48 SNPs analyzed, a total of eight showed an association with weight response after BS after adjusting for age, sex, T2D, HTN, type of surgical technique and initial BMI; five variants showed an association with weight loss and three variants with weight regain. Figure 1 illustrates the mean values of %TWL at nadir and at the end of the follow-up of the variants with significative association according to dominant or recessive model, differentiating for each SNP, the genotype with a risk allele shown in red font. The variant rs10423928 of the GIPR gene and rs1861975 of the DPPIV gene showed associations with %TWL at nadir and at year 6. The variant rs9764 of NPY1R showed an association with %TWL at nadir. The variants rs11100493 of NPY5R, rs1801260 of the CLOCK gene and rs10305439 and rs2143734 of the GLP1R gene showed associations with %TWL at the end of the follow up. The variant rs1801260 of the CLOCK gene, rs10305439 and rs877446 of the GLP1R gene showed significant association with %WR_MWL at the end of the follow up. The mean differences achieved (IC95%; p) are described in Table 3. AIC values for each model in the genotype association study are included in Supplementary Table S1.

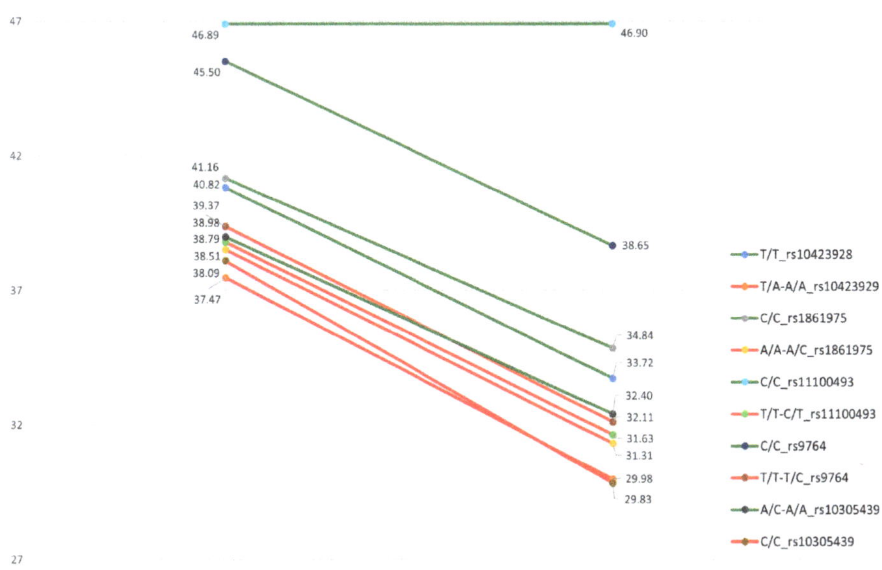

Figure 1. Mean values of %TWL at nadir and at year 6 according to the genetic variants.

Table 3. Variants with significant association with weight response: Mean differences between genotypes (N = 375).

Gene	SNP	%TWL_nadir	%TWL_6y	%WR_MWL	Risk Allele
GIPR	10423928	−3.32 (−5.53–−1.11); 0.0036	−3.55 (−6.33–−0.77); 0.013		A
DPPIV	1861975	2.92 (−0.11–5.72); 0.042	3.92 (0.47–7.36); 0.026		A
NPY1R	9764	4.61 (0.09–9.13); 0.047			T
NPY5R	11100493		22.20 (2.19–42.20); 0.03		T
CLOCK	1801260		1.85 (0.07–3.62); 0.042	−3.27 (−6.42–−0.12); 0.042	A
GLP1R	10305439		2,71 (0.41–5.01); 0.022	−4.88 (−8.84–−0.92); 0.016	C
GLP1R	2143734		−1.76 (−3.46–−0.05); 0.039		G
GLP1R	877446			−5.03 (−9.72–0.34); 0.036	A

Mean difference (IC95%); *p*. TWL, total weight loss; %TWL_nadir, percentage of total weight loss at nadir; %TWL_6y, percentage of total weight loss at year 6; %WR_MWL, percentage of weight regain from the maximum weight loss to year 6. Results adjusted by age, sex, T2D, HTN, type of surgical technique and initial BMI.

TWL, total weight loss. Red lines: risk genotypes, associated with lower %TWL.

With the %EWL phenotype, no variants showed significant association with %EWL at nadir. The number of variants associated with %EWL at the end of the follow-up was reduced to 2, with the same sense of association and varying quantitative differences with respect to %TWL: SNP rs1861975 of DPPIV gene [mean difference %EWL (IC95%) = 10.33 (1.79–18.88); $p = 0.018$]; SNP rs10305439 of the GLP1R gene [mean difference %EWL (IC95%) = 6.45 (0.91–12.00); $p = 0.023$].

The remaining variants showed no significant association with any of the weight response phenotypes analyzed.

3.2. Clustered Risk and Weight Response

Once the risk alleles for each genetic variant and weight response phenotype were identified, three RS-phenotypes (RS_%TWL_nadir, RS_%TWL_6y and RS-%WR_MWL) were calculated. The results of the logistic and linear regression analysis of the RS-phenotype scoring categories and the variables %TWL_nadir, %TWL_6y and %WR_MWL are shown below. All of the results were adjusted by age, sex, T2D, HTN, type of surgical technique and initial BMI. The mean score of the RS_%TWL_nadir was 2.5 ± 1.28 points (0–6 points). No association between RS_%TWL_nadir and %TWL_nadir was found.

The mean score of RS_%TWL_6y was 4.86 ± 1.66 points (0–12 points). A score of ≥7 points was significantly associated with weight loss at the end of the follow-up (Figure 2), with a mean difference in terms of %TWL_6y [Mean difference (IC95%) = −5.37 (−7.97–−3.62); $p = 0.0001$]. Scoring ≥ 7 points was also associated with a significant risk of achieving a %EWL > 50% [OR (95%CI) = 0.46 (0.23–0.90); $p = 0.026$]. Table 4 includes a comparison of the patient profile according to the RS_%TWL_6y scoring categories. No significant differences were found in any of the variables included.

Table 4. Comparative pre-surgery variables according to RS_%TWL_6y scoring categories.

	RS_%TWL_6y Categories		
Variable	**RS < 7 N = 306**	**RS ≥ 7 N = 70**	***p***
BMI_00, kg/m^2	44.65 (6.50)	45.77 (6.98)	0.225
Age, in years	44.79 (12.25)	44.77 (10.86)	0.988
Female gender, n (%)	212 (69.51)	47 (67.1)	0.73
T2D, n (%)	108 (35.4)	26 (37.1)	0.77
HTN, n (%)	141 (46.22)	41 (58.57)	0.06
Restrictive n (%)	52 (17.05)	8 (11.42)	0.25
Mixed, n (%)	164 (53.77)	41 (58.57)	0.45
Malabsorptive, n (%)	89 (29.18)	21 (30)	0.87

Mean (SD) unless otherwise stated. BMI_00, pre-surgery body mass index; T2D, type 2 diabetes; HTN, hypertension; RS, risk score; RS_%TWL_6y, risk score for total weight loss at year 6.

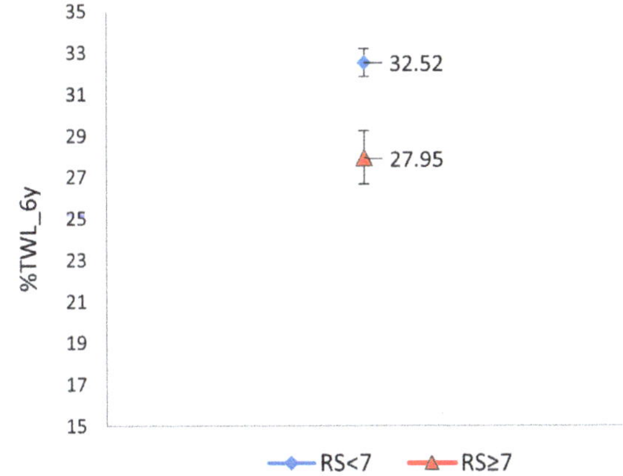

Figure 2. Mean %TWL at year 6 according to RS_%TWL_6y scoring categories.

The mean RS-%WR_MWL score was 3.42 ± 1.46 points (0–12 points). A score of ≥7 points was significantly associated with weight regain, with a mean difference in %WR_MWL [mean difference (IC95%) = 7.06 (2.80–11.31); $p = 0.0012$] and with a significant risk of achieving an %WR_MWL > 20% [OR (95%CI) = 2.01 (1.22–3.31); $p = 0.0059$].

4. Discussion

In our work, the combined effect of genetic variants of GIPR, DPPIV, NPY1R, NPY5R, CLOCK, and GLP1R genes was significantly associated with weight loss and long-term weight regain. The risk score for the associated phenotype %TWL at year 6 included six SNPs, of which only the rs9939973 variant of the FTO gene has been included in previous GRS studies [28]. The RS_%TWL_6y scoring category of seven points or more, which accounts for 18% of the sample, was associated with a mean %TWL at the end of follow-up 5.37 times lower than the mean %TWL of subjects scoring less than seven points ($p = 0.0001$) and 2.17 times more likely to achieve an %EWL less than 50% ($p = 0.026$). The weight loss achieved and maintained at year 6 was similar or even superior to previous studies [29–31] that include a long-term follow-up [32], with 83% of the sample reaching an EWL above 50% at the end of the follow-up.

Most published studies conclude that weight loss appears to be influenced by multiple genetic variants, which interact with each other and with phenotypic traits. The results of the review by Gupta et al. [33] demonstrate that the combination of several genes, as measured by genetic risk scores (GRS) in various studies [15,34,35] may have significant predictive value after surgery. Genetic variants included in the GRS for weight development after BS usually include hypothalamic genes related to monogenic obesity, involved in the regulation of energy homeostasis, mainly the hypothalamic leptin-melanocortin system [36]. In the study by Rinella et al., 17 SNPs with potential clinical utility were identified from the 111 gene variants included, and the combined association with weight loss after BPGYR was studied [37]. De Toro et al. studied the combined effect of 186 SNPs with a polygenic risk score model in patients undergoing biliopancreatic diversion with duodenal switch; however, only 11 variants showed a significant association with %EWL [35]. In the OBEGEN study, a clinical-genetic predictive model of response was obtained by combining three clinical variables (age, type of surgery and the presence of T2D) and nine SNPs out of the fifty analyzed [38]. It should be noted that in all these studies, the ratio of variants with significant associations with weight loss with respect to those included in the methodology ranges between 6 and 20%. Moreover, due to methodological differences in the calculation of the risk score, follow-up after BS, types of surgical techniques and adjustment for covariables performed, no conclusive results concerning the key variants to be included in the GRS models can be obtained.

The phenotype of weight response was %EWL in most studies, with a follow-up of up to four years after BS. In our study, a follow-up of six years, considered long-term, was carried out, and weight regain phenotypes were included. Weight regain measured with respect to maximum weight loss achieved was lower than in previous studies [21,39]. The results of the association study showed that a greater number of significant associations were found with the variable %TWL as a phenotype than with %EWL. Previous findings of the original cohort showed that %TWL enabled better differentiation of weight loss trajectories by surgical technique, age, sex and comorbidities [20]. Other studies suggest that %TWL is the consistent measure for comparing weight loss between cohorts [40,41] as it allows better averaging of individual weight response without reference to ideal BMI.

Our work includes 5 of the 39 genes included in the study by Ciudin et al. [38], together with variants not studied in previous studies concerning risk scores. The 48 SNPs included were chosen for their involvement in the pathophysiology of weight control, at the gastrointestinal or hypothalamic levels [19,42]. There are multiple neuronal circuits involved in the control of appetite regulation and energy expenditure [43,44], which encode neuropeptides synthesized in central and peripheral neurons, together with the endocrine cells of the gastrointestinal tract and other endocrinologically active organs [43,45]. The genetic variants with significant association from GIPR, DPPIV, NPY1R, NPY5R and GLP1R genes included in the risk scores are related to these neural axis circuits.

In the methodology for calculating the RS-associated phenotype, we used an unweighted model previously described in other studies [14,34,38], assigning risk scoring according to the combination of risk alleles of the SNPs identified in the study of the association of each individual variant with weight response. Adjustment variables include potential predictors of long-term weight regain identified in a previous analysis by our group based on the original cohort [20]. As a phenotype for calculating the risk score in our series, we used the quantitative variable %TWL and %WR with respect to the maximum weight loss achieved without establishing a cut-off point, since there is no defined phenotype nor a defined cut-off point [32] for long-term weight response after BS. The %EWL variable with a cut-off point of 50% is the criterion used in most of the GRS studies [14,34,35,37,38]; although in the short term after BS, so it follows that the most significant results with weight response have been obtained when using an extreme phenotype of weight loss. The association found in our sample with this coded phenotype would allow us to categorize the patients of our cohort as "hyper-responder" or "hypo-responder", according to Bonouvrie et al. [27].

The higher magnitude of statistical significance found in our sample when combining several SNPs, pooling risk alleles for a given phenotype is consistent with what has been reported in the literature: weight loss after BS may be influenced by multiple genetic variants that have modest individual effects, but synergistically produce a larger aggregate effect. As such, polygenic risk scores may better capture the genetic architecture of weight loss with BS [33].

Some limitations related to long-term response to BS must be taken into consideration, such as the lack of information on variables with potential impact on weight evolution such as dietary intake and behavior, hormonal disturbances, weight loss medication and the level of physical activity. Adjustments made based on the clinical profile and BMI at the time of the surgery minimize the effect of potential confounding factors. Moreover, the clinical profile of the patient when stratifying according to SR scoring categories was comparable. The selection of genetic variants may miss potential SNPs with an effect on the weight response, for which there is currently no proven evidence. Despite these limitations, our strengths include a high rate of patient retention throughout a long follow-up and having included phenotypes for both weight loss and regain.

In summary, in this large cohort of patients followed up to six years we have identified genetic variants with combined effect in the weight response, some of which have not previously been described. The aggregation of SNPs associated with weight loss and regain in our sample was different, suggesting a distinct grouped risk combination by weight response phenotype.

Supplementary Materials: The following supporting information can be downloaded at: https://www.mdpi.com/article/10.3390/jcm12134288/s1, Table S1: Genotype association study: Akaike Information Criterion (AIC) value for each model. Variants with significant association with weight response variables.

Author Contributions: Conceptualization, M.T.-E., A.B. and M.A.R.-H.; methodology, M.T.-E. and A.B.; formal analysis, M.T.-E. and A.B.; investigation, M.T.-E., A.B., M.A.R.-H., P.M.-M., A.S.-P. and A.J.T.; resources, M.T.-E., A.B., M.A.R.-H., P.M.-M., A.S.-P. and A.J.T.; writing—original draft preparation, M.T.-E. and A.B.; writing—review and editing M.T.-E., A.B., M.A.R.-H., P.M.-M., A.S.-P., A.J.T. and A.L.C.-P.; supervision, A.B. and M.A.R.-H. All authors have read and agreed to the published version of the manuscript.

Funding: This research was funded by Fundación Mutua Madrileña and Fundación Estudios Metabólicos.

Institutional Review Board Statement: All of the procedures performed were in accordance with the 1975 Helsinki declaration and its later amendments or comparable ethical standards for studies involving human participants. The project was approved by the Clinical Research Ethics Committee, Hospital Clinico San Carlos, Madrid, Spain (16 February 2009).

Informed Consent Statement: Informed consent was obtained from all subjects involved in the study.

Data Availability Statement: Not applicable.

Conflicts of Interest: The authors declare no conflict of interest.

References

1. Chang, S.-H.; Stoll, C.R.T.; Song, J.; Varela, J.E.; Eagon, C.J.; Colditz, G.A. The effectiveness and risks of bariatric surgery: An updated systematic review and meta-analysis, 2003–2012. *JAMA Surg.* **2014**, *149*, 275–287. [CrossRef]
2. Sheng, B.; Truong, K.; Spitler, H.; Zhang, L.; Tong, X.; Chen, L. The Long-Term Effects of Bariatric Surgery on Type 2 Diabetes Remission, Microvascular and Macrovascular Complications, and Mortality: A Systematic Review and Meta-Analysis. *Obes. Surg.* **2017**, *27*, 2724–2732. [CrossRef] [PubMed]
3. O'Brien, P.E.; Hindle, A.; Brennan, L.; Skinner, S.; Burton, P.; Smith, A.; Crosthwaite, G.; Brown, W. Long-Term Outcomes After Bariatric Surgery: A Systematic Review and Meta-analysis of Weight Loss at 10 or More Years for All Bariatric Procedures and a Single-Centre Review of 20-Year Outcomes After Adjustable Gastric Banding. *Obes. Surg.* **2019**, *29*, 3–14. [CrossRef] [PubMed]
4. Junquera Bañares, S.; Ramírez Real, L.; Camuñas Segovia, J.; Martín García-Almenta, M.; Llanos Egüez, K.; Álvarez Hernández, J. Evaluación de la calidad de vida, pérdida de peso y evolución de comorbilidades a los 6 años de la cirugía bariátrica. *Endocrinol. Diabetes Nutr.* **2021**, *68*, 501–508. [CrossRef]
5. Maggard, M.A.; Shugarman, L.R.; Suttorp, M.; Maglione, M.; Sugarman, H.J.; Livingston, E.H.; Nguyen, N.T.; Li, Z.; Mojica, W.A.; Hilton, L.; et al. Meta-analysis: Surgical treatment of obesity. *Ann. Intern. Med.* **2005**, *142*, 547–559. [CrossRef] [PubMed]
6. Courcoulas, A.P.; Christian, N.J.; Belle, S.H.; Berk, P.D.; Flum, D.R.; Garcia, L.; Horlick, M.; Kalarchian, M.A.; King, W.C.; Mitchell, J.E.; et al. Weight change and health outcomes at 3 years after bariatric surgery among individuals with severe obesity. *JAMA* **2013**, *310*, 2416–2425. [CrossRef]
7. Capoccia, D.; Guida, A.; Coccia, F.; Guarisco, G.; Testa, M.; Leonetti, F.; Silecchia, G. Weight Regain and Diabetes Evolution After Sleeve Gastrectomy: A Cohort Study with over 5 Years of Follow-Up. *Obes. Surg.* **2020**, *30*, 1046–1051. [CrossRef]
8. Busetto, L.; Dicker, D.; Azran, C. Practical recommendations of the obesity management task force of the European Association for the Study of obesity for the post-bariatric surgery medical management. *Obes. Facts* **2018**, *10*, 597–632. [CrossRef]
9. Nicoletti, C.F.; Cortes-Oliveira, C.; Pinhel, M.A.S.; Nonino, C.B. Bariatric surgery and precision nutrition. *Nutrients* **2017**, *9*, 974. [CrossRef]
10. Boswell, L.; Jiménez, A.; Ortega, E.; Pané, A.; Hollanda, A.D.; Moizé, V.; Andreu, A.; Ibarzabal, A.; Flores, L.; Vidal, J. Genetic background influences weight-loss trajectories on the mid-term after bariatric surgery. *Int. J. Obes.* **2019**, *43*, 1869–1874. [CrossRef]
11. Loos, R.J. The genetics of adiposity. *Curr. Opin. Genet. Dev.* **2018**, *50*, 86–95. [CrossRef] [PubMed]
12. Locke, A.E.; Kahali, B.; Berndt, S.I.; Justice, A.E.; Pers, T.H.; Day, F.R.; Powell, C.; Vedantam, S.; Buchkovich, M.L.; Yang, J.; et al. Genetic studies of body mass index yield new insights for obesity biology. *Nature* **2015**, *518*, 197–206. [CrossRef] [PubMed]
13. Goodarzi, M.O. Genetics of obesity: What genetic association studies have taught us about the biology of obesity and its complications. *Lancet Diabetes Endocrinol.* **2018**, *6*, 223–236. [CrossRef] [PubMed]

14. Still, C.D.; Wood, G.C.; Chu, X.; Erdman, R.; Manney, C.H.; Benotti, P.N.; Petrick, A.T.; Strodel, W.E.; Mirshahi, U.L.; Mirshahi, T.; et al. High allelic burden of four obesity SNPs is associated with poorer weight loss outcomes following gastric bypass surgery. *Obesity* **2011**, *19*, 1676–1683. [CrossRef]
15. Bandstein, M.; Voisin, S.; Nilsson, E.K.; Schultes, B.; Ernst, B.; Thurnheer, M.; Benedict, C.; Mwinyi, J.; Schiöth, H.B. A Genetic Risk Score Is Associated with Weight Loss Following Roux-en Y Gastric Bypass Surgery. *Obes. Surg.* **2016**, *26*, 2183–2189. [CrossRef]
16. Käkelä, P.; Jääskeläinen, T.; Torpström, J.; Ilves, I.; Venesmaa, S.; Pääkkönen, M.; Gylling, H.; Paajanen, H.; Uusitupa, M.; Pihlajamäki, J. Genetic Risk Score Does Not Predict the Outcome of Obesity Surgery. *Obes. Surg.* **2014**, *24*, 128–133. [CrossRef]
17. Aasbrenn, M.; Schnurr, T.M.; Have, C.T.; Svendstrup, M.; Hansen, D.L.; Worm, D.; Balslev-Harder, M.; Hollensted, M.; Grarup, N.; Burgdorf, K.S.; et al. Genetic Determinants of Weight Loss After Bariatric Surgery. *Obes. Surg.* **2019**, *29*, 2554–2561. [CrossRef]
18. Holzer, P.; Reichmann, F.; Farzi, A. Neuropeptide Y, peptide YY and pancreatic polypeptide in the gut-brain axis. *Neuropeptides* **2012**, *46*, 261–274. [CrossRef]
19. Suzuki, K.; Simpson, K.A.; Minnion, J.S.; Shillito, J.C.; Bloom, S.R. The role of gut hormones and the hypothalamus in appetite regulation. *Endocr. J.* **2010**, *57*, 359–372. [CrossRef]
20. Torrego-Ellacuría, M.; Barabash, A.; Larrad-Sainz, A.; Hernández-Nuñez, G.M.; Matía-Martín, P.; Pérez-Ferre, N.; Marcuello, C.; Sánchez-Pernaute, A.; Torres, A.J.; Calle-Pascual, A.L.; et al. Weight Regain Outcomes After Bariatric Surgery in the Long-term Follow-up: Role of Preoperative Factors. *Obes. Surg.* **2021**, *31*, 3947–3955. [CrossRef]
21. King, W.C.; Hinerman, A.S.; Belle, S.H.; Wahed, A.S.; Courcoulas, A.P. Comparison of the Performance of Common Measures of Weight Regain after Bariatric Surgery for Association with Clinical Outcomes. *JAMA* **2018**, *320*, 1560–1569. [CrossRef] [PubMed]
22. Torrego-Ellacuría, M.; Barabash, A.; Matía-Martín, P.; Sánchez-Pernaute, A.; Torres, A.J.; Calle-Pascual, A.L.; Rubio-Herrera, M.A. Influence of CLOCK Gene Variants on Weight Response after Bariatric Surgery. *Nutrients* **2022**, *14*, 3472. [CrossRef] [PubMed]
23. HapMap International Public Project, n.d. Available online: https://www.internationalgenome.org/ (accessed on 1 January 2023).
24. dbSNP, NCBI n.d. Available online: https://www.ncbi.nlm.nih.gov/snp (accessed on 1 January 2023).
25. Ensembl Project, n.d. Available online: http://www.ensembl.org/Homo_sapiens/ (accessed on 1 January 2023).
26. Solé, X.; Guinó, E.; Valls, J.; Iniesta, R.; Moreno, V. SNPStats: A web tool for the analysis of association studies. *Bioinformatics* **2006**, *22*, 1928–1929. [CrossRef] [PubMed]
27. Bonouvrie, D.S.; Uittenbogaart, M.; Luijten, A.A.P.M.; van Dielen, F.M.H.; Leclercq, W.K.G. Lack of Standard Definitions of Primary and Secondary (Non)responders After Primary Gastric Bypass and Gastric Sleeve: A Systematic Review. *Obes. Surg.* **2019**, *29*, 691–697. [CrossRef]
28. Hosseini-Esfahani, F.; Koochakpoor, G.; Mirmiran, P.; Daneshpour, M.S.; Azizi, F. Dietary patterns modify the association between fat mass and obesity-associated genetic variants and changes in obesity phenotypes. *Br. J. Nutr.* **2019**, *121*, 1247–1254. [CrossRef] [PubMed]
29. Jiménez, A.; Ibarzabal, A.; Moizé, V.; Pané, A.; Andreu, A.; Molero, J.; de Hollanda, A.; Flores, L.; Ortega, E.; Lacy, A.; et al. Ten-year outcomes after Roux-en-Y gastric bypass and sleeve gastrectomy: An observational nonrandomized cohort study. *Surg. Obes. Relat. Dis.* **2019**, *15*, 382–388. [CrossRef]
30. Arterburn, D.E.; Johnson, E.; Coleman, K.J.; Herrinton, L.J.; Courcoulas, A.P.; Fisher, D.; Li, R.A.; Theis, M.K.; Liu, L.; Fraser, J.R.; et al. Weight Outcomes of Sleeve Gastrectomy and Gastric Bypass Compared to Nonsurgical Treatment. *Ann. Surg.* **2021**, *274*, e1269–e1276. [CrossRef]
31. Sánchez-Pernaute, A.; Herrera, M.Á.R.; Ferré, N.P.; Rodríguez, C.S.; Marcuello, C.; Pañella, C.; Antoñanzas, L.L.; Torres, A.; Pérez-Aguirre, E. Long-Term Results of Single-Anastomosis Duodeno-ileal Bypass with Sleeve Gastrectomy (SADI-S). *Obes. Surg.* **2022**, *32*, 682–689. [CrossRef]
32. Brethauer, S.A.; Kim, J.; el Chaar, M.; Papasavas, P.; Eisenberg, D.; Rogers, A.; Ballem, N.; Kligman, M.; Kothari, S.; ASMBS Clinical Issues Committee. Standardized outcomes reporting in metabolic and bariatric surgery. *Surg. Obes. Relat. Dis.* **2015**, *11*, 489–506. [CrossRef]
33. Gupta, S.R.; Zhou, Y.; Wadden, T.A.; Berkowitz, R.I.; Chao, A.M. A Systematic Review of Genetic Correlates of Weight Loss After Bariatric Surgery. *Obes. Surg.* **2021**, *31*, 4612–4623. [CrossRef]
34. Ciudin, A.; Fidilio, E.; Ortiz, A.; Pich, S.; Salas, E.; Mesa, J.; Hernández, C.; Simó-Servat, O.; Lecube, A.; Simó, R. Genetic Testing to Predict Weight Loss and Diabetes Remission and Long-Term Sustainability after Bariatric Surgery: A Pilot Study. *J. Clin. Med.* **2019**, *8*, 964. [CrossRef] [PubMed]
35. de Toro-Martín, J.; Guénard, F.; Tchernof, A.; Pérusse, L.; Marceau, S.; Vohl, M.C. Polygenic risk score for predicting weight loss after bariatric surgery. *JCI Insight* **2018**, *3*, 1–12. [CrossRef] [PubMed]
36. Fairbrother, U.; Kidd, E.; Malagamuwa, T.; Walley, A. Genetics of Severe Obesity. *Curr. Diabetes Rep.* **2018**, *18*, 85. [CrossRef] [PubMed]
37. Rinella, E.S.; Still, C.; Shao, Y.; Wood, G.C.; Chu, X.; Salerno, B.; Gerhard, G.S.; Ostrer, H. Genome-wide association of single-nucleotide polymorphisms with weight loss outcomes after Roux-en-Y gastric bypass surgery. *J. Clin. Endocrinol. Metab.* **2013**, *98*, 1131–1136. [CrossRef]
38. Ciudin, A.; Fidilio, E.; Gutiérrez-Carrasquilla, L.; Caixàs, A.; Vilarrasa, N.; Pellitero, S.; Simó-Servat, A.; Vilallonga, R.; Ruiz, A.; de la Fuente, M.; et al. A Clinical-Genetic Score for Predicting Weight Loss after Bariatric Surgery: The OBEGEN Study. *J. Pers. Med.* **2021**, *11*, 1040. [CrossRef]

39. Cooper, T.C.; Simmons, E.B.; Webb, K.; Burns, J.L.; Kushner, R.F. Trends in Weight Regain Following Roux-en-Y Gastric Bypass (RYGB) Bariatric Surgery. *Obes. Surg.* **2015**, *25*, 1474–1481. [CrossRef]
40. de Vries, L.; Van den Broecke, C.; Decruyeneare, A.; Van Nieuwenhove, Y. A SIMPLE Performance Assessment of Bariatric Procedures and Post-operative Weight Regain. *J. Gastrointest. Surg.* **2022**, *26*, 542–549. [CrossRef]
41. Belle, S.H.; Berk, P.D.; Courcoulas, A.P.; Engel, S.; Flum, D.R.; Gourash, W.; Horlick, M.; Hsu, J.Y.; Khandelwal, S.; Mitchell, J.E.; et al. Reporting weight change: Standardized reporting accounting for baseline weight. *Surg. Obes. Relat. Dis.* **2013**, *9*, 782–789. [CrossRef]
42. Hameed, S.; Dhillo, W.S.; Bloom, S.R. Gut hormones and appetite control. *Oral. Dis.* **2009**, *15*, 18–26. [CrossRef]
43. Holzer, P.; Farzi, A. Neuropeptides and the microbiota- Gut-brain axis. *Adv. Exp. Med. Biol.* **2014**, *817*, 196–219. [CrossRef]
44. Murphy, K.G.; Dhillo, W.S.; Bloom, S.R. Gut peptides in the regulation of food intake and energy homeostasis. *Endocr. Rev.* **2006**, *27*, 719–727. [CrossRef] [PubMed]
45. Casimiro, I.; Sam, S.; Brady, M.J. Endocrine implications of bariatric surgery: A review on the intersection between incretins, bone, and sex hormones. *Physiol. Rep.* **2019**, *7*, e14111. [CrossRef] [PubMed]

Journal of
Clinical Medicine

MDPI

Article

Mixed Meal Tolerance Test Versus Continuous Glucose Monitoring for an Effective Diagnosis of Persistent Post-Bariatric Hypoglycemia

Ana M. Ramos-Levi [1,†], Miguel A. Rubio-Herrera [2,3,*,†], Pilar Matía-Martín [2,3], Natalia Pérez-Ferre [2,3], Clara Marcuello [2], Andrés Sánchez-Pernaute [4], Antonio J. Torres-García [4] and Alfonso L. Calle-Pascual [2,3,5]

[1] Departament of Endocrinology and Nutrition, Hospital La Princesa, Instituto de Investigación Princesa, Universidad Autónoma de Madrid, 28049 Madrid, Spain; ana_ramoslevi@hotmail.com
[2] Departament of Endocrinology and Nutrition, Hospital Clínico San Carlos, IdISSC, 28040 Madrid, Spain
[3] Faculty of Medicine, Department of Medicine, Universidad Complutense, 28040 Madrid, Spain
[4] Department of Surgery, Hospital Clínico San Carlos, IdISSC, Faculty of Medicine, Universidad Complutense, 28040 Madrid, Spain
[5] Centro de Investigación Biomédica en Red de Diabetes y Enfermedades Metabólicas Asociadas (CIBERDEM), 28040 Madrid, Spain
* Correspondence: marubioh@gmail.com
† These authors contributed equally to this work.

Citation: Ramos-Levi, A.M.; Rubio-Herrera, M.A.; Matía-Martín, P.; Pérez-Ferre, N.; Marcuello, C.; Sánchez-Pernaute, A.; Torres-García, A.J.; Calle-Pascual, A.L. Mixed Meal Tolerance Test Versus Continuous Glucose Monitoring for an Effective Diagnosis of Persistent Post-Bariatric Hypoglycemia. *J. Clin. Med.* **2023**, *12*, 4295. https://doi.org/10.3390/jcm12134295

Academic Editors: David Benaiges Boix and Alberto Martínez-Castelao

Received: 30 April 2023
Revised: 31 May 2023
Accepted: 24 June 2023
Published: 27 June 2023

Abstract: Gastric bypass determines an increase in incretin secretion and glucose excursions throughout the day and may sometimes entail the development of severe post-bariatric hypoglycemia (PBH). However, there is no consensus on the gold standard method for its diagnosis. In this study, we evaluated the usefulness of a mixed meal tolerance test (MMTT) and continuous glucose monitoring (CGM) for the diagnosis of PBH, defined as glucose levels <54 mg/dL (3.0 mmol/L). We found that hypoglycemia occurred in 60% of patients after the MMTT and in 75% during CGM, and it was predominantly asymptomatic. The MMTT confirmed the diagnosis of PBH in 88.9%of patients in whom surgery had been performed more than three years ago, in comparison to 36.4% in cases with a shorter postsurgical duration. CGM diagnosed nocturnal asymptomatic hypoglycemia in 70% of patients, and daytime postprandial hypoglycemia in 25% of cases. The mean duration of asymptomatic hypoglycemia was more than 30 min a day. Patients with ≥2% of their CGM readings with hypoglycemia exhibited a higher degree of glucose variability than those with <1% of the time in hypoglycemia. Our results show that the MMTT may be a useful dynamic test to confirm the occurrence of hypoglycemia in a large number of patients with persistent and recurrent PBH during long-term follow-up after gastric bypass. CGM, on its part, helps identify hypoglycemia in the real-world setting, especially nocturnal asymptomatic hypoglycemia, bringing to light that PBH is not always postprandial.

Keywords: gastric bypass; post-bariatric hypoglycemia; mixed meal tolerance test; continuous glucose monitoring

1. Introduction

Bariatric surgery (BS) has proven to be a very useful tool for the management of severe obesity since it allows significant long-term weight loss and amelioration, or even resolution of associated comorbidities [1]. Despite its well-known beneficial effects in improving patients' metabolic syndrome and quality of life, BS also entails several controversies, especially regarding weight regain and reappearance of comorbidities [2], an unexplained increase in other causes of mortality [3], and deterioration of bone health [4].

Post-bariatric hypoglycemia (PBH) is one of the most defying challenges that patients and clinicians encounter during the follow-up after BS, but its physiopathology and diagnosis have not been fully established. PBH is characterized by the development of hypoglycemia, usually between one and three hours after a meal, with adrenergic and neuroglucopenic symptoms that improve after the administration of rapidly absorbed carbohydrates (Whipple's triad) [5]. In the literature, this clinical picture has been usually referred to as postprandial hyperinsulinemic hypoglycemia (PHH); but given the frequent occurrence of hypoglycemia not related to a prior meal intake, especially during the night, the term PBH is generally preferred. Several studies have described an increased prevalence two years after Roux-en-Y gastric bypass, but it has also been reported in patients who underwent other types of procedures, such as sleeve gastrectomy, and one anastomosis gastric bypass [6].

There is no generalized consensus on how to effectively diagnose PBH [5]. Indeed, there is wide heterogeneity in the results observed across different studies, mainly due to the specific characteristics of patients included, the diagnostic methods, and the threshold values to define PBH. As a result, the prevalence of PBH has not been consistently established, since it is clearly dependent on the diagnostic method used to identify it. For instance, severe PBH, with associated neuroglucopenic symptoms, has been reported to occur in less than 1% of patients [7,8]. However, its prevalence may grow up to 30% of patients when specific questionnaires are used, [9] and more than 50% when dynamic tests such as an oral glucose tolerance test (OGTT) or a mixed meal tolerance test (MMTT) are used [5].

In an attempt to overcome the associated diagnostic difficulties, and with the availability of new technologies, continuous glucose monitoring (CGM) has been recently used to better evaluate glucose excursions in post-bariatric patients. These devices are easily placed on the patient, well tolerated, easily adjustable, and provide useful information regarding interstitial glucose values and glucose variability throughout the day and night, for several days. In fact, CGM aids in a deeper evaluation of glucose values, because it allows correlation in the setting of the patient's specific lifestyle, for instance, times of meal intake, exercise, etc., and even helps detect asymptomatic periods of hypoglycemia. Thus, overall, it allows a more precise diagnosis of PBH. In addition, CGM may be useful to evaluate the effectiveness of specific dietary or pharmacological treatments [8].

The objective of this study is to evaluate the prevalence of PBH in a series of consecutive patients who underwent RYBG and who report recurrent postprandial hypoglycemia, using the MMTT and CGM for seven days.

2. Materials and Methods

2.1. Participants

We performed a cross-sectional study with 20 patients without known diabetes, aged 23–65 years old, who had undergone bariatric surgery (BS) (specifically, Roux-en-Y gastric bypass) during the period between 2014 and 2019, and who referred hypoglycemic symptoms, according to Whipple's triad. We collected data from their clinical records, including age, sex, body mass index (BMI) before BS and at the time of evaluation, time since BS, and percentage weight loss. Patients were excluded if they were taking any antidiabetic medications since surgery or if they had glycated hemoglobin (HbA1c) levels >6.0% or fasting blood glucose >100 mg/dL.

All patients signed a written informed consent. The study was approved by the Ethics Committee of the Hospital Clinico San Carlos (code CI-11/080E, approved on 21 September 2011), and was in compliance with the Helsinki Declaration.

2.2. Mixed Meal Tolerance Test (MMTT)

Patients underwent a mixed meal tolerance test (MMTT) after a 12 h overnight fast. A peripheral venous catheterization was performed in the forearm to draw repeated blood samples at times 0, 30, 60, 90, 120, 180, and 240 min after intake of the standard beverage. Glucose and insulin levels were analyzed at these different times. The standard product used for the MMTT was TDiet 2.0® (Vegenat Healthcare, Badajoz, Spain), which is a 200 mL

400 kcal beverage containing 45 g of carbohydrates, 20 g of proteins, and 15.5 g of total fat, and was taken in less than 10 min.

2.3. Continuous Glucose Monitoring (CGM)

A CGM device was placed, after an overnight fast, for seven days, with surveillance of glucose levels in interstitial fluid every five minutes, 288 times per day (Medtronic Ipro2, Medtronic, Northridge, CA, USA). Each participant was instructed to calibrate their CGM device at least twice daily. A download of glucose data was performed using Carelink. Glucose variability (GV) was analyzed using standard measures of amplitude and timing, i.e., using mean, median, standard deviation (SD), variation coefficient (CV), minimum, maximum, and percentage of time under target ranges (<54 mg/dL, between 55 and 140 mg/dL, and >140 mg/dL) [10].

The device was placed on the patient by a trained nurse in the outpatient diabetes clinic. Each patient received comprehensive instructions regarding calibration of the CGM device, following the results of conventional capillary glucose monitoring, and according to the manufacturer's instructions. Specifically, patients were trained to perform 4 capillary glucose tests throughout the day, three before each of the three main meals, and one before bedtime, according to the Ipro2 user manual. In addition, patients were asked to perform an additional capillary blood test at night if they woke up by any chance. The trained nurse ensured that instructions were properly understood. All patients performed finger-prick measurements with a glucometer, starting at 12 h after insertion of the CGM device, and every six hours thereafter, during the seven days of the study.

CGM devices provided information regarding the time in which the patient underwent a hypoglycemic event (blood glucose levels <54 mg/dL [3 mmol/L]) for more than 15 min. We collected data on (a) the number of diurnal postprandial hypoglycemic events, occurring between 06:00 and 00:00, after four hours from the last food intake, and (b) the number of nocturnal hypoglycemic events, occurring between 00:00 and 06:00, after four hours from the last meal. The following measurements were recorded: mean interstitial glucose (IG) (mg/dL), mean IG peak (mg(dL), mean IG nadir (mg/dL), standard deviation [SD (mg/dL)], and variation coefficient [CV (%)], percentage of time spent with IG <54 mg/dL, % of the time with IG 55–70 mg/dL, % of the time with IG 71–140 mg/dL and % of the time with IG >140 mg/dl.

Measurements were not obtained at the same time as the MMTT but were not delayed more than a couple of days. The MMTT was performed in the first place, and then, the CGM device was placed, with a time-lapse of just two days.

2.4. Dietary Intake during CGM

To estimate patients' dietary intake, we used a self-reported record of seven consecutive days, which included at least one non-working day. Data were standardized using the EASY-DIET™ software (https://www.easydiet.es), from the Spanish Academy of Nutrition and Diet. Physical activity was quantified using the International Physical Activity Questionnaire (IPAQ) as METs/min/week.

2.5. Laboratory Tests

Plasma glucose levels were measured using the glucose oxidase method. HbA1c was analyzed with a method standardized by the International Federation of Clinical Chemistry and Laboratory Medicine, using ion-exchange high-performance liquid chromatography in gradient, with a Tosoh G8 analyzer (Tosoh Co., Tokyo, Japan). Serum insulin was measured by a chemiluminescence immunoassay in an IMMULITE 2000 Xpi (Siemens, Healthcare Diagnostics, Munich, Germany).

2.6. Statistical Analysis

Continuous variables were summarized as mean ± standard deviation. Categorical variables were expressed as percentages. The incremental area under the curve (iAUC) was calculated using the trapezoidal rule, with the deduction of fasting hormonal levels from subsequent time points.

Comparison between continuous variables was performed using an independent-sample *t*-test. For variables with a skewed distribution, Mann Whitney U-test was used for mean comparisons. The Chi-square test was used to analyze categorical data. Linear regression analysis was used to adjust for potential confounders identified in univariate analysis. Repeated measures ANOVA was conducted for each outcome using "time" (for each of the measurements performed at different times) as a within-subjects factor and "group" (total severe hypoglycemia <1% vs. total severe hypoglycemia >2%) as a between-subjects factor. All statistical analysis was performed using JASP Team (2023, version 0.17.1 computer software).

3. Results

Eighteen women and two men without previously diagnosed diabetes, who had undergone Roux-en-Y gastric bypass and reported repeated postprandial hypoglycemic symptoms, were included in the study. The mean age was 43.0 ± 10.5 years, and the mean presurgical BMI was 43.9 ± 7.1 kg/m^2. At the time of evaluation, the median time from BS was 24 months (IQR 21–51), and the mean BMI was 28.5 ± 3.9 kg/m^2, with a percentage weight loss of 34.2 ± 8.7.

Symptoms of hypoglycemia occurred after one to three hours from the last food intake. The most frequently reported (>90%) symptoms were overall general weakness and dizziness. Tremors and palpitations were reported by 55% of patients. Other neuroglucopenic symptoms, such as sweating, blurred vision, or confusion, were not consistently reported.

3.1. Mixed Meal Tolerance Test

Twelve patients (60%) presented hypoglycemia (glucose values <54 mg/dL [3.0 mmol]) [Hypo group]. Compared with the group without biochemical hypoglycemia (Non-Hypo), glycemia nadir was significantly lower (mean ± SD: 41.9 ± 8.4 mg/dL, for 90–180 min, vs. 70.9 ± 15.5 mg/dL; $p < 0.001$), following prior hyperinsulinemia (mean insulin level 206.2 ± 79.7 µUI/mL during the period of 30–60 min, in the hypo group, than in the non-Hypo group (108.2 ± 47.2 µUI/mL; $p = 0.003$). There were no differences between both groups in age, BMI, time since surgery, HbA1c, C-Peptide, HOMA-IR, and glycemic variability. Only four patients reported severe symptoms of hypoglycemia when their glucose values dropped below 40 mg/dL. When this occurred, the MMTT was stopped (min 90–120), hypoglycemia was treated by oral administration of 15 g of rapidly absorbed carbohydrate, and glucose levels were monitored every 15 min until values were safely above 60 mg/dL. The rest of the patients in the hypo group were either asymptomatic or had mild symptoms of hypoglycemia that did not require discontinuation of the test.

Patients who had undergone surgery more than 36 months before the study (group A) significantly exhibited more hypoglycemic episodes (glucose values < 54 mg/dL) after the MMTT than patients who had undergone surgery less than 36 months ago (group B) (88.9% vs. 36.4%, $p = 0.0281$). In addition, the former group had higher prior peak insulin levels (209.4 ± 82.5 vs. 129.9 ± 73.3 µUI/mL; $p = 0.035$). The area under the curve (AUC) was not significantly different for glucose values between both groups (14,778.3 ± 4021.2 mg × dL × min for group A and 14,754.6 ± 5900.9 mg × dL × min for group B), although differences were observed for the insulin AUC (11,986.7 ± 5476.4 vs. 6269.4 ± 3002.3 µUI × mL × h; $p = 0.020$ (Figure 1).

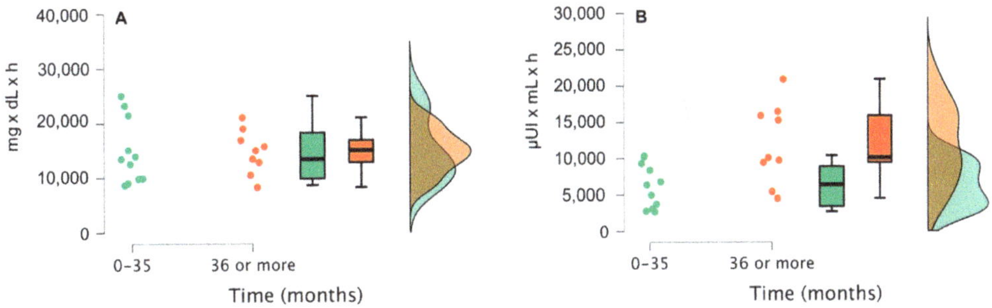

Figure 1. The graph shows glucose (**A**) and insulin (**B**) secretion profiles, according to the time elapsed after bariatric surgery. Individual glucose and insulin AUC values are shown, as well as the boxplot representing the AUC (median and interquartile range). Curves on the right show the results for the MMTT for subjects in whom surgery was performed before (green) or more than (orange) three years ago.

3.2. Continuous Glucose Monitoring (CGM)

The mean number of readings for a median of seven days was 1705.9 ± 204.4. Fifteen patients (75%) presented at least one hypoglycemic episode (glucose reading < 54 mg/dL) for more than 15 min, and 3.1% of the total number of glucose readings. Amongst patients with hypoglycemia, the mean number of episodes was 4.2 ± 2.7 and glucose values were between 54–70 mg/dL for 19.5% of the time. Eight patients (66.7%) had nocturnal hypoglycemia, with a mean number of 42.2 ± 2.7 events. This meant that nocturnal hypoglycemia was recorded in 2.5 ± 2.0% of the total amount of glucose readings, meaning 213.2 ± 188.6 min throughout the six days of CGM.

Only five patients (25%) had diurnal postprandial hypoglycemia, with a mean number of 9.6 ± 30.4 episodes (3.2 ± 2.1% of the total number of readings and 198.0 ± 151.9 min). We did not find significant differences in the number of diurnal or nocturnal hypoglycemic events according to the time elapsed after BS. A median of 1% of CGM readings in hypoglycemia (<54 mg/dL) was considered as the cut-off point to define those subjects with a higher or lower percentage of hypoglycemia during the seven days of CGM recording. So, if patients with severe hypoglycemia in ≤1% of their readings (n = 11) were compared to those with ≥2% of their readings (n = 9), we observed that the latter group exhibited a greater amount of time in overall hypoglycemia, during both day and night and with a higher glucose variability (CV 0.26 ± 0.04 vs. 0.21 ± 0.05; p = 0.039) (Table 1).

Table 1. Clinical and laboratory characteristics after the mixed meal tolerance test (MMTT) and continuous glucose monitoring (CGM) in subjects with different duration in severe hypoglycemia (<54 mg/dL).

Total Severe Hypoglycemia	≤1%	≥2%	p
Age (years)	40.2 ± 6.7	46.4 ± 9.7	0.517
BMI at time of BS (kg/m^2)	47.03 ± 7.1	39.9 ± 5.1	0.033
BMI at time of CGM (kg/m^2)	29.9 ± 3.6	26.8 ± 3.8	0.119
%WL at time of CGM	35.4 ± 10.6	32.7 ± 5.9	0.412
Time from BS (months)	42.6 ± 23	24.1 ± 12.0	0.073
HbA1c (%) at time of CGM	5.56 ± 0.4	5.2 ± 0.4	0.113
C-peptide at time of CGM	1.73 ± 0.78	1.34 ± 0.24	0.227
HOMA-IR at time of CGM	1.24 ± 0.82	1.19 ± 0.72	0.893

Table 1. *Cont.*

Total Severe Hypoglycemia	≤1%	≥2%	*p*
AUC glycemia MMTT (mg × dL × min)	13,548.6 ± 3661.6	16,208.3 ± 6219.1	0.254
AUC insulin MMTT (μUI × mL × min)	9639.6 ± 4424.8	7878.5 ± 5121.8	0.453
Mean BG (mg/dL)	89.5 ± 13.9	75.1 ± 8.8	0.022
Max BG (mg/dL)	175.6 ± 44.1	160.9 ± 23.8	0.518
Min BG (mg/dL)	48.4 ± 5.4	40.4 ± 1.3	0.002
% time in BG <54 mg/dL	0.55 ± 0.52	6.33 ± 4.18	<0.001
% time in BG 55–70 mg/dL	16.7 ± 13.4	33.2 ± 15.4	0.015
% time in BG 71–140 mg/dL	78.1 ± 11.3	58.9 ± 11.3	0.009
% time in BG >140 mg/dL	3.6 ± 6.1	1.56 ± 1.51	0.876
SD (mg/dL)	19.5 ± 6.1	19.3 ± 3.7	0.958
CV (mg/dL)	0.215 ± 0.05	0.261 ± 0.04	0.039
Diurnal hypoglycemias (%)	0.05 ± 0.17	1.73 ± 2.31	0.026
Nocturnal hypoglycemias (%)	0.79 ± 0.49	3.41 ± 1.92	0.009
Nocturnal hypoglycemias (min)	65.0 ± 48.9	295.6 ± 187.8	0.009

BMI: body mass index. BS: bariatric surgery. WL: weight loss. AUC: area under curve. BG: blood glucose. SD: standard deviation. CV: variation coefficient. Multivariate analysis after adjusting for gender, age, presurgical BMI, actual BMI, weight loss, time since surgery, and peak insulin levels in the MMTT did not show significant results for their association with hypoglycemic events.

Multivariate analysis after adjusting for gender, age, presurgical BMI, actual BMI, weight loss, time since surgery, and peak insulin levels in the MMTT, and repeated measures ANOVA for time and group did not show significant results for their association with hypoglycemic events.

3.3. Dietary Intake during CGM

Total dietary intake was not significantly different between patients with fewer hypoglycemia events (<1%) in comparison to those with frequent PBH (≥2%): 969.8 ± 149.6 vs. 1016.1 ± 220.2 kcal; $p = 0.583$. Regarding the distribution of macronutrients, we observed that there was a significantly higher intake of protein (29.9 ± 3.8% vs. 24.6 ± 3.6%; $p = 0.005$), but not a significant difference in the intake of carbohydrates (34.0 ± 3.4% vs. 38.9 ± 11.2, $p = 0.214$) or fat (36.1 ± 3.0% vs. 38.2 ± 11.1%; $p = 0.580$) in patients who had frequent PBH (≥2%). Physical activity was also not different between patients with <1% or ≥2% hypoglycemia events during CGM: 1411.7 ± 845.1 vs. 1449.8 ± 1062.2 MET/min/wk; $p = 0.945$.

4. Discussion

Our study reveals that more than 50% of patients with prior BS and symptoms of PBH do indeed present hypoglycemia, with glucose levels below 54 mg/dL measured in an MMTT and CGM. Even though the clinical relevance and interpretation of hypoglycemia observed with these two diagnostic methods differ, it is a very significant finding, with implications in everyday clinical practice. Interestingly, in our cohort of patients, 60% experienced hypoglycemia after an MMTT, whilst only 20% referred symptoms at the time of glucose values below 40 mg/dL. Patients who experienced postprandial hypoglycemia after the MMTT (Hypo group) in our series had also a significant increase in prior insulin levels (>200 μUI/mL), which doubles levels of patients without postprandial hypoglycemia (non-hypo group).

The underlying mechanism involved in the occurrence of PBH has been associated with the increased gastric emptying observed after Roux-en-Y gastric bypass, entailing an increased glucose absorption, which is accompanied by a significant increase in incretin levels, including GLP-1 [11–13]. In this regard, when GLP-1 is blocked by administration of its antagonist exendine 9–39, there is no hyper-insulinemic response, and hypoglycemia reverts in all patients exhibiting PBH [14]. An imbalance in the counter-regulatory response mediated by glucagon has also been suggested; specifically, lower early peak levels have been observed after MMTT in patients with hypoglycemia, which were unable to counter-regulate the over-elevated levels of insulin [12,13]. Even though this mitigated glucagon response has been consistently reported in several studies, some authors have not observed a significant difference in levels of patients with no PBH after RYGB [15], suggesting that this analytical finding may be inherent to altered post-bariatric surgery physiology, in the setting of sustained weight loss and lower nadir glucose levels, and not a true cause of PBH. Interestingly, in the aforementioned study, the authors found that levels of pancreatic polypeptide (PP) were significantly decreased in patients with PBH, in comparison to the control group. Given the fact that PP is a surrogate marker of parasympathetic input to the pancreas and a marker of autonomic hypoglycemia counter-regulation, in addition to glucagon and catecholamines, the authors speculated a global attenuation of neuro-hormonal responses to insulin-induced hypoglycemia in post-bariatric surgery patients experiencing substantial weight loss [15].

In our study, we observed a higher frequency of hypoglycemia in patients who had undergone BS more than three years ago, in agreement with previous reports [6,16]. A potential explanation for this finding may be related to a greater widening of the gastroyeyunal anastomosis over time, which would enable an increased gastric emptying and a greater incretin and insulin response to equivalent carbohydrate intake. In fact, in patients who underwent BS more than three years ago, peak insulin levels and AUC were much higher than in patients in whom surgery was performed less than 3 years ago.

We remark on the fact that the duration of the MMTT in our series was extended to 240 min because some patients may experience what is known as postprandial delayed hypoglycemia. Indeed, in three of the 12 patients in the Hypo group (25%), the minimum glucose levels were reached after 180 min. This consideration must be taken into account, especially in the specific setting of post-bariatric patients since shorter evaluations of only 120 min after intake of the mixed meal may underestimate the true prevalence of postprandial hypoglycemia during the MMTT and reduce its utility for diagnosis. This issue may turn markedly relevant. For instance, according to Halperin et al., CGM exhibits a higher sensibility and specificity (90% and 50%, respectively) for detecting hypoglycemia than MMTT (33% and 40%, respectively) [17]. Kefur et al. found similar trends favors to CGM [18]. However, Honka et al. presented opposite results; they found a higher sensibility and specificity (77% and 100%, respectively) for the MMT for detecting hypoglycemia [19]. It is worth noting that Halperin et al. [17] performed their MMTT with a mixed meal containing 40 g of carbohydrates, and a duration of only 120 min, which, as previously mentioned, may reduce the test's sensibility. Kefur et al. [18], on their part, used a mixed meal with only 28 g of carbohydrates, which is not enough for detecting hypoglycemia, and, therefore, also reducing their test's sensibility. Using around 50 g of carbohydrate mixed meal and a sufficiently long duration for the test, similar to the one performed in our study, the sensibility and specificity of the MMTT are significantly better than for CGM [6,19]. The composition of the MMTT may also be relevant, but it has not been consistently standardized. Although the total glucose load is lower than in the OGTT, the mixed intake of protein and fat also triggers insulin secretion. In addition, because the usual presentation of the mixed meal is in the format of a liquid preparation, it passes quickly through the gastric pouch and the small intestine, thereby potentially increasing the risk of early dumping and PBH.

From a clinical point of view, CGM seems more attractive than an MMTT to detect hypoglycemia, since it allows the analysis of glucose excursions during day and night, for several days, in relation to real-world patient's everyday life, and even detects asymptomatic and unawareness hypoglycemia, such as nocturnal hypoglycemia, not only postprandial hypoglycemia [20]. In a recent meta-analysis of eight studies including 280 post-bariatric patients, around 50% exhibited diurnal and nocturnal hypoglycemia, according to CGM. Therefore, the authors concluded that CGM is the most efficient and precise method for detecting any form of PBH [6], in agreement with previous studies [17,18]. Another interesting finding of this meta-analysis is that patients with previous RYGB exhibit a greater glucose variability than patients who underwent sleeve gastrectomy (SG); in fact, they noted that diurnal hypoglycemia was more characteristic for post-SG patients, whilst nocturnal hypoglycemia was more frequently observed in post-RYGB patients. In line with these observations, a previous study performed by our group revealed a greater glucose variability in patients with prior RYGB, in comparison to patients in whom their BS preserved the gastric pyloric sphincter [21].

In line with this previous point, when evaluated using CGM, our patients showed a higher frequency of hypoglycemia (75% of patients), with a clear nocturnal and asymptomatic predominance (70%, versus 25% postprandial). This means that post-RYGB patients experience a mean duration of at least 30 min with nocturnal asymptomatic severe hypoglycemia (<54 mg/dL). Unawareness of hypoglycemia may be due to repeated chronic hypoglycemia, which reduces the threshold for detection and triggering of counter-hormonal response [20], or aberrant regulation of glycogenolysis and/or neoglycogenesis during the night [22]. In this scenario, it is advisable to screen patients for nocturnal sweating, poor sleep quality, restless dreams, and morning headaches as potential symptoms linked to nocturnal hypoglycemia [22]. In this regard, for instance, our patients only reported symptoms of hypoglycemia after the MMTT when glucose levels were below 40 mg/dL. The clinical implication of this finding is highly relevant, since repeated unawareness of hypoglycemia may entail deleterious effects on cognitive function [23] and is associated with an increased risk of non-fatal stroke, cardiovascular-related death, and total mortality in patients with diabetes [24,25].

The few studies that evaluate dietary intake and physical activity during CGM have not been able to prove significant differences between patients with or without postprandial hypoglycemia. In fact, there have been no differences either in macronutrient distribution, i.e., in the intake of rapidly absorbed carbohydrates, glycemic index, or glycemic load [20,26]. In agreement with these previous reports, we have not found significant differences in overall dietary intake or physical activity in our cohort of patients, although a very subtle higher intake of protein in patients with frequent PBH. Additional studies are needed to elucidate the relationship between the quantity and quality of carbohydrates and proteins on insulin secretion in post-bariatric patients.

We did not find an association between the observed response of the Hypo and Non-hypo groups to the MMTT, and the frequency of overall hypoglycemia detected with CGM. However, when we stratified patients according to a low prevalence of hypoglycemia ($\leq$1%) versus a high prevalence ($\geq$2%), glucose variability was greater and pre-surgery BMI was lower in patients with a higher frequency of hypoglycemia, similar to what has been previously reported [27]. Accordingly, we did not find differences in glucose and insulin curves after the MMTT between both groups. Interestingly, 82% of the group with <1% hypoglycemia was adequately controlled with diet and alpha-glucosidase inhibitors within a few weeks, whereas 78% of the group with $\geq$2% hypoglycemia required 2 or more drugs to control hypoglycemia symptoms. Some patients even required endoscopic adjustment of gastro-jejunal anastomosis using argon plasma coagulation and/or the Apollo overstitch procedure.

Therefore, we can assume that, from a clinical point of view, the MMTT and CGM retrieve different results in patients that refer to PBH, but these results may complement each other. In this regard, the MMTT is a provocative dynamic test that helps establish the confirmed diagnosis of PBH in 89% of our patients with a longer duration after BS but would be less predictive in patients reporting PBH with a shorter follow-up period after BS.

On the other hand, CGM would serve as an alert for detecting any type of hypoglycemia (postprandial, nocturnal, asymptomatic, symptomatic), in any case, scenario of everyday life, regardless of the time elapsed after BS, the percentage weight loss or the result after the MMTT, confirming the usefulness and convenience of CGM in the real-world setting [6].

A debatable matter regarding CGM is the specific type of device that should be used and the threshold values for defining hypoglycemia. These devices usually measure glucose levels in the interstitial liquid of the subcutaneous adipose tissue and prove an acceptable correlation with plasma glucose levels. In our study, we defined hypoglycemia according to a Joint Position Statement of the American Diabetes Association and the European Association for the Study of Diabetes as glucose levels <54 mg/dL (<3.0 mmol/L), detected by self-monitoring of capillary glucose, continuous glucose monitoring or a laboratory measurement [28]. It is rare that this level is reached under physiological conditions in nondiabetic individuals. Moreover, this threshold was chosen according to the study by Shah et al., performed in healthy non-diabetic individuals wearing CGM for 10 days [29]. They found that 14% of participants had a hypoglycemic event overnight. Overall, 35% of participants spent ≥2% of the time with sensor glucose <70 mg/dL (almost 30 min/d), but only 1% of participants spent ≥2% of time <54 mg/dL. [28]. This could be viewed as the most accurate approximation to the definition of PBH and for decision-making regarding the treatment of critical situations, especially in the setting of patients with diabetes taking glucose-lowering drugs.

However, discrimination of glucose levels in the range of severe hypoglycemia is quite poor for the majority of CGM devices, and this should be taken into account [30]. In fact, one of the most critical aspects of studies evaluating hypoglycemia concerns the accuracy and reliability of interstitial glucose measurements with different devices, which is performed using the mean absolute relative difference (MARD) between CGM readings and paired blood glucose values [31]. The ideal device would have a MARD < 10%, but the mean MARD for the majority of CGM devices is well above that target, and in the range of hypoglycemia, it may even be >20% [32,33]. The majority of studies evaluating PBH have used Medtronic or Dexcom devices, with similar results using different thresholds (<70 mg/dL, <60 mg/dL, or <50 mg/dL) [6]. Another important consideration is the location for placing the device, since there may be noteworthy reading errors if the device is trampled, for instance, if the patient rests on his/her arm, which is the usual site, presumably, due to local blood-flow decreases caused by tissue compression [34]. To avoid this potential confounder, our patients wore the device on the abdomen.

Our study has some limitations. First, we only evaluated patients with a prior history of repeated hypoglycemia after RYGB, without a control group of asymptomatic patients with the same type of BS, which may hinder the potential detection of differences in cases of asymptomatic hypoglycemia. Second, we were unable to perform detailed dietary and exercise recordings to account for all glucose excursions during CGM. Additionally, even though patients calibrated the device according to capillary glucose levels every six hours, calibration was withheld during the patients' night-time rest. Thus, we lack a paired comparison of the accuracy of the correlation of CGM and capillary glucose levels during the periods in the range of hypoglycemia. In any case, we remark on the strengths of our study, which concern the performance of an MMTT with a full evaluation of glucose and insulin curves for 240 min, improved potential detection of hypoglycemia, and the concomitant use of a CGM device for seven days to evaluate all glucose excursions occurring during this period of time.

5. Conclusions

In patients with recurrent symptoms of PBH after RYGB, the MMTT confirms the diagnosis of postprandial hyperinsulinemic hypoglycemia when bariatric surgery was performed more than three years ago. Detection of nocturnal asymptomatic hypoglycemia with CGM jeopardizes the idea that PBH is predominantly postprandial. Additional studies with accurate CGM devices in the range of hypoglycemia are needed to better explore PBH.

Author Contributions: Conceptualization, A.M.R.-L. and M.A.R.-H.; methodology, A.M.R.-L. and M.A.R.-H.; formal analysis, A.M.R.-L. and M.A.R.-H.; investigation, A.M.R.-L., M.A.R.-H., P.M.-M., C.M., N.P.-F., A.S.-P., A.J.T.-G. and A.L.C.-P.; resources, A.M.R.-L., M.A.R.-H., P.M.-M., A.S.-P. and A.L.C.-P.; writing—original draft preparation, A.M.R.-L. and M.A.R.-H.; writing—review and editing A.M.R.-L., M.A.R.-H., P.M.-M., A.S.-P., A.J.T.-G. and A.L.C.-P.; supervision, A.M.R.-L. and M.A.R.-H. All authors have read and agreed to the published version of the manuscript.

Funding: Fundación de Investigación en Nutrición y Metabolismo (FINUMET) and Fundación de Estudios Metabólicos, Madrid, Spain.

Institutional Review Board Statement: All procedures performed were in accordance with the 1975 Helsinki Declaration and its later amendments or comparable ethical standards for studies involving human participants. The project was approved by the Clinical Research Ethics Committee (code CI-11/080E), Hospital Clínico San Carlos, Madrid, Spain.

Informed Consent Statement: Informed consent was obtained from all subjects involved in the study.

Data Availability Statement: Not applicable.

Conflicts of Interest: The authors declare no conflict of interest.

References

1. Hatoum, I.J.; Blackstone, R.; Hunter, T.D.; Francis, D.M.; Steinbuch, M.; Harris, J.L.; Kaplan, L.M. Clinical Factors Associated with Remission of Obesity-Related Comorbidities After Bariatric Surgery. *JAMA Surg.* **2016**, *151*, 130–137. [CrossRef]
2. Torrego-Ellacuría, M.; Barabash, A.; Larrad-Sainz, A.; Hernández-Nuñez, G.M.; Matía-Martín, P.; Pérez-Ferre, N.; Marcuello, C.; Sánchez-Pernaute, A.; Torres, A.J.; Calle-Pascual, A.L.; et al. Weight Regain Outcomes after Bariatric Surgery in the Long-term Follow-up: Role of Preoperative Factors. *Obes. Surg.* **2021**, *31*, 3947–3955. [CrossRef] [PubMed]
3. Neovius, M.; Bruze, G.; Jacobson, P.; Sjöholm, K.; Johansson, K.; Granath, F.; Sundström, J.; Näslund, I.; Marcus, C.; Ottosson, J.; et al. Risk of suicide and non-fatal self-harm after bariatric surgery: Results from two matched cohort studies. *Lancet Diabetes Endocrinol.* **2018**, *3*, 197–207. [CrossRef] [PubMed]
4. Lindeman, K.G.; Greenblatt, L.B.; Rourke, C.; Bouxsein, M.L.; Finkelstein, J.S.; Yu, E.W. Longitudinal 5-Year Evaluation of Bone Density and Microarchitecture after Roux-en-Y Gastric Bypass Surgery. *J. Clin. Endocrinol. Metab.* **2018**, *103*, 4104–4112. [CrossRef] [PubMed]
5. Emous, M.; Ubels, F.L.; Van Beek, A.P. Diagnostic tools for post-gastric bypass hypoglycaemia. *Obes. Rev.* **2015**, *16*, 843–856. [CrossRef] [PubMed]
6. Lupoli, R.; Lembo, E.; Rainone, C.; Schiavo, L.; Iannelli, A.; Di Minno, M.N.; Capaldo, B. Rate of post-bariatric hypoglycemia using continuous glucose monitoring: A meta-analysis of literature studies. *Nutr. Metab. Cardiovasc. Dis.* **2022**, *32*, 32–39. [CrossRef]
7. Sarwar, H.; Chapman, W.H., 3rd; Pender, J.R.; Ivanescu, A.; Drake, A.J., 3rd; Pories, W.J.; Dar, M.S. Hypoglycemia after Roux-en-Y gastric bypass: The BOLD experience. *Obes. Surg.* **2014**, *24*, 1120–1124. [CrossRef]
8. Vilarrasa, N.; Goday, A.; Rubio, M.A.; Caixàs, A.; Pellitero, S.; Ciudin, A.; Calañas, A.; Botella, J.I.; Bretón, I.; Morales, M.J.; et al. Hyperinsulinemic Hypoglycemia after Bariatric Surgery: Diagnosis and Management Experience from a Spanish Multicenter Registry. *Obes. Facts* **2016**, *9*, 41–51. [CrossRef]
9. Lee, C.J.; Clark, J.M.; Schweitzer, M.; Magnuson, T.; Steele, K.; Koerner, O.; Brown, T.T. Prevalence of and risk factors for hypoglycemic symptoms after gastric bypass and sleeve gastrectomy. *Obesity* **2015**, *23*, 1079–1084. [CrossRef]
10. Kovatchev, B.; Cobelli, C. Glucose Variability: Timing, Risk Analysis, and Relationship to Hypoglycemia in Diabetes. *Diabetes Care* **2016**, *39*, 502–510. [CrossRef]
11. Goldfine, A.B.; Mun, E.C.; Devine, E.; Bernier, R.; Baz-Hecht, M.; Jones, D.B.; Schneider, B.E.; Holst, J.J.; Patti, M.E. Patients with Neuroglycopenia after Gastric Bypass Surgery Have Exaggerated Incretin and Insulin Secretory Responses to a Mixed Meal. *J. Clin. Endocrinol. Metab.* **2007**, *92*, 4678–4685. [CrossRef]
12. Tharakan, G.; Behary, P.; Albrechtsen, N.J.W.; Chahal, H.; Kenkre, J.; Miras, A.D.; Ahmed, A.R.; Holst, J.J.; Bloom, S.R.; Tan, T. Roles of increased glycaemic variability, GLP-1 and glucagon in hypoglycaemia after Roux-en-Y gastric bypass. *Eur. J. Endocrinol.* **2017**, *177*, 455–464. [CrossRef]
13. Lobato, C.B.; Pereira, S.S.; Guimarães, M.; Hartmann, B.; Albrechtsen, N.J.W.; Hilsted, L.; Holst, J.J.; Nora, M.; Monteiro, M.P. A Potential Role for Endogenous Glucagon in Preventing Post-Bariatric Hypoglycemia. *Front. Endocrinol.* **2020**, *11*, 608248. [CrossRef]
14. Salehi, M.; Gastaldelli, A.; D'Alessio, D.A. Blockade of Glucagon-like Peptide 1 Receptor Corrects Postprandial Hypoglycemia After Gastric Bypass. *Gastroenterology* **2014**, *146*, 669–680.e2. [CrossRef]
15. Tripyla, A.; Herzig, D.; Reverter-Branchat, G.; Pavan, J.; Schiavon, M.; Eugster, P.J.; Grouzmann, E.; Nakas, C.T.; Sauvinet, V.; Meiller, L.; et al. Counter-regulatory responses to postprandial hypoglycaemia in patients with post-bariatric hypoglycaemia vs surgical and non-surgical control individuals. *Diabetologia* **2023**, *66*, 741–753. [CrossRef]

16. Ostrovsky, V.; Knobler, H.; Lazar, L.O.; Pines, G.; Kuniavsky, T.; Cohen, L.; Schiller, T.; Kirzhner, A.; Zornitzki, T. Persistent post-bariatric-surgery hypoglycemia: A long-term follow-up reassessment. *Nutr. Metab. Cardiovasc. Dis.* **2023**, *33*, 1197–1205. [CrossRef]
17. Halperin, F.; Patti, M.E.; Skow, M.; Bajwa, M.; Goldfine, A.B. Continuous Glucose Monitoring for Evaluation of Glycemic Excursions after Gastric Bypass. *J. Obes.* **2011**, *2011*, 869536. [CrossRef]
18. Kefurt, R.; Langer, F.B.; Schindler, K.; Shakeri-Leidenmühler, S.; Ludvik, B.; Prager, G. Hypoglycemia after Roux-En-Y gastric bypass: Detection rates of continuous glucose monitoring (CGM) versus mixed meal test. *Surg. Obes. Relat. Dis.* **2015**, *11*, 564–569. [CrossRef]
19. Honka, H.; Chuang, J.; D'alessio, D.; Salehi, M. Utility of Continuous Glucose Monitoring vs. Meal Study in Detecting Hypoglycemia After Gastric Bypass. *J. Clin. Endocrinol. Metab.* **2022**, *107*, e2095–e2102. [CrossRef]
20. Lupoli, R.; Lembo, E.; Ciciola, P.; Schiavo, L.; Pilone, V.; Capaldo, B. Continuous glucose monitoring in subjects undergoing bariatric surgery: Diurnal and nocturnal glycemic patterns. *Nutr. Metab. Cardiovasc. Dis.* **2020**, *30*, 1954–1960. [CrossRef]
21. Ramos-Leví, A.M.; Sánchez-Pernaute, A.; Marcuello, C.; Galindo, M.; Calle-Pascual, A.L.; Torres, A.J.; Rubio, M.A. Glucose Variability After Bariatric Surgery: Is Prediction of Diabetes Remission Possible? *Obes. Surg.* **2017**, *27*, 3341–3343. [CrossRef] [PubMed]
22. Lee, D.; Dreyfuss, J.M.; Sheehan, A.; Puleio, A.; Mulla, C.M.; Patti, M.E. Glycemic Patterns Are Distinct in Post-Bariatric Hypoglycemia after Gastric Bypass (PBH-RYGB). *J. Clin. Endocrinol. Metab.* **2021**, *106*, 2291–2303. [CrossRef] [PubMed]
23. Guldstrand, M.; Ahrén, B.; Wredling, R.; Backman, L.; Lins, P.E.; Adamson, U. Alteration of the counterregulatory responses to insulin-induced hypoglycemia and of cognitive function after massive weight reduction in severely obese subjects. *Metabolism* **2003**, *52*, 900–907. [CrossRef] [PubMed]
24. Wei, W.; Zhao, S.; Fu, S.-L.; Yi, L.; Mao, H.; Tan, Q.; Xu, P.; Yang, G.-L. The Association of Hypoglycemia Assessed by Continuous Glucose Monitoring with Cardiovascular Outcomes and Mortality in Patients with Type 2 Diabetes. *Front. Endocrinol.* **2019**, *10*, 536. [CrossRef] [PubMed]
25. Pieber, T.R.; DEVOTE Study Group; Marso, S.P.; McGuire, D.K.; Zinman, B.; Poulter, N.R.; Emerson, S.S.; Pratley, R.E.; Woo, V.; Heller, S.; et al. DEVOTE 3: Temporal relationships between severe hypoglycaemia, cardiovascular outcomes and mortality. *Diabetologia* **2018**, *61*, 58–65. [CrossRef] [PubMed]
26. Hemmingsson, J.U.; Leijonmarck, C.-E.; Klingvall, M. Postbariatric hypoglycemia in symptomatic versus asymptomatic patients: Proposals for clinical assessments. *BMJ Open Diabetes Res. Care* **2022**, *10*, e002572. [CrossRef]
27. Emous, M.; Broek, M.V.D.; Wijma, R.B.; de Heide, L.J.M.; van Dijk, G.; Laskewitz, A.; Totté, E.; Wolffenbuttel, B.H.R.; van Beek, A.P. Prevalence of hypoglycaemia in a random population after Roux-en-Y gastric bypass after a meal test. *Endocr. Connect.* **2019**, *8*, 969–978. [CrossRef]
28. International Hypoglycaemia Study Group. Glucose concentrations of less than 3.0 mmol/L (54 mg/dL) should Be reported in clinical trials: A joint position statement of the American diabetes association and the European association for the study of diabetes. *Diabetologia* **2017**, *60*, 3–6. [CrossRef]
29. Shah, V.N.; DuBose, S.N.; Li, Z.; Beck, R.W.; Petesrs, A.L.; Weinstock, R.S.; Kruger, D.; Tansey, M.; Sparling, D.; Woerner, S.; et al. Continuous Glucose Monitoring Profiles in Healthy Nondiabetic Participants: A Multicenter Prospective Study. *J. Clin. Endocrinol. Metab.* **2019**, *104*, 4356–4364. [CrossRef]
30. Vilarrasa, N.; Bretón, I.; Ballesteros-Pomar, M.; Lecube, A.; Goday, A.; Pellitero, S.; Sánchez, R.; Zugasti, A.; Ciudin, A.; de Hollanda, A.; et al. Recommendations for the diagnosis and treatment of hypoglycaemia after bariatric surgery. *Endocrinol. Diabetes Nutr.* **2022**, *69*, 723–731. [CrossRef]
31. Heinemann, L.; Schoemaker, M.; Schmelzeisen-Redecker, G.; Hinzmann, R.; Kassab, A.; Freckmann, G.; Reiterer, F.; Del Re, L. Benefits and Limitations of MARD as a Performance Parameter for Continuous Glucose Monitoring in the Interstitial Space. *J. Diabetes Sci. Technol.* **2020**, *14*, 135–150. [CrossRef]
32. Freckmann, G.; Pleus, S.; Link, M.; Zschornack, E.; Klötzer, H.-M.; Haug, C. Performance Evaluation of Three Continuous Glucose Monitoring Systems: Comparison of Six Sensors per Subject in Parallel. *J. Diabetes Sci. Technol.* **2013**, *7*, 842–853. [CrossRef]
33. Zhou, Y.; Mai, X.; Deng, H.; Yang, D.; Zheng, M.; Huang, B.; Xu, L.; Weng, J.; Xu, W.; Yan, J. Discrepancies in glycemic metrics derived from different continuous glucose monitoring systems in adult patients with type 1 diabetes mellitus. *J. Diabetes* **2022**, *14*, 476–484. [CrossRef]
34. Mensh, B.D.; Wisniewski, N.A.; Neil, B.M.; Burnett, D.R. Susceptibility of Interstitial Continuous Glucose Monitor Performance to Sleeping Position. *J. Diabetes Sci. Technol.* **2013**, *7*, 863–870. [CrossRef]

Journal of
Clinical Medicine

MDPI

Review

Micronutrients in Pregnancy after Bariatric Surgery: A Narrative Review

Irene Bretón [1,2,*], María D. Ballesteros-Pomar [3], Alfonso Calle-Pascual [2,4,5], Luis Antonio Alvarez-Sala [2,6] and Miguel Angel Rubio-Herrera [2,4]

1 Department of Endocrinology and Nutrition, Hospital General Universitario Gregorio Marañón, Instituto de Investigación Sanitaria Gregorio Marañón, 28007 Madrid, Spain
2 Department of Medicine, Facultad de Medicina, Universidad Complutense, 28040 Madrid, Spain
3 Department of Endocrinology and Nutrition, Complejo Asistencial Universitario de León, 24008 León, Spain
4 Department of Endocrinology and Nutrition, Hospital Clínico Universitario San Carlos, Instituto de Investigación Sanitaria del Hospital Clínico San Carlos, 28040 Madrid, Spain
5 Centro de Investigación Biomédica en Red de Diabetes y Enfermedades Metabólicas Asociadas (CIBERDEM), 28029 Madrid, Spain
6 Department of Internal Medicine, Hospital General Universitario Gregorio Marañón, 28007 Madrid, Spain
* Correspondence: irenebreton@gmail.com

Abstract: Bariatric surgery is increasingly used in women of childbearing age due to the rising prevalence of obesity and the effectiveness and availability of this treatment. Pregnancy in women with previous bariatric surgery deserves special attention. Weight loss induced by surgery reduces the risks that obesity poses to pregnancy. But on the other hand, decreased intake and malabsorption may increase the risk of malnutrition and micronutrient deficiency and negatively affect maternal and foetal health. The aim of this narrative review is to provide an updated analysis of the impact of different bariatric surgery techniques on mineral and micronutrient nutritional status during pregnancy and the possible effect on maternal–foetal health.

Keywords: bariatric; pregnancy; micronutrient deficiency

Citation: Bretón, I.; Ballesteros-Pomar, M.D.; Calle-Pascual, A.; Alvarez-Sala, L.A.; Rubio-Herrera, M.A. Micronutrients in Pregnancy after Bariatric Surgery: A Narrative Review. *J. Clin. Med.* **2023**, *12*, 5429. https://doi.org/10.3390/jcm12165429

Academic Editor: Giuseppe Nisi

Received: 12 June 2023
Revised: 14 August 2023
Accepted: 16 August 2023
Published: 21 August 2023

1. Introduction

Obesity is the most common metabolic disease in our environment and is associated with numerous medical and psychosocial complications and a clear deterioration in the quality of life. People with obesity have an increased risk of overall mortality and of developing other pathologies, such as type 2 diabetes, arterial hypertension, dyslipidaemia, respiratory diseases, and neoplasms, among others [1,2].

Obesity directly affects reproductive function in both males and females through complex and not fully understood mechanisms. In women, obesity increases the risk of infertility and is a poor prognostic factor when assisted reproduction techniques are used [3,4]. Both pregestational maternal obesity and excessive weight gain are associated with an increased risk of maternal–foetal complications, both short- and long-term [5–7] (Table 1). The risk of developing these complications is high, more than double that of normal-weight women [8]. It is estimated that 24.9% of the risk of any complication can be attributed to maternal overweight, and this attributable risk reaches 31.6% in the case of a large-for-gestational-age newborn (LBW) [8]. In morbidly or extremely obese women, the risk of complications during pregnancy and delivery is even higher [9,10].

Table 1. Clinical consequences of maternal obesity and excess weight gain in pregnancy.

Clinical Consequences of Maternal Obesity and Excess Weight Gain in Pregnancy	
Maternal	
Pre-conception	Higher risk of type 2 diabetes, high blood pressure, and infertility.
Pregnancy	Previous metabolic diseases, gestational diabetes, hypertension, deep vein thrombosis, pulmonary thromboembolism, depression.
Delivery	Higher risk of complications, instrumental delivery, caesarean, higher anaesthetic risk.
Postpartum	Infection, depression, failure in breastfeeding, weight retention, obesity
Newborn and infant	
	Macrosomia, large-for-gestational-age newborn, prematurity, shoulder dystocia, birth defects, neonatal hypoglycaemia.
Long term	
	Higher risk of obesity, metabolic complications. Higher vascular risk for both the mother and offspring.

Bariatric surgery results in significant and sustained weight loss in people with severe obesity and can decrease the risk of mortality and induce the remission or improvement of most comorbidities. The increase in the prevalence of obesity and the efficacy of bariatric surgery are leading to the increasing use of this treatment, especially in women of child-bearing age.

Pregnancy in women with previous BS deserves special consideration. Weight loss induced by surgery reduces the risks that obesity implies for pregnancy. However, due to its effect on nutrient intake and absorption, it can also have adverse consequences on maternal and foetal health. Among them, vitamin and mineral deficiencies are especially frequent and require a protocolised evaluation and treatment.

The aim of this narrative review is to provide an updated analysis of the impact of different bariatric surgery techniques on mineral and micronutrient nutritional status during pregnancy and the possible effect on maternal–foetal health.

2. Bariatric Surgery and Pregnancy

Bariatric surgery (BS) includes a set of surgical techniques used in patients with severe forms of obesity, with an aim to achieve weight loss, maintained over time, in order to improve associated diseases and the quality of life. Various bariatric surgery techniques have been described [11]. Based on their main mechanism of action, they are usually classified into three main groups: restrictive: vertical banded gastroplasty, adjustable gastric banding, and gastrectomy; mixed: gastric bypass; and malabsorptive: biliopancreatic diversion and its variants. The most frequently used BS procedures are Roux-Y gastric bypass (RYGB) and sleeve gastrectomy (SG); biliopancreatic diversion (BPD) and gastric banding (GB), widely used a decade ago, have been displaced by the first two [12] (Figure 1).

The mechanisms by which BS induces weight loss and improvements in metabolic diseases are complex and not fully understood [13,14]. Decreased intake and malabsorption, when present, are ultimately responsible for weight loss and improvements in obesity-related complications, but surgery is also able to induce changes in digestive hormones, such as ghrelin or GLP-1, among others, which are involved in the regulation of energy expenditure, insulin sensitivity and secretion, modification of the microbiota [15], or the physiology of bile acids [16,17]. Several studies have shown that, in patients with severe obesity, bariatric surgery decreases the risk of mortality and can achieve the remission or improvement of most comorbidities [18,19]. However, these procedures are not without risks. Among these, vitamin and mineral deficiencies are particularly common and require protocolised assessment, preventive supplementation, and treatment [20,21]. Figure 2 shows the preferred sites of the absorption of minerals and micronutrients.

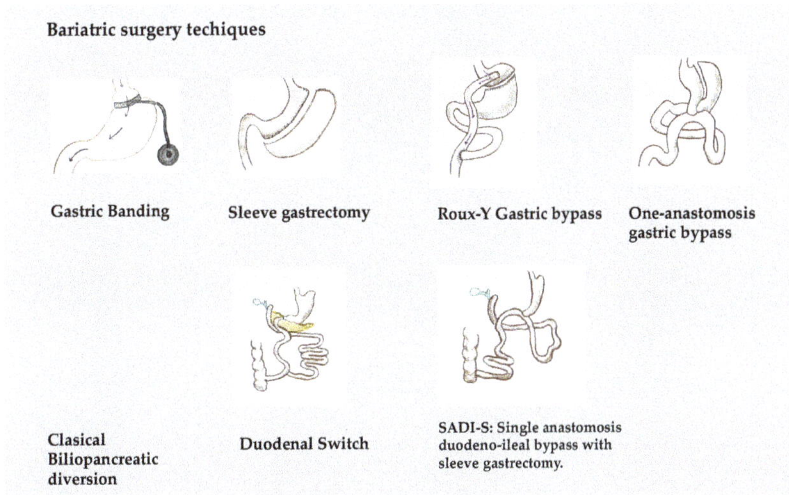

Figure 1. Main bariatric surgical techniques.

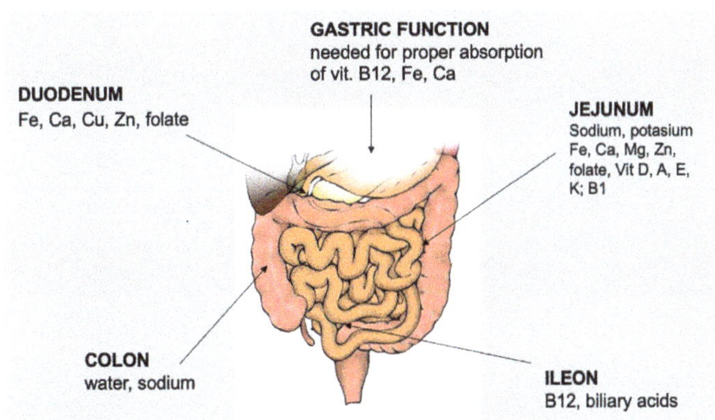

Figure 2. Main sites of absorption of minerals and micronutrients.

The risk of mineral and micronutrient deficiencies after bariatric surgery depends on the patient's dietary intake and on the anatomical and functional changes induced by the surgery itself. Malabsorption is frequent in techniques that exclude the duodenum and first jejunal loops and/or with a long biliopancreatic limb. It should be noted that in some techniques that are usually not considered "malabsorptive", such as Roux-Y gastric bypass, the length of the limbs can vary considerably, and the biliopancreatic limb can be 150–200 cm or more. In these cases, although the malabsorption of proteins and other macronutrients is not frequent, the risk of a deficiency of micronutrients absorbed in the duodenum and first jejunal loops, such as iron, calcium, or copper, is greatly increased. Steatorrhea further decreases the absorption of calcium and liposoluble vitamins. Bariatric surgery induces changes in several gastrointestinal hormones, such as GLP-1, which has been linked to decreased food intake, improved glucose metabolism, and other lesser-known effects, such as the modulation of the sense of taste [22]. No specific role in micronutrient absorption after BS has been described so far. Table 2 summarises the main mechanisms leading to micronutrient deficiencies following different bariatric surgery techniques.

Table 2. Main micronutrient deficiencies after bariatric surgery.

Surgical Technique	Physiopathological Factors	Most Affected Micronutrients
Gastric banding	Decrease intake Food intolerance (meat, milk)	All micronutrients, especially those with low body stores (thiamine) Iron, zinc, calcium, vit D
Sleeve gastrectomy	Decrease intake Food intolerance (meat, milk) Gastrectomy	All micronutrients, especially those with low body stores (thiamine) Iron, zinc, calcium, vit D Vitamin B12, iron, calcium
Roux-Y gastric bypass	Decrease intake Food intolerance (meat, milk) Gastrectomy Duodenal/jejunal exclusion	All micronutrients, especially those with low body stores (thiamine) Iron, zinc, calcium, vit D Vitamin B12, iron, calcium Iron, calcium, zinc, copper, liposoluble vitamins
Biliopancreatic diversion duodenal switch SADI-S	Decrease intake Food intolerance (meat, milk) Gastrectomy Duodenal/jejunal exclusion Steatorrhea	All micronutrients, especially those with low body stores (thiamine) Iron, zinc, calcium, vit D Vitamin B12, iron, calcium Iron, calcium, zinc, copper, liposoluble vitamins Calcium, liposoluble vitamins

Scientific societies have provided recommendations for clinical and nutritional follow-up after bariatric surgery and proposals for preventive micronutrient supplementation, according to the type of surgical technique [23,24] (Table 3).

Table 3. Proposal of micronutrient recommendations in pregnancy after bariatric surgery.

Micronutrient	SG/RYGB	BPD and Other Malabsorptive Procedures
Folate	400–8008 μg/d 800–1000 μg/d in women of childbearing age	
Vitamin B12	350–1000 μg/d (oral or sublingual) 1000 μg/month IM-SC)	
Thiamine	12 mg/d Increase to 100–300 mg if low intake, nausea/vomiting	
Vitamin D	3000 UI/d (Vit D > 30 ng/mL)	A higher dose is usually needed
Vitamin A	800–3000 μg/d	3000 μg/d (10.000 UI)
Vitamin E	15 mg/d	90 mg/d
Vitamin K	50–120 μg/d	300 μg/d
Iron	SG: male or non-menstruating: 18 mg/d Menstruating female or RYGB/BPD: 45–60 mg/d	
Calcium	1200–1500 mg/d	1800–2400 mg/d
Magnesium	350 mg/d	350 mg/d
Zinc	SG: 8–11 mg/d RYGB: 8–22 mg/d	16–22 mg/d
Copper	SG: 1 mg/d RYGB 2 mg/d	2 mg/d

The increasing number of BS procedures being performed today, especially in women of childbearing age, makes post-surgery gestation a topic of great interest. Several systematic reviews and meta-analyses that evaluate the effect of BS on maternal and foetal outcomes have been published. Bariatric surgery can decrease the risk of obesity-related complications in pregnancy [25–27]. However, it may also have adverse consequences on maternal–foetal health [28–34]. Galazis et al. published a meta-analysis that includes 17 studies and provides results depending on the characteristics of the control group [25]. Thus, it is observed that the benefits of BS in reducing the risk of complications are more evident when maternal–foetal outcomes are compared with those of women with severe obesity. When the control group includes women with obesity, but the BMI is adjusted to pre-pregnancy, a decreased risk of LGA, but an increased risk of preterm delivery and a small-for-gestational-age (SGA) newborn, is observed. In this case, no increase or a decrease in the risk of GD, preeclampsia, the need for caesarean section, or neonatal complications is observed. The meta-analysis performed by Kwong et al. provides data on the effect of BS on maternal–foetal complications when compared with a group with similar BMI before BS and before gestation. The results of this meta-analysis indicate that, when compared with women with equal pregestational BMI, prior BS decreases the risk of high birth weight and increases the risk of low birth weight (<2500 g), SGA, the need for caesarean section, and prematurity. No changes in the risk of GD or preeclampsia or neonatal complications were observed [27]. There was a significant increase in the risk of perinatal mortality, congenital anomalies, preterm birth, and neonatal ICU admission, with a birth weight more than 200 g lower than those born to mothers without prior BS [35].

There is little information on the most appropriate interval between bariatric surgery and pregnancy and on the risk of complications of early gestation [36–38]. Clinical guidelines recommend delaying pregnancy for 12–18 months after BS, until weight loss has stabilised and dietary intake is adequate, to prevent nutritional deficiencies [31,32,39,40]. Although studies that have evaluated early pregnancies have not consistently observed an increase in complications [36,37,41], a closer clinical follow-up is recommended in these cases.

3. Micronutrients, Pregnancy, and Bariatric Surgery

Maternal nutritional factors are of great importance for foetal development. Energy and nutrient requirements increase during gestation to allow for adequate embryonic and foetal development and the necessary changes in the mother for pregnancy and lactation. A balanced diet, which provides enough energy, usually contains enough essential micronutrients. However, during pregnancy, requirements are often not met by food-based diets, and in these situations, specific supplementation is necessary to prevent deficiencies [42]. Micronutrients are essential for foetal development (Table 4). There is no unanimous agreement on preventive supplementation during pregnancy, which will depend on the characteristics of the pregnant woman and the risk of deficiency in her environment [43–47].

Previous bariatric surgery, especially if there is significant malabsorption, can increase the risk of malnutrition and micronutrient deficiencies during pregnancy, with adverse consequences for the mother and newborn [29–34]. There are several factors that may favour the risk of micronutrient deficiency in pregnancy after bariatric surgery, including decreased intake, gastrectomy, and malabsorption, as has been described before. There are few data on dietary intake in pregnant women with previous barbaric surgery. Available information suggests that it may be insufficient in essential nutrients [44]. In general, malabsorptive techniques are associated with a higher risk of complications in pregnancy after BS, especially maternal anaemia and low-birth-weight babies [45]. Anyway, it should be noted that patients who undergo malabsorptive BS have a higher pre-surgical BMI and that pregnancy in women with a BMI over 50 kg/m^2 presents a very high risk of complications [46]. There are other risk factors for micronutrient deficiency that should not be overlooked. Veganism increases the risk of vitamin B12, iron, and zinc deficiencies. Drug–nutrient interaction therapy should be considered; for example, proton-pump inhibitors can decrease vitamin B12, iron, and magnesium absorption. Smoking and consumption of alcoholic beverages, well-recognised causes of pregnancy complications and alterations in foetal development, can also induce micronutrient deficiencies [47]. The evaluation of the nutritional status of vitamins and minerals should consider the reference serum values during pregnancy [48].

Table 4. Clinical consequences of micronutrient deficiency during pregnancy.

Micronutrient	Clinical Consequences of Deficiency for Maternal–Foetal Health
Folate	Neural tube defects, miscarriage, abruptio placentae, prematurity
Vitamin B12	Abortion, prematurity, growth retardation, neural tube defects, cognitive impairment
Thiamine	Risk of thiamine deficiency in hyperemesis gravidarum
Vitamin D	Gestational diabetes, preeclampsia, low birth weight, long-term complications
Vitamin A	Foetal malformations, pulmonary dysplasia, anaemia
Vitamin E	Preeclampsia, neural tube defects, cognitive impairment, haemolytic disease of the newborn
Vitamin K	Periventricular and intraventricular haemorrhage
Iron	Increased maternal and foetal morbidity and mortality, miscarriage, decreased weight and foetal development
Zinc	Delayed foetal growth and maturation, prematurity
Copper	Abortion, prematurity, low weight
Selenium	Preeclampsia
Iodine	Alteration in the development of central nervous system, mental retardation

This section describes the main micronutrient deficiencies in pregnancy after bariatric surgery. For each micronutrient, its physiology, its relationship with pregnancy, the effect of bariatric surgery, and data on its deficiency in pregnancy after bariatric surgery are described.

3.1. Folate

Folic acid and folate are precursors of the coenzyme tetrahydrofolate, which is involved in the transfer of one-carbon groups in the metabolism of amino acids and nucleic acids. It also participates as a donor in the methylation of homocysteine to methionine. Folate deficiency alters DNA synthesis and cell division and induces megaloblastic anaemia, leukopenia, thrombopenia, and other alterations [49]. Folate stores are not high: the body's folate content ranges from 5 to 10 mg [49]. The main dietary sources of folate are vegetables, fruits, cereals, eggs, and fortified foods. Absorption occurs preferentially in the proximal third of the small intestine, being lower in patients with atrophic gastritis or intestinal resection. Folate requirements range from 300 to 400 µg/day, according to various guidelines and recommendations [50]. It is recommended that women of childbearing age receive a dose of 400 mg, in addition to that provided by food [50].

Folic acid is a relevant micronutrient during pregnancy and is essential for neural tube development [51]. Folate requirements increase in pregnancy by 50% because of increased maternal plasma volume, uterine and placental size, and foetal development. Maternal folate intake is related to newborn weight [52]. Most organisations recommend a total folate intake of 600 µg/day [50]. Folate deficiency during pregnancy is associated with neural tube defects (NTDs), with clinical manifestations of varying degrees of severity. In the brain, it can cause anencephaly and encephalocele, situations incompatible with life. In the spinal cord, it causes spina bifida syndrome, an isolated cleft of the spine, meningocele, and myelo-meningocele. In 90% of cases, they appear as isolated malformations. Folate deficiency has also been linked to recurrent miscarriage, placental abruption, and prematurity [53], probably related to a toxic effect of homocysteine on the embryo and alterations in placental vascularisation [54]. Pregnant women with obesity are at increased risk of NTDs. Obesity may lead to decreased plasma folate levels and increased erythrocyte uptake [55]. Folate requirements during pregnancy are generally not met by the diet. Folate supplementation, alone or in combination with vitamins and minerals, reduces the risk of NTDs [56]. However, it has no clear effect on other malformations or on other clinical variables of pregnancy [57]. Most guidelines recommend preventive supplementation with 400 mcg/day, starting 4 weeks before conception and lasting until at least week 12 of gestation. In women at high risk of neural tube defects, including women with obesity, a higher dose of 1–4 mg/day is recommended [58]. It should be kept in mind that doses higher than 1 mg/day may mask symptoms of vitamin B12 deficiency.

The prevalence of folate deficiency after bariatric surgery is highly variable in different series. Although folate absorption occurs primarily in the proximal intestine, there is an intestinal adaptation that allows it to be absorbed throughout the intestine after a bowel resection. For this reason, the prevalence of folate deficiency after BS is lower than for other water-soluble vitamins and is generally easily prevented with a multivitamin [59]. Anyway, deficiency has been reported in up to 44–65% of patients after restrictive techniques [60,61] and 8–47% after mixed techniques [59,62]. However, other authors have not observed deficiencies after RYGB or BPD [63]. A systematic review of the literature did not reveal an increase in folate deficiency after BS [64].

Data on the prevalence of folate deficiency throughout gestation after BS are very scarce. Very few cases of NTDs have been reported [65,66]. This is striking, considering the increasing number of such pregnancies and the fact that obesity itself increases the risk of NTDs. Regarding the prevalence of folate deficiency, the reference serum levels for pregnancy should be noted. In a prospective study of 49 patients with malabsorptive BS, 4% had levels below 2.52 ng/mL in the first trimester [67]. In another retrospective study analysing 39 pregnancies (including 9 miscarriages), decreased levels were observed in 16% of pregnancies in the first trimester [68]. In a retrospective multicentre study in Spain, folate deficiency was observed in 5.4% of pregnancies [69].

3.2. Vitamin B12

Vitamin B12 is present in animal tissues. Its absorption is very complex: it first needs to be freed from dietary proteins via the action of gastric acid and pepsin and then binds to haptocorrins, glycoproteins present in salivary and gastric secretions. The absorption of vitamin B12 occurs specifically in the distal ileum. Vitamin B12 is excreted via the bile and undergoes enterohepatic circulation [70]. Vitamin B12 deficiency results in megaloblastic anaemia, and, in severe cases, leukopenia and thrombopenia may occur. In addition, vitamin B12 deficiency has neurological effects, with paraesthesias and the involvement of the posterior cords of the spinal cord, which can sometimes occur in the absence of anaemia [70].

Vitamin B12 deficiency during pregnancy is associated with an increased risk of prematurity, miscarriage, intrauterine growth retardation and low birth weight, neural tube defects, and impaired cognitive development [71,72].

The complexity of vitamin B12 absorption makes vitamin B12 deficiency very common in any clinical situation involving the gastrointestinal tract, including bariatric surgery [73]. In mixed and malabsorptive techniques, deficiency is very common; it affects more than 75% of cases and increases as time passes after BS, when the body's stores of this vitamin are depleted, so prophylactic supplementation is recommended [73,74]. In general, it is recommended that vitamin B12 be administered intramuscularly (1000 µg/30–90 days) [75,76]. Oral or sublingual administration at high doses (more than 350 mg/day) also normalises plasma levels [75].

Clinical vitamin B12 deficiency during pregnancy after BS is rare but can cause serious problems in the newborn or infant, even in the absence of maternal symptoms [77–79]. Vitamin B12 requirements during pregnancy or lactation after BS are not established. Guidelines recommend a similar pattern to that in the non-pregnant population [76]. A recent study evaluated the levels of several micronutrients in the cord blood of 56 NBs of mothers with a history of BS compared to a group of NBs of healthy mothers. In the case of vitamin B12, decreased levels were observed in 14% vs. 2% ($p < 0.05$) [80]. Another study evaluated plasma vitamin B12 levels in 150 pregnancies after different BS techniques. Vitamin B12 levels did not decrease throughout gestation. An asymptomatic decrease in plasma levels (<130 pg/mL) was observed in 11.7% in the BPD group, 15.6 after RYGB, and 11% after SG; in eight patients, it was below 100 pg/mL [81]. Preventive vitamin B12 supplementation recommendations should be followed after BS and maintained throughout pregnancy. The dose included in ordinary or usual pregnancy multivitamins is not sufficient.

3.3. Thiamine

Thiamine is a water-soluble vitamin involved in carbohydrate metabolism, such as glycolysis, as a cofactor of the enzyme pyruvate dehydrogenase, and the pentose pathway. It is present in many foods and is absorbed primarily in the proximal small intestine. Body stores are very low, which increases the risk of clinical deficiency if intake is inadequate [82]. Thiamine deficiency is promoted by decreased intake, vomiting, intravenous glucose administration, refeeding, or ethanol intake and results in a clinical picture with ophthalmoplegia, nystagmus, confusion, and peripheral neuropathy. Laboratory data (plasma thiamine levels or transketolase activity) confirm the deficiency. Magnetic resonance imaging is of particular interest, as it characteristically identifies a hyperintense T2 signal in the periaqueductal white matter [83]. Treatment should be initiated immediately, even if it is based solely on clinical suspicion, by administering high doses of thiamine (300–500 mg/day parenterally), followed by 50–100 mg/day orally for months [84].

Thiamine requirements increase during pregnancy and lactation [85]. Hyperemesis gravidarum is a recognised cause of thiamine deficiency and is probably underdiagnosed [86]. The recommended daily intake during normal pregnancy and lactation is 1.4 mg/day [87].

Thiamine deficiency is a complication of bariatric surgery, which can have serious consequences and lead to irreversible neurological damage [88,89]. It has been described with all surgical techniques: most have been identified in patients with nausea and vomiting, poor oral tolerance, or poor compliance with supplementation. Diagnosis should be made early, as the delay can lead to irreversible neurological damage and, in the case of pregnancy, can have serious consequences for the mother and foetus [90]. It is recommended that all patients receive ≥12 mg/day of thiamine after BS [23]; supplementation should be maintained throughout life [91]. This dose should be increased in case of any risk of deficiency, such as anorexia, low intake, vomiting, or refeeding (50–300 mg/day).

There are few data in the literature on thiamine deficiency during pregnancy in women with previous BS. So far, one case of clinical deficiency has been described in a post-RYGB pregnancy with hyperemesis gravidarum [92]. Asymptomatic low thiamine serum levels in the third trimester have been observed in 17% of patients, being more frequent in malabsorptive techniques [67]. In another study evaluating serum levels in 57 pregnancies, decreased serum levels were observed in 45.5, 15.4, and 20% in the three trimesters of gestation, respectively [93]. In both studies, normal ranges for the non-pregnant population were used.

3.4. Calcium and Vitamin D

Calcium is an essential nutrient in human physiology that is involved in several metabolic pathways. Vitamin D-dependent calcium absorption takes place mainly in the duodenum and first jejunal loops; calcium requirements depend on the nutritional status of this vitamin. Vitamin D has multiple functions in the body: it promotes the absorption of calcium, phosphorus, and magnesium in the intestine, which allows for adequate bone mineralisation, stimulates innate and adaptive immunity, inhibits cell proliferation, and stimulates cell differentiation. The Endocrine Society proposes a serum level >30 ng/mL [94].

Vitamin D deficiency (VDD) is common in the general population and in pregnancy and can have adverse consequences on maternal and foetal health [95]. Vitamin D is involved in placental function, and its deficiency has been linked to insulin resistance and GD and to preeclampsia [96]. It is also involved in the development of the foetal nervous system, immune function, and lung maturation. VDD has been associated with an increased risk of low birth weight in some studies, but others have not observed this association. A meta-analysis including 12 studies with 19,027 patients found that vitamin D below 20 ng/mL is associated with an increased risk of SGA (birth weight percentile < 10), with an OR of 1.41, 95% CI 1.14, 1.75, 1.75 [97]. Women with deficient VitD levels had a higher preeclampsia rate compared to women with replete VitD levels (OR 1.50, 95% CI 1.05–2.14) [98]. Vitamin D below 16 ng/dL has been associated with a higher risk of C-section, and a level below 14 ng/dL has been associated with a higher risk of prematurity [99].

Bariatric surgery can induce calcium deficiency due to low dietary intake and malabsorption. Vitamin D deficiency is very common in morbidly obese patients. Bariatric surgery, especially when malabsorptive techniques are used, favours vitamin D deficiency, which is observed in more than 70% of cases. Long-term follow-up studies have also shown that VDD prevalence is high and is generally associated with increased PTH levels, which may have consequences for bone health. A systematic review of the literature confirms that hyperparathyroidism persists in the long term, despite calcium and vitamin D supplementation [100]. Several prevention and treatment guidelines have been described, which in general include regular monitoring, calcium supplementation, especially in techniques that exclude the duodenum, and vitamin D supplementation at the necessary dose, depending on the surgical technique [101]. The ASMBS recommends supplementing all patients with calcium (BPD 1800–2400 mg/day; RYGB, SG, and GB 1200–1500 mg/day) and vitamin D to maintain plasma levels above 30 ng/mL, generally 3000 IU/day [23,75].

Vitamin D deficiency is prevalent in pregnancy after bariatric surgery, although data in the literature are limited. In a study conducted in Brazil in 46 pregnancies after RYGB, 70% had levels below 20 ng/mL in all three trimesters. Hypocalcaemia was reported in 15% of cases in the first and second trimesters and in 20% in the third trimester and an increased PTH in 32.6% of pregnancies in the third trimester [102]. These data were confirmed in another retrospective study evaluating 42 pregnant women with a history of RYGB, also conducted in Brazil, which observed an inadequacy of vitamin D levels of up to 90 [103]. Bariatric multivitamins can prevent vitamin D deficiency during pregnancy in women with previous RYGB [104] As bariatric surgery increases the risk of vitamin D deficiency, pregnancy in women with BS may pose a risk to bone health if not adequately supplemented.

3.5. Vitamin A

Vitamin A, present in foods as retinol or retinyl esters or as provitamins in the form of carotenoids, plays an important role in cell growth and differentiation, vision, immunity, and reproduction. The main dietary sources are liver, dairy, and fish oils, as well as coloured vegetables in the case of provitamin A carotenoids. Vitamin A deficiency (VAD) is very prevalent in developing countries and is a public health problem [105]. A diagnosis is considered when plasma levels are below 20 μg/dL [106]. Retinol is bound to prealbumin and retinol-binding protein (RBP), and serum levels may not always indicate vitamin A nutritional status [107].

Vitamin A is an essential nutrient in embryonic and foetal development for lung and sense organ maturation [108]. VAD during pregnancy is associated with an increased risk of low birth weight, prematurity, lung disease (bronchopulmonary dysplasia), an increased risk of infection in the newborn, and mortality in the neonatal period. In addition, vitamin A deficiency decreases iron mobilisation and increases the risk of anaemia [109]. It is estimated that there are approximately 19 million pregnant women with vitamin A deficiency [110]. The WHO recommends universal vitamin A supplementation during pregnancy in regions with a high prevalence of deficiency and night blindness [111]. During gestation, an intake of 700 μg/day is recommended [112]. High intakes of vitamin A (>3000 μg/day or >10,000 IU/day) during pregnancy are associated with an increased risk of malformations and should be avoided [112].

Bariatric surgery is nowadays one of the leading causes of clinical vitamin A deficiency in developed countries. The prevalence of decreased vitamin A serum levels in malabsorptive techniques can reach 60% [113]. In gastric bypass, a prevalence of 11% has been reported, and it is associated with visual symptoms such as xerophthalmia or night vision impairment [114]. In a prospective study in GBP patients, decreased levels were observed in 37.5%, 50.8%, and 52.9% preoperatively, at 30 days, and at 180 days, respectively [115]. Clinical vitamin A deficiency, manifested by visual and skin changes, is less common. Several clinical cases have been reported, especially after BPD [116–120]; the prevalence of clinical deficiency can reach 2.8–10% in some series. The ASMBS recommends supplementation with 5000–10,000 IU/day in malabsorptive BS [6,23,75].

Vitamin A deficiency may have adverse effects on pregnancy after bariatric surgery [121]. Some cases of malformations, such as microphthalmia, and other foetal complications secondary to maternal VAD have been reported. The first case of clinical vitamin A deficiency during gestation, 13 years after BPD, was published in 2002 [122]. Subsequently, other cases were published [123–125], most of them in patients with malabsorptive bariatric surgery and poor clinical follow-up. Regarding the adequacy of serum levels to reference values, Studies have shown discordant results regarding the adequacy of vitamin A serum levels. In a study conducted in Brazil in 30 pregnant women after RYGB, the prevalence of VAD (<30 μg/dL) reached 90%; 86.7% developed night blindness. No association was observed with maternal anaemia, which affected 73.3% of women. No data on pre-pregnancy VAD are provided in this study [126]. The prevalence of decreased serum levels in other countries has ranged from 20 to 60. No relationship has been observed between the different techniques or with maternal and foetal complications [93]. In a case–control study in France, a higher percentage of vitamin A levels in cord blood below the 2.5th percentile was observed in pregnancies after RYGB. It should be noted that in this study, the percentage of low birth weight for gestational age was high (23% vs. 3% in the control group) [80].

3.6. Vitamin E

Vitamin E is a fat-soluble vitamin with an antioxidant function and is mainly found in animal fats and oils. Its deficiency, which is very rare, leads to ataxia and other neurological symptoms, as well as to increased red blood cell fragility and haemolytic anaemia [127,128].

Vitamin E is necessary for proper foetal and early childhood development [128]; a dietary intake of 12 mg per day during pregnancy is recommended [129]. Supplementation with vitamin E and other micronutrients contributes to the prevention of neural tube defects, and a relationship between plasma levels and cognitive function has been observed [130,131]. Vitamin E has also been linked to problems in pregnancy involving oxidative damage, such as preeclampsia. Anyway, there is no evidence to recommend universal vitamin E supplementation to reduce the risk of maternal–foetal complications [132].

Vitamin E deficiency after BS is rare and occurs mainly in malabsorptive diseases, and it takes several years to develop clinical manifestations [133]. Probably for this reason, publications on clinical vitamin E deficiency after bariatric surgery are limited [134]. The ASMBS recommends preventive supplementation in all patients after BS at a dose of 15 mg/day [21,23]. A higher dose is usually needed in BPD. Plasma tocopherol levels are dependent on circulating lipids, and an adjustment for total lipids or plasma cholesterol is recommended [128]. In a study published in Spain, 8.7% and 21.4% of patients with RYGB and BPD, respectively, were found to have vitamin E/cholesterol levels lower than 5 mg/d [135].

Data on the nutritional status of vitamin E in pregnancy after BS are very limited. So far, only one study has been published examining this issue. In a prospective multicentre study of 49 patients, 2% were found to have serum levels below 500 μg/dL in the first trimester. No cases were observed in the second and third trimester [67]. A decrease (below the 2.5th percentile) of vitamin E in cord blood has been observed in cord blood in pregnancy after RYGB compared to a control group (16% vs. 3%) [80].

3.7. Vitamin K

Vitamin K is involved in the synthesis of clotting factors and is mainly present in animal fats and oils [136]. It also plays an important role in bone health [137]. Vitamin K deficiency during pregnancy has been related to a higher risk of periventricular and intraventricular haemorrhage, especially in mothers on treatment with anti-epileptic drugs or with malabsorptive conditions [138].

Decreased vitamin K levels have been reported after BS, especially after malabsorptive techniques, and are usually asymptomatic [139]. Data on the nutritional status of vitamin K throughout gestation in women with previous BS are scarce. Some cases of neonatal intracranial haemorrhage have been reported, probably secondary to vitamin K deficiency [140], even after restrictive techniques [141]. A prospective study of 49 post-BS gestational patients and 27 controls found that plasma vitamin K levels were decreased in the first trimester (<0.8 nmol/L) in both groups and were significantly lower in the BS group. Prothrombin time was normal in both groups, although significantly longer in the BS group. Coagulation factors were normal [142].

3.8. Iron

Iron is involved in the structure and function of haemoglobin, myoglobin, and enzymes of the respiratory chain. It is absorbed in the duodenum and early jejunal tract and requires an acidic gastric pH [143]. It is found in food in two different forms: as part of the heme group (meat and meat products) and in the non-heme form (legumes, nuts, vegetables), with the former being much more bioavailable. Iron deficiency is very common and causes anaemia, alterations in the mucous membranes, and asthenia, among other symptoms [144]. Obesity itself alters the iron nutritional status, as it constitutes a state of low-grade inflammation, which increases the synthesis of acute-phase reactants, including hepcidin, which decreases iron absorption and also decreases the mobilisation of iron from endogenous stores [145]. Iron intake recommendations depend on its bioavailability in food; EFSA recommends 16 mg/day for women of childbearing age [50].

Iron-deficiency anaemia is one of the most common complications of pregnancy and is a public health problem in many countries. Iron requirements increase during pregnancy because of the increase in total red blood cell volume, up to 20–25% by the end of pregnancy. It is estimated that up to 1200 mg of additional iron is used during pregnancy [146]. Although intestinal absorption also increases, iron intake from food does not appear to be sufficient to maintain adequate iron nutritional status throughout pregnancy, especially if there is a pre-pregnancy iron deficiency state [146]. Anaemia in pregnancy increases maternal morbidity and mortality, hinders foetal growth and maturation, and is associated with an increased risk of low birth weight and alterations in neurocognitive development. In the long term, it promotes obesity and metabolic problems in offspring, including increased vascular risk [146]. The diagnosis of anaemia is established if plasma haemoglobin is less than 11 g/dL in the first and third trimesters and 10.5 g/dL in the second trimester [147]. Iron deficiency during pregnancy is mainly diagnosed based on the determination of plasma ferritin: in general, a cut-off point of 30 µg/L is established [148]. The WHO recommends supplementation with 30–60 mg of elemental iron in all pregnancies [149].

Iron-deficiency anaemia is one of the most frequent nutritional complications of bariatric surgery due to reduced intake and malabsorption, mainly secondary to the modification of gastric pH or the exclusion of the duodenum and proximal jejunum, in addition to possible digestive or menstrual losses [150,151]. The prevalence of iron deficiency and iron-deficiency anaemia ranges from 20 to 70% after RYGB and from 10 to 50% after SG and can require parenteral administration in 2–10% [152]. Preventive supplementation is recommended in techniques that exclude the duodenum at a dose of 40–60 mg/day, especially in high-risk cases (after surgery, women of childbearing age, pregnancy, etc.) [75]. The iron content of conventional multivitamins is not sufficient.

Several studies have found that a history of bariatric surgery increases the risk of iron-deficiency anaemia during pregnancy and that this complication is more common with a longer time after surgery [54,88,153,154]. The prevalence of anaemia ranges from 17 to 70%, with 10–16% requiring intravenous iron and 3–17% requiring transfusion [54]. There is no agreement on the most appropriate pattern of iron supplementation in pregnancy after BS. The recommended dosage ranges from 40 to 600 mg/day, according to different authors [76,154–156], but this recommendation is not based on studies specifically designed to evaluate this issue. It should be noted that intravenous iron administration is not indicated during the first trimester of pregnancy [151]. Iron-deficiency anaemia prevention during pregnancy in women with previous BS needs a close follow-up, which should start before conception. The multivitamins designed for pregnancy do not include enough iron for pregnancy after BS.

3.9. *Magnesium*

Magnesium is an intracellular cation that is part of the bone structure, contributing to proper mineralisation, and is involved as a cofactor of numerous enzymes in muscle contraction, gland secretion, and nerve transmission [157]. Approximately 45% is absorbed in the small intestine via a paracellular diffusion mechanism; a smaller fraction is absorbed in the ileum via transporters (TRPM6 and TRPM7). Magnesium absorption is stimulated by vitamin D and PTH. The plasma Mg concentration is primarily regulated by renal elimination, where approximately 70% of filtered magnesium is reabsorbed [158]. The main sources of magnesium are cereals, nuts, and dairy products. The most characteristic symptoms of magnesium deficiency are anorexia, muscle cramps, rhabdomyolysis, hyperreflexia, convulsions, confusional syndrome, and paralytic ileus. It is not easy to assess the nutritional status of Mg, as it is mainly an intracellular element, and plasma levels may remain within normal limits even when deficiency is present [159]. For this reason, some authors propose raising the reference value for plasma Mg to levels above 2 mg/dL [159].

Magnesium is an important element for pregnancy [160]. Magnesium sulphate is used in the treatment of patients with preeclampsia [161]; it can induce placental vasodilatation, decreases umbilical artery tone, attenuates the effect of endothelin I and angiotensin II on placental vascularisation, and decreases IL-β secretion in placental tissue [162,163]. Plasma Mg levels decrease progressively throughout gestation; this decrease is greater in women with preterm labour [164]. However, no decrease in plasma magnesium has been observed in patients with preeclampsia [164]. The effect of magnesium supplementation on the course and complications of pregnancy is controversial, and the effect probably depends on patient characteristics and maternal magnesium nutritional status [165,166]. There is no evidence to recommend magnesium supplementation to prevent the risk of preeclampsia or other pregnancy complications in healthy women [94,166]. Magnesium intake recommendations do not increase in pregnancy.

Bariatric surgery increases the risk of magnesium deficiency because of decreased intake and malabsorption. However, and probably due to the difficulty in diagnosis, information on magnesium nutritional status after BS is very scarce [76]. There are few data on magnesium deficiency in pregnancy after BS, and, in general, no decrease in serum levels has been observed [93,167].

Considering the difficulty in assessing the nutritional status of magnesium, its importance in gestation, the deficit in magnesium intake in our environment and the possible effect of BS, this is an issue that should be given greater attention in the future. Most multivitamins include a magnesium dosage lower than the recommendations.

3.10. *Zinc*

Zinc is an element involved in the function of more than 200 enzymes, including carbonic anhydrase, DNA polymerase and RNA polymerase. It is directly involved in replication and transcription and plays important roles in growth, foetal nervous system development, and immune response. Zinc is present in foods of animal origin and in cereals and legumes. The recommended intake of zinc is 8–12 mg/day for males and females, respectively [168]. Zinc deficiency is very common in developing countries and has very important clinical consequences: retarded growth and sexual maturation, asthenia, dermatitis, hypogonadism, altered sense of taste, and other general manifestations [169]. Zinc deficiency is generally related to decreased intake or availability. It has also been described in numerous clinical conditions associated with malabsorption, such as short bowel syndrome, inflammatory bowel disease, and coeliac disease [170].

Zinc is directly involved in foetal growth and development, especially in the nervous system, and in the immune response [171]. There is active transport in the placenta, so levels in the cord blood are higher than in the mother's blood [172]. In animals, zinc deficiency leads to an increased risk of miscarriage, placental abnormalities, congenital malformations, and intrauterine growth retardation [171,173]. In humans, decreased plasma zinc levels have been associated with decreased birth weight and preeclampsia in some studies, but not in others [174,175]. In a recently published meta-analysis, a significant pooled correlation was found between umbilical cord blood zinc concentrations and birth weight (r: 0.09, 95% CI: 0.04 to 0.15) [176].

Zinc deficiency is common in BS patients, even before surgery [21], especially in mixed or malabsorptive techniques [88]. Most cases are asymptomatic, although low intake and Zn deficiency have been linked to alopecia after BS [177]. The ASMBS, recommends assessing nutritional status prior to BS, keeping in mind that plasma levels may fall in relation to obesity itself. In addition, preventive supplementation is recommended in all patients, with a dose that depends on the surgical technique used: malabsorptive techniques: 16–22 mg/day; gastric bypass: 8–22 mg/day; and restrictive techniques: 8–11 mg/day [21,23].

Data on the nutritional status of zinc and its clinical consequences for pregnancy after bariatric surgery are limited. In a study of 30 patients with a history of RYGB, 20% showed decreased plasma levels in the first and third trimesters, with no relation to maternal anthropometry or newborn weight [178]. Another study, conducted in 56 patients, describes plasma zinc levels of 13.1 ± 2.6, 11.5 ± 1.7, and 10.7 ± 1.4 µmol.

L in the three trimesters, respectively. They found no cases of deficiency, no differences between the different techniques, and no effects on maternal and foetal outcomes [93]. In a prospective study in 87 women [179], zinc deficiency (<0.51 mg/L) was found in 8.0%, all after RYGB (18.9% vs. 0% in SG; $p = 0.02$), and preterm birth occurred in 100% of these cases. The usual multivitamins do not provide sufficient zinc for pregnancy after bariatric surgery, especially in the case of malabsorptive techniques. It is also necessary to consider that the pharmacological use of some nutrients, such as iron, decreases the bioavailability of zinc from food and that a high dose of zinc decreases the absorption of copper.

3.11. Copper

Copper is an essential element that acts as a ligand for numerous proteins and enzymes (superoxide dismutase, ferroxidase, amino oxidase, cytochrome-C oxidase, etc.). It is involved in antioxidant protection, in the transport of iron and other metals, and in the metabolism of amino acids. It is absorbed in the stomach and duodenum, and gastric acid contributes to the release of Cu from food. Copper requirements according to the RDA are 900 µg/day in adults. In pregnant and breastfeeding women, the requirements increase, and more than 1000 µg/day is necessary [168]. Copper is an essential element in brain development [180] and has been linked to neurodegenerative diseases [181]. Copper deficiency leads to a clinical picture with haematological (anaemia, leukopenia, or pancytopenia) and neurological (myelopathy and peripheral neuropathy) manifestations [182].

Copper deficiency can have negative effects on embryonic and foetal development [183]. Copper is involved in the normal functioning of numerous enzymes, so its deficiency alters ATP production, lipid peroxidation, hormone activation, and angiogenesis and causes pulmonary and skeletal alterations. Genetic alterations in copper metabolism lead to alterations in embryonic and foetal development that may increase mortality. Menken's disease is transmitted in an X-linked recessive manner and usually results in the death of the child before the age of 5 years after presenting with clinical signs of neuronal and connective tissue degeneration. Studies have shown that, in normal gestations, copper levels increase progressively throughout pregnancy [184] due to an increase in ceruloplasmin secondary to gestational hyperestrogenism and a decrease in biliary copper excretion [185]. Maternal copper deficiency increases the risk of prematurity and low-birth-weight infants, and a decrease in cord blood copper has been observed in low-birth-weight infants [183]. Copper deficiency during pregnancy has also been associated with an increased risk of the premature rupture of membranes and preterm birth [186].

Copper deficiency is rare in the Western population but has been increasing in recent years as a consequence of drug treatment and especially in relation to bariatric surgery [182,187]. Its prevalence is estimated at 9.6% after RYGB [188]. Copper deficiency is a recognised cause of neurological impairment after BS, especially with techniques that exclude the duodenum, the main site of absorption [189]. Several studies have observed a decrease in plasma copper levels after bariatric bypass surgery [190]. Clinical copper deficiency is less common but can be severe; several cases have been reported, mainly after malabsorptive techniques, with neurological impairment and/or anaemia [191,192]. It is recommended that all patients receive copper supplementation, at a dose depending on the surgical technique used [21,23]: in patients with SG or GB, 1 mg/day, and in patients with RYGB or BPD, 2 mg/day, in the form of copper sulphate or gluconate. Zinc treatment may decrease copper absorption [193]. Cu supplementation of 1–2 mg for every 8–15 mg of zinc is recommended [21].

There are no data on plasma copper levels in pregnancy after BS or the possible impact on the course and complications of pregnancy. No cases of clinical copper deficiency during pregnancy after BS have been reported. Decreased plasma copper levels in pregnant women with a history of bariatric surgery could have adverse consequences on foetal development or increase the risk of complications. Although there are no specific recommendations on Cu supplementation in pregnancy after BS, these women should receive at least similar supplementation to that recommended in BS in general [75,76]. This dose is safe in pregnancy and does not reach the maximum tolerable intake (10 mg/day) [182]. It should be noted that most multivitamins designed for pregnancy do not provide copper.

3.12. Selenium

Selenium plays an important role in maintaining redox balance through selenoproteins such as glutathione peroxidase (GSH) [194]. Plasma values above 70 µg/L optimise GSH function [195]. It is absorbed in the upper sections of the small intestine, mainly in the duodenum. Se intake and nutritional status are highly dependent on the geographical area. The EFSA recommends an intake of selenium in the adult population of 70 µg/day for men and women, and a similar amount is recommended during pregnancy. During breastfeeding, on the other hand, considering the Se content in breast milk, an intake of 85 µg/day is recommended, similar to that for non-pregnant women [196].

A decrease in selenium levels and GSH peroxidase activity has been observed in pregnancy [107] and has been linked to some complications, such as preeclampsia [197,198]. In a recently published systematic review that included 26 studies with 1855 preeclampsia cases compared with 3728 healthy pregnant controls, the level of selenium was significantly lower in cases of preeclampsia compared with the controls (SMD = −0.85; 95% confidence interval: −1.46, −0.25; $p < 0.01$). A decrease in serum Se has been observed throughout gestation [199], with no association with the risk of SGA [200].

There are few data on the nutritional status of selenium in relation to bariatric surgery. Several cases of cardiomyopathy secondary to selenium deficiency after bariatric surgery have been reported [201,202], which have improved after specific supplementation. In patients who are candidates for BS, decreased selenium serum levels have been observed compared to a control group [203]. A decrease has also been described after BS [204], which can be prevented by micronutrient supplementation [205]. Although Se deficiency may be more frequent in techniques that exclude the duodenum, decreased levels have also been reported after sleeve gastrectomy [206]. In a systematic review and meta-analysis that included nine studies with a total of 1174 patients, selenium deficiency prevalence was 16% and 2% at 1- and 2-year follow-ups after BS, respectively [207]. Symptoms included weakness, myopathy and cardiomyopathy, loss of muscle mass, erythematous desquamating eruption, lethargy, dyspnoea, and bilateral lower extremity pitting oedema.

The prevalence of selenium deficiency in pregnancy after BS was evaluated in a retrospective study including 57 singleton pregnancies [93]. Selenium serum levels were low in 77.8%, 22.2%, and 50.0% in the first, second, and third trimesters, respectively. In a prospective study in 87 women [179], selenium deficiency (<60 µg/L) was found in 17.2%: 21.6% after RYGB and 14.0% after SG ($p = 0.36$). A selenium deficit in the second trimester in women with a history of BS was negatively correlated with birthweight and with birthweight z-score [179].

3.13. Iodine

Iodine is an essential element whose main function is its participation in the synthesis of thyroid hormones. It is a critical nutrient in cellular metabolism and in the development of the nervous system in the prenatal and postnatal periods [208]. The main sources of iodine are dairy products, fish, eggs, and, above all, fortified foods such as iodised salt. Iodine deficiency is a major public health problem and one of the preventable causes of stunted growth and impaired neurological development [208].

Iodine requirements increase during pregnancy and lactation, and an intake of 200–250 µg/day is recommended. All women of childbearing age should ensure an adequate iodine intake at least one year before pregnancy. The intake of iodine in food and iodised salt is generally sufficient to meet these requirements. However, considering the risk of iodine deficiency for foetal development, iodine supplementation should be recommended in cases where there is a risk of insufficient intake [209].

Very few studies have been published on the impact of barbaric surgery on iodine absorption or metabolism. So far, three studies have been published. Urinary iodine excretion had not changed 6 months after malabsorptive BS, nor had autoimmunity or thyroid gland volume [210]. Another study compared the nutritional status of iodine in three groups of women: morbidly obese, patients after bariatric surgery with at least 18 months of follow-up after bariatric surgery, and a normal-weight control group. Obese women had a significantly lower urinary iodine concentration (UIC, µg/g creatinine) in comparison with non-obese women (96.6 [25.8–267.3] vs. 173.3 [47.0–493.6] µg/g; $p < 0.001$), with a lower proportion of subjects with an adequate iodine status (46.6 vs. 83.3%, $p < 0.001$). Mean UIC was higher in women with previous BS in comparison with women with obesity (131.9 [62.9–496.4] vs. 96.6 [25.8–267.3] µg/g; $p < 0.001$). No difference in UIC was found between RYGB and SG. UIC was negatively correlated with BMI ($r = -0.278$, $p < 0.001$). Multiple linear regression analyses showed that BMI was independently associated with UIC ($beta = -0.312$, $p < 0.001$; R (2) = 0.166). In this study, women consuming iodised salt were excluded [211]. The SOS study investigators evaluated 188 patients after RYGB and 188 after SG, at least 10 years after BS, compared with a control group, and did not observe a higher prevalence of iodine deficiency [212]. BS has not been shown to impair iodine absorption or metabolism or to induce iodine deficiency, so specific supplementation recommended after bariatric surgery does not need to include iodine in iodine-sufficient countries, and ensuring that the dietary intake of iodine in food and iodised salt is sufficient.

No studies have been published evaluating the iodine nutritional status during pregnancy in women with previous BS. In agreement with previously described studies, in these women, the same recommendation of iodine intake can be made as in the general pregnant population, 200–250 µg/day.

There is no agreement on the most appropriate preventive micronutrient supplementation during gestation in women with previous bariatric surgery, and, due to the paucity of data, recommended doses are generally based on expert opinion. Table 5 includes a summary of these recommendations [31–33,154,213].

Table 5. Summary of micronutrient recommendations in pregnancy after bariatric surgery.

Micronutrient	Dose	Comment
Folate	800–1000 μg	Higher dose in women with obesity (1–5 mg)
Vitamin B12	1000–2000 μg/1–3 months, i.m.	Can also be administered orally (>350–500 μg/d)
Thiamine	12 mg	Increase to 100–300 mg if low intake, nausea/vomiting
Vitamin D	2000–4000 UI	Vitamin D > 30 ng/mL
Vitamin A	800–1500 μg	A dose below 3000 μg (10.000 UI) is safe in pregnancy; the retinol form of vitamin A should be avoided
Vitamin E	15 mg	Monitoring in malabsorptive techniques
Vitamin K	50–120 μg/d	Higher risk of deficiency in premature newborns
Iron	100–200 mg	Ferritin > 30 mg/L, gradual increase of dose; i.v. iron is not recommended in first term
Calcium	1500–2400 mg	Increase dietary intake; separated from iron supplement
Magnesium	350 mg	Multivitamins usually contain a lower dose
Zinc	12–30 mg	Can decrease copper absorption
Copper	1–2 mg	Separated from zinc supplements
Selenium	50–60 μg	Monitor in malabsorptive techniques
Iodine	200–250 μg	The same dose as that in normal pregnancy

4. Conclusions

Obesity increases the risk of complications during gestation, such as gestational diabetes, preeclampsia, or macrosomia. Bariatric surgery may reduce these risks but may induce mineral and micronutrient deficiencies, which can have adverse consequences for the short- and long-term health of the mother and her offspring. This narrative review of the literature enables us to offer some recommendations to optimise the follow-up of pregnancy in women with previous bariatric surgery [28–34] (Table 6). Further studies are needed to identify the factors that promote micronutrient deficiencies during pregnancy after bariatric surgery, the effects on maternal and foetal health and long-term outcomes, and the most effective preventive treatment.

Table 6. Pregnancy after bariatric surgery: summary of recommendations.

Pregnancy in Women with Previous Bariatric Surgery: Summary of Recommendations
Appropriate selection of the bariatric surgical technique. Non-malabsorptive techniques should, in general, be preferred.
Appropriate follow-up after bariatric surgery, with the necessary supplementation to prevent and treat possible nutritional deficiencies.
Preferably, the onset of pregnancy should be delayed by 12–18 months after bariatric surgery. Pre-conceptional clinical and nutritional assessment is recommended.
Follow-up during pregnancy should be carried out by a multidisciplinary team.
Close monitoring of the patient if oral tolerance is inadequate or vomiting occurs. It is advisable to increase the thiamine dose to 100–300 mg/day.
Monitoring of maternal weight gain and intrauterine growth. Consider oral nutritional supplements and/or pancreatic enzymes.
Preventive supplementation with minerals and micronutrients, at the necessary dose, depending on the type of bariatric surgery and clinical and analytical evolution.
Iodine recommendations are similar to those for women who have not undergone bariatric surgery.
Screening for gestational complications, following specific protocols. In the case of gestational diabetes, it is recommended to avoid oral glucose overload.
Monitoring for the occurrence of surgical complications, such as internal hernia, a serious but rare clinical condition that requires a specific diagnostic approach and treatment.
Encourage lactation with a close clinical and nutritional follow-up.

Author Contributions: Writing—Review and editing—was performed by all authors (I.B., M.D.B.-P., A.C.-P., L.A.A.-S. and M.A.R.-H.). All authors have read and agreed to the published version of the manuscript.

Funding: This research received no external funding.

Institutional Review Board Statement: Not applicable.

Data Availability Statement: Not applicable.

Conflicts of Interest: The authors declare no conflict of interest.

References

1. Mechanick, J.I.; Hurley, D.L.; Garvey, W.T. Adiposity-Based Chronic Disease as a new Diagnostic Term: The American Association of Clinical Endocrinologists and American College of Endocrinology Position Statement. *Endocr. Pract.* **2016**, *23*, 372–378. [CrossRef] [PubMed]
2. Garvey, W.T.; Mechanick, J.I.; Brett, E.M.; Garber, A.J.; Hurley, D.L.; Jastreboff, A.M.; Nadolsky, K.; Pessah-Pollack, R.; Plodkowski, R.; Reviewers of the AACE/ACE Obesity Clinical Practice Guidelines. American association of clinical endocrinologists and american college of endocrinology comprehensive clinical practice guidelines for medical care of patients with obesity—Executive Summary. *Endocr. Pract.* **2016**, *22*, 1–203. [CrossRef]
3. Rittenberg, V.; Seshadri, S.; Sunkara, S.K.; Sobaleva, S.; Oteng-Ntim, E.; El-Toukhy, T. Effect of body mass index on IVF treatment outcome: An updated systematic review and meta-analysis. *Reprod. Biomed. Online* **2011**, *23*, 421–439. [CrossRef] [PubMed]
4. Bellver, J.; Busso, C.; Pellicer, A.; Remohí, J.; Simón, C. Obesity and assisted reproductive technology outcomes. *Reprod. Biomed. Online* **2006**, *12*, 562–568. [CrossRef] [PubMed]
5. Yu, Z.; Han, S.; Zhu, J.; Sun, X.; Ji, C.; Guo, X. Pre-Pregnancy Body Mass Index in Relation to Infant Birth Weight and Offspring Overweight/Obesity: A Systematic Review and Meta-Analysis. *PLoS ONE* **2013**, *8*, e61627. [CrossRef] [PubMed]
6. Marchi, J.; Berg, M.; Dencker, A.; Olander, E.K.; Begley, C. Risks associated with obesity in pregnancy, for the mother and baby: A systematic review of reviews. *Obes. Rev.* **2015**, *16*, 621–638. [CrossRef]
7. Goldstein, R.F.; Abell, S.K.; Ranasinha, S.; Misso, M.; Boyle, J.A.; Black, M.H.; Li, N.; Hu, G.; Corrado, F.; Rode, L.; et al. Association of Gestational Weight Gain with Maternal and Infant Outcomes: A Systematic Review and Meta-analysis. *JAMA* **2017**, *317*, 2207–2225. [CrossRef]
8. Santos, S.; Voerman, E.; Amiano, P.; Barros, H.; Beilin, L.; Bergström, A.; Charles, M.; Chatzi, L.; Chevrier, C.; Chrousos, G.; et al. Impact of maternal body mass index and gestational weight gain on pregnancy complications: An individual participant data meta-analysis of European, North American, and Australian cohorts. *BJOG* **2019**, *126*, 984–995. [CrossRef]
9. Martin, A.; Krishna, I.; Ellis, J.; Paccione, R.; Badell, M. Super obesity in pregnancy: Difficulties in clinical management. *J. Perinatol.* **2014**, *34*, 495–502. [CrossRef]
10. Crane, J.M.; Murphy, P.; Burrage, L.; Hutchens, D. Maternal and Perinatal Outcomes of Extreme Obesity in Pregnancy. *J. Obstet. Gynaecol. Can.* **2013**, *35*, 606–611. [CrossRef]
11. Arterburn, D.E.; Courcoulas, A.P. Bariatric surgery for obesity and metabolic conditions in adults. *BMJ* **2014**, *349*, g3961. [CrossRef] [PubMed]
12. Angrisani, L.; Santonicola, A.; Iovino, P.; Ramos, A.; Shikora, S.; Kow, L. Bariatric Surgery Survey 2018: Similarities and Disparities Among the 5 IFSO Chapters. *Obes. Surg.* **2021**, *31*, 1937–1948. [CrossRef]
13. Batterham, R.L.; Cummings, D.E. Mechanisms of Diabetes Improvement Following Bariatric/Metabolic Surgery. *Diabetes Care* **2016**, *39*, 893–901. [CrossRef] [PubMed]
14. Hutch, C.R.; Sandoval, D.A. Physiological and molecular responses to bariatric surgery: Markers or mechanisms underlying T2DM resolution? *Ann. N. Y. Acad. Sci.* **2017**, *1391*, 5–19. [CrossRef]
15. Davies, N.K.; O'Sullivan, J.M.; Plank, L.D.; Murphy, R. Altered gut microbiome after bariatric surgery and its association with metabolic benefits: A systematic review. *Surg. Obes. Relat. Dis.* **2019**, *15*, 656–665. [CrossRef]
16. Penney, N.C.; Kinross, J.; Newton, R.C.; Purkayastha, S. The role of bile acids in reducing the metabolic complications of obesity after bariatric surgery: A systematic review. *Int. J. Obes.* **2015**, *39*, 1565–1574. [CrossRef]
17. Vítek, L.; Haluzík, M. The role of bile acids in metabolic regulation. *J. Endocrinol.* **2016**, *228*, R85–R96. [CrossRef]
18. Syn, N.L.; E Cummings, D.; Wang, L.Z.; Lin, D.J.; Zhao, J.J.; Loh, M.; Koh, Z.J.; Chew, C.A.; Loo, Y.E.; Tai, B.C.; et al. Association of metabolic–bariatric surgery with long-term survival in adults with and without diabetes: A one-stage meta-analysis of matched cohort and prospective controlled studies with 174 772 participants. *Lancet* **2021**, *397*, 1830–1841. [CrossRef]
19. Wiggins, T.; Guidozzi, N.; Welbourn, R.; Ahmed, A.R.; Markar, S.R. Association of bariatric surgery with all-cause mortality and incidence of obesity-related disease at a population level: A systematic review and meta-analysis. *PLOS Med.* **2020**, *17*, e1003206. [CrossRef]
20. Amaya García, M.J.; Vilchez López, F.J.; Campos Martín, C.; Sánchez Vera, P.; Pereira Cunill, J.L. Micronutrientes en Cirugía Bariátrica. *Nutr. Hosp.* **2012**, *27*, 349–361. [CrossRef]

21. Parrott, J.; Frank, L.; Rabena, R.; Craggs-Dino, L.; Isom, K.A.; Greiman, L. American Society for Metabolic and Bariatric Surgery Integrated Health Nutritional Guidelines for the Surgical Weight Loss Patient 2016 Update: Micronutrients. *Surg. Obes. Relat. Dis.* **2019**, *13*, 727–741. [CrossRef] [PubMed]
22. Jensterle, M.; Rizzo, M.; Janez, A. Glucagon-Like Peptide 1 and Taste Perception: From Molecular Mechanisms to Potential Clinical Implications. *Int. J. Mol. Sci.* **2021**, *22*, 902. [CrossRef] [PubMed]
23. Mechanick, J.I.; Apovian, C.; Brethauer, S.; Garvey, W.T.; Joffe, A.M.; Kim, J.; Kushner, R.F.; Lindquist, R.; Pessah-Pollack, R.; Seger, J.; et al. Clinical practice guidelines for the perioperative nutrition, metabolic, and nonsurgical support of patients undergoing bariatric procedures—2019 update: Cosponsored by American Association of Clinical Endocrinologists/American College of Endocrinology, The Obesity Society, American Society for Metabolic & Bariatric Surgery, Obesity Medicine Association, and American Society of Anesthesiologists. *Surg. Obes. Relat. Dis.* **2020**, *16*, 175–247. [CrossRef] [PubMed]
24. O'Kane, M.; Parretti, H.M.; Pinkney, J.; Welbourn, R.; Hughes, C.A.; Mok, J.; Walker, N.; Thomas, D.; Devin, J.; Coulman, K.D.; et al. British Obesity and Metabolic Surgery Society Guidelines on perioperative and postoperative biochemical monitoring and micronutrient replacement for patients undergoing bariatric surgery—2020 update. *Obes. Rev.* **2020**, *21*, e13087. [CrossRef]
25. Galazis, N.; Docheva, N.; Simillis, C.; Nicolaides, K.H. Maternal and neonatal outcomes in women undergoing bariatric surgery: A systematic review and meta-analysis. *Eur. J. Obstet. Gynecol. Reprod. Biol.* **2014**, *181*, 45–53. [CrossRef]
26. Yi, X.Y.; Li, Q.F.; Zhang, J.; Wang, Z.H. A meta-analysis of maternal and fetal outcomes of pregnancy after bariatric surgery. *Int. J. Gynaecol. Obstet.* **2015**, *130*, 3–9. [CrossRef]
27. Kwong, W.; Tomlinson, G.; Feig, D.S. Maternal and neonatal outcomes after bariatric surgery; a systematic review and meta-analysis: Do the benefits outweigh the risks? *Am. J. Obstet. Gynecol.* **2018**, *218*, 573–580. [CrossRef]
28. Badreldin, N.; Kuller, J.; Rhee, E.; Brown, L.; Laifer, S. Pregnancy Management After Bariatric Surgery. *Obstet. Gynecol. Surv.* **2016**, *71*, 361–368. [CrossRef]
29. Harreiter, J.; Schindler, K.; Bancher-Todesca, D.; Göbl, C.; Langer, F.; Prager, G.; Gessl, A.; Leutner, M.; Ludvik, B.; Luger, A.; et al. Management of Pregnant Women after Bariatric Surgery. *J. Obes.* **2018**, *2018*, 4587064. [CrossRef]
30. González, I.; Lecube, A.; Rubio, M.; García-Luna, P.P. Pregnancy after bariatric surgery: Improving outcomes for mother and child. *Int. J. Women's Health* **2016**, *8*, 721–729. [CrossRef]
31. Shawe, J.; Ceulemans, D.; Akhter, Z.; Neff, K.; Hart, K.; Heslehurst, N.; Štotl, I.; Agrawal, S.; Steegers-Theunissen, R.; Taheri, S.; et al. Pregnancy after bariatric surgery: Consensus recommendations for periconception, antenatal and postnatal care. *Obes. Rev.* **2019**, *20*, 1507–1522. [CrossRef] [PubMed]
32. Alamri, S.H.; Abdeen, G.N. Maternal Nutritional Status and Pregnancy Outcomes Post-bariatric Surgery. *Obes. Surg.* **2022**, *32*, 1325–1340. [CrossRef] [PubMed]
33. Huang, B.; Yo, J.H.; Gandhi, S.; Maxwell, C. Micronutrient screening, monitoring, and supplementation in pregnancy after bariatric surgery. *Obstet. Med.* **2022**, *15*, 151–159. [CrossRef]
34. Guthrie, T.M.; Dix, C.F.; Truby, H.; Kumar, S.; de Jersey, S.J. A Systematic Review Investigating Maternal Nutrition During Pregnancy After Bariatric Surgery. *Obes. Surg.* **2023**, *33*, 1857–1865. [CrossRef] [PubMed]
35. Akhter, Z.; Rankin, J.; Ceulemans, D.; Ngongalah, L.; Ackroyd, R.; Devlieger, R.; Vieiram, R.; Heslehurst, N. Investigating the association between pregnancy following bariatric surgery and adverse perinatal outcomes: A systematic review and meta-analysis. *PLoS Med.* **2018**, *125*, e1002866.
36. Cooper, N.; Fiennes, A.; Hashemi, M.; Adamo, M.; El-Kalaawy, M. Pregnancy in first 12 months after bariatric surgery. *Surg. Obes. Relat. Dis.* **2010**, *6*, 234. [CrossRef]
37. Johansson, K.; Cnattingius, S.; Näslund, I.; Roos, N.; Lagerros, Y.T.; Granath, F.; Stephansson, O.; Neovius, M. Outcomes of Pregnancy after Bariatric Surgery. *N. Engl. J. Med.* **2015**, *372*, 814–824. [CrossRef] [PubMed]
38. Heusschen, L.; Krabbendam, I.; van der Velde, J.M.; Deden, L.N.; Aarts, E.O.; Merién, A.E.R.; Emous, M.; Bleumink, G.S.; Lutgers, H.L.; Hazebroek, E.J. A Matter of Timing—Pregnancy After Bariatric Surgery. *Obes. Surg.* **2021**, *31*, 2072–2079. [CrossRef] [PubMed]
39. Harrison, R.K.; Berkelhammer, C.; Suarez, V.; Kay, H.H. Managing Malnourishment in Pregnancy after Bariatric Surgery. *J. Obstet. Gynaecol. Can.* **2018**, *40*, 211–214. [CrossRef]
40. Karmon, A.; Sheiner, E. Pregnancy after bariatric surgery: A comprehensive review. *Arch. Gynecol. Obstet.* **2008**, *277*, 381–388. [CrossRef]
41. Beiglböck, H.; Mörth, E.; Reichardt, B.; Stamm, T.; Itariu, B.; Harreiter, J.; Eichelter, J.; Prager, G.; Kautzky-Willer, A.; Wolf, P.; et al. The Timing of Pregnancies After Bariatric Surgery has No Impact on Children's Health—A Nationwide Population-based Registry Analysis. *Obes. Surg.* **2023**, *33*, 149–155. [CrossRef]
42. Mensink, G.B.M.; Fletcher, R.; Gurinović, M.; Huybrechts, I.; Lafay, L.; Serra-Majem, L.; Szponar, L.; Tetens, I.; Verkaik-Kloosterman, J.; Baka, A.; et al. Mapping low intake of micronutrients across Europe. *Br. J. Nutr.* **2013**, *110*, 755–773. [CrossRef]
43. Das, J.K.; Salam, R.A.; Kumar, R.; Bhutta, Z.A. Micronutrient fortification of food and its impact on woman and child health: A systematic review. *Syst. Rev.* **2013**, *23*, 2–67. [CrossRef]
44. Maslin, K.; James, A.; Brown, A.; Bogaerts, A.; Shawe, J. What Is Known About the Nutritional Intake of Women during Pregnancy Following Bariatric Surgery? A Scoping Review. *Nutrients* **2019**, *11*, 2116. [CrossRef]

45. Lecube, A.; de Hollanda, A.; Calañas, A.; Vilarrasa, N.; Rubio, M.A.; Breton, I.; Goday, A.; Vidal, J.; Iglesias, P.; Fernández-Soto, M.L.; et al. Trends in Bariatric Surgery in Spain in the Twenty-First Century: Baseline Results and 1-Month Follow Up of the RICIBA, a National Registry. *Obes. Surg.* **2015**, *26*, 1836–1842. [CrossRef] [PubMed]
46. Alanis, M.C.; Goodnight, W.H.; Hill, E.G.; Robinson, C.J.; Villers, M.S.; Johnson, D.D. Maternal super-obesity (body mass index $\geq$ 50) and adverse pregnancy outcomes. *Acta Obstet. Gynecol. Scand.* **2010**, *89*, 924–930. [CrossRef] [PubMed]
47. Cogswell, M.E.; Weisberg, P.; Spong, C. Cigarette smoking, alcohol use and adverse pregnancy outcomes: Implications for micronutrient supplementation. *J. Nutr.* **2003**, *133* (Suppl. S1), 1722S–1731S. [CrossRef] [PubMed]
48. Abbassi-Ghanavati, M.; Greer, L.G.; Cunningham, F.G. Pregnancy and Laboratory Studies. *Obstet. Gynecol.* **2009**, *114*, 1326–1331. [CrossRef]
49. Bailey, L.B.; Stover, P.J.; McNulty, H.; Fenech, M.F.; Gregory, J.F., III.; Mills, J.L.; Pfeiffer, C.M.; Fazili, Z.; Zhang, M.; Ueland, P.M.; et al. Biomarkers of Nutrition for Development—Folate Review. *J. Nutr.* **2015**, *145*, 1636S–1680S. [CrossRef]
50. EFSA Panel on Dietetic Products; Nutrition and Allergies (NDA). Scientific Opinion on Dietary Reference Values for iron. *EFSA J.* **2015**, *13*, 4254. [CrossRef]
51. MRC Vitamin Study Research Group. Prevention of neural tube defects: Results of the Medical Research Council Vitamin Study. *Lancet* **1991**, *338*, 131–137. [CrossRef]
52. Shaw, G.M.; Carmichael, S.L.; Nelson, V.; Selvin, S.; Schaffer, D.M. Occurrence of Low Birthweight and Preterm Delivery among California Infants before and after Compulsory Food Fortification with Folic Acid. *Public Health Rep.* **2004**, *119*, 170–173. [CrossRef] [PubMed]
53. Rodríguez, L.; Médico, M. Suplementos en embarazadas: Controversias, evidencias y recomendaciones. *Inf. Ter. Sist. Nac. Salud.* **2010**, *34*, 117–128.
54. Rottenstreich, A.; Elazary, R.; Goldenshluger, A.; Pikarsky, A.J.; Elchalal, U.; Ben-Porat, T. Maternal nutritional status and related pregnancy outcomes following bariatric surgery: A systematic review. *Surg. Obes. Relat. Dis.* **2019**, *15*, 324–332. [CrossRef]
55. Mojtabai, R. Body mass index and serum folate in childbearing age women. *Eur. J. Epidemiol.* **2004**, *19*, 1029–1036. [CrossRef]
56. De-Regil, L.M.; Peña-Rosas, J.P.; Fernández-Gaxiola, A.C.; Rayco-Solon, P. Effects and safety of periconceptional oral folate supplementation for preventing birth defects. *Cochrane Database Syst. Rev.* **2015**, *2015*, CD007950. [CrossRef]
57. Lassi, Z.S.; Salam, R.A.; Haider, B.A.; Bhutta, Z.A. Folic acid supplementation during pregnancy for maternal health and pregnancy outcomes. *Cochrane Database Syst. Rev.* **2013**, *3*, CD006896. [CrossRef] [PubMed]
58. Moussa, H.N.; Nasab, S.H.; A Haidar, Z.; Blackwell, S.C.; Sibai, B.M.; Srikrishnan, A.; Dash, P.; Divieto, C.; Sassi, M.P.; Abdelhafiz, A.H.; et al. Folic acid supplementation: What is new? Fetal, obstetric, long-term benefits and risks. *Futur. Sci. OA* **2016**, *2*, FSO116. [CrossRef] [PubMed]
59. E Brolin, R.; Gorman, R.C.; Milgrim, L.M.; A Kenler, H. Multivitamin prophylaxis in prevention of post-gastric bypass vitamin and mineral deficiencies. *Int. J. Obes.* **1991**, *15*, 661–667.
60. MacLean, L.D. Nutrition following intestinal bypass and gastric operations for morbid obesity. *Can. J. Surg.* **1984**, *27*, 134–135.
61. Gasteyger, C.; Suter, M.; Calmes, J.M.; Gaillard, R.C.; Giusti, V. Changes in Body Composition, Metabolic Profile and Nutritional Status 24 Months after Gastric Banding. *Obes. Surg.* **2006**, *16*, 243–250. [CrossRef]
62. Aasheim, E.T.; Björkman, S.; Søvik, T.T.; Engström, M.; E Hanvold, S.; Mala, T.; Olbers, T.; Bøhmer, T. Vitamin status after bariatric surgery: A randomized study of gastric bypass and duodenal switch. *Am. J. Clin. Nutr.* **2009**, *90*, 15–22. [CrossRef] [PubMed]
63. Skroubis, G.; Sakellaropoulos, G.; Pouggouras, K.; Mead, N.; Nikiforidis, G.; Kalfarentzos, F. Comparison of Nutritional Deficiencies after Rouxen-Y Gastric Bypass and after Biliopancreatic Diversion with Roux-en-Y Gastric Bypass. *Obes. Surg.* **2002**, *12*, 551–558. [CrossRef]
64. Weng, T.-C.; Chang, C.-H.; Dong, Y.-H.; Chang, Y.-C.; Chuang, L.-M. Anaemia and related nutrient deficiencies after Roux-en-Y gastric bypass surgery: A systematic review and meta-analysis. *BMJ Open* **2015**, *5*, e006964. [CrossRef] [PubMed]
65. Moliterno, J.A.; DiLuna, M.L.; Sood, S.; Roberts, K.E.; Duncan, C.C. Gastric bypass: A risk factor for neural tube defects? *J. Neurosurg. Pediatr.* **2008**, *1*, 406–409. [CrossRef]
66. Pelizzo, G.; Calcaterra, V.; Fusillo, M.; Nakib, G.; Ierullo, A.M.; Alfei, A.; Spinillo, A.; Stronati, M.; Cena, H. Malnutrition in pregnancy following bariatric surgery: Three clinical cases of fetal neural defects. *Nutr. J.* **2014**, *13*, 59. [CrossRef]
67. Devlieger, R.; Guelinckx, I.; Jans, G.; Voets, W.; Vanholsbeke, C.; Vansant, G. Micronutrient Levels and Supplement Intake in Pregnancy after Bariatric Surgery: A Prospective Cohort Study. *PLoS ONE* **2014**, *9*, e114192. [CrossRef] [PubMed]
68. Bebber, F.E.; Rizzolli, J.; Casagrande, D.S.; Rodrigues, M.T.; Padoin, A.V.; Mottin, C.C.; Repetto, G. Pregnancy after Bariatric Surgery: 39 Pregnancies Follow-up in a Multidisciplinary Team. *Obes. Surg.* **2011**, *21*, 1546–1551. [CrossRef]
69. González, I.; Rubio, M.A.; Cordido, F.; Bretón, I.; Morales, M.J.; Vilarrasa, N.; Monereo, S.; Lecube, A.; Caixàs, A.; Vinagre, I.; et al. Maternal and Perinatal Outcomes After Bariatric Surgery: A Spanish Multicenter Study. *Obes. Surg.* **2014**, *25*, 436–442. [CrossRef]
70. O'leary, F.; Samman, S. Vitamin B12 in Health and Disease. *Nutrients* **2010**, *2*, 299–316. [CrossRef]
71. Finkelstein, J.L.; Layden, A.J.; Stover, P.J. Vitamin B-12 and Perinatal Health. *Adv. Nutr. Int. Rev. J.* **2015**, *6*, 552–563. [CrossRef]
72. Rogne, T.; Tielemans, M.J.; Chong, M.F.-F.; Yajnik, C.S.; Krishnaveni, G.V.; Poston, L.; Jaddoe, V.W.V.; Steegers, E.A.P.; Joshi, S.; Chong, Y.-S.; et al. Associations of Maternal Vitamin B12 Concentration in Pregnancy with the Risks of Preterm Birth and Low Birth Weight: A Systematic Review and Meta-Analysis of Individual Participant Data. *Am. J. Epidemiol.* **2017**, *185*, 212–223. [CrossRef]

73. Majumder, S.; Soriano, J.; Cruz, A.L.; Dasanu, C.A. Vitamin B12 deficiency in patients undergoing bariatric surgery: Preventive strategies and key recommendations. *Surg. Obes. Relat. Dis.* **2013**, *9*, 1013–1019. [CrossRef] [PubMed]
74. Smelt, H.J.M.; Pouwels, S.; Smulders, J.F. Different Supplementation Regimes to Treat Perioperative Vitamin B12 Deficiencies in Bariatric Surgery: A Systematic Review. *Obes. Surg.* **2017**, *27*, 254–262. [CrossRef] [PubMed]
75. Mechanick, J.; Youdim, A.; Jones, D.; Timothy Garvey, W.; Hurley, D.L.; Mc Mahon, M. AACE/TOS/ASMBS Bariatric Surgery Clinical Practice Guidelines. *Endocr. Pract.* **2013**, *19*, 1–36.
76. Busetto, L.; Dicker, D.; Azran, C.; Batterham, R.L.; Farpour-Lambert, N.; Fried, M.; Hjelmesæth, J.; Kinzl, J.; Leitner, D.R.; Makaronidis, J.M.; et al. Obesity Management Task Force of the European Association for the Study of Obesity Released "Practical Recommendations for the Post-Bariatric Surgery Medical Management". *Obes. Surg.* **2018**, *28*, 2117–2121. [CrossRef] [PubMed]
77. Grange, D.K.; Finlay, J.L. Nutritional Vitamin B_{12} Deficiency in a Breastfed Infant Following Maternal Gastric Bypass. *Pediatr. Hematol. Oncol.* **1994**, *11*, 311–318. [CrossRef]
78. Wardinsky, T.D.; Montes, R.G.; Friederich, R.L.; Broadhurst, R.B.; Sinnhuber, V.; Bartholomew, D. Vitamin B12 Deficiency Associated With Low Breast-Milk Vitamin B12 Concentration in an Infant Following Maternal Gastric Bypass Surgery. *Arch. Pediatr. Adolesc. Med.* **1995**, *149*, 1281–1284. [CrossRef]
79. Celiker, M.Y.; Chawla, A. Congenital B12 deficiency following maternal gastric bypass. *J. Perinatol.* **2009**, *29*, 640–642. [CrossRef]
80. Gascoin, G.; Gerard, M.; Sallé, A.; Becouarn, G.; Rouleau, S.; Sentilhes, L.; Coutant, R. Risk of low birth weight and micronutrient deficiencies in neonates from mothers after gastric bypass: A case control study. *Surg. Obes. Relat. Dis.* **2017**, *13*, 1384–1391. [CrossRef]
81. Mead, N.C.; Sakkatos, P.; Sakellaropoulos, G.C.; Adonakis, G.L.; Alexandrides, T.K.; Kalfarentzos, F. Pregnancy outcomes and nutritional indices after 3 types of bariatric surgery performed at a single institution. *Surg. Obes. Relat. Dis.* **2014**, *10*, 1166–1173. [CrossRef]
82. Sriram, K.; Manzanares, W.; Joseph, K. Thiamine in Nutrition Therapy. *Nutr. Clin. Pract.* **2012**, *27*, 41–50. [CrossRef] [PubMed]
83. Ashraf, V.; Prijesh, J.; Praveenkumar, R.; Saifudheen, K. Wernicke's encephalopathy due to hyperemesis gravidarum: Clinical and magnetic resonance imaging characteristics. *J. Postgrad. Med.* **2016**, *62*, 260–263. [CrossRef]
84. Frank, L.L. Thiamin in Clinical Practice. *J. Parenter. Enter. Nutr.* **2015**, *39*, 503–520. [CrossRef]
85. Kareem, O.; Nisar, S.; Tanvir, M.; Muzaffer, U.; Bader, G.N. Thiamine deficiency in pregnancy and lactation: Implications and present perspectives. *Front. Nutr.* **2023**, *10*, 1080611. [CrossRef]
86. Di Gangi, S.; Gizzo, S.; Patrelli, T.S.; Saccardi, C.; D'antona, D.; Nardelli, G.B. Wernicke's encephalopathy complicating hyperemesis gravidarum: From the background to the present. *J. Matern. Neonatal Med.* **2012**, *25*, 1499–1504. [CrossRef] [PubMed]
87. Finglas, P.M. Dietary Reference intakes for thiamin, riboflavin, niacin, vitamin B6, folate, vitamin B12, pantothenic acid, biotin and choline. *Trends Food Sci. Technol.* **2000**, *11*, 296–297. [CrossRef]
88. Jans, G.; Matthys, C.; Bogaerts, A.; Lannoo, M.; Verhaeghe, J.; Van der Schueren, B.; Devlieger, R. Maternal Micronutrient Deficiencies and Related Adverse Neonatal Outcomes after Bariatric Surgery: A Systematic Review. *Adv. Nutr. Int. Rev. J.* **2015**, *6*, 420–429. [CrossRef]
89. Kröll, D.; Laimer, M.; Borbély, Y.M.; Laederach, K.; Candinas, D.; Nett, P.C. Wernicke Encephalopathy: A Future Problem Even After Sleeve Gastrectomy? A Systematic Literature Review. *Obes. Surg.* **2016**, *26*, 205–212. [CrossRef]
90. Ngene, N.C.; Moodley, J. Clinical awareness for health care professionals: Fatal encephalopathy complicating persistent vomiting in pregnancy. *S. Afr. Med. J.* **2016**, *106*, 792–794. [CrossRef]
91. Bahardoust, M.; Eghbali, F.; Shahmiri, S.S.; Alijanpour, A.; Yarigholi, F.; Valizadeh, R.; Madankan, A.; Pouraskari, A.B.; Ashtarinezhad, B.; Farokhi, H.; et al. B1 Vitamin Deficiency After Bariatric Surgery, Prevalence, and Symptoms: A Systematic Review and Meta-analysis. *Obes. Surg.* **2022**, *32*, 3104–3112. [CrossRef] [PubMed]
92. Saab, R.O.; El Khoury, M.I.; Jabbour, R.A. Wernicke encephalopathy after Roux-en-Y gastric bypass and hyperemesis gravidarum. *Surg. Obes. Relat. Dis.* **2013**, *9*, e105–e107. [CrossRef]
93. Holick, M.F.; Binkley, N.C.; Bischoff-Ferrari, H.A.; Gordon, C.M.; Hanley, D.A.; Heaney, R.P.; Murad, M.H.; Weaver, C.M. Evaluation, Treatment, and Prevention of Vitamin D Deficiency: An Endocrine Society Clinical Practice Guideline. *Med. J. Clin. Endocrinol. Metab.* **2011**, *96*, 1911–1930. [CrossRef] [PubMed]
94. Wagner, C.L.; Hollis, B.W. The Implications of Vitamin D Status During Pregnancy on Mother and her Developing Child. *Front. Endocrinol.* **2018**, *9*, 500. [CrossRef]
95. Bodnar, L.M.; Catov, J.M.; Simhan, H.N.; Holick, M.F.; Powers, R.W.; Roberts, J.M. Maternal Vitamin D Deficiency Increases the Risk of Preeclampsia. *J. Clin. Endocrinol. Metab.* **2007**, *92*, 3517–3522. [CrossRef]
96. Wei, S.-Q.; Qi, H.-P.; Luo, Z.-C.; Fraser, W.D. Maternal vitamin D status and adverse pregnancy outcomes: A systematic review and meta-analysis. *J. Matern.-Fetal Neonatal Med.* **2013**, *26*, 889–899. [CrossRef] [PubMed]
97. Hu, K.-L.; Zhang, C.-X.; Chen, P.; Zhang, D.; Hunt, S. Vitamin D Levels in Early and Middle Pregnancy and Preeclampsia, a Systematic Review and Meta-Analysis. *Nutrients* **2022**, *14*, 999. [CrossRef] [PubMed]
98. Perez-Ferre, N.; Torrejon, M.J.; Fuentes, M.; Fernandez, M.D.; Ramos, A.; Bordiu, E.; del Valle, L.; Rubio, M.A.; Bedia, A.R.; Montañez, C.; et al. Association of Low Serum 25-Hydroxyvitamin D Levels in Pregnancy with Glucosehomeostasis and Obstetric And Newborn Outcomes. *Endocr. Pract.* **2012**, *18*, 676–684. [CrossRef] [PubMed]

99. Switzer, N.J.; Marcil, G.; Prasad, S.; Debru, E.; Church, N.; Mitchell, P.; Billington, E.O.; Gill, R.S. Long-term hypovitaminosis D and secondary hyperparathyroidism outcomes of the Roux-en-Y gastric bypass: A systematic review. *Obes. Rev.* **2017**, *65*, 560–566. [CrossRef]
100. Chakhtoura, M.T.; Nakhoul, N.; Akl, E.A.; Mantzoros, C.S.; El Hajj Fuleihan, G.A. Guidelines on vitamin D replacement in bariatric surgery: Identification and systematic appraisal. *Metabolism* **2016**, *65*, 586–597. [CrossRef] [PubMed]
101. Medeiros, M.; Matos, A.C.; Pereira, S.E.; Saboya, C.; Ramalho, A. Vitamin D and its relation with ionic calcium, parathyroid hormone, maternal and neonatal characteristics in pregnancy after roux-en-Y gastric bypass. *Arch. Gynecol. Obstet.* **2016**, *293*, 539–547. [CrossRef]
102. Cruz, S.; de Matos, A.C.; da Cruz, S.P.; Pereira, S.; Saboya, C.; Ramalho, A. Maternal Anthropometry and Its Relationship with the Nutritional Status of Vitamin D, Calcium, and Parathyroid Hormone in Pregnant Women after Roux-en-Y Gastric Bypass. *Obes. Surg.* **2018**, *28*, 3116–3124. [CrossRef] [PubMed]
103. World Health Organization. *Global Prevalence of Vitamin A Deficiency in Populations at Risk 1995–2005: WHO Global Database on Vitamin A Deficiency*; WHO Iris: Geneva, Switzerland, 2009; p. 55. Available online: https://apps.who.int/iris/handle/10665/44110 (accessed on 15 August 2023).
104. Snoek, K.; van de Woestijne, N.; Willemsen, S.; Klaassen, R.; Galjaard, S.; Laven, J.; Steegers-Theunissen, R.; Schoenmakers, S. The Impact of Preconception Gastric Bypass Surgery on Maternal Micronutrient Status before and during Pregnancy: A Retrospective Cohort Study in the Netherlands between 2009 and 2019. *Nutrients* **2022**, *14*, 736. [CrossRef] [PubMed]
105. OMS. Concentraciones en suero de retinol para establecer la prevalencia de la carencia de vitamina A a escala poblacional. In *Sistema de Información Nutricional Sobre Vitaminas y Minerales*; Organización Mundial de la Salud: Geneva, Switzerland, 2011.
106. Rubio, M.A.; Cuesta, M.; Pelaz, L.; Pérez, C.; Torrejón, M.J.; Cabrerizo, L.; Matía, P.; Pérez-Ferre, N.; Sánchez-Pernaute, A.; Torres, A. Fat-soluble vitamin deficiencies after bariatric surgery could be misleading if they are not appropriately adjusted. *Nutr. Hosp.* **2014**, *30*, 118–123. [CrossRef]
107. Rayman, M.P.; Bode, P.; Redman, C.W.G. Low selenium status is associated with the occurrence of the pregnancy disease preeclampsia in women from the United Kingdom. *Am. J. Obstet. Gynecol.* **2003**, *189*, 1343–1349. [CrossRef]
108. Oliveira, J.M.; Michelazzo, F.B.; Stefanello, J.; Rondó, P.H. Influence of iron on vitamin A nutritional status. *Nutr. Rev.* **2008**, *66*, 141–147. [CrossRef]
109. WHO. *Guideline: Vitamin A Supplementation in Pregnant Women*; World Health Organization: Geneva, Switzerland, 2011; pp. 1–30.
110. McCauley, M.E.; van den Broek, N.; Dou, L.; Othman, M. Vitamin A supplementation during pregnancy for maternal and newborn outcomes. *Cochrane Database Syst. Rev.* **2015**, *10*, CD008666. [CrossRef]
111. EFSA NDA Panel. Scientific Opinion on Dietary Reference Values for biotin. *EFSA J.* **2015**, *12*, 3580. [CrossRef]
112. Slater, G.H.; Ren, C.J.; Siegel, N.; Williams, T.; Barr, D.; Wolfe, B.; Dolan, K.; A Fielding, G. Serum fat-soluble vitamin deficiency andabnormal calcium metabolism after malabsorptivebariatric surgery. *J. Gastrointest. Surg.* **2004**, *8*, 48–55. [CrossRef]
113. Eckert, M.J.; Perry, J.T.; Sohn, V.Y.; Boden, J.; Martin, M.J.; Rush, R.M.; Steele, S.R. Incidence of low vitamin A levels and ocular symptoms after Roux-en-Y gastric bypass. *Surg. Obes. Relat. Dis.* **2010**, *6*, 653–657. [CrossRef]
114. Pereira, S.; Saboya, C.; Chaves, G.; Ramalho, A. Class III Obesity and its Relationship with the Nutritional Status of Vitamin A in Pre- and Postoperative Gastric Bypass. *Obes. Surg.* **2009**, *19*, 738–744. [CrossRef] [PubMed]
115. Vales Montero, M.; Chavarría Cano, B.; Martínez Ginés, M.L.; Díaz Otero, F.; Velázquez Pérez, J.M.; Cuerda Compes, M.C.; Bretón Lesmes, I. Deficiencia clínica de vitamina A tras bypass gástrico: Descripción de un caso clínico y revisión de la literatura. *Nutr. Hosp.* **2016**, *33*, 404. [CrossRef]
116. Ocón, J.; Cabrejas, C.; Altemir, J.; Moros, M. Phrynoderma. *J. Parenter. Enter. Nutr.* **2012**, *36*, 361–364. [CrossRef]
117. Fok, J.S.; Li, J.Y.Z.; Yong, T.Y. Visual deterioration caused by vitamin A deficiency in patients after bariatric surgery. *Eat. Weight. Disord.—Stud. Anorexia, Bulim. Obes.* **2012**, *17*, e144–e146. [CrossRef] [PubMed]
118. Ramos-Leví, A.M.; Pérez-Ferre, N.; Sánchez-Pernaute, A.; García, A.J.T.; Herrera, M.A.R. Torres Garcia, and M. a Rubio Herrera, "Severe vitamin A deficiency after malabsortive bariatric surgery. *Nutr. Hosp.* **2013**, *28*, 1337–1340. [CrossRef] [PubMed]
119. Stroh, C.; Weiher, C.; Hohmann, U.; Meyer, F.; Lippert, H.; Manger, T. Vitamin A Deficiency (VAD) After a Duodenal Switch Procedure: A Case Report. *Obes. Surg.* **2009**, *20*, 397–400. [CrossRef]
120. Chagas, C.B.; Saunders, C.; Pereira, S.; Silva, J.; Saboya, C.; Ramalho, A. Vitamin A Deficiency in Pregnancy: Perspectives after Bariatric Surgery. *Obes. Surg.* **2012**, *23*, 249–254. [CrossRef]
121. Huerta, S.; Rogers, L.M.; Li, Z.; Heber, D.; Liu, C.; Livingston, E.H. Vitamin A deficiency in a newborn resulting from maternal hypovitaminosis A after biliopancreatic diversion for the treatment of morbid obesity. *Am. J. Clin. Nutr.* **2002**, *76*, 426–429. [CrossRef]
122. Smets, K.J.; Barlow, T.; Vanhaesebrouck, P. Maternal vitamin A deficiency and neonatal microphthalmia: Complications of biliopancreatic diversion? *Eur. J. Pediatr.* **2006**, *165*, 502–504. [CrossRef]
123. Breton, J.O.; Sallan, L. Maternal and neonatal complications in a pregnant woman with biliopancreatic diversion. [Spanish] TT—Complicaciones maternas y neonatales en una mujer gestante con derivacion biliopancreatica. *Nutr. Hosp. Organo Of. Soc. Esp. Nutr. Parenter. Y Enter.* **2010**, *25*, 120–122.
124. Mackie, F.L.; Cooper, N.S.; Whitticase, L.J.; Smith, A.; Martin, W.L.; Cooper, S.C. Vitamin A and micronutrient deficiencies post-bariatric surgery: Aetiology, complications and management in a complex multiparous pregnancy. *Eur. J. Clin. Nutr.* **2018**, *72*, 1176–1179. [CrossRef] [PubMed]

125. Cruz, S.; Matos, A.; Da Cruz, S.P.; Pereira, S.; Saboya, C.; Ramalho, A. Relationship between the Nutritional Status of Vitamin A per Trimester of Pregnancy with Maternal Anthropometry and Anemia after Roux-en-Y Gastric Bypass. *Nutrients* **2017**, *9*, 989. [CrossRef] [PubMed]
126. Hazart, J.; Le Guennec, D.; Accoceberry, M.; Lemery, D.; Mulliez, A.; Farigon, N.; Lahaye, C.; Miolanne-Debouit, M.; Boirie, Y. Maternal Nutritional Deficiencies and Small-for-Gestational-Age Neonates at Birth of Women Who Have Undergone Bariatric Surgery. *J. Pregnancy* **2017**, *2017*, 4168541. [CrossRef] [PubMed]
127. Niki, E.; Traber, M.G. A History of Vitamin E. *Ann. Nutr. Metab.* **2012**, *61*, 207–212. [CrossRef] [PubMed]
128. Traber, M.G. Vitamin E Inadequacy in Humans: Causes and Consequences. *Adv. Nutr. Int. Rev. J.* **2014**, *5*, 503–514. [CrossRef]
129. Institute of Medicine; Food and Nutrition Board; Panel on Dietary Antioxidants and Related Compounds; Subcommittee on Upper Reference Levels of Nutrients; Subcommittee on Interpretation and Uses of Dietary Reference Intakes; Standing Committee on the Scientific Evaluation of Dietary Reference Intakes. *Dietary Reference Intakes for Vitamin C, Vitamin E, Selenium, and Carotenoids*; National Academies Press (US): Washington, DC, USA, 2000. [CrossRef]
130. Chen, K.; Zhang, X.; Wei, X.-P.; Qu, P.; Liu, Y.-X.; Li, T.-Y. Antioxidant vitamin status during pregnancy in relation to cognitive development in the first two years of life. *Early Hum. Dev.* **2009**, *85*, 421–427. [CrossRef]
131. Koscik, R.L.; Lai, H.J.; Laxova, A.; Zaremba, K.M.; Kosorok, M.R.; Douglas, J.A.; Rock, M.J.; Splaingard, M.L.; Farrell, P.M. Preventing early, prolonged vitamin E deficiency: An opportunity for better cognitive outcomes via early diagnosis through neonatal screening. *J. Pediatr.* **2005**, *147*, S51–S56. [CrossRef]
132. Hovdenak, N.; Haram, K. Influence of mineral and vitamin supplements on pregnancy outcome. *Eur. J. Obstet. Gynecol. Reprod. Biol.* **2012**, *164*, 127–132. [CrossRef]
133. Sitrin, M.D.; Lieberman, F.; Jensen, W.E.; Noronha, A.; Milburn, C.; Addington, W. Vitamin E Deficiency and Neurologic Disease in Adults with Cystic Fibrosis. *Ann. Intern. Med.* **1987**, *107*, 51–54. [CrossRef]
134. Wilson, R.D.; Audibert, F.; Brock, J.-A.; Carroll, J.; Cartier, L.; Gagnon, A.; Johnson, J.-A.; Langlois, S.; Murphy-Kaulbeck, L.; Okun, N.; et al. Pre-conception Folic Acid and Multivitamin Supplementation for the Primary and Secondary Prevention of Neural Tube Defects and Other Folic Acid-Sensitive Congenital Anomalies. *J. Obstet. Gynaecol. Can.* **2015**, *37*, 534–549. [CrossRef] [PubMed]
135. Bastos Maia, S.; Rolland Souza, A.S.; Costa Caminha, M.d.F.; Lins da Silva, S.; Callou Cruz, R.d.S.B.L.; Carvalho dos Santos, C.; Batista Filho, M. Vitamin A and Pregnancy: A Narrative Review. *Nutrients* **2019**, *11*, 681. [CrossRef]
136. Harshman, S.G.; Saltzman, E.; Booth, S.L. Vitamin K. *Curr. Opin. Clin. Nutr. Metab. Care* **2014**, *17*, 531–538. [CrossRef] [PubMed]
137. Pearson, D.A. Bone Health and Osteoporosis: The Role of Vitamin K and Potential Antagonism by Anticoagulants. *Nutr. Clin. Pract.* **2007**, *22*, 517–544. [CrossRef]
138. Shahrook, S.; Ota, E.; Hanada, N.; Sawada, K.; Mori, R. Vitamin K supplementation during pregnancy for improving outcomes: A systematic review and meta-analysis. *Sci. Rep.* **2018**, *8*, 11459. [CrossRef] [PubMed]
139. Homan, J.; Ruinemans-Koerts, J.; Aarts, E.; Janssen, I.M.; Berends, F.J.; de Boer, H. Management of vitamin K deficiency after biliopancreatic diversion with or without duodenal switch. *Surg. Obes. Relat. Dis.* **2016**, *12*, 338–344. [CrossRef]
140. Van Mieghem, T.; Van Schoubroeck, D.; Depiere, M.; Debeer, A.; Hanssens, M. Fetal Cerebral Hemorrhage Caused by Vitamin K Deficiency After Complicated Bariatric Surgery. *Obstet. Gynecol.* **2008**, *112*, 434–436. [CrossRef] [PubMed]
141. Bersani, I.; De Carolis, M.P.; Salvi, S.; Zecca, E.; Romagnoli, C.; De Carolis, S. Maternal–neonatal vitamin K deficiency secondary to maternal biliopancreatic diversion. *Blood Coagul. Fibrinolysis* **2011**, *22*, 334–336. [CrossRef]
142. Jans, G.; Guelinckx, I.; Voets, W.; Galjaard, S.; Van Haard, P.M.; Vansant, G.M.; Devlieger, R. Vitamin K1 monitoring in pregnancies after bariatric surgery: A prospective cohort study. *Surg. Obes. Relat. Dis.* **2014**, *10*, 885–890. [CrossRef]
143. Aron-Wisnewsky, J.; O Verger, E.; Bounaix, C.; Dao, M.C.; Oppert, J.-M.; Bouillot, J.-L.; Chevallier, J.-M.; Clément, K. Nutritional and Protein Deficiencies in the Short Term following Both Gastric Bypass and Gastric Banding. *PLoS ONE* **2016**, *11*, e0149588. [CrossRef]
144. DeLoughery, T.G. Iron Deficiency Anemia. *Med. Clin. N. Am.* **2017**, *101*, 319–332. [CrossRef]
145. Aigner, E.; Feldman, A.; Datz, C. Obesity as an Emerging Risk Factor for Iron Deficiency. *Nutrients* **2014**, *6*, 3587–3600. [CrossRef]
146. Hamamy, H.; Alwan, N.A. Maternal Iron Status in Pregnancy and Long-Term Health Outcomes in the Offspring. *J. Pediatr. Genet.* **2015**, *4*, 111–123. [CrossRef]
147. Spanish Ministry of Health. *Grupo de Trabajo de la Guía de Práctica Clínica de Atención en el Embarazo y Puerperio*; A Tención en el e Mbarazo y P Uerperio; Spanish Ministry of Health: Madrid, Spain, 2014; p. 397.
148. Breymann, C. Iron deficiency and anaemia in pregnancy: Modern aspects of diagnosis and therapy. *Eur. J. Obstet. Gynecol. Reprod. Biol.* **2005**, *123*, S3–S13. [CrossRef]
149. World Health Organization. *Guideline: Daily Iron and Folic Acid Supplementation in Pregnant Women*; World Health Organization: Geneva, Switzerland, 2012.
150. Muñoz, M.; Rosado, E.L. Iron Deficiency and Anaemia in Bariatric Surgical patients: Causes, Diagnosis and Proper Management. *Nutr. Hosp.* **2009**, *24*, 640–654. [CrossRef] [PubMed]
151. Jericó, C.; Bretón, I.; de Gordejuela, A.G.R.; de Oliveira, A.C.; Rubio, M.; Tinahones, F.J.; Vidal, J.; Vilarrasa, N. Diagnóstico y tratamiento del déficit de hierro, con o sin anemia, pre y poscirugía bariátrica. *Endocrinol. Y Nutr.* **2016**, *63*, 32–42. [CrossRef]
152. Steenackers, N.; Van der Schueren, B.; Mertens, A.; Lannoo, M.; Grauwet, T.; Augustijns, P.; Matthys, C. Iron deficiency after bariatric surgery: What is the real problem? *Proc. Nutr. Soc.* **2018**, *77*, 445–455. [PubMed]

153. Nomura, R.M.Y.; Dias, M.C.G.; Igai, A.M.K.; Paiva, L.V.; Zugaib, M. Anemia During Pregnancy after Silastic Ring Roux-en-Y Gastric Bypass: Influence of Time to Conception. *Obes. Surg.* **2011**, *21*, 479–484. [CrossRef]
154. Falcone, V.; Stopp, T.; Feichtinger, M.; Kiss, H.; Eppel, W.; Husslein, P.W.; Prager, G.; Göbl, C.S. Pregnancy after bariatric surgery: A narrative literature review and discussion of impact on pregnancy management and outcome. *BMC Pregnancy Childbirth* **2018**, *18*, 507. [CrossRef]
155. Hezelgrave, N.L.; Oteng-Ntim, E. Pregnancy after Bariatric Surgery: A Review. *J. Obes.* **2011**, *2011*, 501939. [CrossRef]
156. Dalfrà, M.G.; Busetto, L.; Chilelli, N.C.; Lapolla, A. Pregnancy and foetal outcome after bariatric surgery: A review of recent studies. *J. Matern. Neonatal Med.* **2012**, *25*, 1537–1543. [CrossRef]
157. Gröber, U.; Schmidt, J.; Kisters, K. Magnesium in Prevention and Therapy. *Nutrients* **2015**, *7*, 8199–8226. [CrossRef]
158. De Baaij, J.H.F.; Hoenderop, J.G.J.; Bindels, R.J. Magnesium in Man: Implications for Health and Disease. *Physiol. Rev.* **2015**, *95*, 1–46. [CrossRef] [PubMed]
159. Costello, R.B.; Elin, R.J.; Rosanoff, A.; Wallace, T.C.; Guerrero-Romero, F.; Hruby, A.; Lutsey, P.L.; Nielsen, F.H.; Rodriguez-Moran, M.; Song, Y.; et al. Perspective: The Case for an Evidence-Based Reference Interval for Serum Magnesium: The Time Has Come. *Adv. Nutr.* **2016**, *7*, 977–993. [CrossRef]
160. Lager, S.; Powell, T.L. Regulation of Nutrient Transport across the Placenta. *J. Pregnancy* **2012**, *2012*, 179827. [CrossRef] [PubMed]
161. Amaral, L.M.; Wallace, K.; Owens, M.; LaMarca, B. Pathophysiology and Current Clinical Management of Preeclampsia. *Curr. Hypertens. Rep.* **2017**, *19*, 61. [CrossRef]
162. Holcberg, G.; Sapir, O.; Hallak, M.; Alaa, A.; Shorok, H.-Y.; David, Y.; Katz, M.; Huleihel, M. Selective Vasodilator Effect of Magnesium Sulfate in Human Placenta. *Am. J. Reprod. Immunol.* **2004**, *51*, 192–197. [CrossRef] [PubMed]
163. Dhariwal, N.K.; Lynde, G.C. Update in the Management of Patients with Preeclampsia. *Anesthesiol. Clin.* **2017**, *35*, 95–106. [CrossRef]
164. Dalton, L.M.; Fhloinn, D.M.N.; Gaydadzhieva, G.T.; Mazurkiewicz, O.M.; Leeson, H.; Wright, C.P. Magnesium in pregnancy. *Nutr. Rev.* **2016**, *74*, 549–557. [CrossRef]
165. Makrides, M.; Crosby, D.D.; Shepherd, E.; A Crowther, C. Magnesium supplementation in pregnancy. *Cochrane Database Syst. Rev.* **2014**, *2019*, CD000937. [CrossRef]
166. Shepherd, E.; Salam, R.A.; Manhas, D.; Synnes, A.; Middleton, P.; Makrides, M.; Crowther, C.A. Antenatal magnesium sulphate and adverse neonatal outcomes: A systematic review and meta-analysis. *PLOS Med.* **2019**, *16*, e1002988. [CrossRef]
167. Gimenes, J.C.; Nicoletti, C.F.; de Souza Pinhel, M.A.; de Oliveira, B.A.P.; Júnior, W.S.; Marchini, J.S.; Nonino, C.B. Pregnancy After Roux en Y Gastric Bypass: Nutritional and Biochemical Aspects. *Obes. Surg.* **2017**, *27*, 1815–1821. [CrossRef]
168. Trumbo, P.; A Yates, A.; Schlicker, S.; Poos, M. Dietary Reference Intakes. *J. Am. Diet. Assoc.* **2001**, *101*, 294–301. [CrossRef] [PubMed]
169. Prasad, A.S. Discovery of Human Zinc Deficiency: Its Impact on Human Health and Disease. *Adv. Nutr. Int. Rev. J.* **2013**, *4*, 176–190. [CrossRef] [PubMed]
170. Roohani, N.; Hurrell, R.; Kelishadi, R.; Schulin, R. Zinc and its importance for human health: An integrative review. *J. Res. Med. Sci.* **2013**, *18*, 144–157.
171. Wilson, R.L.; Grieger, J.A.; Bianco-Miotto, T.; Roberts, C.T. Association between Maternal Zinc Status, Dietary Zinc Intake and Pregnancy Complications: A Systematic Review. *Nutrients* **2016**, *8*, 641. [CrossRef] [PubMed]
172. Walker, J.B.; Houseman, J.; Seddon, L.; McMullen, E.; Tofflemire, K.; Mills, C.; Corriveau, A.; Weber, J.-P.; LeBlanc, A.; Walker, M.; et al. Maternal and umbilical cord blood levels of mercury, lead, cadmium, and essential trace elements in Arctic Canada. *Environ. Res.* **2006**, *100*, 295–318. [CrossRef]
173. King, J.C. Determinants of maternal zinc status during pregnancy. *Am. J. Clin. Nutr.* **2000**, *71*, 1334S–1343S. [CrossRef]
174. Hanachi, P.; Norrozi, M.; Moosavi, R.M. The Correlation of Prenatal Zinc Concentration and Deficiency with Anthropometric Factors. *J. Fam. Reprod. Health* **2014**, *8*, 21–26.
175. Shen, P.-J.; Gong, B.; Xu, F.-Y.; Luo, Y. Four trace elements in pregnant women and their relationships with adverse pregnancy outcomes. *Eur. Rev. Med. Pharmacol. Sci.* **2015**, *19*, 4690–4699. [PubMed]
176. Atazadegan, M.A.; Heidari-Beni, M.; Riahi, R.; Kelishadi, R. Association of selenium, zinc and copper concentrations during pregnancy with birth weight: A systematic review and meta-analysis. *J. Trace Elem. Med. Biol.* **2022**, *69*, 126903. [CrossRef]
177. Rojas, P.; Gosch, M.; Basfi-Fer, K.; Carrasco, F.; Codoceo, J.; Inostroza, J.; Valencia, A.; Adjemian, D.; Rojas, J.; Díaz, E.; et al. Alopecia in women with severe and morbid obesity who undergo bariatric surgery. *Nutr. Hosp.* **2011**, *26*, 856–862. [CrossRef] [PubMed]
178. Chagas, C.; Saunders, C.; Pereira, S.; Silva, J.; Saboya, C.; Ramalho, A. Vitamin A status and its relationship with serum zinc concentrations among pregnant women who have previously undergone Roux-en-Y gastric bypass. *Int. J. Gynecol. Obstet.* **2016**, *133*, 94–97. [CrossRef]
179. Ducarme, G.; Planche, L.; Abet, E.; du Roure, V.D.; Ducet-Boiffard, A. A Prospective Study of Association of Micronutrients Deficiencies during Pregnancy and Neonatal Outcome among Women after Bariatric Surgery. *J. Clin. Med.* **2021**, *10*, 204. [CrossRef]
180. Scheiber, I.F.; Mercer, J.F.; Dringen, R. Metabolism and functions of copper in brain. *Prog. Neurobiol.* **2014**, *116*, 33–57. [CrossRef]
181. Tiffany-Castiglioni, E.; Hong, S.; Qian, Y. Copper handling by astrocytes: Insights into neurodegenerative diseases. *Int. J. Dev. Neurosci.* **2011**, *29*, 811–818. [CrossRef]

182. Altarelli, M.; Ben-Hamouda, N.; Schneider, A.; Berger, M.M. Copper Deficiency: Causes, Manifestations, and Treatment. *Nutr. Clin. Pract.* **2019**, *34*, 504–513. [CrossRef] [PubMed]
183. Uriu-Adams, J.Y.; Scherr, R.E.; Lanoue, L.; Keen, C.L. Influence of copper on early development: Prenatal and postnatal considerations. *Biofactors* **2010**, *36*, 136–152. [CrossRef]
184. Zhang, Z.; Yuan, E.; Liu, J.; Lou, X.; Jia, L.; Li, X.; Zhang, L. Gestational age-specific reference intervals for blood copper, zinc, calcium, magnesium, iron, lead, and cadmium during normal pregnancy. *Clin. Biochem.* **2013**, *46*, 777–780. [CrossRef] [PubMed]
185. Alebic-Juretic, A.; Frkovic, A. Plasma copper concentrations in pathological pregnancies. *J. Trace Elem. Med. Biol.* **2005**, *19*, 191–194. [CrossRef]
186. Keen, C.L.; Uriu-Hare, J.Y.; Hawk, S.N.; Jankowski, M.; Daston, G.P.; Kwik-Uribe, C.L.; Rucker, R.B. Effect of copper deficiency on prenatal development and pregnancy outcome. *Am. J. Clin. Nutr.* **1998**, *67*, 1003S–1011S. [CrossRef]
187. Saltzman, E.; Karl, J.P. Nutrient Deficiencies After Gastric Bypass Surgery. *Annu. Rev. Nutr.* **2013**, *33*, 183–203. [CrossRef]
188. Gletsu-Miller, N.; Broderius, M.; Frediani, J.K.; Zhao, V.M.; Griffith, D.P.; Davis, S.S., Jr.; Sweeney, J.F.; Lin, E.; Prohaska, J.R.; Ziegler, T.R. Incidence and prevalence of copper deficiency following roux-en-y gastric bypass surgery. *Int. J. Obes.* **2012**, *36*, 328–335. [CrossRef]
189. Kumar, P.; Hamza, N.; Madhok, B.; De Alwis, N.; Sharma, M.; Miras, A.D.; Mahawar, K.K. Copper Deficiency after Gastric Bypass for Morbid Obesity: A Systematic Review. *Obes. Surg.* **2016**, *26*, 1335–1342. [CrossRef]
190. Balsa, J.A.; Botella-Carretero, J.I.; Gómez-Martín, J.M.; Peromingo, R.; Arrieta, F.; Santiuste, C.; Zamarrón, I.; Vázquez, C. Copper and Zinc Serum Levels after Derivative Bariatric Surgery: Differences between Roux-en-Y Gastric Bypass and Biliopancreatic Diversion. *Obes. Surg.* **2011**, *21*, 744–750. [CrossRef]
191. Btaiche, I.F.; Yeh, A.Y.; Wu, I.J.; Khalidi, N. Neurologic Dysfunction and Pancytopenia Secondary to Acquired Copper Deficiency Following Duodenal Switch. *Nutr. Clin. Pract.* **2011**, *26*, 583–592. [CrossRef] [PubMed]
192. Griffith, D.P.; Liff, D.A.; Ziegler, T.R.; Esper, G.J.; Winton, E.F. Acquired Copper Deficiency: A Potentially Serious and Preventable Complication Following Gastric Bypass Surgery. *Obesity* **2009**, *17*, 827–831. [CrossRef]
193. Rowin, J.; Lewis, S.L. Copper deficiency myeloneuropathy and pancytopenia secondary to overuse of zinc supplementation. *J. Neurol. Neurosurg. Psychiatry* **2005**, *76*, 750–751. [CrossRef]
194. Pieczyńska, J.; Grajeta, H. The role of selenium in human conception and pregnancy. *J. Trace Elem. Med. Biol.* **2014**, *29*, 31–38. [CrossRef] [PubMed]
195. Combs, J.G.F. Biomarkers of Selenium Status. *Nutrients* **2015**, *7*, 2209–2236. [CrossRef] [PubMed]
196. EFSA Panel on Dietetic Products, Nutrition and Allergies (NDA). Scientific Opinion on Dietary Reference Values for selenium. *EFSA J.* **2014**, *12*, 3846. [CrossRef]
197. Xu, M.; Guo, D.; Gu, H.; Zhang, L.; Lv, S. Selenium and Preeclampsia: A Systematic Review and Meta-analysis. *Biol. Trace Elem. Res.* **2016**, *171*, 283–292. [CrossRef]
198. Hamdan, H.Z.; Hamdan, S.Z.; Adam, I. Association of Selenium Levels with Preeclampsia: A Systematic Review and Meta-analysis. *Biol. Trace Elem. Res.* **2023**, *201*, 2105–2122. [CrossRef] [PubMed]
199. Álvarez, S.I.; Castañón, S.G.; Ruata, M.L.C.; Aragüés, E.F.; Terraz, P.B.; Irazabal, Y.G.; González, E.G.; Rodríguez, B.G. Updating of normal levels of copper, zinc and selenium in serum of pregnant women. *J. Trace Elem. Med. Biol.* **2007**, *21*, 49–52. [CrossRef]
200. Bermúdez, L.; García-Vicent, C.; López, J.; Torró, M.I.; Lurbe, E. Assessment of ten trace elements in umbilical cord blood and maternal blood: Association with birth weight. *J. Transl. Med.* **2015**, *13*, 291. [CrossRef]
201. Boldery, R.; Fielding, G.; Rafter, T.; Pascoe, A.L.; Scalia, G.M. Nutritional Deficiency of Selenium Secondary to Weight Loss (Bariatric) Surgery Associated with Life-Threatening Cardiomyopathy. *Heart Lung Circ.* **2007**, *16*, 123–126. [CrossRef]
202. Massoure, P.-L.; Camus, O.; Fourcade, L.; Simon, F. Bilateral leg oedema after bariatric surgery: A selenium-deficient cardiomyopathy. *Obes. Res. Clin. Pract.* **2017**, *11*, 622–626. [CrossRef]
203. Alasfar, F.; Ben-Nakhi, M.; Khoursheed, M.; Kehinde, E.O.; Alsaleh, M. Selenium Is Significantly Depleted Among Morbidly Obese Female Patients Seeking Bariatric Surgery. *Obes. Surg.* **2011**, *21*, 1710–1713. [CrossRef] [PubMed]
204. Freeth, A.; Prajuabpansri, P.; Victory, J.M.; Jenkins, P. Assessment of Selenium in Roux-en-Y Gastric Bypass and Gastric Banding Surgery. *Obes. Surg.* **2012**, *22*, 1660–1665. [CrossRef]
205. Papamargaritis, D.; Aasheim, E.T.; Sampson, B.; le Roux, C.W. Copper, selenium and zinc levels after bariatric surgery in patients recommended to take multivitamin-mineral supplementation. *J. Trace Elem. Med. Biol.* **2015**, *31*, 167–172. [CrossRef] [PubMed]
206. Eltweri, A.M.; Bowrey, D.J.; Sutton, C.D.; Graham, L.; Williams, R.N. An audit to determine if vitamin b12 supplementation is necessary after sleeve gastrectomy. *Springerplus* **2013**, *2*, 218. [CrossRef] [PubMed]
207. Shahmiri, S.S.; Eghbali, F.; Ismaeil, A.; Gholizadeh, B.; Khalooeifard, R.; Valizadeh, R.; Rokhgireh, S.; Kermansaravi, M. Selenium Deficiency After Bariatric Surgery, Incidence and Symptoms: A Systematic Review and Meta-Analysis. *Obes. Surg.* **2022**, *32*, 1719–1725. [CrossRef]
208. Hatch-McChesney, A.; Lieberman, H.R. Iodine and Iodine Deficiency: A Comprehensive Review of a Re-Emerging Issue. *Nutrients* **2022**, *14*, 3474. [CrossRef] [PubMed]
209. Nazeri, P.; Shariat, M.; Azizi, F. Effects of iodine supplementation during pregnancy on pregnant women and their offspring: A systematic review and meta-analysis of trials over the past 3 decades. *Eur. J. Endocrinol.* **2021**, *184*, 91–106. [CrossRef]
210. Michalaki, M.; Volonakis, S.; Mamali, I.; Kalfarentzos, F.; Vagenakis, A.G.; Markou, K.B. Dietary iodine absorption is not influenced by malabsorptive bariatric surgery. *Obes Surg.* **2014**, *24*, 1921–1925. [CrossRef] [PubMed]

211. Lecube, A.; Zafon, C.; Gromaz, A.; Fort, J.M.; Caubet, E.; Baena, J.A.; Tortosa, F. Iodine Deficiency Is Higher in Morbid Obesity in Comparison with Late after Bariatric Surgery and Non-obese Women. *Obes. Surg.* **2014**, *25*, 85–89. [CrossRef]
212. Manousou, S.; Carlsson, L.M.S.; Eggertsen, R.; Hulthén, L.; Jacobson, P.; Landin-Wilhelmsen, K.; Trimpou, P.; Svensson, P.-A.; Nyström, H.F. Iodine Status After Bariatric Surgery—A Prospective 10-Year Report from the Swedish Obese Subjects (SOS) Study. *Obes. Surg.* **2018**, *28*, 349–357. [CrossRef] [PubMed]
213. Cheah, S.; Gao, Y.; Mo, S.; Rigas, G.; Fisher, O.; Chan, D.L.; Chapman, M.G.; Talbot, M.L. Fertility, pregnancy and post partum management after bariatric surgery: A narrative review. *Med. J. Aust.* **2022**, *216*, 96–102. [CrossRef] [PubMed]

MDPI
St. Alban-Anlage 66
4052 Basel
Switzerland
www.mdpi.com

Journal of Clinical Medicine Editorial Office
E-mail: jcm@mdpi.com
www.mdpi.com/journal/jcm

www.ingramcontent.com/pod-product-compliance
Lightning Source LLC
Chambersburg PA
CBHW041015270926
51850CB00024B/198
9783036594583